ADVANCED TEXTBOOK ON TRADITIONAL CHINESE MEDICINE AND PHARMACOLOGY

Vol. III

- Internal Medicine

NEW WORLD PRESS   BEIJING, CHINA

First Edition   1996

Written by Wang Shousheng
Translated by Jin Huide
Edited by Chen Keji

Copyright by NEW WORLD PRESS, Beijing, China.
All rights reserved. No part of this book may be
reproduced in any form or by any means without
permission in writing from the publisher.

ISBN 7-80005-296-6

Published by New World Press
24 Baiwanzhuang Road, Beijing 100037, China

Distributed by
China International Book Trading Corporation
35 Chegongzhuang Xilu, Beijing 100044, China
P.O. Box 399, Beijing, China

Printed in the People's Republic of China

Members of the Editorial Board

Cai Jingfeng	Jiang Jian	Yang Weiyi
Chao Guci	Li Anbang	Yu Xiaodan
Chen Daojin	Li Fei	Yu Yongjie
Chen Keji	Li Liangyu	Zeng Shouzeng
Chen Xianqing	Li Lixia	Zhang Dianpu
Cheng Xizhen	Li Yanwen	Zhang Guoliang
Dong Lianrong	Liu Darong	Zhang Haoliang
Fang Boying	Liu Yanchi	Zhang Kai
Fang Tingyu	Liu Xuehua	Zhang Ruifu
Fu Shiyuan	Luo Yikuan	Zhang Xinchun
Fu Weikang	Ou Ming	Zhou Jingping
Hou Can	Qian Chenghui	Zhou Xuesheng
Huang Yabei	Sun Meizhen	Zhen Zhiya
Huang Yuezhong	Wang Lufen	Zuo Yanfu
Hui Jiyuan	Xu Yizhi	

FOREWORD

In order to promote international exchange in the field of traditional Chinese medicine and to meet the needs of increasingly large numbers of foreign students studying traditional Chinese medicine, the Foreign Affairs Bureau of the State Education Commission and the Department of Traditional Chinese Medicine under the Ministry of Public Health (now the State Administration of Traditional Chinese Medicine and Pharmacy) held a meeting in Guangzhou in April 1986 to examine and approve textbooks of traditional Chinese medicine for foreign students. Eight textbooks for use by foreign students were examined during the meeting, including *Basic Theory of Traditional Chinese Medicine* and *The History of Traditional Chinese Medicine* compiled by the Beijing College of Traditional Chinese Medicine, *Traditional Chinese Internal Medicine* and *The Chinese Language* compiled by the Shanghai College of Traditional Chinese Medicine, *Chinese Pharmacy* and *The Science of Traditional Chinese Prescriptions* compiled by the Nanjing College of Traditional Chinese Medicine, and *Traditional Chinese Diagnosis* and *The Science of Acupuncture and Moxibustion* compiled by the Guangzhou College of Traditional Chinese Medicine.

The four colleges of traditional Chinese medicine involved in the compilation of the textbooks have been teaching foreign students for five to ten years, during which time they have accumulated a great deal of experience. Most of the editors have experience in compiling textbooks in the fields of study used nationwide by full-time colleges of traditional Chinese medicine. Many of these textbooks have long been used in teaching foreign students. As a result, they are both comprehensive and applicable.

This series of textbooks draws on the contents of the fourth and fifth editions of national textbooks used by full-time colleges of traditional Chinese medicine and takes into consideration the fact that foreign students have a relatively short time for classroom studies and that there are differences in cultures and traditions. Such aspects as the depth and range of the contents, and the scientific, ideological and advanced level of the textbooks have been carefully considered. Efforts have been made to shorten and simplify while preserving the essence of traditional Chinese medicine and its systematic theories.

The publication of these textbooks marks a great achievement in the dissemination of traditional Chinese medicine. Training foreign students is an important way of spreading traditional Chinese medicine throughout the world. We hope that teachers and students will comment on any shortcomings they discover in this series of textbooks so that we may alter and improve subsequent editions.

State Administration of Traditional
Chinese Medicine and Pharmacy
1991

INTERNAL MEDICINE

CONTENTS

PART ONE   INTRODUCTION 5
  Definition and Scope 5
  Main Contents 5
  Aim and Methods 5
  Development 6
  Commonly Used Methods of Treatment 7

PART TWO   THE TREATMENT OF DISEASES 15
  The Common Cold 15
  Cough 25
  Lung Abscess 33
  Asthma 40
  Dyspnea 48
  Pulmonary Tuberculosis 55
  Retention of Phlegm and Fluid 66
  Spontaneous Sweating and Night Sweating 72
  Hemorrhagic Syndrome 78
  Palpitation 95
  Chest *Bi*-Syndrome 101
  Insomnia 109
  Jue-Syndrome (Syncope) 115
  Stagnation Syndrome 122
  Manic-Depressive Syndrome 128
  Epilepsy 136
  Epigastric Pain 141
    Appendix I   Acid Regurgitation 146
    Appendix II   Gastric Upset 146
  Dysphagia 151
  Vomiting 157
    Appendix   Regurgitation 161
  Hiccup 166
  Diarrhea 172
  Dysentery 180
  Abdominal Pain 188
  Constipation 195
  Parasitosis 203
  Hypochondriac Pain 208
  Jaundice 214
  Abdominal Masses 225
  Tympanites 230
  Headache 240
  Vertigo 248
  Apoplexy 255
  Goiter 266
  Malaria 271
  Edema 278
  Stranguria 287

Appendix Cloudy Urine	291
Retention of Urine	294
Lumbago	300
Diabetes	306
Spermatorrhea	312
Appendix Impotence	315
Tinnitus and Deafness	317
Bi-Syndrome	323
Wei-Syndrome	330
Fever due to Internal Disorders	339
Consumptive Disease	350
Index of Medical Formulae	365
Additional Formulae	392

PART ONE   INTRODUCTION

I. Definition and Scope

Traditional Chinese internal medicine (TCIM for short) studies etiology, pathogenesis, distinction of syndromes and treatment of diseases that fall into the category of internal medicine according to the theories of traditional Chinese medicine. As the basis for other clinical subjects, it plays a major role in traditional Chinese medicine.

Diseases which can be treated by traditional Chinese medicine are generally divided into two categories: those caused by external pathogenic factors and those caused by internal damage. The former refers to exogenous febrile diseases caused by cold, wind-heat, summer-heat, and damp-heat as described in *Treatise on Cold Diseases* and *Studies on Seasonal Febrile Diseases*. They are distinguished according to the theories of six meridians, *wei* (defensive), *qi*, *ying* (nutrient) and *xue* (blood) systems, as well as triple *jiao*. The latter refers to diseases of the meridians and *zang-fu* organs as described in *Synopsis of Prescriptions of the Golden Chamber*. These diseases are classified in line with the pathological changes in the *zang-fu*, *qi*, blood and body fluids, and the meridians as well. In spite of their differences, the two categories are mutually related in that internal damage enables exogenous pathogenic factors to invade more easily, and the invasion by exogenous pathogenic factors aggravates internal damage. Nevertheless, this book focuses on diseases due to internal damage.

II. Main Contents

Included in this book are fundamental theories of traditional Chinese internal medicine, common diseases, and the rules governing their distinction and treatment. Part One focuses on commonly used methods of treatment. Part Two deals with 45 common diseases, with each discussing under the headings of "etiology and pathogenesis," "differentiation and treatment," "comments," and "case studies." For some of the diseases, "differential diagnosis" is added. Also introduced in this part are descriptions from medical classics and important theories guiding clinical work.

III. Aim and Methods

Since preclinical subjects such as the fundamentals of traditional Chinese medicine, as well as the theories of diagnosis, Chinese materia medica and prescription are the foundations of traditional Chinese internal medicine, it is advisable to review and apply them constantly. Some diseases are mutually related, thus one may serve as reference for studying the other. Moreover, it is necessary to combine the theory with clinical practice. Diseases should be analyzed according to the doctrines of traditional Chinese medicine before syndromes are differentiated and given treatment.

IV. Development

It has been a long process getting TCIM formed and developed, during which medical scholars have fought unremittingly against diseases and established theories, thus making valuable contributions to humanity.

The earliest records of these diseases, including heart disease, headaches, gastrointestinal disease, and parasitosis, were first found in the inscriptions on bones and tortoise shells during the late period of the Shang Dynasty (1,500-1,000 B.C.), when medicinal decoction and liquor were employed as treatments. The branching of medicine in the Zhou Dynasty (1,000-221 B.C.) produced a kind of doctor called "yiyi" or internist in modern times.

A monumental book, *The Inner Canon of the Yellow Emperor*, was compiled in the Spring and Autumn and Warring States period (770-221 B.C.). This detailed medical classic, which describes etiology and pathogenesis, diagnosis and the principles of treatment, had far-reaching influence on the development of medicine later.

By compiling the experiences of his predecessors and combining them with his own, Zhang Zhongjing of the Han Dynasty (206 B.C.-220 A.D.) wrote *Treatise on Cold Diseases and Miscellaneous Disorders*. The book consists of two sections; one of them focuses on interpreting exogenous febrile diseases according to the theory of the six meridians, while the other dedicates to miscellaneous disorders due to internal damage from pathological changes in *zang-fu* organs. He introduced the theoretical system of determining treatment based on distinction of syndromes, i.e., analysis of pathogenesis, determination of treatment principles, formulation of prescriptions, and selection of medicinal herbs.

The Classic of Sphygmology by Wang Shuhe of the Jin Dynasty (265-420 A.D.) has helped to diagnose diseases of internal medicine. *A Handbook of Prescriptions for Emergencies* by Ge Hong of the same dynasty is a collection of simple yet effective prescriptions. For example, Sargassum and Thallus Laminariae seu Eckloniae were used to treat goiter in China then, but this methed was to be learned by Europeans over a thousand years later.

The Pathogenesis and Manifestations of Diseases by Chao Yuanfang of the Sui Dynasty (581-618 A.D.) is a special book on pathogenesis, devoting much of its space to a detailed description of diseases of internal medicine. *Essentially Treasured Prescriptions* and *Clandestine Essentials from the Imperial Library* are two works compiled in the Tang Dynasty (618-907 A.D.), which enriched and diversified methods of treatment. *Imperial Benevolent Prescriptions of the Taiping Period* and *Imperial Medical Encyclopedia* of the Northern Song Dynasty (960-1127 A.D.) are two books on medical prescriptions published under the auspices of the imperial court. *Treatise on the Tripartite Pathogenesis of Diseases* of the Southern Song Dynasty (1127-1279 A.D.) expounds further on the etiology of traditional Chinese internal medicine.

Unique contributions were made to traditional Chinese medicine by doctors living in the Jin (ruling the northern part of China from 1115 to 1234 A.D.) and Yuan dynasties (1271-1368 A.D.). Liu Wansu initiated the theory of "fire-heat," advocating the prescription of naturally "cool" herbs in the treatment. Zhang Congzheng was particularly good at eliminating pathogenic factors by promoting sweating, vomiting and purgation. Li Dongyuan emphasized the importance of the spleen and stomach in the treatment of diseases due to internal damage. Zhu Danxi established the theory that *yang* is usually redundant while *yin* is ever deficient, and the nourishment of *yin* was his primary principle of treatment. All these provided TCIM with rich theories and experiences.

A Summary of Internal Medicine by Xue Ji of the Ming Dynasty (1368-1644 A.D.) was the first medical book in China to incorporate the term of "internal medicine" in its title. *Collection of Experiences of Famous Physicians in the Ming Dynasty* by Wang Lun summed up the consensus which prevailed in the field of internal medicine at that time: "Employ Zhang Zhongjing's method in the treatment of diseases caused by external pathogenic factors; employ Li Dongyuan's method in the treatment of diseases due to internal damage; employ Liu Wansu's method in the treatment of acute febrile diseases; and employ Zhu Danxi's method in the treatment of miscellaneous diseases." Many internal diseases are described in *Standard for Diagnosis and Treatment* by Wang Kentang, *A Complete Collection of Jingyue's Treatise* by Zhang Jiebin, and *Determination of Treatment Based on Analysis of Symptoms, Tracing Causative Factors, and Feeling the Pulse* by Qin Jingming. *A Complete Collection of Jingyue's Treatise*, in particular, presents a unique view to the determination of treatment based on distinction of syndromes, thus contributing much to the development of traditional Chinese internal medicine.

One of the great achievements of the Qing Dynasty (1644-1911 A.D.) in traditional Chinese internal medicine was the further development of the theory on seasonal febrile diseases. Major figures who made contributions to the development of this theory included Ye Tianshi, Xue Shengbai, Wu Jutong and Wang Mengying; their works forged a new chapter in traditional Chinese internal medicine. The Qing Dynasty also spawned a rich collection of medical books, and those on internal medicine were too numerous to be mentioned one by one. Among them were *Encyclopedia of the Qing Dynasty: Section on Medicine*, *Golden Mirror of Orthodox Medical Lineage*, *Zhang's Medical Treatise* and *Shen's Treatise on the Importance of Life Preservation*. In addition, there were short yet practical books, such as *A Supplement to Diagnosis and Treatment*, *Insight into Medicine*, *Diagnosis and Treatment of Classified Syndromes*, *Supplementary Notions of Medical Experience*, *Easy Understanding of Medicine*, and *Correction of Medical Classics*.

In conclusion, traditional Chinese internal medicine has undergone a long course of development with the natural progression of history and advances in medicine.

V. Commonly Used Methods of Treatment

1. To Relieve Exterior Syndrome

This treatment may help to eliminate pathogenic factors by opening the pores and promoting perspiration. Thus it is also known as the diaphoretic method.

Indications:

(1) To eliminate superficial pathogenic factors

This method relieves exterior syndrome by eliminating pathogenic factors on the body surface. Since exterior syndrome can be caused by cold or heat, herbs that are naturally acrid and warm or acrid and cool are used to produce a diaphoretic effect.

(2) To let out skin eruptions

The early stage of measles with delayed or incomplete skin eruptions is treated by dispelling toxins. Herbs that are acrid and cool in nature are used; naturally acrid and warm herbs are contraindicated.

(3) To eliminate dampness

The diaphoretic method is also employed for wind-cold complicated with dampness, and *bi*-syndrome due to wind-dampness.

(4) To relieve edema

The diaphoretic method relieves edema by dispelling retained water and promoting the dispersing function of the lung. Thus it is suitable for treating edema of the excess type complicated with exterior syndrome.

Precautions:

(1) It is contraindicated in cases of severe vomiting, severe diarrhea, stranguria, skin infection and hemorrhaging.

(2) It should be discontinued as soon as pathogenic factors are dispelled, since excessive sweating may consume *yin* and *yang*.

(3) The diaphoretic method differs in different seasons, geographic areas, and the condition of individual patients. For instance, mild diaphoretics are prescribed in summer but potent diaphoretics in winter. A large dose of diaphoretic is prescribed for the cold climates of northwest China, and a smaller dose for the warm climates of southeast China. Slow-acting diaphoretics are advisable for patients with weak constitutions, and potent ones for patients with strong constitutions.

(4) This method should be combined with other methods of treatment if the exterior syndrome is complicated by other disorders. For instance, regulating *qi* is combined with relieving exterior syndrome in cases of *qi* stagnation; resolving retained fluid is adopted in cases where phlegm and fluid are retained; strengthening *qi* is essential in cases of *qi* deficiency; similarly, assisting *yang* is employed in cases of *yang* deficiency; nourishing blood is recommended in cases of blood deficiency; and nourishing *yin* is applied in cases of *yin* deficiency.

2. To Eliminate Heat

This method of treatment employs naturally cool herbs to relieve heat syndrome.

Indications:

(1) To disperse heat in the *qi* system

This method is indicated when the *qi* system is affected by pathogenic factors involving excessive heat in the interior. Its manifestations are fever, aversion to heat, absence of chills, perspiration, thirst, restlessness, yellow tongue coating, and a bounding and large pulse, or rapid pulse.

(2) To disperse heat in the *ying* system and cool the blood

It is indicated when the *ying* system is affected by pathogenic heat with symptoms of delirium; and when the *xue* system is affected by pathogenic heat with manifestations of crimson tongue, rapid pulse, hematemesis, epistaxis and skin eruption.

(3) To disperse heat and toxins

It is indicated for various diseases due to heat and toxins, such as infectious epidemic diseases, acute febrile diseases, and abscesses of internal organs due to fire and toxins.

(4) To disperse heat in the *zang-fu* organs

It is indicated for interior heat syndromes of *zang-fu* organs resulting from pathogenic heat or hyperfunction of the *zang-fu* organs.

Precautions:

(1) This method is contraindicated for cold syndromes characterized by false heat symptoms. This occurs when there is an excess of *yin*, and when the deficient *yang* rises to the surface due to the decrease of fire from the gate of life (*mingmen*).

(2) It is contraindicated for fever caused by impeded *yang-qi* due to persistent pathogenic factors affecting the body surface, and weak constitution due to stagnation of cold in the *zang-fu* organs. The method should be applied with caution in cases of asthenic fever caused by a deficiency of *qi* and blood.

(3) Since heat inevitably consumes *yin*, then *qi*. To treat such disorders, this method is often combined with the method of nourishing *yin* and strengthening *qi*. Bitter and cold herbs for dispersing heat are generally dry in property, and readily consume *yin* fluid. Therefore, this method is not advisable for prolonged administration.

(4) If vomiting follows the oral administration of heat-clearing herbs, ginger juice, which is naturally acrid and warm, should be added in small doses, and naturally cool herbs should be taken orally

while still hot. In this respect, this method contradicts standard practice.

3. To Promote Purgation
This is a method to pass dry stools, relieve stagnation, eliminate excess heat and dispel retained water.

Indications:

This treatment is indicated for interior syndromes of the excess type. Different methods of purgation are adopted appropriate to the manifestations.

(1) Purgation with cold herbs

This is meant to pass dry stools and eliminate excess heat, and it is indicated for interior-heat syndromes of the excess type.

(2) Purgation with warm herbs

This is intended to warm the interior, eliminate cold and relieve excess conditions, and it is indicated for interior-cold syndromes of the excess type characterized by stagnation of cold in the *zang-fu* organs.

(3) Purgation with moisturizing herbs

This is indicated for constipation due to consumption of fluid by heat, prolonged illness, old age, or postpartum deficiency of blood.

(4) Purgation with herbs that dispel water

This is indicated for fluid retention in the chest and hypochondrium, edema and ascites.

Precautions:

(1) The purgation method is contraindicated for cases in which the pathogenic factors are on the body surface of between the exterior and interior, or the large intestine is not stagnated in syndromes of *Yangming fu* organ. Potent purgatives should not be used in cases of constipation due to consumption of fluid in the elderly, or deficiency of *yang-qi* in patients with weak constitutions. In addition, this method should be used cautiously in cases of pregnancy or during menstruation.

(2) The purgation method should be discontinued as soon as pathogenic factors are dispelled, since over use may damage the body's resistance.

4. To Harmonize
This treatment means to harmonize *Shaoyang*, strengthen the resistance, eliminate pathogenic factors, and regulate the functions of the internal organs.

Indications:

(1) To harmonize *Shaoyang*

This is indicated for *Shaoyang* syndromes marked by the retention of pathogenic factors between the exterior and interior of the body. Its manifestations are alternating chills and fever, a feeling of distress and fullness in the chest and hypochondrium, restlessness, nausea, a bitter taste in the mouth, a dry throat, thin coating on the tongue, and taut pulse.

(2) To harmonize the liver and spleen

This is indicated for cases of disharmony between the liver and spleen. The symptoms include mental depression, stuffiness in the chest, pain in the hypochondrium and abdomen, and diarrhea.

(3) To regulate the stomach and intestines

This is indicated for functional disturbances of the stomach and intestines due to stagnation of cold and heat along with abnormal ascent and descent of *qi*. Such cases are manifested by sensations of distention and fullness in the epigastrium and abdomen, nausea, vomiting, abdominal pain, increased borborygmus, and diarrhea.

Precautions:

(1) Generally, this method is not used if pathogenic factors remain on the body surface and have not yet entered *Shaoyang*, or if they have already reached the interior of the body, presenting an excess syndrome or a cold-syndrome of the deficiency type.

(2) The *Shaoyang* syndrome, with pathogenic factors invading the area between the exterior and interior of the body, may affect either the exterior or the interior more, and may be characterized either by cold or heat. The method of treatment should change according to actual conditions.

5. To Warm the Interior

This treatment is used to eliminate pathogenic cold and invigorate *yang-qi*.

Indications:

(1) To warm the middle *jiao* and eliminate cold

This is indicated for direct affection of the *zang-fu* organs by external pathogenic cold, as well as internal cold produced by the deficiency of *yang*. The symptoms include a cold feeling in the body, cold limbs, a sensation of cold and pain in the epigastrium and abdomen, nausea, vomiting, diarrhea, a pale tongue with white coating, and a deep and slow pulse.

(2) To warm the meridians and disperse cold

This is indicated for blocked meridians due to pathogenic cold and retarded blood circulation. The symptoms include a sensation of cold and pain in the four limbs, dark purple skin, cyanosis, a tongue with petechiae, and a thready and unsmooth pulse.

(3) To restore *yang* and prevent collapse

This is indicated for cases manifesting the weakening of *yang-qi* and excess of *yin* cold in the interior, marked by cold limbs, aversion to cold, lying with the body curled up, diarrhea with undigested food in the stool, profuse sweating with a cold sensation in the body, and a fainting pulse.

Precautions:

(1) This treatment is prohibited in cases of heat-syndromes with false cold symptoms; flaring of internal fire with the symptoms of hematemesis, hematuria and bloody stool; constitutional deficiency of *yin* indicated by a red tongue and dry throat; and diarrhea with exhausted *yin* fluid due to accumulation of heat in the large intestines and accompanied by loss of consciousness, shortness of breath, emaciation, and dark complexion.

(2) Potent warm herbs should only be prescribed for severe cold syndromes, and the milder ones for less severe cases. This is because warm and hot herbs are usually dry in nature, and their excessive use may consume blood and body fluids, thus producing dryness and heat. Potent warm herbs are only used in large doses for restoring *yang* in emergency cases.

(3) Warm herbs are only used if the cold syndromes are not of the deficiency type. Sweet and warm herbs are combined in the treatment of cold syndromes of the deficiency type.

6. To Tonify

This treatment is designed to enrich *yin* and blood and invigorate *yang* and *qi*, and also repairs deficiency in the *zang-fu* organs.

Indications:

(1) To tonify *qi*

This is indicated for cases of *qi* deficiency marked by lassitude, shortness of breath, dyspnea on exertion, pale complexion, poor appetite, loose stool, and a weak pulse or a large feeble pulse.

(2) To enrich blood

This is indicated for cases of blood deficiency with dizziness, blurring of vision, tinnitus, deafness, palpitation, insomnia, pale complexion, and a thready and rapid or thready and unsmooth pulse.

(3) To replenish *yin*

This is indicated for cases of *yin* deficiency with dry mouth and throat, restlessness, insomnia, constipation, hectic fever, night sweating, a red tongue with scanty coating, and a thready and rapid pulse.

(4) To invigorate *yang*

This is indicated for cases of *yang* deficiency with aversion to cold, cold limbs, sweating with a cold sensation in the body, dyspnea, soreness and weakness in the lumbus and knees, diarrhea, edema, a swollen and pale tongue, and a deep and slow pulse.

Precautions:

(1) This treatment is prohibited in cases of excesses with false deficiency symptoms.

(2) There is no absolute division between the improvement of *qi* and blood tone, although each has its own emphasis. Since *qi* rules blood, the purpose of enriching blood is often achieved through invigorating *qi*. In treating cases of blood deficiency due to profuse blood loss, it is even more necessary to invigorate *qi* in order to prevent a total collapse.

(3) There is no absolute division between replenishing *yin* and invigorating *yang*. Zhang Jingyue says, "Those who are good at invigorating *yang* seek *yang* from *yin*, and those who are good at replenishing *yin* seek *yin* from *yang*."

(4) Different methods of tonification are used when deficiency involves different *zang-fu* organs. For the five *zang* organs, primary attention should be given to the spleen and kidneys.

(5) In cases of *yang* deficiency with cold symptoms, the tonifying effect is achieved by prescribing sweet and warm herbs, and heat-clearing and moisturizing herbs are not advisable. In cases of *yin* deficiency with heat signs, the tonifying effect is achieved by using sweet and cool herbs, and acrid and dry herbs should not be applied.

7. To Disperse

This method is meant to disperse the retention of pathogenic factors of the excess type.

Indications:

(1) To disperse food stagnation

This is indicated for dyspepsia with symptoms of distress in the chest and epigastrium, belching, acid regurgitation, abdominal distention, and diarrhea.

(2) To disperse stones

This is indicated for stones in the biliary and urinary tracts.

(3) To disperse goiter and masses

This method treats goiter and masses by resolving phlegm, softening hardness, and dispersing stagnation.

(4) To relieve edema

This reduces edema by promoting diuresis.

Precautions:

(1) This treatment is not as violent as purgation, but it is one of the methods of eliminating pathogenic factors. It is therefore necessary first of all to acquire a clear understanding of the relative strength of the body's anti-pathogenic *qi* and the pathogenic factors before it is adopted.

(2) For cases with dyspepsia due to splenic deficiency, invigorating the spleen should be combined with the dispersal of stagnant food.

(3) In the treatment of edema due to splenic deficiency, the spleen should be invigorated. Otherwise, it is impossible to promote diuresis.

(4) Edema due to renal deficiency involves renal *yang*. To warm and invigorate renal *yang* is vital in relieving edema.

8. To Regulate *Qi*
This treats derangement of *qi*.
Indications:
(1) To promote the circulation of *qi*
This is indicated for cases of *qi* stagnation due to the stagnation of hepatic *qi*.
(2) To conduct *qi* downward
This is indicated for the unhealthy *qi*, which is caused by the dysfunction of the lung and stomach.
Precautions:
(1) Deficient and excess conditions should be clarified before this treatment is adopted. If the method of circulating *qi* is used to treat a case for which the proper treatment should be invigorating *qi*, *qi* will be even more deficient. Conversely, if invigorating *qi* is employed in a case of *qi* stagnation, *qi* will be even more stagnant.
(2) Since herbs that regulate *qi* are mostly aromatic, dry, bitter and warm in nature, the method of regulating *qi* should be applied with caution if the stagnation of *qi* is complicated by the consumption of *yin* fluid.

9. To Regulate Blood
This means to treat retention of stagnant blood in the interior and various hemorrhagic diseases by regulating the blood.
Indications:
(1) To activate blood circulation and remove blood stasis
This is indicated for cases of retarded blood circulation and retention of stagnant blood in the interior.
(2) To check bleeding
This is indicated for various hemorrhagic diseases, such as hemoptysis, epistaxis, hematemesis, hematuria and hemafecia.
Precautions:
(1) Since stagnation of *qi* leads to stagnation of blood, and circulation of *qi* leads to circulation of blood, activating blood circulation and removing blood stasis can be combined with regulating *qi* to enhance the therapeutic effects.
(2) Since blood circulates when warm and coagulates when cold, this treatment can be combined with warming the meridians and dispersing cold to strengthen the effect.
(3) This treatment is prohibited for pregnant women.
(4) Hemorrhagic diseases may be caused by extravasated blood movement due to heat in the blood or by the failure of *qi* to control blood. In the former case, the treatment should be cooling the blood to check bleeding. In the latter, the principle should be improving *qi* circulation to control blood.
(5) Care should be taken not to cause retention of stagnant blood when bleeding is checked. In case of massive bleeding, the blood flow can be checked as an emergency measure. However, a proper amount of herbs that activate blood circulation and remove blood stasis are often added to prevent retention of stagnant blood when bleeding is not severe.

10. To Promote Astringency

This treatment arrests abnormal discharges by promoting astringency.

Indications:

(1) To constrict the body surface and arrest sweating

This is indicated for weakness of the body surface with excess sweating, i.e., spontaneous sweating and night sweating.

(2) To constrict the intestines and check diarrhea

This is indicated for deficiency of spleen *yang* and *yang* deficiency of the spleen and kidneys marked by long-standing diarrhea or dysentery, and incontinence of feces.

(3) To arrest spermatorrhea and enuresis

This is indicated for nocturnal and spontaneous emission due to deficiency of kidney *qi* and weakness of the seminal gate, as well as for frequent urination and nocturnal enuresis due to deficiency of kidney *qi* with impaired function of the urinary bladder in controlling urine.

Precautions:

(1) This treatment arrests abnormal discharges resulting from weak resistance. Therefore, it is not indicated for sweating in a febrile disease, the early stages of dysentery, diarrhea due to improper diet, and nocturnal emission caused by a disturbance of fire.

(2) Since this is only a symptomatic treatment, causative treatment should also be given at the same time. For example, spontaneous sweating due to *yang* deficiency is treated by combining sweat-checking with *qi*-tonifying; night sweating due to *yin* deficiency is treated by combining sweat-checking with nourishing *yin*.

11. To Restore Consciousness

This is a method to treat loss of consciousness by reopening the blocked upper orifices.

Indications:

(1) To restore consciousness with cold herbs

This is indicated for invasion of the pericardium by heat with symptoms such as loss of consciousness, fever, flushed face, restlessness, thirst, a red tongue, and a rapid pulse.

(2) To restore consciousness with warm herbs

This restores consciousness by warming and circulating *qi*, reopening the orifices, eliminating turbid pathogenic factors, and resolving phlegm. It is indicated for the excess syndrome of wind stroke, as well as for *jue*-syndrome due to disorders in *qi* circulation and retention of phlegm with symptoms of falling-down fits, loss of consciousness, lockjaw, a white tongue coating, and a slow pulse.

Precautions:

(1) This is mostly applicable to the excess-syndrome strokes. However, other methods of treatment should also be employed according to the actual conditions, e.g., dispersing heat, relieving constipation, cooling the liver, suppressing wind, resolving phlegm, and eliminating turbid pathogenic factors.

(2) Patent medicine for restoring consciousness are all made into pills or powder, for they are handy to apply as first aid. The recently developed injections produce even quicker results. Since herbs that restore consciousness contain fragrant volatile ingredients, they should not be decocted over fire.

12. To Relieve Spasm

This method relieves convulsion, dizziness, tremor and deviation of the mouth and eye by calming the liver, suppressing and eliminating wind and removing obstructions in the collaterals.

Indications:

(1) To clear heat and suppress wind

This is indicated for wind that stirs up extreme heat characterized by high fever, loss of consciousness and convulsion.

(2) To calm the liver and suppress wind

This is indicated for hyperfunction of liver *yang* and stirring of liver wind marked by dizziness, blurring of vision, fainting, deviation of the mouth and eye and hemiplegia in severe cases.

(3) To nourish blood and suppress wind

This is indicated for cases in which pathogenic heat causes damage to *yin*, which in turn gives rise to blood deficiency that fails to nourish the tendons and muscles, resulting in *yang* deficiency marked by tremor of fingers and contracture of the tendons and muscles.

(4) To eliminate wind and relieve convulsion

This is indicated for cases in which wind-phlegm blocks the collaterals with symptoms of muscular spasm, convulsion and deviation of the mouth and eye.

Precautions:

(1) There is a distinction between internal wind and external wind. External wind should be dispersed. The method of eliminating wind and relieving convulsion is used in the treatment of external wind. Internal wind should be calmed down. Methods of dispersing heat and calming wind, soothing the liver and calming wind, and nourishing blood and calming wind are used in treating cases due to internal wind. But, external wind may stir up internal wind, and internal wind may be complicated by external wind. In treatment, both should be taken into consideration at the same time.

(2) Since herbs that eliminate wind are all warm and dry in nature, they should be used with caution in cases of fluid deficiency, *yin* deficiency, or hyperactivity of *yang* with heat signs.

The twelve methods of treatment listed above can be used separately or in combination. A single method can be adopted at certain stages of a disease or in the treatment of certain prominent symptoms. Usually, several methods of treatment are used in combination, e.g., sweating and purgation, warming and clearing, purgation and tonification, dispersing and tonification, dispersing heat and restoring consciousness, restoring consciousness and relieving spasm, warming the interior and promoting astringency, etc.

PART TWO   THE TREATMENT OF DISEASES

I. The Common Cold

The common cold results from the attack of the body by external pathogenic wind, and is manifested principally as headache, nasal stuffiness with discharge, sneezing, chilliness, and fever.

This disease may occur throughout the year, but more often in winter or spring. Due to climate changes in the four seasons and different pathogenic factors, the common cold can be divided into two categories — cases caused by wind-cold and by wind-heat. They are often complicated by dampness in rainy seasons, and summer-heat in summer. The common cold, severe cold, influenza, and cold due to weak resistance are distinguished in terms of the strength of the patient's resistance and the severity of the pathogenic factors. Mild cases are generally referred to as the common cold; severe cases are called the severe common cold; serious contagious cases fall into the category of influenza. In addition, there is a category of the common cold due to weak resistance.

The pathogenesis of the common cold involves the attack of the lung and body surface by external pathogenic factors. For this reason, it is treated by relieving the exterior syndrome and eliminating pathogenic factors. The common cold due to weak resistance is treated by combining the method of strengthening resistance with the method of eliminating pathogenic factors.

Etiology and Pathogenesis

The common cold is caused by the invasion of external pathogenic wind, which usually associates with seasonal or non-seasonal pathogenic factors.

1. External Factors

The seasonal factors include warmth (heat) in spring, summer-heat in summer, dampness in late summer, dryness in autumn, and cold in winter. Non-seasonal pathogenic factors refer to abnormal weather changes, e.g., cold weather in spring, cool in summer, hot in autumn, and warm in winter. These factors may exceed the human body's adaptability, and succeed in invasion, thus causing common cold or influenza.

2. Internal Causes

(1) Improper life style and ill-timed clothing

If the normal life style is disturbed, if the clothes are not changed according to the climate, or if strain and stress take place, the skin and interspace of the muscles will become loose, impairing their functions of circulating *qi* and blood and preventing external pathogenic factors. The common cold thus ensues. *Basic Questions* says, "When a person remains calm and quiet, and lives a regular life, the pores stay closed, and he can withstand an attack from pathogenic wind even if it comes in a powerful way."

(2) Weakness of resistance

This may result from old age, congenital deficiency doubled by lack of proper care after birth, prolonged or severe illnesses, all of which may weaken the body's defensive *qi*. Since the lung dominates the body surface, controls the skin and hair, warms and nourishes the interspace of the muscles by spreading defensive *qi*, the flourishing of the lung *qi* implies proper functioning of defensive *qi* in resisting attacks by pathogenic factors. On the contrary, the deficiency of lung *qi* hampers the function of defensive *qi*, and thus allows the affection of the body by pathogenic factors. The common cold then follows.

If a person has *yang* deficiency, he will suffer from wind-cold easily. A person with *yin* deficiency is susceptible to wind-heat and dryness-heat. In case of excessive dampness from phlegm, he is likely to be affected by external dampness.

The lung and body surface are affected in cases of the common cold. This is because the lung is at the top of all the *zang-fu* organs, with the functions of dominating *qi* and respiration, and of controlling the skin and hair. It opens into the nose and is linked to passage of *qi* through the throat. Since wind is characterized by lightness in weight, more often than not it affects first the upper part of the body.

The attack of the body surface by external pathogenic factors hinders the smooth circulation of defensive *qi*. The struggle between the body's anti-pathogenic *qi* and the pathogenic factors gives rise to recurrent chilliness and fever. The invasion of the lung by external pathogenic factors damages the lung's dispersing and descending function, thereby producing cough and nasal stuffiness. Since influenza is the result of violent attacks of seasonal pathogenic and pestilential factors, it presents prominent systemic symptoms.

Differential Diagnosis

1. Febrile Diseases due to Invasion of Cold and Seasonal Febrile Diseases

There are many similarities between the common cold, *Taiyang* syndrome in febrile diseases due to invasion of cold, and the syndromes of the *wei* system or the upper *jiao* in seasonal febrile diseases. But, treatment and prognosis for them are different. *A Complete Collection of Jingyue's Treatise* distinguishes them by saying, "The common cold is due to invasion of external pathogenic factors. If they are extreme and penetrate deep into the body, and then permeate all the meridians and collaterals, a febrile disease results. If the pathogenic factors are mild and only affect the body surface, they result in the common cold (invasion by wind)." The severity of the disease, and the ways of transmission are the two points which help to differentiate them clinically. The common cold is mild and involves the lung and body surface. However, in febrile diseases due to invasion of cold, and seasonal febrile diseases, the pathological conditions are severe, and pathogenic factors go from the surface of the body to the interior. Febrile diseases due to cold are transmitted through the six meridians, while seasonal febrile diseases undergo the four stages of *wei*, *qi*, *ying*, and *xue*, or pass through the upper, middle and lower *jiao*.

2. Influenza

Influenza is characterized by the abrupt and simultaneous onset of chilliness and fever, general aching, lassitude, cough, and sore throat. Its pathological conditions are relatively severe, and the disease is epidemic, spreading widely through a part of population, old or young, men or women, in an area for a period of time. The *Pathogenesis and Manifestations of Diseases* says, "Influenza results from the invasion of the body by contagious pathogenic factors, when the weather changes abnormally, but the affected does not change clothes according to the temperature."

Distinction and Treatment

The clinical manifestations of the common cold at the early stage include nasal stuffiness with discharge, sneezing, headache, and aversion to wind, followed by fever, cough and itching in the throat or sore throat. The disease usually lasts 5-10 days. The principle of treatment is to promote the lung's dispersing function, and relieve the exterior syndrome. The latter is done by means of inducing perspiration with acrid and warm herbs in cases of wind-cold, or by means of dispersing heat with acrid and cool herbs in cases of wind-heat. The recipes should be modified in treating cases complicated by dampness, summer-heat, or dryness. If the pathological conditions are severe or complicated, strong herbs that are acrid and warm, or acrid and cool in nature are recommended, or both the exterior syndrome and interior syndrome are relieved simultaneously.

Generally, influenza falls into the category of the common cold caused by wind-heat. If the pathogenic factors have been transmitted to the interior of the body, influenza is then diagnosed and treated as a seasonal febrile disease.

The common cold due to weak body resistance should be differentiated in terms of whether *qi*, *xue*, *yin*, or *yang* is deficient. Treatment is determined accordingly. For such cases, the method of relieving exterior syndrome is often combined with the method of benefiting *qi*, assisting *yang*, nourishing blood, or replenishing *yin*, respectively.

It is not advisable to disperse invading pathogenic factors on the body surface too violently, because excessive perspiration can consume fluid and weaken body resistance. Nor is it advisable to use tonics too early, because early application of tonics may allow the pathogenic factors to stay in the body and further transmit to the interior. The exclusive application of diaphoretics is undesirable in the treatment of the common cold due to weak resistance, because it can cause profuse sweating, which may cause damage to the body's primordial *qi*, or produce side effects such as epistaxis, hemoptysis, etc.

1. The Common Cold due to Wind-cold

Clinical manifestations: nasal stuffiness with clear discharge, sneezing, itching in the throat, coarse voice, coughing with thin and white sputum, aversion to cold, fever, headache, general aching, absence of sweating in severe cases, a thin and white tongue coating, and a superficial, or superficial and tense pulse.

Analysis: Invasion of the lung and body surface by external pathogenic wind-cold impairs the lung's function in dispersing and lowering water. This explains nasal stuffiness with clear discharge, itching in the throat, a coarse voice, and coughing. Cold consumes the body's *yang-qi*, and weakens body resistance against pathogenic factors. This subsequently gives rise to chilliness, fever, absence of sweating, headache, and general aching. Thin and white tongue coating, and a superficial pulse are both signs of invasion of the body surface by wind-cold. A tense pulse is the result of excessive pathogenic cold.

Treatment: To relieve exterior syndrome with acrid and warm herbs, promote the lung's dispersive function, and eliminate cold.

Prescription: In the treatment of mild cases of the common cold due to wind-cold, Decoction of Allii Fistulosi and Sojae Preparatum (290) is prescribed, adding such herbs as Semen Armeniacae Amarum, Folium Perillae, Herba Schizonepetae, and Radix Ledebouriellae. Bulbus Allii Fistulosi warms and circulates *yang-qi*, and disperses cold; Semen Sojae Preparatum expels pathogenic wind-cold from the body surface by inducing perspiration; Semen Armeniacae Amarum and Folium Perillae promote the lung's dispersive function and resolve phlegm; and Herba Schizonepetae and Radix Ledebouriellae strengthen the dispersive effect with their acrid and warm nature.

If chilliness and fever are severe, and are accompanied by headache, general aching and absence of sweating, this suggests a severe case of common cold due to wind-cold. For such a case, the prescription is Anti-Phlogistic Powder of Schizonepetae and Ledebouriellae (197), which disperses pathogenic wind-cold from the body surface, promotes the lung's dispersive function, resolves phlegm, and relieves coughing. In this prescription, Herba Schizonepetae and Radix Ledebouriellae, both acrid and warm in nature, disperse wind-cold; Radix Bupleuri and Herba Menthae expel pathogenic factors from the exterior of the body, and relieve fever; Rhizoma Chuanxiong activates blood circulation, disperses wind, and relieves headache; Radix Peucedani, Radix Platycodi, Fructus Aurantii, Poria, and Radix Glycyrrhizae promote the lung's dispersive function, regulate *qi*, resolve phlegm, and stem coughing; and Rhizoma seu Radix Notopterygii and Radix Angelicae Pubescentis eliminate wind, disperse cold and expel dampness, and they are also important in relieving headache and general aching.

Herbs that dry dampness such as Rhizoma Atractylodis and Cortex Magnoliae Officinalis, are added if the common cold due to wind-cold is complicated with dampness. This is manifested by a heavy sensation in the head, lassitude, stuffiness in the chest, nausea, poor appetite, lack of taste in the mouth, loose stool or diarrhea, and a white and sticky tongue coating. *Erchen* Decoction (3) can be used in combination in cases of coughing with profuse sputum. Rhizoma Cyperi, and Caulis Perillae are added to soothe the liver and regulate *qi* when invasion of wind-cold is complicated with stagnation of *qi* with the symptoms of stuffiness in the chest, and pain in the chest and hypochondrium.

2. The Common Cold due to Wind-heat

Clinical manifestations: Fever, slight aversion to wind and cold, sweating, headache, nasal stuffiness with turbid discharge, thirst, congested and sore throat, coughing with yellow and thick sputum, a thin and yellow tongue coating, and a superficial and rapid pulse.

Analysis: This syndrome is due to direct invasion of wind-heat, or to invasion of wind-cold which subsequently turns to heat after staying in the body for some time. Invasion of the lung inhibits the flow of defensive *qi*, and causes fever and slight aversion to wind and cold. Since wind-heat is a *yang* pathogenic factor, its attack of the body surface loosens the interspace of the skin and muscles. It thereby causes fever more pronounced than chilliness, accompanied by sweating which, however, does not eliminate the pathogenic factors. The pathogenic factor of *yang* easily consumes *yin* fluid, and this explains the thirst. The upward disturbance of wind-heat causes headache, nasal stuffiness with turbid discharge, and congested and sore throat. Attack of the lung by wind-heat pollutes its clean and moist environment, and subsequently results in coughing with yellow and thick sputum. A yellow and sticky tongue coating, and a superficial and rapid pulse are all signs suggesting attack of the lung and body surface by wind-heat.

Treatment: To relieve exterior syndrome with acrid and cool herbs, disperse heat, and disperse wind.

Prescription: Powder of Lonicerae and Forsythiae (287) or its modified forms are applied. In this prescription, Flos Lonicerae and Fructus Forsythiae disperse heat and remove toxins, and expel pathogenic factors from the body surface with their acrid and cool property; Herba Menthae, Spica Schizonepetae and Semen Sojae Preparatum disperse wind and heat, and expel pathogenic factors from the body surface; Radix Platycodi, Radix Glycyrrhizae and Fructus Arctii ease the throat, relieve swelling, promote the lung's dispersive function, and resolve phlegm; and Herba Lophatheri and Rhizoma Phragmitis disperse heat with their sweet and cool property, promote the generation of body fluids, and relieve thirst. If serious headache is present, Folium Mori, and Flos Chrysanthemi are added to disperse heat in the head and eyes. In cases of coughing with profuse sputum, Semen Armeniacae Amarum, Bulbus Fritillariae Cirrhosae and Pericarpium Trichosanthis are added to stop coughing, and resolve phlegm. If congested and sore throat is pronounced, Radix Isatidis, Lasiosphaera seu Calvatia, and Radix Scrophularia are added to disperse heat, eliminate toxins, and ease the throat.

In the treatment of severe cases of the common cold due to wind-heat manifested as persistent high fever, chilliness or chills, headache, dryness of the nose and throat, thirst or preference for cold drinks, restlessness, and a red tongue with thin and yellow coating, such herbs as Radix Puerariae, Radix Scutellariae, Gypsum Fibrosum, Rhizoma Anemarrhenae and Radix Trichosanthis are added to Powder of Lonicerae and Forsythiae (287). Radix Puerariae expels pathogenic factors from the muscles; Radix Scutellariae, and Gypsum Fibrosum disperse heat; Rhizoma Anemarrhenae, and Radix Trichosanthis induce the production of body fluids and relieve thirst.

If the cases of wind-heat are complicated by dampness, showing such symptoms as a heavy sensation in the head, lassitude, stuffiness in the chest, nausea, yellow urine, and a yellow and sticky tongue coating, aromatics that resolve dampness are added, such as Herba Agastaches, Herba Eupatorii and Flos Magnoliae Officinalis. Alternatively, Semen Armeniacae Amarum, Semen Amomi Rotundus and Semen Coicis can be added to disperse heat and resolve dampness.

If the common cold occurs in summer, summer-heat and dampness are often the causes to complicate it. The clinical manifestations include high fever, sweating which does not bring down the fever, sluggishness of the body, lassitude, thirst, scanty and deep yellow urine, a yellow and sticky tongue coating, and a soft and rapid pulse. Clearing away summer-heat and eliminating dampness through urination is accomplished by prescribing Decoction of Elsholtziae with Modification (311). In this prescription, Herba Elsholtziae relieves exterior syndrome, disperses cold and dampness; Flos Lonicerae and Fructus Forsythiae eliminate heat and toxins; Flos Lablab Album expels summer-heat and resolves dampness; and Cortex Magnoliae Officinalis dries out dampness and relieves fullness. Herbs that eliminate summer-heat and resolve dampness and available during a particular season can be added, such as Folium Nelumbinis (fresh), Herba Agastaches (fresh), and Exocarpium Citrulli, as well as Six-to-One Powder (54).

Pathogenic dryness is usually associated with the common cold in autumn. The clinical manifestations then include fever, slight aversion to wind and cold, headache, dryness of the mouth, lips and throat, thirst, coughing with no sputum or with sputum that is difficult to expectorate, a red tongue or a red and thorny tongue with thin and dry coating, and a slightly rapid pulse. For the treatment of such cases, Decoction of Mori and Armeniacae Amarum (256) or its modified forms are prescribed.

3. The Common Cold due to Weak Resistance

People in old age, with a weak constitution, and after a serious illness, mostly have a weak resistance, and therefore, they are susceptible to the common cold. Deficiency of *yang-qi* makes it impossible to eliminate pathogenic factors from the body; and deficiency of *yin* blood implies lack of sweat source, making it impossible to eliminate pathogenic factors. For this reason, the common cold of this type is usually stubborn. Conditions commonly seen include the common cold due to *qi* deficiency, blood deficiency, *yin* deficiency, and *yang* deficiency. Usually, the principle of treatment is to strengthen resistance, eliminate pathogenic factors, and deal with the cause and the secondary symptoms simultaneously.

(1) The common cold due to *qi* deficiency

Clinical manifestations: Chilliness, fever, headache, nasal stuffiness or clear nasal discharge, coughing with white and thin sputum, lassitude, dislike of speaking, a thin and white tongue coating, and a superficial and weak pulse.

Analysis: Constitutional *qi* deficiency means weakness of resistance. Attack of the body surface by pathogenic wind-cold impairs the lung's dispersive function, resulting in chilliness, fever, headache, nasal stuffiness, cough with white and thin sputum, and a superficial pulse. Deficiency of lung *qi* is the cause of lassitude, shortness of breath, and dislike of speaking.

Treatment: To benefit *qi* and relieve exterior syndrome.

Prescription: Modified Decoction of Ginseng and Perillae (189). In this prescription, Radix Ginseng, Poria and Radix Glycyrrhizae benefit *qi*, strengthen resistance, and eliminate pathogenic factors; Folium Perillae and Radix Puerariae disperse wind and relieve exterior syndrome; and Radix Peucedani, Radix Platycodi, Pericarpium Citri Reticulatae, Fructus Aurantii and Rhizoma Pinelliae promote the lung's dispersive function, regulate *qi* flow, resolve phlegm and cure coughing. If *qi* deficiency is serious, Radix Astragali is added. In treating cases of *qi* deficiency with spontaneous sweating complicated by the attack of pathogenic wind, the treatment should focus on benefiting *qi*, consolidating the body surface, checking sweating and eliminating wind. In this case, Jade Screen Powder (73) should be prescribed with modifications. In this prescription, Radix Astragali replenishes *qi* and consolidates the body surface; Radix Ledebouriellae helps Radix Astragali to replenish *qi* and eliminate wind; and Rhizoma Atractylodis Macrocephalae invigorates the spleen. Patients with chronic disorders and *qi* deficiency easily catch cold; this may in turn aggravate the chronic disorders. In this case, long-standing administration of Jade Screen Powder (73) strengthens resistance and thus prevents the common cold.

(2) The common cold due to *yang* deficiency

Clinical manifestations: Mild fever, severe chilliness, headache, general aching, pale complexion, cold limbs, low voice, a swollen tongue with thin and white coating, and a deep and weak pulse.

Analysis: *Yang-qi* deficiency deprives the body surface of warmth and nourishment, and thus causes exterior cold-syndrome, which is aggravated by invasion of external pathogenic wind-cold. For this reason, fever is less significant than chilliness. Cold limbs, low voice, a pale and swollen tongue and a deep and weak pulse are all signs of *yang-qi* deficiency. Headache and general aching are manifestations of exterior syndrome caused by the attack of external pathogenic wind-cold.

Treatment: To assist *yang* and relieve exterior syndrome.

Prescription: Modified Pill of Ginseng and Aconiti Lateralis Preparata for Restoration (192). In this prescription, Radix Aconiti Lateralis Preparata and Ramulus Cinnamomi assist *yang*; Radix Ginseng, Radix Astragali and Radix Glycyrrhizae Preparata benefit *qi* and strengthen *yang*; and Rhizoma seu Radix Notopterygii, Radix Ledebouriellae and Herba Asari relieve exterior syndrome and disperse cold. In cases of chilliness, absence of sweating and mild fever, Decoction of Ephedrae, Aconiti and Asari (274) can be modified and prescribed. In this prescription, Radix Aconiti Lateralis Preparata warms the meridians and assists *yang*; Herba Ephedrae causes perspiration and relieves exterior syndrome; and Herba Asari disperses *Shaoyang* cold and relieves exterior syndrome of *Taiyang*. This prescription is more appropriate for mild cases of the common cold due to *yang* deficiency.

(3) The common cold due to blood deficiency

Clinical manifestations: Headache, low-grade fever, mild chilliness, pale complexion, pale lips and nails, palpitation, dizziness, a pale tongue with thin and white coating, a thready and soft, or superficial and weak pulse.

Analysis: *Yin* blood deficiency may result from illness or bleeding. If blood fails to go upward and nourish the face, pale complexion and lips will result. When blood cannot sufficiently nourish the heart and brain, palpitation and dizziness will follow. Attack of external pathogenic factors causes fever, chilliness, and headache. A pale tongue, and a thready or superficial and weak pulse are signs of blood deficiency complicated by attack of external pathogenic factors.

Treatment: To nourish blood and relieve exterior syndrome.

Prescription: Modified Decoction of Seven Ingredients Containing Allii Fistulosi (291). In this prescription, Bulbus Allii Fistulosi, Semen Sojae Preparatum, Radix Puerariae and Rhizoma Zingiberis Recens relieve exterior syndrome and eliminate pathogenic factors; and Radix Rehmanniae and Radix Ophiopogonis nourish blood and replenish *yin*. The only way to expel pathogenic factors on the body surface is to cause sweating. Since sweat and blood have the same origin, no sweat can be produced in cases of blood deficiency. In this circumstance, medicinal herbs that nourish blood are used in combination with those that relieve exterior symptoms. In cases with high fever, Flos Lonicerae and Fructus Forsythiae are added to disperse heat.

If common cold is complicated by deficiency of both *qi* and blood, Pill of Dioscoreae (327) is prescribed. In this prescription, Rhizoma Dioscoreae, Radix Ginseng, Rhizoma Atractylodis Macrocephalae, Poria and Radix Glycyrrhizae Preparata replenish *qi*; Radix Angelicae Sinensis, Radix Rehmanniae, Radix Paeoniae Alba and Rhizoma Chuanxiong enrich blood; Semen Sojae Germinatum, Radix Ledebouriellae, Radix Bupleuri and Ramulus Cinnamomi relieve exterior syndrome and eliminate pathogenic factors. This prescription can relieve exterior syndrome without damaging *qi* and blood, and replenish *qi* and blood without hindering the elimination of pathogenic factors.

(4) The common cold due to *yin* deficiency

Clinical manifestations: Headache, fever, mild chilliness, absence of sweating or slight sweating, dizziness, restlessness, thirst, dryness of the throat, a hot sensation in the palms and soles, non-productive cough, a red tongue with exfoliated coating or none at all, and a thready and rapid pulse.

Analysis: *Yin* deficiency produces internal heat, which is the cause of dizziness, thirst, dryness in the throat, a hot sensation in the palms and soles, restlessness, and absence of sweating or slight sweating. This also explains a red tongue with exfoliated coating or none at all, and a thready and rapid pulse. Fever, mild chilliness, headache and cough are manifestations of exterior syndrome caused by the attack of external pathogenic factors.

Treatment: To nourish *yin* and relieve exterior syndrome.

Prescription: Modified Decoction of Polygonati Odorati (114). In this prescription, Rhizoma Polygonati Odorati nourishes *yin* and promotes the production of body fluids without causing the retention of pathogenic factors; Bulbus Allii Fistulosi, Semen Sojae Preparatum and Radix Platycodi induce perspiration and relieve exterior syndrome; Radix Cynanchi Atrati clears away asthenic heat and expels pathogenic factors from the body; and Radix Glycyrrhizae and Fructus Jujubae harmonize the middle *jiao* with their sweet and moist property and help Rhizoma Polygonati Odorati to promote the production of body fluids. If the exterior syndrome is serious, a small amount of Herba Schizonepetae and Herba Menthae can be added to eliminate wind and relieve exterior syndrome. In cases of coughing with difficulty in expectoration, Fructus Arctii and Pericarpium Trichosanthis can be added to ease the throat and resolve phlegm. In cases with restlessness and thirst, Herba Lophatheri, Radix Trichosanthis and Rhizoma Phragmitis can be added to disperse heat, calm the patient, promote the generation of body fluids, and relieve thirst.

Remarks

Common cold is due to the attack of the body by external pathogenic factors. Its popular name is *shangfeng* or "damage by wind" in literal translation.

In differentiating syndromes of wind-cold and wind-heat, the following points should be made clear: Which is more pronounced, chilliness or fever? Is thirst present? Is the throat congested and sore? What is the condition of the pulse and tongue coating? The common cold due to wind-cold generally exhibits prominent chilliness, mild fever, clear nasal discharge, absence of thirst, absence of sore throat, a thin and white tongue coating, and a superficial and tense pulse. The common cold due to wind-heat characteristically exhibits high fever which can be persistent, turbid nasal discharge, thirst, congested and sore throat, a thin and yellow tongue coating, and a superficial and rapid pulse. Influenza has an abrupt onset, and spreads rapidly and widely among people in a geographic area for a period of time. It falls into the category of the severe common cold due to wind-heat.

Influenza is treated by relieving exterior syndrome with herbs that are acrid and cool in property. The dosage of herbs that disperse heat and eliminate toxins should be increased, e.g., Rhizoma Dryopteris Crassirhizomae, Radix Isatidis, Folium Isatidis, etc. in treating influenza. If the pathogenic factors have gone into the interior of the body, influenza is then diagnosed and treated as a seasonal febrile disease.

Case Studies

Name: Jiang XX; Sex: Male; Age: 36.

First visit: The clinical manifestations included fever, headache, chilliness, absence of sweating, nasal stuffiness, cough, stuffiness and pain in the chest, sore joints, a white and moist tongue coating, and a superficial and tense pulse. The body temperature was 40.2°C.

Anti-Phlogistic Powder of Schizoneperae and Ledebouriellae (197) was prescribed to eliminate pathogenic factors through sweating. The following prescription was formulated:

Herba Schizonepetae	4.5 g;
Radix Ledebouriellae	4.5 g;
Rhizoma seu Radix Notopterygii	4.5 g;
Radix Bupleuri	4.5 g;
Radix Peucedani	4.5 g;
Fructus Aurantii	4.5 g;
Radix Platycodi	4.5 g;
Poria	9 g;
Herba Menthae	3 g;
Radix Glycyrrhizae	1.5 g;
Rhizoma Zingiberis Recens	2 slices.

Second visit: The patient sweated profusely after taking this decoction. Fever subsided, and body temperature was 36.8°C. But he still complained of coughing with sticky sputum, and soreness and weakness of the limbs and body. Treatment aimed at dispersing wind-cold, promoting the lung's dispersive function and resolve phlegm. The new prescription consisted of the following herbs:

Caulis Perillae	4.5 g;
Radix Peucedani	4.5 g;
Rhizoma Pinelliae (prepared with ginger)	9 g;
Poria	9 g;
Radix Platycodi	3 g;
Pericarpium Citri Reticulatae	4.5 g;
Ramulus Mori	12 g.

Explanation: This is a case of the common cold due to wind-cold. Anti-Phlogistic Powder of Schizoneperae and Ledebouriellae (197), acrid and warm in nature, was prescribed to induce sweating, through which pathogenic factors were eliminated. Coughing with sticky sputum was present at his second visit. Powder of Armeniacae Amarum and Perillae (145) was then prescribed to disperse wind-cold, promote the lung's dispersive function and resolve phlegm. Ramulus Mori was used to disperse wind and clear the collaterals in the treatment of soreness and weakness of the limbs and body.

Name: Li XX; Date: Spring of 1954.

The clinical manifestations included dizziness, fever, general aching, deep yellow urine, constipation, thirst, a thick and sticky tongue coating, and a superficial and bounding pulse. The treatment was to disperse heat, resolve dampness and relieve exterior syndrome. The following prescription was formulated:

Herba Menthae	4.5 g;
Flos Lonicerae	9 g;
Fructus Forsythiae	9 g;
Radix Scutellariae	9 g;
Herba Lophatheri	9 g;
Talcum	9 g;

Folium Isatidis	9 g;
Fructus Gardeniae	9 g;
Fructus Aurantii Immaturus	6 g;
Radix Curcumae	4.5 g;
Fructus Trichosanthis	30 g.

After taking this decoction, the patient began to sweat. Then fever subsided, thirst was relieved, urine became slightly yellowish in color, and the pulse calmed down. But the patient still complained of dizziness, poor appetite and lassitude. So Folium Isatidis was removed from the prescription; the dosage of Fructus Aurantii Immaturus was decreased by 1/4, and that of Fructus Trichosanthis by 1/5.

Explanation: This is a case of the common cold due to wind-heat. The treatment was to relieve exterior syndrome with acrid and cool herbs. Flos Lonicerae, Fructus Forsythiae and Herba Menthae eliminate wind-heat and promote the lung's dispersive function. Fever, absence of chilliness, deep yellow urine, constipation, and a superficial and bounding pulse were all consequences of excessive heat, for which Fructus Gardeniae, Radix Scutellariae, Folium Isatidis and Fructus Trichosanthis were prescribed. A thick and sticky tongue coating suggested complication by dampness, for which Talcum, Herba Lophatheri, Radix Curcumae and Fructus Aurantii Immaturus were used.

Name: Song XX; Sex: Male; Age: 55.

First visit (April 20, 1960): The patient was weak and susceptible to the common cold. The recent attack occurred a month ago, and did not respond to medication. The clinical manifestations included headache, chilliness, aversion to wind, spontaneous sweating, lassitude, painful joints, a pale tongue with no coating, and a deep, slow and weak pulse. Both urination and defecation were normal. The diagnosis was the common cold due to *yang* deficiency. The treatment was to warm *yang* and benefit *qi*. The prescription was based on Jade Screen Powder (73):

Radix Astragali	15 g;
Radix Ledebouriellae	3 g;
Rhizoma Atractylodis Macrocephalae	9 g;
Radix Aconiti Lateralis Preparata	9 g.

Radix Aconiti Lateralis Preparata was decocted 30 minutes before the other herbs. The decoction was taken warm twice.

Second visit: Aversion to wind disappeared, chilliness and headache improved, but spontaneous sweating was still present. The overall impression of the pulse was taut and retarded, the left side deep and weak, and the right side deep and slow. The tongue coating was white and sticky. All this was due to *yang* deficiency complicated by internal dampness. The method of warming *yang* and eliminating dampness was adopted. The following prescription was given:

Radix Astragali (crude)	12 g;
Rhizoma Atractylodis Macrocephalae	9 g;
Radix Aconiti Lateralis Preparata	3 g;
Semen Coicis	15 g;
Herba Artemisiae Scopariae	9 g;
Ramulus Mori (stir-baked)	30 g.

Third visit: All the symptoms considerably improved, and the patient felt much comfortable than before. He still had a feeling of mild chilliness. The pulse was retarded and forceful. Ramulus Mori was thus removed from the prescription, and 2 g of Rhizoma Alpiniae Officinarum was added to warm stomach *yang*.

Last visit: Chilliness disappeared. The pulse was deep and slow on the right side, taut and retarded on the left. The method of warming *yang* and invigorating middle *jiao* continued. Some medicinal pills were recommended to relieve the remaining symptoms gradually. They included 6 g of Bolus of Aconiti Lateralis Preparata for Regulating Middle *Jiao* (163), to be taken in the morning; and 6 g of Pill for Strengthening Middle *Jiao* and Benefiting *Qi* (154), to be taken in the evening.

Explanation: Constitutional *yang* deficiency means weak body resistance, which explains susceptibility to the common cold. Since the recent attack was not relieved by sweating, Jade Screen Powder (73) plus Radix Aconiti Lateralis Preparata was prescribed to warm *yang*, benefit *qi*, consolidate the body surface and harmonize the *ying* (nutrient) and *wei* (defensive) *qi*. The method of warming *yang* and eliminating dampness was adopted next. The treatment concluded by warming *yang* and strengthening middle *jiao*. The exclusive application of diaphoretics in the treatment of such a disease would make the body surface even weaker, and defensive *qi* even more deficient. Thus, different herbs should be used for different manifestations of the same disease.

II. Cough

As a common symptom of the respiratory system, cough often results from lung disorders. When pathological changes of other *zang-fu* organs have affected the lung, cough also occurs. The Chinese word for cough is "*kesou*." "*Ke*" and "*sou*" had the same meaning before the Song Dynasty. In the Jin Dynasty, a physician by the name of Liu Hejian held that the production of coughing sound with no sputum expectorated was called "*ke*," the presence of sputum in the throat which can be spat out was called "*sou*," and the combination of the coughing sound with the sputum that can be spat out was referred to as "*kesou*." As a matter of fact, it is very difficult to tell one from the other. Currently, a general distinction is made between productive and non-productive cough.

There have been different ways of classifying cough since ancient times. *Basic Questions* named coughing after the *zang-fu* organs affected, e.g., lung cough, spleen cough, heart cough, liver cough, kidney cough, and gallbladder cough. Ten types of cough were described in *Pathogenesis and Manifestations of Diseases*, and they were also principally named after the affected *zang-fu* organs. But the naming of cough in relation to pathogenic factors, such as cough due to wind and cough due to cold, first appeared in this book. There were also classifications of cough according to its time of occurrence and its characteristics, e.g., prolonged cough, morning cough, whooping cough and nocturnal cough. All these classifications are too complicated, and are of little practical significance. It was not until the Ming Dynasty that the physician Zhang Jingyue proposed two categories: cough due to attack of external pathogenic factors, and cough due to internal damage. This classification is much more accurate than earlier ones.

The causes of cough were attributed to attack of the lung system by pathogenic factors and to functional disturbance of *zang-fu* organs in *Basic Questions*. *A Complete Collection of Jingyue's Treatise* says, "Coughing presents many syndromes, all of which are caused by lung disorders." *Medicine in Three-Word Verses* says, "The lung is located on top of the internal organs. It becomes empty on exhalation, and full on inhalation. It agrees only with normal lung *qi*, and does not tolerate external pathogenic *qi*. Interference of external pathogenic *qi* in the lung leads to cough. The lung also agrees with the clear *qi* of the *zang-fu* organs, and does not tolerate pathogenic *qi* of *zang-fu* organs. Disturbance of the lung by this pathogenic *qi* causes cough, too."

Cough is commonly seen in infections of the upper respiratory tract, acute and chronic bronchitis, bronchiectasis, and pulmonary tuberculosis.

Etiology and Pathogenesis
Cough results from attack of the lung system by external pathogenic factors, or from dysfunction of other *zang-fu* organs affecting the lung.
1. Attack by External Pathogenic Factors
It is generally acknowledged that attack of the body by any of the six external pathogenic factors may cause cough. Clinical observation, however, has shown that cough is caused by the attack of wind, cold, dryness and heat more often than summer-heat and dampness.

The lung dominates *qi* flow and performs the respiratory function. As a canopy of the five *zang* organs, it connects the throat, opens into the nose, and controls the skin and hair. The six external pathogenic factors attack the body via the nose and throat or the skin and hair. The lung is the first internal organ to be affected, and this impairs the lung's dispersive and descending function, thereby hindering lung *qi*, polluting the clean, moist environment of the lung and producing sputum. In order to expectorate sputum and eliminate pathogenic factors, coughing soon occurs. Since the attacking pathogenic factors vary with the seasons and there are individual differences of constitution, cough manifests syndromes of wind-cold, wind-heat, and dryness-heat.

2. Dysfunction of *Zang-Fu* Organs

Weakness of the lung itself, and disorders of other *zang-fu* organs can all cause cough. The common causes are as follows:

(1) Dysfunction of the spleen in transportation and transformation

The spleen digests food and transports the nutritious essence to the lung, where it is distributed to various parts of the body. Dysfunction of the spleen in transportation and transformation produces turbid phlegm, which is then stored in the lung, blocking *qi* passage and impairing the lung's dispersive and descending function. Consequently, cough occurs. Hence the saying among ancient physicians in traditional Chinese medicine, "The spleen is the source of the production of phlegm, and the lung is the organ where phlegm is stored."

(2) Invasion of the lung by liver fire

The theory of the five elements holds that metal acts on wood; and wood counteracts metal when metal is in a state of deficiency. The theory of meridians relates the liver to the lung by saying, "The liver meridian passes through the hypochondrium on both sides, and then enters the lung." Therefore, hyperactivity of the liver and weakness of the lung may combine to result in a pathological condition that is called attack of the lung by liver fire. Acted on by liver fire, the fluid of the lung turns to phlegm, which then hinders lung *qi* and impairs the lung's dispersive and descending function. As a result, cough occurs.

(3) Lung deficiency

This refers to deficiency of lung *yin* or lung *qi*. The lung prefers a moist environment and dislikes dryness. Deficiency of lung *yin* means dryness in the lung, which then impairs its dispersive and descending function. Deficiency of lung *qi* also impairs the function of the lung and causes cough. Cough due to lung deficiency is usually accompanied by signs of spleen and kidney deficiency. This is because, according to the theory of the five elements, the lung is the son of the spleen and the mother of the kidneys. Disorders of the son consume *qi* of the mother, and disorders of the mother affect the son. Inability of the kidneys to receive *qi* gives rise to the shortness of breath on exertion. The presence of this symptom suggests a more serious pathological condition.

To conclude, dysfunction of the lung is the root cause of cough, no matter whether the immediate cause is the attack of external pathogenic factors or disorders of other organs, because both of them produce cough by impairing the lung's dispersive and descending function.

Distinction and Treatment

First of all, cough due to the attack of external pathogenic factors should be differentiated from cough due to the internal damage. The former is marked by an abrupt onset of frequent spells of cough, short duration of disease and rapid recovery following proper treatment. Fever and headache are the accompanying symptoms. All this suggests syndromes of the excess type. Cough due to the internal damage is characterized by a slow onset, long duration, dysfunction of other *zang-fu* organs and difficult cure, presenting syndromes of the deficiency type, or deficiency complicated by excess.

Two methods are available for the treatment of cough. The method of expelling pathogenic factors and releasing the flow of lung *qi* is used for cough due to the attack of external pathogenic factors. It is not advisable to use bitter and cold herbs, moistening herbs, astringents and antitussives at the early stage of treatment, because these herbs, especially astringents and antitussives, are not conducive to the elimination of pathogenic factors from the body surface. In cases of cough due to the internal damage, the method of regulating *zang-fu* organs is adopted. This includes invigorating the spleen and resolving phlegm, clearing heat in the liver and suppressing fire, strengthening the kidneys' function in receiving *qi*, and nourishing lung *yin* and replenishing lung *qi*. Since cough due to the internal damage often manifests primary deficiency and secondary excess, both the cause and the symptoms should be considered in treatment.

1. Cough due to the Invasion of External Pathogenic Factors

(1) Cough due to wind-cold

Clinical manifestations: Cough with moderate amount of thin and white sputum, non-productive cough at the initial stage, tightness and stuffiness in the chest, nasal stuffiness with clear discharge, sneezing, chilliness, fever, general aching, a sensation of distention in the head, headache, a thin and white tongue coating, and a superficial or superficial and tense pulse.

Analysis: Invasion of the lung system by pathogenic wind-cold impairs the lung's dispersive and descending function and hinders the flow of lung *qi*. This explains cough and nasal stuffiness with clear discharge. Since white color suggests cold, both sputum and nasal discharge in this syndrome are thin and white. Cold is marked by stagnation and obstruction, and so retention of wind-cold in the chest gives rise to tightness and stuffiness there. Attack of the body surface by wind-cold hinders defensive *qi*, and thereby causes chilliness, fever, general aching, a sensation of distention in the head and headache. A thin and white tongue coating, and a superficial or superficial and tense pulse are the result of the attack of the body surface by wind-cold.

Treatment: To disperse wind-cold and release circulation of lung *qi*.

Prescription: Modified Powder of Armeniacae Amarum and Perillae (145). In this prescription, Folium Perillae and Rhizoma Zingiberis Recens disperse wind-cold; Radix Peucedani, Semen Armeniacae Amarum, Radix Platycodi and Radix Glycyrrhizae promote the lung's dispersive function, resolve phlegm, and check cough; and Fructus Aurantii, Rhizoma Pinelliae, Pericarpium Citri Reticulatae and Poria regulate *qi*, dry out dampness and resolve phlegm.

If the invasion of the body surface by wind-cold gives rise to chilliness, fever, severe cough with profuse sputum and a distressed sensation in the chest, accompanied by shortness of breath, general dreariness and absence of sweating, the method of relieving exterior syndrome, dispersing cold, promoting the lung's dispersive function and resolving phlegm is then adopted. The applicable prescriptions include Powder of Inulae (185) and Three Crude Drugs Decoction (18). In these prescriptions, Herba Ephedrae, Herba Schizonepetae and Radix Peucedani disperse wind-cold; Herba Ephedrae, Semen Armeniacae Amarum and Rhizoma Pinelliae strengthen the pulmonary function, resolve phlegm, and check cough; and Herba Inulae resolves phlegm and relieves the distressed sensation in the chest.

If retention of phlegm-heat in the lung, which gives rise to cough, shortness of breath and yellow and sticky sputum, combines with the attack of external pathogenic wind-cold, which produces fever, chilliness or chills, absence of sweating, general aching, nasal stuffiness and possibly clear nasal discharge, the syndrome is then cold on the exterior and heat in the interior. This is conventionally referred to as "cold wrapping up fire," and is most commonly seen in late autumn and early winter. The treatment is to disperse wind-cold, promote the lung's dispersive function, and disperse heat by prescribing Decoction of Ephedrae, Armeniacae Amarum, Gypsum Fibrosum and Glycyrrhizae (272). In the treatment of serious cases manifesting an absence of sweating along with restlessness, Great Blue Dragon Decoction (23) is used to induce perspiration, relieve the exterior syndrome, disperse heat and ease restlessness. If there is pronounced heat in the lung, Cortex Mori, Cortex Lycii, and Radix Scutellariae are added.

(2) Cough due to wind-heat

Clinical manifestations: Cough with thick or yellow and thick sputum which is difficult to expectorate, turbid nasal discharge, sore throat, thirst, fever, sweating which does not bring down the fever, headache, slight chilliness, a thin and yellow tongue coating, and a superficial and rapid pulse.

Analysis: Invasion of the lung by wind-heat produces cough. Consumption of body fluids by heat is the cause of thirst and yellow, thick sputum which is difficult to expectorate. Disturbance of the upper orifices by wind-heat results in turbid nasal discharge, headache and sore throat. The struggle between the pathogenic factors and the body's anti-pathogenic *qi* on the body surface induces fever. Since wind-heat is a pathogenic factor of the *yang* type, its attack of the body surface opens the pores and thereby causes slight chilliness and sweating. A thin and yellow tongue coating and a superficial and rapid pulse also suggest the attack of the body surface by wind-heat.

Treatment: To eliminate wind, disperse heat, promote the lung's dispersive function and resolve phlegm.

Prescription: Decoction of Mori and Chrysanthemi (257). In this prescription, Folium Mori and Flos Chrysanthemi eliminate wind, relieve exterior syndrome and expel wind-heat from the body surface; Fructus Forsythiae and Herba Menthae disperse heat, eliminate toxins and expel pathogenic factors from the body surface with their acrid and cool property; Radix Platycodi, Radix Glycyrrhizae and Semen Armeniacae Amarum disperse heat, ease the throat, check cough and resolve phlegm; and Rhizoma Phragmitis clears heat and produces body fluids.

If there is retention of phlegm-heat in the lung originally, the attack of wind-heat will aggravate cough. Other symptoms include yellow, sticky and thick sputum, asthmatic breathing, fever or a burning sensation of the skin on palpation, especially in the afternoon. If there is slight chilliness, Powder for Expelling Lung Heat (174) is prescribed along with additional drugs to clear heat from the lung, check cough and soothe asthma. In this prescription, Cortex Mori clears heat in the lung; and Cortex Lycii disperses phlegm-heat in the lung. The added drugs include Radix Platycodi and Fructus Arctii for promoting the lung's dispersive function and eliminating phlegm, and Semen Armeniacae Amarum and Bulbus Fritillariae Cirrhosae for resolving phlegm and checking cough. If there is severe heat in the lung, Radix Scutellariae and Rhizoma Anemarrhenae are added to strengthen the effect in clearing heat.

(3) Cough due to dryness-heat

Clinical manifestations: Non-productive cough, or cough with scanty and sticky sputum which is difficult to expectorate, or severe cough with chest pain and blood-tinged sputum, dryness of the nose and throat, aversion to wind, fever, a tongue with red tip and border, yellow and dry tongue coating, a thready and rapid pulse.

Analysis: Cough due to dryness-heat often occurs in the dry season like autumn. Attack of the lung by pathogenic dryness-heat consumes lung fluid and hinders lung *qi*. This is the cause of non-productive cough, cough with sticky sputum which is difficult to expectorate, or severe cough with chest pain. Damage to the vessels of the lung leads to blood-tinged sputum. Since the lung opens into the nose, and the throat is the passageway for *qi*, attack by dryness-heat gives rise to dryness of the nose and throat. Attack of the body surface by dryness-heat hinders defensive *qi*, and thereby causes aversion to wind and fever. A tongue with red tip and border, yellow and dry coating, and a thready and rapid pulse all suggest dryness-heat.

Treatment: To disperse heat in the lung, moisten dryness and check cough.

Prescription: Modified Decoction of Mori and Armeniacae Amarum (256). In this prescription, Folium Mori mildly disperses dryness-heat; Semen Armeniacae Amarum moistens the lung and checks cough; Radix Adenophorae, Exocarpium Pyri and Fructus Gardeniae produce body fluids, moisten dryness and disperse heat; Semen Sojae Preparatum eliminates wind and promotes the lung's dispersive function; and Bulbus Fritillariae Thunbergii disperses heat in the lung, resolves phlegm and checks cough. A proper amount of Pericarpium Trichosanthis, Radix Trichosanthis and Rhizoma Phragmitis can be added to moisten the lung and disperse heat.

If dryness-heat and wind-cold combine to cause cough, the condition is then referred to as "cool-dryness." In addition to non-productive cough and dryness of the nose and throat, this syndrome also presents marked chilliness, fever, headache, absence of sweating, and a thin, white and dry tongue coating. In this case, herbs that eliminate wind and promote the lung's dispersive function should be combined with herbs that moisten the lung and resolve phlegm. The prescription is Decoction of Mori and Armeniacae Amarum (256), which is added with Herba Schizonepetae, Radix Ledebouriellae, Folium Perillae, Radix Peucedani and Fructus Arctii.

Frequent non-productive cough with a sensation of fullness and pain in the chest more pronounced behind the sternum, blood-tinged sputum, asthmatic breathing, thirst and a red tongue with scanty coating all result from the consumption of *yin* following damage of the lung by dryness-heat. The treatment is to disperse heat and moisten dryness primarily, and to nourish the lung and produce fluids secondarily. Modified Decoction for Clearing Away Dryness and Treating Lung Disorders (285) is recommended. In this recipe, Folium Mori and Gypsum Fibrosum clear away dryness-heat from the lung and stomach; Colla Corii Asini, Radix Ophiopogonis, and Semen Cannabis disperse heat and moisten the lung; Radix Ginseng and Radix Glycyrrhizae benefit *qi* and produce body fluids; and Semen Armeniacae Amarum and Folium Eriobotryae resolve phlegm and check coughing.

If wind-cold and wind-heat are indistinguishable, or if the cough has lasted for a long time, or if it relapses with itching in the throat, difficulty in expectoration and absence of pronounced exterior syndrome, modified Powder for Relieving Cough (45) is then prescribed. In this prescription, Radix Asteris and Rhizoma Cynanchi Stauntonii improve the circulation of lung *qi*, resolve phlegm and check cough; Exocarpium Citri Rubrum, Radix Platycodi and Radix Glycyrrhizae promote the lung's dispersive function, ease the throat, conduct the unhealthy *qi* downward and resolve phlegm; and Herba Schizonepetae eliminates pathogenic factors. This prescription exerts warm and cool effects simultaneously, and is most suitable for a retention of residual pathogenic factors and the blockage of the *qi* passage by turbid phlegm due to impaired pulmonary function.

2. Cough due to the Internal Damage

(1) Attack of the lung by phlegm-dampness

Clinical manifestations: Cough with profuse thin and white sputum, a sensation of distention in the chest and epigastrium, poor appetite, listlessness, lassitude, loose stool, a white and sticky tongue coating, and a soft and smooth pulse.

Analysis: Deficiency of spleen *qi* implies dysfunction of the spleen in transportation and transformation. Food therefore cannot be transformed into nutritious essence. This subsequently produces dampness and phlegm, whose attack on the lung is the cause of cough with profuse thin and white sputum. Retention of phlegm-dampness in the lung and stomach leads to a sensation of distention there, and poor appetite. Listlessness, lassitude, and loose stool are the consequences of deficient spleen *qi*. A white and sticky tongue coating and a soft and smooth pulse all suggest phlegm-dampness.

Treatment: To invigorate the spleen, dry out dampness, resolve phlegm and check cough.

Prescription: Rhizoma Atractylodis, Cortex Magnoliae Officinalis, Radix Asteris and Flos Farfarae are added to *Erchen* Decoction (3). In this recipe, Rhizoma Atractylodis and Poria invigorate the spleen and dry out dampness; Pericarpium Citri Reticulatae and Cortex Magnoliae Officinalis regulate *qi* and ease the chest; Rhizoma Pinelliae, Radix Asteris, Flos Farfarae and Radix Glycyrrhizae resolve phlegm and check cough. Modified Decoction of Six Mild Drugs (55) is also applicable. If there are pronounced signs of cold, herbs that warm the lung and disperse cold are added, such as Herba Asari, Rhizoma Zingiberis and Ramulus Cinnamomi.

If phlegm-dampness has turned to heat, manifesting cough with thick and yellow sputum, a yellow and sticky tongue coating, and a smooth and rapid pulse, accompanied by epigastric and abdominal distention, lassitude and poor appetite, the method of regulating *qi*, eliminating dampness, dispersing heat in the lung and resolving phlegm will then be adopted. This is done by prescribing *Erchen* Decoction (3), added with Cortex Mori, Bulbus Fritillariae Cirrhosae, Fructus Trichosanthis and Radix Scutellariae.

(2) Invasion of the lung by liver fire

Clinical manifestations: Non-productive cough, frequent feeling of a stream of air going upward to the throat, hypochondriac pain on both sides when coughing, blood-tinged sputum or even hemoptysis in violent coughing, irritability, red face and eyes, a thin and yellow tongue coating with little moisture, and a taut and rapid pulse.

Analysis: Liver fire consumes lung fluid, and thereby causes non-productive cough. Damage to the vessels of the lung gives rise to blood-tinged sputum or hemoptysis. The liver meridian passes through the hypochondrium on both sides, and then enters the lung. Invasion of the lung by liver fire produces cough and hypochondriac pain at the same time. Hyperactive liver fire causes irritability along with red face and eyes. A thin and yellow tongue coating with little moisture, and a taut and thready pulse all suggest hyperactivity of the liver and consumption of fluid due to heat in the lung.

Treatment: To disperse heat in the liver, reduce fire, moisten the lung and resolve phlegm.

Prescription: Modified Combination of Powder of Indigo Naturalis and Concha Meretricis seu Cyclinae (321) and Decoction for Clearing Away Heat in the Lung and Resolving Phlegm (279). In this recipe, Indigo Naturalis and Fructus Gardeniae disperse heat in the liver and reduce fire; and Radix Scutellariae and Cortex Mori disperse heat in the lung. The elimination of heat in the lung ensures a clean and moist environment for the lung, thereby alleviating the cough. Concha Meretricis seu Cyclinae, Fructus Trichosanthis, Bulbus Fritillariae Cirrhosae, Rhizoma Anemarrhenae and Radix Ophiopogonis strengthen the antitussive effect by dispersing heat, resolving phlegm, moistening the lung and producing body fluids. In cases of blood-tinged sputum or hemoptysis, herbs that check bleeding are added, such as Cacumen Platyeladi, Rhizoma Imperatae, Herba Agrimoniae, and Radix Notoginseng, etc.

(3) Cough due to deficiency of the lung

Both deficiency of lung *yin* and deficiency of lung *qi* may cause cough. Cough due to lung *qi*-deficiency is mostly accompanied by asthmatic breathing; it will be discussed in the section "Asthma." Cough due to lung *yin*-deficiency is introduced here.

Clinical manifestations: A slow onset of cough with little sputum or blood-tinged sputum, or even hemoptysis, dryness in the mouth and throat, afternoon fever, malar flush, a hot sensation in the palms and soles, insomnia, night sweating, emaciation, lassitude, listlessness, a red tongue with exfoliated coating or none at all, and a thready and rapid pulse.

Analysis: Deficiency of *yin* fluid in the lung means lack of nourishment, and this inevitably impairs the lung's dispersive and descending function and produces cough. Deficiency of lung *yin* also produces internal heat, which is the cause of dryness of the mouth and throat. Damage to the vessels of the lung by heat explains blood-tinged sputum and hemoptysis. Afternoon fever, malar flush, a hot sensation in the palms and soles, insomnia, and night sweating are all induced by hyperactivity of fire due to *yin* deficiency. A red tongue with exfoliated coating or none at all, and a thready and rapid pulse are all heat signs due to *yin* deficiency.

Treatment: To nourish *yin*, disperse heat in the lung, resolve phlegm and check cough.

Prescription: Modified Decoction of Adenophorae and Ophiopogonis (150). In this prescription,

Radix Adenophorae, Rhizoma Polygonati Odorati, Radix Ophiopogonis and Radix Trichosanthis nourish *yin*, produce body fluids, moisten the lung and check cough; Semen Lablab Album and Radix Glycyrrhizae invigorate the spleen and harmonize the middle *jiao*. Bulbus Fritillariae Cirrhosae, Semen Armeniacae Amarum, Fructus Trichosanthis and Fructus Aristolochiae are added to disperse heat in the lung, resolve phlegm and check cough.

If *yin* deficiency produces internal heat that impairs the vessels of the lung and thereby causes blood-tinged sputum or hemoptysis, Decoction of Colla Corii Asini for Invigorating Lung (153) is applied. In this recipe, Colla Corii Asini nourishes *yin*, invigorates the lung, replenishes blood and checks bleeding; Fructus Aristolochiae, Fructus Arctii and Semen Armeniacae Amarum resolve phlegm and check cough; and Fructus Oryzae Glutinosae and Radix Glycyrrhizae invigorate the spleen and lung. In cases of afternoon fever and malar flush due to hyperactivity of deficiency fire, such herbs as Radix Stellariae, Cortex Lycii and Radix Scutellariae are added.

Lingering cough due to internal damage, accompanied by dyspnea, is treated by strengthening the kidneys' ability to receive *qi*. The recommended herbal drugs include Radix Ginseng, Gecko, Radix Rehmanniae Preparata and Fructus Schisandrae.

Remarks

Improper or delayed treatment may change cough due to attack of the external pathogenic factors into cough due to the internal damage. External pathogenic factors may easily affect the *zang-fu* organs. When the weather changes suddenly or in a cold season, if the body resistance is weak, this can aggravate cough, and possibly develop it into dyspnea, palpitation, edema and tympanites. Therefore, patients with cough due to the internal damage should avoid catching cold. They should also avoid smoking and alcohol, and do proper physical exercises to build up health. In the meantime, they should take medication to treat the underlying cause of the disease during the remission stage, according to the principle "to treat the underlying cause in chronic cases."

Cough at the initial stage is relieved by easing the circulation of lung *qi*; astringents and antitussives are not used. This is because these drugs may "close the door and keep the enemy in the house." Early administration of astringents and antitussives will make it impossible to expectorate sticky sputum, thus aggravating the pathological condition. Nevertheless, a proper amount of astringents and antitussives can be prescribed for the treatment of long-standing cough in which lung *qi* is damaged and pathogenic factors have been eliminated. The drugs for such cases include Fructus Schisandrae, Pericarpium Papaveris, and Fructus Chebulae.

Since the dysfunction of lung *qi* produces phlegm in both types of cough, expectorants must be used to support treatment. In cases of heat-phlegm, use Fructus Trichosanthis, Bulbus Fritillariae Cirrhosae, Rhizoma Belamcandae, Concretio Silicae Bambusae, Concha Meretricis seu Cyclinae and Pumex. In cases of dryness-phlegm, use Exocarpium Pyri, Radix Adenophorae, Radix Trichosanthis, Semen Armeniacae Amarum and Radix Stemonae. For dampness-phlegm, apply Rhizoma Pinelliae, Exocarpium Citri Rubrum, Rhizoma Arisaematis and Semen Sinapis Albae.

Case Studies

Name: Yi XX; Sex: Male; Age: 60; Date: February 9, 1958.

First visit: For three to four years, the patient suffered from bronchitis, which was worse in winter. Currently, he complained of cough with profuse white sputum. Since this was worse at night, he could only sleep for three to four hours. He also noted poor appetite and loose stool with four to five bowel movements a day. The tongue coating was white and sticky, and the pulse was retarded and smooth.

All this was due to *yang* deficiency with retention of dampness in the spleen. The treatment was to warm up the spleen and eliminate dampness. Decoction of Six Mild Drugs (55) and Decoction of Poria, Cinnamomi, Atractylodis Macrocephalae, and Glycyrrhizae (170) were prescribed with additional drugs:

Radix Codonopsis	9 g;
Rhizoma Atractylodis Macrocephalae	6 g;
Poria	9 g;
Radix Glycyrrhizae Preparata	3 g;
Rhizoma Pinelliae Preparata	9 g;
Exocarpium Citri Rubrum	6 g;
Ramulus Cinnamomi	4.5 g;
Fructus Schisandrae	1.5 g;
Rhizoma Zingiberis	3 g;
Fructus Jujubae	4 pieces.

Second visit: Cough and sleep improved. He could sleep for five to six hours before cough occurred again. Sputum decreased in amount and could be spat out. Appetite also improved. He had two to three bowel movements a day with unformed stool. The pulse was weak at the "*cun*" position, taut at the "*guan*" position, and deep at the "*chi*" position on both sides. The sticky tongue coating was less obvious. The same treatment was adopted. Three grams of Radix Aconiti Lateralis Preparata were added to the previous prescription; this herb should be decocted first.

To consolidate the therapeutic results, the following prescription was given:

Radix Ginseng or Radix Codonopsis	15 g;
Rhizoma Atractylodis Macrocephalae	15 g;
Rhizoma Zingiberis	9 g;
Radix Glycyrrhizae Preparata	15 g;
Radix Aconiti Lateralis Preparata	30 g;
Semen Myristicae (roasted)	15 g;
Fructus Chebulae (roasted)	15 g;
Fructus Schisandrae	15 g;
Fructus Psoraleae	30 g;
Exocarpium Citri Rubrum	15 g;
Rhizoma Dioscoreae	30 g;
Semen Euryales	30 g;
Fructus Amomi	15 g.

All these herbs were ground into powder and made into pills with honey, as large as seeds of the Chinese parasol tree, to be taken with warm water, 6 g each time.

Explanation: This cough is due to internal damage. The clinical manifestations of cough with profuse white sputum, poor appetite, loose stool, a white and sticky tongue coating, and a retarded and smooth pulse all suggest *yang* deficiency with retention of dampness in the spleen. The pill prescription is based on Decoction of Aconiti Lateralis Preparata for Regulating Middle *Jiao* (163) and Pill of Four Miraculous Drugs (94) to regulate the spleen and kidneys.

III. Lung Abscess

Lung abscess is manifested principally as cough, chest pain, fever and foul sputum, and in severe cases, spitting of purulent bloody sputum.

The medical classic *Synopsis of Prescriptions of the Golden Chamber* recommends Decoction of Platycodi (235) and Decoction of Lepidii seu Descurainiae and Jujubae for Purging Lung-Heat (294) to treat lung abscess. Another medical classic, *Essentially Treasured Prescriptions for Emergencies*, prescribes Rhizoma Phragmitis, Semen Coicis, Semen Benincasae and Semen Persicae; this was subsequently known as Decoction of Phragmitis (30).

Suppurative infections of the lungs in Western medicine, such as pulmonary abscess, suppurative pneumonia, pulmonary gangrene and suppurative infection due to bronchiectasis, can all be differentiated and treated according to the following descriptions.

Etiology and Pathogenesis

Lung abscess is due to retention of heat in the lung. In *Synopsis of Prescriptions of the Golden Chamber*, Zhang Zhongjing says, "Attack of the lung by external pathogenic wind gives rise to cough... Excessive heat produces stagnant blood, which accumulates to form pus to be spat like rice porridge." In *Zhang's Medical Treatise*, Zhang Shiwan explains lung abscess by saying, "Lung abscess is due to the invasion by wind-cold, which stays in the lung, and then turns to heat." The main cause of lung abscess is therefore the attack by external pathogenic wind-heat, or by wind-cold which then turns to heat. Retention of heat in the lung produces stagnant blood and causes necrosis of tissues; thus suppuration ensues.

The formation of lung abscess is also closely related to the internal factors. For example, some people have excessive phlegm-heat constitutionally. Drinking excessive alcohol or eating too much highly flavored food can also produce phlegm-heat in the body. If this combines with external wind-heat, heat will accumulate in the lung.

Presenting itself mainly as excess syndrome due to the retention of heat in the lung, lung abscess develops in four stages. First, attack of the lung by the external pathogenic wind-heat impairs the lung's dispersive and descending function. Second, excessive phlegm-heat in the lung damages blood vessels and causes stagnant blood to form abscess. Third, excessive heat causes stagnation of blood and necrosis of tissues, thus resulting in the perforation of abscess. Fourth, the elimination of pathogenic factors and restoration of the body resistance result in a gradual recovery.

Distinction and Treatment

In differentiation, primary attention should be given to the quantity, smell, color and quality of sputum. Patients with lung abscess usually expectorate large amounts of foul, yellowish green or yellow purulent sputum. *An Introduction to Medicine*, a classic on traditional Chinese medicine, says, "The foul, purulent and bloody expectoration sinks in water." *Continued Flaring of Medical Lamp* describes the method of distinguishing pus and sputum by saying, "The patient with lung abscess has a dull pain in the chest and brings up foul sputum. When spat into water, pus sinks to the bottom, while sputum floats on the surface."

Generally speaking, lung abscess manifests heat syndrome and excess syndrome. Further distinction is made by reference to the four stages in its development. The initial stage, with the attack of the lung by external pathogenic wind-heat, reveals an exterior excess syndrome. The abscess formation stage, marked by the accumulation of excessive heat in the lung, manifests a heat excess syndrome. The abscess perforation stage, principally exhibits an excess syndrome which may be complicated by a deficiency syndrome. The convalescent stage, characterized by the gradual elimination of heat and recovery of body resistance, generally shows a deficiency syndrome. In chronic cases of persistent heat, which consumes lung *qi* and lung *yin* following the perforation of the abscess, a deficiency syndrome complicated by excess syndrome ensues.

Since there is retention of heat and stagnant blood, and suppuration in lung abscess, the treatment aims at dispersing heat, eliminating toxins, removing blood stasis and draining pus. Specifically, wind-heat and heat in the lung are dispersed in the initial stage, and phlegm is resolved. At the abscess-formation stage, heat is dispersed, toxins eliminated and blood stasis removed. Pus is drained, heat dispersed and toxins eliminated at the perforation stage. Finally, at the convalescent stage, the flow of *qi* is improved and *yin* nourished. In the treatment of chronic cases, body resistance is strengthened and pathogenic factors eliminated by adding medicinal herbs that disperse heat and eliminate toxins and those that benefit *qi* flow and nourish *yin*.

1. Initial Stage

Clinical manifestations: Chilliness, fever or high fever, cough with scanty and sticky sputum, chest pain aggravated by coughing, difficult breathing, dryness of the throat, a thin and yellow tongue coating, and a superficial, smooth and rapid pulse.

Analysis: The struggle between the invading pathogenic wind-heat and the body's anti-pathogenic *qi* leads to chilliness and fever. Presence of pathogenic heat causes high fever. Attack of the lung by heat impairs the lung's dispersive function and thereby causes cough, chest pain and difficult breathing. Consumption of lung fluid by heat explains scanty and sticky sputum and dryness of the throat. A thin and yellow tongue coating and a superficial, smooth and rapid pulse all suggest the attack of pathogenic wind and retention of phlegm-heat.

Treatment: To disperse wind-heat, disperse heat in the lung and resolve phlegm.

Prescription: Powder of Lonicerae and Forsythiae (287) along with medicines that clear heat and eliminate toxins, such as Herba Houttuyniae. In this prescription, Flos Lonicerae, Fructus Forsythiae, Rhizoma Phragmitis and Herba Lophatheri disperse wind-heat, clear heat and eliminate toxins; and Herba Menthae, Herba Schizonepetae, Semen Sojae Preparatum, Fructus Arctii and Radix Platycodi disperse wind and promote the lung's dispersive function. The additional Herba Houttuyniae strengthens the formula's effect of dispersing heat and eliminating toxins.

In cases of cough with profuse sputum, Fructus Trichosanthis, Bulbus Fritillariae Cirrhosae and Semen Armeniacae Amarum are added to resolve phlegm and check cough. In cases of headache, Fructus Viticis, Flos Chrysanthemi and Folium Mori are added to disperse wind-heat and disperse heat in the head and eyes. In cases of chest pain, Radix Curcumae, Semen Persicae and Radix Paeoniae Rubra are added to remove blood stasis and relieve pain. In cases where dryness consumes body fluids, Radix Adenophorae, Radix Ophiopogonis, Radix Asparagi and Radix Trichosanthis are added to moisten the lung and produce fluid. If coughing is severe, Decoction of Ephedrae, Armeniacae Amarum, Gypsum Fibrosum and Glycyrrhizae (272) is then added to disperse heat in the lung and relieve dyspnea. The administration of all these herbal medicines are based on Powder of Lonicerae and Forsythiae (287) and Decoction of Mori and Chrysanthemi (257).

2. Abscess-Formation Stage

Clinical manifestations: High fever, sweating, chills, stuffiness and pain in the chest, shortness of breath, cough with purulent and foul sputum, dryness of the mouth and throat, restlessness, a yellow and sticky tongue coating, and a smooth and rapid pulse.

Analysis: Excessive internal heat and the struggle between the body's anti-pathogenic *qi* and pathogenic factors lead to high fever and chills. Dissipation of body fluids due to pathogenic heat causes profuse sweating. Retention of phlegm-heat in the lung results in unhealthy lung *qi*, and thereby develops cough and shortness of breath. Accumulation of stagnant blood and heat forms abscesses, eliciting purulent and foul sputum. Blockage of the collaterals of the lung by phlegm-heat causes chest pain. Consumption of fluid by heat explains dryness of the mouth and throat. Excessive heat disturbs the mind, causing restlessness. A yellow and sticky tongue coating and a smooth and rapid pulse suggest retention of phlegm-heat in the lung and accumulation of heat inside.

Treatment: To disperse heat, eliminate toxins, remove blood stasis and disperse stagnation.

Prescription: Decoction of Phragmitis (30) with additional drugs. In this prescription, Rhizoma Phragmitis promotes the lung's dispersive function and disperses heat; and Semen Coicis, Semen Benincasae and Semen Persicae resolve turbid phlegm, remove blood stasis and disperse stagnation. Herbal medicines that disperse heat and eliminate toxins are added, such as Flos Lonicerae, Fructus Forsythiae, Folium Isatidis and Herba Houttuyniae. If sputum is extremely foul, Bolus of Calculus Bovis for Clearing Away Heat and Detoxification (308) is added to disperse heat in the *ying* system, eliminate toxins and remove blood stasis. In cases of chest pain, Olibanum and Myrrha are added to improve blood circulation and relieve pain. In cases of constipation, Radix et Rhizoma Rhei and Fructus Aurantii Immaturus are added to promote bowel movement and disperse heat. In cases of cough with profuse turbid sputum, Fructus Trichosanthis, Cortex Mori and Semen Lepidii seu Descurainiae are added to clear away phlegm-heat from the lung.

3. Abscess-Perforation Stage

Clinical manifestations: Cough with purulent, bloody and extremely foul sputum, distress, fullness and pain in the chest, dyspnea, or orthopnea in severe cases, feverish sensation, flushed face, restlessness, thirst, a red or crimson tongue with yellow and sticky coating, and a smooth, and rapid pulse.

Analysis: Perforation of the lung abscess leads to cough with foul, purulent and bloody sputum. Retention of pus in the lung blocks its collaterals and hinders the flow of lung *qi*; this explains distress, fullness and pain in the chest, dyspnea or orthopnea. Retention of heat in the interior produces a feverish sensation and flushed face. Consumption of body fluids leads to restlessness and thirst. A red or crimson tongue with yellow and sticky coating and a smooth and rapid pulse all suggest retention of excess heat.

Treatment: To drain pus, disperse heat and eliminate toxins.

Prescription: Decoction of Platycodi (235) is used in combination with Decoction of Phragmitis (30), and to be added with such herbs as Flos Lonicerae, Fructus Forsythiae, Herba Patriniae, Radix Fagopyri and Herba Houttuyniae. In cases of *qi* deficiency accompanied by sweating, Radix Astragali is added to invigorate lung *qi* and promote pus drainage. In cases of fluid consumption marked by the dry mouth, Radix Adenophorae, Radix Ophiopogonis and Bulbus Lilii are added to nourish *yin* and promote the generation of body fluids. In cases of hemoptysis, Rhizoma Imperatae, Nodus Nelumbinis Rhizomatis, Cortex Moutan and Radix Rehmanniae are added to cool the blood and check bleeding.

4. Convalescent Stage

Clinical manifestations: Gradual subsidence of the feverish sensation, improvement of cough, decreased quantity of purulent sputum, but continuing lassitude, poor appetite, a red tongue, and a thready, rapid and weak pulse.

Analysis: Residual phlegm-heat explains productive cough and decreased quantity of purulent sputum. *Qi*, blood and body fluid have not yet recovered; this is the cause of lassitude and poor appetite. A red tongue and a thready, rapid and weak pulse all suggest *qi* and *yin* deficiency.

Treatment: To invigorate the spleen and the lung, benefit *qi* and nourish *yin*.

Prescription: Modified Powder of Ginseng, Poria and Atractylodis Macrocephalae (190) and Decoction of Adenophorae and Ophiopogonis (150). In this prescription, Radix Ginseng, Rhizoma Atractylodis Macrocephalae, Poria, Semen Lablab Album, Semen Coicis and Rhizoma Dioscoreae benefit *qi*, invigorate the spleen, produce body fluids and nourish *yin*; Radix Adenophorae, Radix Ophiopogonis, Radix Trichosanthis and Rhizoma Polygonati Odorati nourish *yin* and produce body fluids; and Radix Platycodi conducts the effect of drugs to the lungs to invigorate the spleen and lung, benefit the flow of *qi* and nourish *yin*.

Prolonged cough with a small quantity of purulent and bloody sputum, afternoon fever, restlessness, dryness of the mouth and throat, spontaneous and night sweating, shortness of breath, emaciation, a crimson tongue with scanty coating and a feeble, rapid pulse all suggest deficiency of both *qi* and *yin*, weakness of resistance and retention of residual heat. Herbal drugs that drain pus and eliminate toxins are added to those that benefit *qi* and nourish *yin*. The prescription is Decoction of Platycodi and Armeniacae Amarum (234).

Remarks

Observing the quality, quantity, color and smell of sputum is vital in understanding the development of lung abscesses. It is white or yellow, sticky, odorless and in small quantity at the initial stage; its quantity increases, and it becomes yellowish-green, thick and foul at the abscess-formation stage. It is purulent, bloody and extremely foul, and its quantity obviously increases at the perforation stage; and it is yellow or thin and clear, less smelly and in decreased quantity at the convalescent stage.

Drugs that disperse heat and eliminate toxins should be used from the beginning to the end of the treatment. Efforts should be made to keep the bowels open, because the lung and the large intestine are related externally and internally, and free bowel motion promotes the lung's dispersive and descending function, and helps eliminate pathogenic heat.

Proper treatment contributes to rapid recovery at the initial stage of lung abscess which is also expected before pus is produced at the abscess-formation stage, because the lung abscess becomes stubborn when pus is formed. *Synopsis of Prescriptions of the Golden Chamber* says, "Early stages of lung abscess are curable, but the formation of pus will lead to death." The perforation stage is thus a turning point, and it is necessary to observe closely the pathological changes at this stage. The prognosis is still good if the symptoms alleviate gradually and convalescence ensues. But it is unfavorable if spitting of purulent, bloody and extremely foul sputum persists, accompanied by reduced energy, fever and anorexia; the recurrence of turbid and foul sputum and other symptoms suggest the chronic nature. Every effort should be made to treat lung abscess at its formative stage. Persistent spitting of purulent, bloody and foul sputum following perforation could be accompanied by scaly skin, constipation, hoarse voice, difficult breathing with open mouth, and cyanosis of nails and lips. These are all critical signs which should not be neglected. Lung abscess in old people, children, people with weak constitution, and alcoholics is stubborn.

The diagnosis of lung abscess should be established as early as possible, and proper treatment should be given without delay. Tonics and astringents should not be used too early.

Case Studies

A patient with his/her background unknown.

The patient suffered from lung abscess with symptoms of fever, cough with foul sputum, and a rapid and large pulse. The pathogenesis was an attack of the skin and hair by external pathogenic wind complicated by the damage to the blood vessels from heat. Decoction of Ephedrae, Armeniacae Amarum, Gypsum Fibrosum and Glycyrrhizae (272) was prescribed to disperse heat. Succus Coicis Radix was taken with the decoction.

Lung abscess was complicated by exterior syndrome, which was severe and relieved first by using the above prescription. Decoction of Phragmitis (30) was then prescribed. The herbs included Semen Benincasae, Radix Platycodi, Poria, Herba Houttuyniae, Semen Coicis, Radix Glycyrrhizae, Semen Citrulli, Radix Curcumae, Rhizoma Belamcandae, Bulbus Fritillariae Cirrhosae, Folium Eriobotryae, Rhizoma Phragmitis, Semen Persicae and Semen Armeniacae Amarum.

When the disease was about to be resolved, hemoptysis was likely to occur. This should not be considered tuberculosis because it was due to physical exertion which had damaged the vessels of the delicate lung. If there was an unpleasant smell, drugs that cool blood could be added to those dispersing heat in the lung. The prescription then consists of Semen Coicis, Semen Benincasae, Flos Lonicerae, Cortex Mori, Herba Houttuyniae, Folium Eriobotryae, Rhizoma Imperatae, and Rhizoma Phragmitis.

It was 25 days since the lung abscess appeared. The damage to the vessels of the lung resulted in blood loss, and other symptoms were also pronounced. Radix Coicis, Cortex Moutan, Radix Glycyrrhizae, Semen Benincasae, Folium Mori, Semen Persicae, Bulbus Fritillariae Cirrhosae, Radix Platycodi, Rhizoma Belamcandae, Folium Eriobotryae, Radix Notoginseng, Rhizoma Imperatae, Rhizoma Phragmitis and Succus Nelumbinis Rhizomatis were prescribed.

Explanation: Fever and a rapid and large pulse at the beginning suggested the attack of the body surface by external pathogenic wind-heat. Cough with foul sputum was due to the retention of pathogenic heat in the lung. The treatment was to relieve exterior syndrome and disperse heat in the lung with acrid and cool drugs. The Decoction of Ephedrae, Armeniacae Amarum, Gypsum Fibrosum and Glycyrrhizae (272) was therefore prescribed. When the exterior syndrome subsided, cough with foul and purulent sputum became the main symptom; this was treated with Decoction of Phragmitis (30).

Lung abscess inevitably damages the lung and its vessels, thereby causing hemoptysis. The doctor must pay attention to this. The last two prescriptions, combining drugs that cool the blood with those dispersing heat in the lung, are recommended for such conditions. This example shows that the treatment should conform to the pathogenesis, and that different drugs are applied at different stages.

Name: Shao XX; Sex: Female; Age: 19; Occupation: Student.

This patient was admitted four days after she noted fever and chest pain. Over the previous two months, she had cough with white or white-blue sputum. Four days ago, she began to suffer from fever, cough with yellow sputum and chest pain on the right side, which became more dreadful when coughing and respiring. Examination at the time of admission on March 12, 1965 showed that the body temperature was 36.5°C. Percussion on the right upper chest revealed a dull resonance. Increased vocal fremitus and moist rales were heard, and there were also scattered pulmonary rales on the left side. The total white blood cell accounted to 14,700, of which the neutrophils accounted for 81%. X-rays revealed the impression of lung abscess on the right side. Bacillus tubercle was not found in the sputum. This established the diagnosis as lung abscess.

First visit (March 12): In addition to the above symptoms, she also had a flushed face, anorexia, epistasis, a red tongue with thin coating, and a thready and rapid pulse. She had been constipated for the previous four months. All this was due to the attack of the lung by wind-heat. Treatment aimed to promote the lung's dispersive function and clear away wind-heat. The prescription consisted of the following herbs:

Folium Mori	9 g;
Cortex Mori	9 g;
Semen Coicis (raw)	12 g;
Fructus Trichosanthis	30 g;
Bulbus Fritillariae Thunbergii	9 g;
Semen Benincasae	12 g;
Radix Paeoniae Rubra	12 g;
Flos Lonicerae	12 g;
Radix Platycodi	6 g;
Rhizoma Imperatae	30 g;
Rhizoma Phragmitis	30 g.

One dose was prescribed.

Second visit (March 13): The patient had a temperature of 39.5°C, cough, chest pain, grayish-brown and foul sputum, thirst, epistasis, a red tongue with thin and yellow coating, and a thready and rapid pulse. All this was due to the attack of the lung by wind-heat leading to the formation of lung abscess. Treatment aimed to disperse heat, relieve toxins, resolve phlegm and drain pus. The following herbs were prescribed:

Flos Lonicerae	30 g;
Fructus Forsythiae	12 g;
Semen Benincasae	15 g;
Semen Coicis (raw)	12 g;
Semen Persicae	9 g;
Radix Scutellariae	9 g;
Fructus Gardeniae (raw)	9 g;
Herba Houttuyniae	30 g;
Rhizoma Phragmitis (fresh)	60 g.

Three doses were prescribed.

Third visit (March 16): Fever subsided, and the body temperature was 37°C. The remaining symptoms included cough with foul sputum, chest pain, thirst, deep yellow urine, a yellow and sticky tongue coating at the root, and a thready and rapid pulse. The same treatment was employed. The prescription included three doses of the following herbs:

Flos Lonicerae	30 g;
Radix Platycodi	12 g;
Semen Benincasae	30 g;
Radix Scutellariae	9 g;
Herba Houttuyniae	30 g;
Bulbus Fritillariae Cirrhosae	6 g;
Bulbus Fritillariae Thunbergii	6 g;
Semen Coicis (raw)	30 g;
Radix Glycyrrhizae (raw)	9 g;
Semen Armeniacae Amarum	9 g;
Semen Persicae	9 g;
Rhizoma Imperatae	30 g;

Rhizoma Phragmitis	30 g.

After three doses, afternoon fever subsided, and both cough with foul sputum and chest pain improved. Similar prescription continued until March 25.

Fourth visit (March 26): Sputum considerably decreased in quantity, and its foul smell disappeared. Appetite improved and body weight increased. The X-ray also showed a great improvement. The tongue coating was thin and the pulse thready. All this showed that there were residual pathogenic factors in the body, and the body resistance was weak. Further treatment aimed to eliminate these pathogenic factors and at the same time strengthen the body resistance. Three doses of the following prescription were administered:

Radix Astragali (raw)	9 g;
Radix Adenophorae (fresh)	9 g;
Rhizoma Atractylodis Macrocephalae (stir-baked)	9 g;
Semen Benincasae	15 g;
Semen Armeniacae Amarum	9 g;
Semen Coicis (raw)	12 g;
Herba Houttuyniae	30 g;
Radix Platycodi	4.5 g;
Radix Glycyrrhizae	4.5 g;
Rhizoma Phragmitis (fresh)	30 g.

After the three doses, the patient was discharged from hospital, but she continued the treatment as an outpatient.

Explanation: Lung abscess is marked by cough with purulent and foul sputum. Since the patient did not have purulent and foul sputum on admission, the diagnosis of the attack of the lung by windheat was established. Lung abscess was not confirmed until the second visit. The above prescriptions were based on Decoction of Phragmitis (30), which disperses heat, resolves phlegm, activates blood circulation and drains pus. The additional Radix Platycodi and Bulbus Fritillariae Thunbergii aimed to resolve phlegm and drain pus. Large amounts of drugs that disperse heat and eliminate toxins were added, including Herba Houttuyniae, Fructus Gardeniae, Radix Scutellariae, Flos Lonicerae and Fructus Forsythiae. When fever had subsided, the treatment focused on both eliminating the remaining pathogenic factors and strengthening body resistance. Radix Astragali, Rhizoma Atractylodis Macrocephalae and Radix Adenophorae were then added to invigorate the spleen and nourish the lung.

IV. Asthma

Asthma is a disease marked by recurrent attacks of paroxysmal dyspnea with wheezing. Wheezing is a high-pitched sound that rattles in the throat during breathing, resembling whistling, snoring or sawing. *Synopsis of Prescriptions of the Golden Chamber* describes wheezing as a sound made by a frog in the throat. It also says, "Retention of phlegm above the diaphragm produces the symptoms of productive cough, asthma, lumbago, watering eyes and violent movement of the body." Regarding the treatment of asthma, it recommends Decoction of Belamcandae and Ephedrae (249).

No distinction was made between asthma and dyspnea before the Jin and Yuan dynasties. It was not until the publication of *Orthodox Medical Record* by Yu Tuan of the Ming Dynasty that they were distinguished. The book states, "Asthma is named after its sound, and dyspnea is named after its breath." *A Guide to Clinical Practice with Case Records* differentiates the two by saying, "When the pathogenic factors have been eliminated, dyspnea is relieved and will not recur. Since the pathogenic factors of asthma are hidden inside the body and lung, asthma tends to recur in the following years."

Bronchial asthma and asthmatic bronchitis in Western medicine may be differentiated and treated according to the following descriptions.

Etiology and Pathogenesis

Asthma with wheezing is a chronic illness with frequent episodes. It often occurs at the junction of autumn and winter, spring and summer. Retention of phlegm in the lung is the main cause, while affection by the external pathogens, improper diet, emotional upset, strain and stress are all the inducing factors. The pathogenesis is the upward movement of phlegm along with the unhealthy *qi* through a narrowed airway. Although the disease mainly infects the lung, the spleen and kidneys are also affected.

1. Main Cause

Retention of phlegm in the lung is the main cause. It originates from splenic deficiency, namely, from the impairment of the spleen's transport and transformative function. Since the production of phlegm is also related to the attack by external pathogenic factors, improper diet and prolonged illness, there is a distinction between cold-phlegm and heat-phlegm.

(1) Cold-phlegm

Constant exposure to wind-cold enables pathogenic cold to penetrate the lung. Overeating raw and cold food produces cold fluid, which is stored in the lung and forms cold-phlegm. The cold fluid is likely to be stirred by the external pathogenic factors, resulting in short breath and wheezing. Cold-phlegm usually occurs after a prolonged illness or *yang* deficiency, and manifests complicated pathological conditions.

(2) Heat-phlegm

Overeating sour, salty, sweet or greasy food impairs splenic function and thereby produces phlegm, which gradually turns into heat. Both heat and phlegm accumulate in the pulmonary system. Phlegm long-retained in the lung may also turn to heat, and the resulting heat-phlegm gives rise to shortness of breath and wheezing when induced by the external factors. Consumption of *yin* after a prolonged illness or excess *yang* inside the human body often cause heat-phlegm.

2. Inducing Factors

External pathogenic factors such as wind, cold, summer-heat and dampness, along with overeating sour, salty, sweet, greasy, raw and cold food or sea food, and emotional upset or strain and stress, can all impair the lung's dispersive and descending function and then stir the phlegm hidden in the lung. These factors often combine to induce asthma. The sudden change of weather is most closely related to the occurrence of this disease.

Recurrent attacks of asthma over a long period of time consume lung qi and inevitably affect the spleen and kidneys. Deficiency of the spleen implies splenic dysfunction, which causes the production and accumulation of phlegm. Moreover, in cases of splenic deficiency, the lung is deprived of nourishment, and thus lung qi becomes even more deficient, which in turn weakens defensive qi. The external pathogenic factors will then penetrate the defensive system of the body, inducing new attacks of asthma. Under normal circumstance, the kidneys dominate the reception of qi. When the kidneys are deficient, however, the function is impaired. In cases of kidney $yang$-deficiency, $yang$ fails to resolve water, and thereby causes the overflow of water and dampness. Yin deficiency produces fire. Both conditions may affect the lung and subsequently give rise to chronic asthmatic attacks; a severe case may last for a long time. In a severe case of asthma marked by recurrent attacks, heart $yang$ is depleted and heart fluid let out. As a result, critical signs of profuse sweating and cold limbs occur.

Differential Diagnosis
Asthma is marked by a wheezing sound rattling in the throat during the attack, indicating respiratory tract is diseased. It is inevitably accompanied by dyspnea.

Dyspnea occurs in various acute and chronic diseases. It is marked by the shortness of breath, breathing with open mouth, raised shoulders, and flapping of the ala nasi. Here the air sacs are diseased. Dyspnea is not necessarily accompanied by asthma.

Distinction and Treatment
The onset of asthma is often abrupt. There may be prodromal symptoms in some cases, e.g., itching of the nose or throat, sneezing, and stuffiness in the chest. After that, a new attack occurs with the sensation of a blockage in the throat, and dyspnea gradually follows, accompanied by prolonged expiration, wheezing sounds in the throat, difficulty in producing expectoration, and a small amount of white and sticky sputum. Severe cases exhibit the symptoms of breathing with open mouth and raised shoulders, a distended sensation in the eyes, orthopnea, restlessness, pale complexion, cyanosis of the lips and nails, cold sweating on the forehead, and occasionally chilliness and fever. If the sticky sputum can be coughed out at this moment, stuffiness in the chest, wheezing and dyspnea will be relieved, and respiration will be free from obstruction.

The early stage of asthma is characterized by exterior syndromes. The treatment focuses on promoting the lung's dispersive function, regulating qi flow and dispelling phlegm so as to eliminate the pathogenic factors. Since phlegm can be complicated by either cold or heat, asthma should be distinguished between heat-asthma and cold-asthma. In a prolonged case with recurrent attacks, the body resistance is weakened. The treatment should focus on nurturing the lung and kidneys, invigorating the spleen and stomach, resolving phlegm and benefiting qi to eliminate pathogenic factors and strengthen the body resistance. During the remission stage, the principle of nurturing the lung, invigorating the spleen and strengthening the kidneys is applied to reinforce the body resistance.

1. During the Attack
(1) Asthma due to cold
Clinical manifestations: Short breath, dyspnea, wheezing, fullness and stuffiness in the chest, orthopnea, cough with white and sticky or thin and frothy sputum, a yellowish-blue complexion, ab-

sence of thirst, or thirst with preference for hot drinks, a white and slippery tongue coating, and a superficial and tense or taut and smooth pulse. The accompanying symptoms include headache, fever, chilliness and absence of sweating.

Analysis: Retention of cold-phlegm in the lung and attack by the external pathogenic wind-cold combine to cause blockage of the air passage by phlegm, giving rise to the shortness of breath, orthopnea and wheezing. Retention of cold-phlegm in the lung blocks *yang-qi* in the chest, which causes stuffiness in the chest and a yellowish-blue complexion. Absence of thirst suggests absence of heat signs. Attack of the pulmonary system by the pathogenic cold inhibits normal distribution of body fluids; this explains thirst with preference for hot drinks. A white and slippery tongue coating, and a superficial and tense pulse are all signs of cold phlegm. Headache, chilliness and fever are all the manifestations of the exterior syndrome due to the attack by wind-cold.

Treatment: To warm the lung, disperse cold, dispel phlegm and ease the throat.

Prescription: Decoction of Belamcandae and Ephedrae (249) or Small Blue Dragon Decoction (33). In the former, Rhizoma Belamcandae promotes the lung's dispersive function, dispels phlegm, and eases the throat; Herba Ephedrae releases lung *qi* and relieves asthma; Herba Asari and Rhizoma Zingiberis Recens, acrid in taste, disperse wind-cold; and Radix Asteris, Flos Farfarae and Rhizoma Pinelliae warm and moisten the lung, send the unhealthy *qi* downward and resolve phlegm. In the latter, Herba Ephedrae promotes the lung's dispersive function and relieves asthma; Ramulus Cinnamomi and Herba Asari disperse cold and relieve the exterior syndrome; Radix Paeoniae Alba assists Ramulus Cinnamomi in harmonizing nutrient *qi* and defensive *qi*; Rhizoma Zingiberis and Rhizoma Pinelliae warm the organs and resolve phlegm; and Fructus Schisandrae prevents *qi* consumption.

The former recipe is better at moistening the lung, resolving phlegm, easing the throat and checking cough. The latter is good for relieving asthma with external and internal cold.

If asthma still exists when the exterior syndrome has been relieved, the combined administration of Three Crude Drugs Decoction (18) and Decoction Containing Three Kinds of Seed for the Aged (15) is recommended. In this combined formula, Herba Ephedrae, Semen Armeniacae Amarum and Radix Glycyrrhizae promote the lung's dispersive function and relieve asthma; Fructus Perillae sends unhealthy *qi* downward and dispels phlegm; Semen Sinapis Albae relaxes the diaphragm and dispels phlegm; and Semen Raphani promotes digestion and resolves phlegm.

In protracted cases marked by *yang* deficiency with symptoms of asthmatic breathing, pale complexion, sweating, cold limbs, lassitude, shortness of breath, a pale and swollen tongue and a deep and weak pulse, Decoction of Perillae for Keeping *Qi* Downward (142) is prescribed. Here, Fructus Perillae sends the unhealthy *qi* downward and relieves asthma; Rhizoma Pinelliae, Radix Peucedani and Cortex Magnoliae Officinalis send the unhealthy *qi* downward and resolve phlegm; Pericarpium Citri Reticulatae and Radix Glycyrrhizae regulate *qi* of the middle *jiao*; and Cortex Cinnamomi warms the kidneys and assists its reception of *qi*. Since all these herbs are warm and dry in nature, Radix Angelicae Sinensis should also be used to nourish the blood and moisten dryness. Lignum Aquilariae Resinatum is added to strengthen the formula's effect in sending unhealthy *qi* downward and relieving asthma.

(2) Asthma due to heat

Clinical manifestations: Short breath, dyspnea, rattling sound in the throat, breathing with raised shoulders, paroxysmal choking cough with thick, sticky and yellow sputum which is difficult to expectorate, stuffiness in the chest, irritability, sweating, thirst, a red tongue with yellow and sticky coating, and a smooth and rapid pulse. Occasionally the exterior syndromes such as headache, fever and aversion to wind are present.

Analysis: Heat-phlegm in the lung when stirred by the pathogenic factors makes lung *qi* stagnant. Both phlegm and stagnant *qi* block the air passage, giving rise to short breath, asthmatic breathing with raised shoulders, and rattling sound in the throat. Heat in the lung consumes fluid, and thereby makes sputum thick, sticky and difficult to expectorate. The effort to bring out such sputum leads to paroxysmal choking cough. Excessive heat consumes body fluids, which is the cause of thirst. Disturbance of the mind by heat-phlegm gives rise to stuffiness in the chest and irritability. A red tongue with yellow and sticky coating, and a smooth and rapid pulse are all signs of excess heat-phlegm inside the body. The attack by the external pathogenic wind-cold explains the exterior syndromes, such as headache, fever and aversion to wind.

Treatment: To promote the lung's dispersive function, disperse heat, resolve phlegm, and send the unhealthy *qi* downward.

Prescription: Modified Decoction for Relieving Edema with Pinelliae (296). In this prescription, Herba Ephedrae and Gypsum Fibrosum release lung *qi*, relieve asthma and disperse heat; Rhizoma Pinelliae and Rhizoma Zingiberis Recens resolve phlegm and send the unhealthy *qi* downward; and Radix Glycyrrhizae and Fructus Jujubae harmonize the middle *jiao*. To dispel phlegm, regulate *qi*, and relieve asthma, Rhizoma Belamcandae, Semen Armeniacae Amarum, Fructus Perillae and Semen Lepidii seu Descurainiae are added.

In cases with excessive phlegm-heat, Radix Scutellariae, Cortex Mori, Herba Houttuyniae and Succus Bambusae are added to disperse heat in the lung and resolve phlegm.

If asthma remains and is accompanied by cough with sticky and yellow sputum even when the exterior syndrome has been relieved, Decoction for Relieving Asthma (179) is then prescribed. Here, Herba Ephedrae promotes the lung's dispersive function and relieves asthma; Fructus Perillae, Semen Armeniacae Amarum and Rhizoma Pinelliae resolve phlegm and send the unhealthy *qi* downward; Cortex Mori, Radix Scutellariae and Flos Farfarae disperse heat and promote the lung's descending function; Radix Glycyrrhizae harmonizes the effects of all the other herbs; and Semen Ginkgo is added for relieving asthma and consolidating lung *qi* by preventing Herba Ephedrae from consuming of the lung *qi*.

Both prescriptions consist of herbs which are cold and hot in nature, because asthma due to heat results from either the external cold that induces heat-phlegm or cold-phlegm that turns into heat. It is not advisable to use only herbs cool and cold in nature.

Protracted cases marked by sticky and scanty sputum, emaciation, dryness of the throat, shortness of breath, night sweating, restlessness, a red tongue with little moisture and thin yellow coating, and a thready and rapid pulse as a result of the *yin* deficiency suggest a deficiency syndrome complicated by the excess syndrome. In such a case, Radix Adenophorae, Bulbus Fritillariae Cirrhosae, Cortex Mori and Gecko are added to the Decoction of Ophiopogonis (140) to nourish *yin*, disperse heat, invigorate the lung and kidneys, resolve phlegm and relieve asthma.

2. At the Remission Stage

Frequent attacks of asthma inevitably lead to weak body resistance, which in turn allows relapse. The treatment thus focuses on strengthening the body resistance as soon as the acute attack is over. Since the lung, spleen and kidneys are all affected by the disease, they should all be strengthened during the remission stage.

(1) Lung deficiency

The lung is a delicate organ, which dominates *qi*, governs respiration and controls the skin and body hair. Lung deficiency means weakness of defensive *qi*, which allows the external pathogenic factors to invade. A new attack of asthma often occurs when there is a sudden change in weather. Lung deficiency manifests itself as aversion to cold, sweating on exertion during the remission stage, sneezing, nasal stuffiness and clear nasal discharge during the attack. Treatment for this is to invigorate the lung and consolidate the defensive *qi*. The prescription is Jade Screen Powder (73) or Decoction of

Cinnamomi and Astragali (230). Both are effective in strengthening the body resistance and reducing the incidence of common cold.

(2) Splenic deficiency

The spleen transforms and transports food essence. Deficiency of *qi* of the middle *jiao* implies splenic dysfunction. As a result, food cannot be transformed and turbid phlegm is produced instead, which is stored in the lung. Once induced by the external pathogenic factors, the phlegm causes asthmatic attacks. Asthma due to splenic deficiency usually manifests cough with profuse sputum, poor appetite, a distressed sensation in the epigastric region, lassitude, loose stool, or diarrhea and abdominal pain after eating greasy food or sea food. Treatment for such a case is to invigorate the spleen and resolve phlegm. Decoction of Six Mild Drugs (55) or Powder of Ginseng, Poria and Atractylodis Macrocephalae (190) is recommended.

(3) Renal deficiency

Protracted asthma inevitably affects the kidneys, and thereby gives rise to the deficiency of kidney *qi* and impairs its reception of *qi*. The lung dominates *qi*, but the root of *qi* lies in the kidneys. Kidney *qi*-deficiency therefore also weakens the function of the lung. Renal deficiency usually manifests the shortness of breath which is aggravated by exertion. Other symptoms are lumbago, weak limbs, aversion to cold, lassitude, dizziness, tinnitus, night sweating and a hot sensation in the palms and soles. Treatment for such a case is to invigorate the kidneys to improve the reception of *qi*. Pill for Invigorating Kidney *Qi* (182) is applied in cases of kidney *yang*-deficiency. If there is mild edema in the lower legs and dysuria, *Jisheng* Pill for Invigorating Kidney *Qi* (206) is recommended. *Duqi* Pill of Seven Ingredients (10) or Pill of Ophiopogonis, Schisandrae and Rehmanniae Preparata (141) is prescribed in cases of kidney *yin*-deficiency.

These prescriptions are recommended for patients who present typical symptoms during the remission stage. For those who do not have such symptoms, however, the recommended herbs include Radix Codonopsis, Radix Astragali, Semen Juglandis, Placenta Hominis and Gecko.

The application of certain medicinal cakes on such acupoints as *Bailao* (Extra), which is located two *cun* (a length unit which is about three centimeters) above and one *cun* lateral to *Dazhui* (DU 14), *Feishu* (BL 13) and *Gaohuang* (BL 43), effectively produces therapeutic results. This method resolves phlegm, eliminates pathogenic factors and benefits *qi*. If asthma with wheeze is due to cold, Semen Sinapis Albae Cake (105) is applied, as recorded in *Zhang's Medical Treatise*. If asthma is due to heat, Fructus Aristolochiae Compound Cake (212) is used.

Children's asthma is curable if proper treatment is applied and various inducing factors are avoided. This is because both the kidney *qi* and lung *qi* in children develop with age. But in adults asthma with frequent attacks as a result of kidney *qi*-deficiency is very stubborn. Cold invasion complicated by *yang* deficiency is the common pathogenesis of this disease, and *yin* deficiency often stems from *yang* deficiency. Therefore, asthma marked by the *yin* deficiency is even more stubborn than that by *yang* deficiency. A critical condition is characterized by the collapse of cardiac and renal *yang*. Its clinical manifestations include asthmatic breathing with open mouth, raised shoulders, flapping of ala nasi, palpitation, restlessness, sweating, cold limbs, blue complexion and cyanosis. Treatment is to fortify primordial *qi*, prevent collapse and consolidate kidney *qi*. Prescriptions include Decoction of Ginseng and Aconiti Lateralis Preparata (188), Pill of Stannum Nigrum (300) and Powder of Ginseng and Gecko (191). Western medicine should be taken at the same time for emergency case. Symptomatic treatment is important during acute attacks of asthma, and every effort should be made to control the symptoms. In the remission stage, causative treatment should be adopted to consolidate the therapeutic results. The patient should be asked to take part in such exercises as *taijiquan* (*taiji* shadow boxing), jogging and *qigong* (breathing exercises) to build up health. Patients should avoid catching cold or being exposed to irritant gas or dust, as well as eating raw, cold, greasy and spicy food and sea food. In addition, patients must give up smoking, and avoid getting fatigue and excited. All this is meant to strengthen the body resistance and prevent new attacks of asthma.

Remarks

Asthma is characterized by paroxysmal rale and dyspnea. Contributing to it are usually the principal and inducing factors, with the former referring to the retention of phlegm (cold-phlegm and heat-phlegm) in the lung, and the latter meaning exogenous pathogens like wind-cold, wind-heat and dampness as well as digestion, emotion and physique. Its basic pathological changes often take place in the lung, with expectoration leading to the shortness of breath. If this disease occurs frequently, the lung, spleen and kidneys will become ill; when this disease is serious, the heart *yang* will get damaged.

Asthma is divided into two types: cold and heat. The cold type manifests the following syndromes, the shortness of breath and wheeze in the throat, white or frothy phlegm being produced when coughing, thirst, and flowing and tense pulse. The heat type manifests the shortness of breath, thick and ropy sputum, cough with difficulty, thirst and slippery pulse. When asthma is relieved, the deficiency of the lung, spleen or kidneys will appear.

Asthma is an excess syndrome when it occurs, so the treatment of the disease should lay emphasis on expelling pathogenic factors. If it is of the cold type, attention should be given to warming the lung and expelling cold on the one hand and eliminating phlegm for resuscitation on the other. Decoction of Belamacandae and Ephedrae (249) and Small Blue Dragon Decoction (33) can be administered. As for the heat type, the main treatment is to ventilate the lung, disperse heat, resolve phlegm and check the unhealthy *qi* with the administration of Decoction for Relieving Edema with Pinelliae (296) and Decoction for Relieving Asthma (179). When asthma is alleviated, Jade Screen Powder (73) and Decoction of Cinnamomi and Astragali (230) are used to treat the deficiency of the lung, Decoction of Six Mild Drugs (55) and Powder of Ginseng to treat the deficiency of the spleen as well as Powder of Ginseng, Poria and Atractyloids Macrocephalae (190) and *Duqi* Pill of Seven Ingredients (10) to treat the deficiency of the kidneys.

Case Studies

Name: Wang XX; Sex: Male; Age: 23; Occupation: Worker.
Chief complaint: Relapse of asthma for nearly one month.
Case history: He got asthma for eight years. Severe attacks occurred frequently, regardless of climatic changes or food, but more often at night. Western drugs were administered, which were effective only for a while. On admission, he presented cough, asthmatic breathing, gurgling with sputum in the throat, coarse breathing, orthopnea, lassitude and poor appetite. One month before admission, he received an injection of aminophylline and adrenalin, as well as perirenal block therapy, without satisfactory results.

Examination: Body temperature was 37°C. The heart rate was 80/min., and respiration rate 25/min. The patient was normally developed and moderately nourished. He looked seriously ill, with pale complexion. The tongue coating was white. Wheezing was heard on both sides of the lungs. The heart was normal. The liver and spleen were not palpable; the abdomen was flat and soft.

Diagnosis: Bronchial asthma (Western medicine); asthma due to cold (Traditional Chinese Medicine).

Treatment: To warm and resolve phlegm and fluid, disperse cold and relieve asthma.
Prescription:

Herba Ephedrae (honey prepared)	3 g;
Ramulus Cinnamomi	3 g;
Herba Asari	3 g;
Fructus Schisandrae	3 g;
Rhizoma Zingiberis Preparata	4.5 g;
Radix Paeoniae Alba	12 g;
Rhizoma Pinelliae (ginger prepared)	9 g;
Radix Glycyrrhizae Preparata	3 g.

Cough and asthmatic breathing stopped after the first dose, and treatment was stopped the next day. But asthma occurred again on the third day with symptoms of asthmatic breathing with raised shoulders, gurgling with sputum in the throat and insomnia for the whole night. The tongue coating was white and the pulse rapid. The same treatment was adopted. The following herbs were prescribed:

Herba Ephedrae	6 g;
Herba Asari	3 g;
Rhizoma Zingiberis Preparata	3 g;
Rhizoma Pinelliae (ginger prepared)	9 g;
Semen Ginkgo	9 g;
Radix Glycyrrhizae Preparata	3 g;
Endocarpium Citri Reticulatae	4.5 g;
Cortex Mori	9 g;
Semen Lepidii seu Descurainiae	6 g;
Polyporus	12 g;
Poria	12 g.

In addition, *Zijin* Pill was administered, 0.15 g each day, half each time with cold boiled water.

After two doses, the asthma considerably improved. Oral administration of another nine doses of the same prescription resulted in complete relief. The patient was then discharged.

Explanation: Small Blue Dragon Decoction (33) was prescribed at his first visit to resolve retained cold-phlegm. The addition of Semen Lepidii seu Descurainiae, Polyporus, Poria and Cortex Mori at the second visit was based on the fact that there was disturbance of retained fluid and unhealthy *qi* complicated by accumulation of heat.

Name: Shen XX; Sex: Male; Age: 29; Occupation: Peasant.

The patient complained of asthma with loud wheezing for ten days, which was even worse at night. Other symptoms included orthopnea, expectoration of a small amount of white and thick sputum, a feeling of suffocation in the chest, low fever, a tongue with exfoliated coating on the left side, thin and white coating on the right side, yellow and sticky coating at the root, and a smooth and rapid pulse. The pathogenesis was pathogenic cold turning into heat, which combined with phlegm blocking the air passage. Treatment aimed to promote the lung's dispersive and descending function, disperse heat, dispel phlegm and relieve asthma. The following drugs were prescribed:

Herba Ephedrae Preparata	4.5 g;
Radix Glycyrrhizae	4.5 g;
Semen Armeniacae Amarum	12 g;
Fructus Perillae	12 g;

Semen Lepidii seu Descurainiae	12 g;
Gypsum Fibrosum	30 g;
Cortex Mori	30 g;
Herba Houtuyniae	30 g;
Fructus Jujubae	6 pieces;
Radix Platycodi	9 g;
Semen Ginkgo	9 g;
Radix Peucedani Preparata	15 g;
Bombyx Batryticatus	15 g;
Lumbricus	15 g.

After six doses, the asthma was relieved, cough markedly reduced, and defecation and urination were normal. But there was no improvement of lassitude and poor appetite. Attempts were then made to invigorate *qi*, nourish *yin* and strengthen the lung and spleen.

Explanation: Pathogenic cold is the principal inducing factor of asthmatic attacks. It is likely to turn into heat if there is *yin* deficiency and *yang* excess. A tongue with exfoliated coating on the left side and thin and white coating on the right is a sign of invasion by pathogenic cold complicated by the *yin* deficiency. Expectoration of thick sputum, a smooth and rapid pulse, and a yellow and sticky tongue coating at the root are all signs of heat, suggesting that pathogenic cold has already turned into heat. The prescription was based on Decoction for Relieving Asthma (179), aiming at relieving the acute symptoms. The effect was consolidated by invigorating *qi* and nourishing *yin*.

A patient surnamed Liu complained of bronchial asthma for over ten years.

His constitution was weak. During the attack, he presented a pale complexion, breathing with staring eyes and raised shoulders, cold limbs, and a deep, feeble and soft pulse. The pathogenesis was renal dysfunction in the reception of *qi*. The prescription consisted of Pill for Invigorating Kidney *Qi* (182) combined with Fructus Psoraleae and Lignum Aquilariae Resinatum. The symptoms were relieved after four doses.

Explanation: When body resistance is weak and the invading pathogenic factors are not pronounced, asthma is due to the renal dysfunction. This case exhibited kidney *yang*-deficiency. Pill for Invigorating Kidney *Qi* (182) warms kidney *yang*, and Fructus Psoraleae and Lignum Aquilariae Resinatum assist the kidneys in the reception of *qi*.

V. Dyspnea

Dyspnea is clinically marked by the short breath, orthopnea, breathing with raised shoulders and flapping of ala nasi, cyanosis of lips and a purple tongue. Persistent dyspnea may lead to prostration. Dyspnea often appears as the main symptom in some acute and chronic diseases, suggesting that the disease has reached a severe stage.

The *Inner Canon of the Yellow Emperor* explicitly describes various symptoms of dyspnea, and relates the pathogenesis to the retention of pathogenic factors in the upper part of the body. It also states that the lung is seriously diseased, and the heart, liver, spleen and kidneys are also affected. *Synopsis of Prescriptions of the Golden Chamber* summarizes that dyspnea is due to the attack by external pathogenic factors. Dyspnea due to the internal damage was recognized by medical scholars of the Jin and Yuan dynasties. For example, *Danxi's Experience on Medicine* says, "Emotional upsets, violent exercises after voracious eating, disharmony of the *qi* of *zang* organs..., and weak constitution with deficiency of both the spleen and kidneys can all cause dyspnea." *A Complete Collection of Jingyue's Treatise* classifies dyspnea into two types, the deficiency and excess. *A Guide to Clinical Practice with Case Records* differentiates dyspnea by saying, "It suggests an excess syndrome if the lung is affected; it implies a deficiency syndrome if the kidneys are diseased." Generally speaking, dyspnea due to the attack of the lung by pathogenic factors is of the excess type, and the treatment should focus on eliminating pathogenic factors and regulating *qi*. Dyspnea due to the deficiency of essence and *qi* is of the deficiency type, and the treatment should concentrate on invigorating the lung and kidneys.

Dyspnea resulting from bronchitis in the aged, pneumonia, emphysema, pulmonary tuberculosis, pleurisy, pneumosilicosis, and various heart troubles may be differentiated and treated according to the following descriptions.

Etiology and Pathogenesis

Dyspnea has many causes, e.g., the attack by the six external pathogenic factors, improper diet, emotional upsets, and weak body resistance following a protracted illness.

1. Attack by External Pathogenic Factors

Attack of the lung by external pathogenic wind-cold impairs the lung's dispersive and descending function, and thereby causes unhealthy lung *qi*, resulting in dyspnea. Wind-cold can turn into heat, which hinders the flow of lung *qi*, and subsequently leads to dyspnea. Attack of the lung by wind-heat, or retention of heat in the lung complicated by the surface cold, may damage the lung and cause the unhealthy lung *qi*; this is another cause of dyspnea. Finally, since the attack by pathogenic summer-heat consumes *qi* and *yin* of the body, therefore the combination of lung *qi*-deficiency and pathogenic heat produces dyspnea.

2. Retention of Excessive Turbid Phlegm

Turbid phlegm results from the malfunction of the spleen. Since the spleen is in charge of sending the clear upward and the turbid downward, therefore it doesn't function well and produces excessive phlegm when it is affected. This may follow overeating greasy, sweet, raw and cold food, or excessive alcoholic drinking. Once turbid phlegm is produced, it will be stored in the lung, blocking lung *qi* and giving rise to dyspnea. If the internal phlegm-dampness turns into fire, or if excessive lung fire consumes body fluid, resulting in the formation of turbid phlegm, then the combination of phlegm and fire in the lung will cause dyspnea.

3. Emotional Upsets

Mental depression and anxiety can all cause *qi* to stagnate; emotional irritation damages the liver and causes liver *qi* to move upward, thus preventing lung *qi* from descending. In either condition, the disturbed circulation of lung *qi* causes dyspnea.

4. Weakness of the Lung and Kidneys

Long-standing coughing damages the lung, and results in lung *qi*-deficiency. Too much sweating due to overwork consumes *qi* and *yin* of the lung. In either condition, the lung fails to dominate *qi*, and dyspnea ensues.

Long-standing coughing also spreads the disease from the lung to the kidneys, an instance of disorder of the mother affecting the son, which results in both pulmonary and renal deficiency. Excessive sexual activity damages the kidneys by consuming kidney essence, and thus impairs the kidneys' function in receiving *qi*. In both conditions, more *qi* exits than that enters, and the unhealthy *qi* leads to dyspnea.

Deficient *qi* of the middle *jiao* deprives lung *qi* of nourishment, and thereby weakens respiration and gives rise to dyspnea. Kidney *yang*-deficiency fails to control fluid, which may disturb the lung and heart, resulting in unhealthy lung *qi* and heart *yang*-deficiency. A deficiency syndrome is thereby complicated by an excess syndrome.

In summary, dyspnea are of two types, the excess and deficiency. Attack by the external pathogenic factors, retention of excessive turbid phlegm and emotional upsets cause dyspnea of the excess type. Weakness of the lung and kidneys gives rise to dyspnea of the deficiency type. In both cases, the lung and kidneys are mainly affected, the liver and spleen involved, and the heart is subsequently affected. Specifically, the lung is responsible for dyspnea of the excess type, and both the lung and kidneys are responsible for the dyspnea of the deficiency type.

In severe dyspnea, both the lung and kidneys are in a state of deficiency, so is heart *yang*. The heart meridian goes to the lung, and the kidney meridian goes to the heart. The condition of heart *yang* is closely related to congenital renal *qi* and the clean *qi* inhaled by the lung. Pulmonary and renal deficiency causes heart *yang*-deficiency, and thus impairs blood circulation. Weak circulation produces blood stasis with symptoms of tachycardia, green-purple complexion, cyanosis of the lips, and a purple tongue. Sweat is the fluid of the heart, and if heart *yang* and heart *qi* are deficient, the heart may fail to bring its fluid under control. Hence, excessive sweating occurs, which makes heart *yang* even more deficient, and prostration is likely to occur then.

Distinction and Treatment

It is most important to clarify the excess and deficiency syndromes of dyspnea. The excess type is clinically marked by long breath, preference for exhalation, coarse breathing sounds and a rapid and forceful pulse; all of these occur abruptly. The treatment should concentrate on eliminating pathogenic factors from the lung and regulating the lung *qi*. The deficiency type is clinically marked by the shortness of breath, preference for deep inhalation, weak breathing sounds, a feeble and weak or superficial, large and empty pulse; all of these occur gradually, and become worse on exertion. The lung, kidneys and spleen should be treated by strengthening their functions in dominating and receiving *qi*. A complicated case with both deficiency and excess syndromes should be differentiated as to which predominates, and then the proper treatment could be applied accordingly.

1. Dyspnea of Excess Type

(1) Attack of the lung by wind-cold

Clinical manifestations: Asthmatic breathing, shortness of breath, stuffiness in the chest, cough with thin and white sputum, a thin and white tongue coating, and a superficial and tense pulse. The accompanying symptoms at the early stage include chilliness, fever, headache, absence of sweating, absence of thirst, and general aching.

Analysis: Attack of the lung by wind-cold blocks the air passage, thus asthmatic breathing, shortness of breath and stuffiness in the chest occur. The reaction of the body to the blockage of air passage is the cough with thin and white sputum. The accompanying symptoms are all the consequences of the attack by wind-cold.

Treatment: To disperse cold, promote the lung's dispersive function and relieve dyspnea.

Prescription: Decoction of Ephedrae (273) with additional drugs. Here, Herba Ephedrae and Ramulus Cinnamomi, acrid and warm in nature, induce sweating, disperse cold and relieve dyspnea; Semen Armeniacae Amarum and Radix Glycyrrhizae ease *qi* circulation and resolve phlegm. The additional Fructus Perillae, Semen Sinapis Albae and Exocarpium Citri Rubrum strengthen the effect of sending unhealthy *qi* downward and resolve phlegm.

If dyspnea is not relieved by sweating, or if dyspnea is caused by disharmony of nutrient and defensive *qi*, Modified Decoction of Cinnamomi, Magnoliae Officinalis and Armeniacae Amarum (226) is prescribed.

In the treatment of a complicated case with both cold and heat syndromes marked by chilliness, general aching, dyspnea, fullness in the chest, restlessness and a yellow-white tongue coating, Great Blue Dragon Decoction (23) or Decoction for Relieving Edema with Pinelliae (296) is prescribed to eliminate wind-cold on the body surface and disperse heat inside the body. In cases with yellow sputum, Radix Scutellariae, Cortex Mori and Herba Houttuyniae are added to disperse heat.

(2) Invasion of the lung by wind-heat

Clinical manifestations: Asthmatic breathing, shortness of breath and flapping of ala nasi, cough with thick and yellow sputum which is difficult to expectorate, or blood-tinged or rosy sputum, chest pain, stuffiness in the chest, and thirst. The accompanying symptoms at the early stage include mild chilliness, persistent fever which does not subside after sweating, a thin and yellow tongue coating, and a superficial and rapid pulse.

Analysis: Attack of the lung by wind-heat consumes body fluid to form phlegm, which blocks the air passage and gives rise to asthmatic breathing and shortness of breath. Since the lung has its orifice in the nose, heat in the lung forces lung *qi* to go upward, thus flapping of ala nasi occurs. Since wind-heat is a pathogenic factor of the *yang* type, therefore it causes thick and yellow sputum which is difficult to expectorate. Excess heat damages the lung vessels and gives rise to chest pain and blood-tinged sputum. Rusty sputum is the result of a combination of phlegm and blood. Consumption of body fluids is the cause of restlessness and thirst. Fever, mild chilliness, thirst and sweating are all symptoms of the exterior syndrome due to the attack by wind-heat. A thin and yellow tongue coating, and a superficial and rapid pulse are all signs of the attack of the lung by wind-heat.

Treatment: To disperse heat, relieve exterior syndrome, promote the lung's dispersive function and relieve dyspnea.

Prescription: Decoction of Ephedrae, Armeniacae Amarum, Gypsum Fibrosum and Glycyrrhizae (272) with additional drugs. In this prescription, Gypsum Fibrosum is used as a principal drug to disperse heat in the lung with its acrid and cold property; Herba Ephedrae, acrid and warm in nature, promotes the lung's dispersive function and relieves dyspnea; Semen Armeniacae Amarum, and Radix Glycyrrhizae resolve phlegm and check cough. The additional Folium Mori, Flos Chrysanthemi, Cortex Mori, Radix Scutellariae and Fructus Trichosanthis aim at eliminating wind, dispersing heat and resolving phlegm. This prescription can be combined with the Powder of Lonicerae and Forsythiae (287).

In cases of rusty or blood-tinged sputum accompanied by chest pain, Decoction of Phragmitis (30) and Decoction for Mild Phlegm-Heat Syndrome in the Chest (37) are used together to disperse heat in the lung, resolve phlegm, remove blood stasis and relieve stagnation.

Prolonged exposure to blazing sun on hot days or working in a hot room with poor ventilation can cause abrupt onset of dizziness, stuffiness in the chest, dyspnea, sweating, fever, lassitude, scanty and deep yellow urine and a soft pulse. These syndromes are the result of consumption of *qi* and fluid by summer-heat. In such cases, White Tiger Decoction with Ginseng (103) and a proper amount of Six-to-One Powder (54) are prescribed to clear away summer-heat, benefit *qi* and produce fluid.

(3) Turbid phlegm blocking the lung

Clinical manifestations: Asthmatic breathing with dyspnea, cough with profuse and sticky sputum which is difficult to expectorate, a feeling of suffocation in the chest, nausea, poor appetite, stickiness and lack of taste in the mouth, a white and sticky tongue coating, and a smooth pulse.

Analysis: Upward disturbance of turbid phlegm blocks air passages and impairs the lung's descending function. Thus asthmatic breathing with dyspnea, cough with profuse sputum and a feeling of suffocation occur. Disturbance of the spleen and stomach by turbid phlegm leads to nausea, poor appetite, stickiness and lack of taste in the mouth. A white and sticky tongue coating and a smooth pulse are signs of retention of turbid phlegm in the interior.

Treatment: To dry dampness, resolve phlegm, send the unhealthy *qi* downward and relieve dyspnea.

Prescription: Modified Decoction Containing Three Kinds of Seed for the Aged (15) and *Erchen Decoction* (3). Here, Rhizoma Pinelliae, Pericarpium Citri Reticulatae, and Poria dry up dampness and resolve phlegm; and Semen Sinapis Albae, Fructus Perillae and Semen Raphani resolve phlegm, send the unhealthy *qi* downward and relieve dyspnea. In a severe case, Three Crude Drugs Decoction (18) is prescribed to strengthen the antidyspneic effect. If signs of dampness are pronounced, Rhizoma Atractylodis and Cortex Magnolicae Officinalis are added to dry it up, invigorate the spleen and circulate *qi*. In the treatment of excessive phlegm-heat with symptoms of cough with yellow and thick sputum, dyspnea, shortness of breath, flushed face, restlessness, thirst, scanty and deep yellow urine, a yellow and sticky tongue coating, and a smooth and rapid pulse, Rhizoma Anemarrhenae and Fructus Trichosanthis are added to the Decoction of Mori (255) to dispel phlegm and reduce fire. In cases with profuse sputum and orthopnea, Semen Lepidii seu Descurainiae and Radix et Rhizoma Rhei are added to relieve dyspnea by sending lung *qi* downward and purging phlegm-fire. In chronic cases of phlegm-heat retention marked by asthmatic breathing, shortness of breath, orthopnea and mental vagueness, the above prescription for dispelling phlegm and reducing fire is combined with Pill of Lapis Chlorite Usta for Expelling Phlegm (323).

(4) Stagnation of *qi* damaging the lung

Clinical manifestations: The patient normally has mental depression or worry. The attack is often induced by mental irritation and is marked by an abrupt onset of dyspnea, an uncomfortable feeling in the throat, chest pain, and numbness of the hands, feet and lips. Insomnia and palpitation may also occur. The tongue coating is thin and the pulse is taut.

Analysis: Long-standing mental depression or worry leads to stagnation of *qi*. Mental irritation causes liver *qi* to attack the lung, and thereby impairs the lung's descending function. The ascent of lung *qi* causes an uncomfortable feeling in the throat, dyspnea and chest pain. Disturbance of the heart and mind leads to insomnia and palpitation. A thin tongue coating and a taut pulse indicate *qi* stagnation.

Treatment: To relieve stagnation, send the unhealthy *qi* downward and relieve dyspnea.

Prescription: Modified Decoction of Six Grinding Ingredients (57). In this prescription, Semen Arecae, Fructus Aurantii Immaturus and Radix Aucklandiae circulate *qi*; Lignum Aquilariae Resinatum sends the unhealthy *qi* downward and relieves dyspnea; and Radix Linderae eases the circulation of liver *qi*. Since most drugs in the prescription are aromatic, circulating *qi* effectively, they are only suitable to patients with strong build and sufficient *qi*. If the patient's constitution is weak, Radix Aucklandiae, Radix et Rhizoma Rhei and Fructus Aurantii Immaturus are removed from the prescription, and Radix Ginseng is added. All the drugs should be ground to juice to be taken with water, or cooked for a while to be taken warm. If palpitation and insomnia are present, Semen Ziziphi Spinosae, Semen Platyeladi, Caulis Polygoni Multiflori and Radix Polygalae are added to soothe the heart and calm the mind.

2. Dyspnea of Deficiency Type

(1) Lung deficiency

Clinical manifestations: Asthmatic breathing, shortness of breath, weak speech and coughing, spontaneous sweating, aversion to wind, dryness of the throat, thirst, flushed face, a light red tongue, and a weak pulse.

Analysis: Lung deficiency implies an impaired domination of *qi*, which explains asthmatic breathing, shortness of breath, weak speech and coughing. Lung *qi*-deficiency means weak defensive *qi*, which is the cause of spontaneous sweating and aversion to wind. Lung *yin*-deficiency produces dryness of the throat, thirst, and flushed face. A light red tongue and a weak pulse are both signs of *qi* and *yin* deficiency.

Treatment: To invigorate the lung and relieve dyspnea.

Prescription: Modified Decoction for Invigorating Lung (158). In this prescription, Radix Ginseng and Radix Astragali invigorate lung *qi*; Cortex Mori and Radix Asteris reduce heat in the lung, relieve dyspnea and check cough; and Radix Rehmanniae Preparata and Fructus Schisandrae consolidate the lung and strengthen the kidneys in receiving *qi*. In the treatment of lung deficiency complicated by cold with dilute sputum, aversion to cold and absence of thirst, Quartz Album and Stalactitum are prescribed to warm the lung, assist *yang*, resolve phlegm and relieve dyspnea. In cases with sweating on exertion, Jade Screen Powder (73) is prescribed. If *yang* deficiency predominates, Bolus for Regulating Middle *Jiao* (258) is recommended. If *yin* deficiency is more pronounced, Powder for Restoring Pulse Beating (96) and Decoction of Lilii for Strengthening the Lung (116) are used in combination. If both the lung and spleen are affected, and *qi* of the middle *jiao* collapses with symptoms of poor appetite, loose stool, and a bearing-down sensation in the abdomen, Decoction for Strengthening the Middle *Jiao* and Benefiting *Qi* (154) is used to strengthen both the lung and spleen, and restore the collapsed *qi*. If an elderly and weak patient with *qi* deficiency has a recent attack of dyspnea following the attack by the external pathogenic factors, treatment should focus on eliminating pathogenic factors, then on resolving turbid phlegm, and finally on replenishing *qi* and resolving phlegm.

(2) Kidney deficiency

Clinical manifestations: Prolonged dyspnea which is worse on exertion, more expiration than inspiration, emaciation, lassitude, sweating, cold limbs, cyanosis, a pale tongue, and a deep and thready pulse.

Analysis: Prolonged dyspnea, emaciation and lassitude all suggest pulmonary disorders affecting the kidneys. Renal dysfunction in receiving *qi* is the cause of more expiration than inspiration and dyspnea worse on exertion. Kidney *yang*-deficiency means weak defensive *yang* in the body, which explains sweating. Failure of *yang-qi* to warm the exterior produces cold limbs and cyanosis. A pale tongue, and a deep and thready pulse are signs of *yang-qi* deficiency.

Treatment: To invigorate the kidneys and promote inspiration.

Prescription: Pill for Invigorating Kidney *Qi* (182) is the main prescription applied. In this prescription, the ingredients of the Pill of Six Drugs Containing Rehmanniae Preparata (56) invigorate kidney *yin*; Radix Aconiti Lateralis Preparata and Cortex Cinnamomi warm and invigorate kidney *yang*. When *yang* is accepted by *yin*, *qi* in the kidneys is consolidated and dyspnea relieved. In case of edema of the legs with dysuria, Radix Achyranthis Bidentatae and Semen Plantaginis are added to formulate the *Jisheng* Pill for Invigorating Kidney *Qi* (206). In serious cases, Radix Ginseng, Fructus Schisandrae, Semen Juglandis, Fructus Psoraleae, and Gecko are added to invigorate lung *qi* and kidney *qi*. If kidney *yin*-deficiency is pronounced with symptoms of the dry throat and mouth, flushed face and cold feet during dyspnea, a red tongue and a thready pulse, *Duqi* Pill of Seven Ingredients (10) and Powder for Restoring Pulse Beating (96) are combined to nourish *yin* and promote inspiration. Herbs acrid and dry in nature are not advisable.

Coexistence of deficiency and excess syndromes is commonly seen, for instance, excessive phlegm and stagnant *qi* accumulating in the upper part of the body and deficiency of kidney *qi* in the lower part. It manifests dyspnea aggravated by exertion, cough with profuse sputum, stuffiness in the chest, lumbago, cold limbs, frequent urination, a sticky tongue coating and a deep, thready and smooth pulse. For such cases, the treatment is to resolve phlegm, send the unhealthy *qi* downward, warm the kidneys and promote inspiration. Decoction of Perillae for Keeping *Qi* Downward (142) is recommended. Here, Fructus Perillae sends the unhealthy *qi* downward and relieves dyspnea; Rhizoma Pinelliae, Radix Peucedani and Cortex Magnoliae Officinalis send the unhealthy *qi* downward and resolve phlegm; Pericarpium Citri Reticulatae and Radix Glycyrrhizae regulate *qi* of the middle *jiao*; Cortex Cinnamomi warms the kidneys and strengthens its function in receiving *qi*; and Radix Angelicae Sinensis nourishes blood and moistens dryness.

Another example is the invasion of the heart and lung by harmful water due to the *yang* deficiency. This syndrome manifests dyspnea, cough, palpitation, orthopnea, dysuria, edema of the limbs, a pale and swollen tongue, and a deep and thready pulse. Treatment aims to warm the kidneys and circulate fluids by means of *Zhenwu* Decoction (223) with some modifications.

If dyspnea continues for a long time, deficiency of *qi* in the lung and kidneys affects the heart, and blood circulation is affected, presenting cyanosis of the lips, tongue and fingers, and a knotted and intermittent pulse, drugs that activate blood circulation and remove blood stasis are added to the prescription that replenishes *qi* and blood. The additional herbs include Radix Salviae Miltiorrhizae, Rhizoma Chuanxiong, Radix Paeoniae Rubra and Ligni Dalbergiae Odoriferae. In cases of persistent dyspnea which leads to collapse of heart *yang*, Radix Ginseng, Radix Aconiti Lateralis Preparata, Os Draconis, and Concha Ostreae should be administered immediately, and Pill of Stannum Nigrum (300) is also taken orally to rescue *yang*, check sweating and relieve collapse.

Remarks

Hindrance of lung *qi* causes dyspnea of the excess type. It can be resolved by eliminating pathogenic factors and easing the circulation of *qi*; this is relatively easier to do. Deficiency of *qi* and weak internal organs cause dyspnea of the deficiency type, which cannot be replenished effectively in a short period of time. This deficiency syndrome is likely to be complicated by the external pathogenic factors; it is much more difficult to cure. When a state of collapse occurs, emergency treatment with Western medicine should be applied.

Case Studies

Name: Lu Yushui; Sex: Male; Age: 26.
Etiology: Chronic cough complicated by the attack of cold.
Clinical manifestations: The disease started with fever, chilliness, headache, nasal stuffiness, cough with profuse sputum and nausea. The condition became worse gradually, and subsequently orthopnea ensued. A deep and tense pulse and a white and slippery tongue coating were observed.

Pathogenesis: Attack of the lung by pathogenic cold impairs the lung's dispersive function and thereby results in cough and dyspnea.

Treatment: To warm and disperse pathogenic cold and promote the lung's dispersive function by means of Small Blue Dragon Decoction (33) with some modifications.

Prescription:

Herba Ephedrae	9 g;
Ramulus Cinnamomi	9 g;
Rhizoma Zingiberis	4.5 g;
Radix Paeoniae Alba	9 g;
Semen Armeniacae Amarum	6 g.

Herba Ephedrae was cooked in water with foam removed, and then the other ingredients were added to form a decoction. Two doses were prescribed.

Explanation: Cough with profuse sputum and nausea suggests the retention of fluid in the chest. This case of prolonged dyspnea with acute exacerbation is different from that due to attack of the lung by cold. The application of Small Blue Dragon Decoction (33) will disperse wind-cold on the body surface, and resolve phlegm and retained fluid in the interior.

Name: Zhang Fengxiang; Sex: Male; Age: 40.

Chief complaint: Abrupt onset of coughing, chest pain and shortness of breath.

Examination: The pulse was bounding and large, especially at the "*cun*" position on the right side. Other manifestations included a burning sensation in the muscles and skin, lassitude, dyspnea interfering sleep, cough with sticky and thick sputum tinged with blood, a bitter taste in the mouth, poor appetite, thirst, chest pain, constipation, and dark urine.

Diagnosis: Cough and dyspnea due to attack of the lung by pathogenic heat. Movement of heat from the lung to the large intestine causes constipation. Downward movement of fire and heat leads to dark urine.

Prescription: Decoction of Scutellariae for Clearing Heat in the Lung added with Radix Stemonae, Folium Eriobotryae, Radix Scrophulariae, Bulbus Lilii and Fructus Kaki Pruina.

After the first dose, breathing was calmed down and cough alleviated. All the symptoms were relieved after the second dose.

Explanation: All the symptoms suggested the dyspnea due to heat. Decoction of Scutellariae for Clearing Away Heat in the Lung was the proper prescription. If constipation is present, Radix et Rhizoma Rhei can be added to disperse heat in the lung through the large intestine.

VI. Pulmonary Tuberculosis

Pulmonary tuberculosis is a chronic infectious disease marked by emaciation, cough, hemoptysis, hectic fever and night sweating. The pathogenesis is the weak body resistance caused by the attack of tubercle bacillus. The lung is diseased. Although *yin* deficiency is the syndrome mostly witnessed clinically, the syndromes of *qi* and *yin* deficiency, *yin* deficiency leading to hyperactivity of fire, and *yin* and *yang* deficiency are also found when the disease progresses. The basic principle of treatment is to nourish *yin*, reduce fire, strengthen resistance and kill tubercle bacillus.

This disease has been dealt with for a long time by traditional Chinese medicine. According to *Basic Questions*, its main symptoms are emaciation, fullness in the chest, dyspnea, and chest pain spreading to the shoulders and fever. Its infectiousness is described in *A Handbook of Prescriptions for Emergencies* of the Jin Dynasty as follows: "When the patient dies, the disease passes on to the other family members until all of them die." *Essentially Treasured Prescriptions for Emergencies* of the Tang Dynasty lists it as a disease of the lung. *Prescriptions of Universal Benevolence for Curing All People* points out its etiological factor as "lung worm." Zhu Danxi, a famous physician of the Yuan Dynasty, stresses that *yin* deficiency is its pathogenesis, and the principle of treatment should be nourishing *yin* and reducing fire.

Etiology and Pathogenesis
1. Attack of Tubercle Bacillus

Contact with, eating or living together with, or looking after patients with pulmonary tuberculosis can all lead to direct attack of the lung by tubercle bacillus via the mouth and nose. Tubercle bacillus spreads via air-borne contact and infection. If the body resistance is weak, pulmonary tuberculosis will occur.

2. Deficiency of *Qi* and Blood

Congenital deficiency or lack of proper care after birth leads to the *qi* and blood deficiency or deficiency of *yin* essence. Improper lifestyle, excessive worry and anger, indulgence in alcohol and sexual activity all consume *qi*, blood and body fluid. Prolonged cough due to frequent attack by the external pathogenic factors damages lung *qi*. Poor recuperation following a protracted or serious illness weakens the anti-pathogenic *qi*. All this makes the attack of tubercle bacillus possible.

The internal and external causes are mutually related. The attack of tubercle bacillus consumes *qi*, blood and *yin* essence, resulting in weak body-resistance; this in turn makes the attack of tubercle bacillus possible. People with strong body-resistance do not suffer, even if they are in direct contact with patients. Therefore, the internal cause is decisive while the external cause is conditional.

The disease affects the lung at the early stage, then the spleen and kidneys, and possibly all five *zang* organs in severe cases. Attack of the lung by tubercle bacillus makes lung *qi* deficient and fire hyperactive. This damages the vessels of the lung and gives rise to non-productive cough, hemoptysis and dry throat. Lung deficiency means impaired body fluid distribution, depriving the kidneys of nourishment. Deficiency of kidney *yin* and disturbance of fire of the deficiency type produce hectic fever, nocturnal emission and amenorrhea. In severe cases, they give rise to hyperactivity of the heart and liver fire, which flares upward and further consumes lung *yin*. As a result, night sweating, insomnia, restlessness, irritability and pain at the costal and hypochondriac region occur. Lung deficiency consumes spleen *qi*, resulting in the shortness of breath, lassitude, poor appetite and loose stool. *Yin* deficiency affects *yang* in severe cases, and produces splenic and renal *yang*-deficiency with symptoms of edema, cold limbs, dyspnea, and dark purple lips and tongue.

In summary, the disease first affects the lung (*yin* deficiency); then the lung and spleen (*qi* and *yin* deficiency); then the lung and kidneys (*yin* deficiency and hyperactivity of fire), and possibly also the heart and liver. Finally, *yin* deficiency affects *yang*, exhibiting consumption of primordial *qi* and deficiency of both *yin* and *yang*. Considering the disease as a whole, *yin* deficiency is the principal pathogenesis.

Differential Diagnosis

Lung abscess and pulmonary tuberculosis are both characterized by cough, fever and sweating. However, the onset of lung abscess is abrupt, and its duration is not long. Its main manifestations are cough with profuse, foul and purulent sputum, high fever, sweating, and a smooth and rapid pulse. These syndromes result from the attack of heat complicated by blood stagnation, belonging to the excess-heat type. Treatment aims to disperse heat, eliminate toxins, drain pus and dispel phlegm.

The onset of pulmonary tuberculosis is slow, and its duration is long. The main manifestations are dry cough with little sputum, low fever, hectic fever, night sweating, and a thready and rapid pulse. These syndromes belong to the deficiency-heat type. Treatment aims to nourish *yin*, disperse heat, strengthen the body resistance and kill tubercle bacillus.

Distinction and Treatment

Pulmonary tuberculosis generally has a long duration and develops gradually. But there are a few cases with abrupt onset, which develop rapidly. Mild cases do not exhibit the main symptoms systematically, and some of them are even free from subjective signs, while all the symptoms may appear in severe cases. Generally, the disease begins with mild cough, lassitude, poor appetite, afternoon fever, and occasionally a small amount of blood streaks in the sputum. Then the cough becomes worse, and symptoms related to *yin* deficiency develop, such as dry cough with little sputum, thirst, hectic fever, malar flush, night sweating, insomnia, stuffiness and pain in the chest, restlessness, irritability, emaciation, nocturnal emission, amenorrhea and hemoptysis. If the disease is not properly treated, critical signs marked by the deficiency of both *yin* and *yang* will follow, e.g., emaciation, withered hair, scaly skin, a hoarse voice, loose stool, and edema of the body and limbs. *An Introduction to Medicine* summarizes the main symptoms as hectic fever, night sweating, cough, hemoptysis, nocturnal emission, and diarrhea. Some of the above symptoms present in mild cases, while in severe cases, all the six symptoms appear. This summary emphasizes the involvement of the lung, spleen and kidneys.

The fundamental principle of treatment is to make up for the deficiency while killing tubercle bacillus. Drugs that kill tubercle bacillus include Radix Stemonae, Rhizoma Bletillae, Rhizoma Coptidis, Bulbus Allii, Spica Prunellae and Herba Andrographitis. The lung, spleen and kidneys should be nourished at the same time. To achieve this, attention should focus on the nourishment of *yin* and the reduction of fire. The treatment for lung is dispersing heat and providing nourishment. Drugs that disperse heat with bitter and cold property should not be used in case of possible damage to the spleen and stomach. For instance, Rhizoma Coptidis, Cortex Phellodendri and Radix Gentianae should be used with caution. Only when the spleen and stomach function properly can the lung be well nourished. The spleen is treated by invigorating and regulating the middle *jiao*. Drugs that resolve phlegm with acrid and dry property should be avoided, such as Rhizoma Atractylodis, Rhizoma Arisaematis, Semen Sinapis Albae and Rhizoma Typhonii, because they damage lung *yin*. The treatment for the kidneys is to nourish *yin*, reduce fire, and invigorate the transportation of the spleen and stomach. Thus the kidney fire is kept under control and kidneys are free from any damage. For these purposes, Ramulus Cinnamomi, Radix Aconiti Lateralis Preparata and Rhizoma Zingiberis are not prescribed in large doses.

1. Deficiency of Lung *Yin*

Clinical manifestations: Dry cough with scanty sputum or blood-tinged sputum, chest pain, hectic fever, malar flush, dry throat and mouth, a red tongue with thin, dry and yellow coating, and a thready and rapid pulse.

Analysis: The lung is affected by tubercle bacillus which impairs the lung *yin* and its descending function; thus lung *qi* runs upward, resulting in cough. Deficiency of lung *yin* produces internal heat, which consumes body fluids and produces scanty sputum. Prolonged cough damages the vessels of the lung, resulting in hemoptysis and chest pain. Failure of body fluids to moisten causes dry throat and mouth. Hectic fever, malar flush, a red tongue with thin, dry and yellow coating, and a thready and rapid pulse are all signs of heat due to the *yin* deficiency.

Treatment: To nourish *yin* and moisten the lung.

Prescription: Modified Decoction of Lilii for Strengthening Lung (116). In this prescription, Bulbus Lilii and Radix Ophiopogonis moisten the lung and produce body fluids; Radix Scrophulariae, Radix Rehmanniae and Radix Rehmanniae Preparata nourish *yin* and disperse heat; Radix Angelicae Sinensis and Radix Paeoniae Alba produce moisture and nourish the blood; and Radix Platycodi, Radix Glycyrrhizae and Bulbus Fritillariae Cirrhosae disperse heat in the lung, resolve phlegm and check cough. The additional Folium Mahoniae and Radix Stemonae clear away the heat of the deficiency type and kill tubercle bacillus.

If deficiency of lung *yin* is pronounced, Radix Adenophorae, Herba Dendrobii and Radix Trichosanthis are added. In cases of hemoptysis, Rhizoma Bletillae, Colla Corii Asini, Ophicalcitum and Herba Agrimoniae are added to check bleeding. In cases of chest pain, Radix Curcumae, Rhizoma Corydalis and Semen Persicae are added to regulate *qi*, activate meridians and relieve pain. In cases of hectic fever and malar flush, Carapax et Plastrum Testudinis, Radix Cynanchi Atrati, Herba Artemisiae Annuae and Cortex Lycii are added to nourish *yin* and disperse heat.

2. Deficiency of Both *Qi* and *Yin*

Clinical manifestations: Paroxysmal cough, hemoptysis, hectic fever, night sweating, malar flush, pale complexion, lassitude, sweating on slight exertion, shortness of breath, feeble voice, anorexia, a red tongue with thin coating or no coating, and a thready and weak pulse.

Analysis: Deficiency of lung *yin* produces internal heat, which damages the lung vessels; this explains cough, hemoptysis, hectic fever, malar flush and night sweating. Deficiency of lung *qi* will further damage the spleen *qi* (a diseased "child" organ may get its "mother" organ involved), causing ill function of the spleen which results in anorexia. Deficiency of lung and spleen *qi* explains lassitude, sweating on slight exertion, shortness of breath, feeble voice and pale complexion. A red tongue with thin coating or no coating and a thready and weak pulse are all signs of simultaneous *qi* and *yin* deficiency.

Treatment: To benefit *qi* and nourish *yin*.

Prescription: Modified Moon Brilliance Pill (61). Here, Radix Adenophorae, Radix Ophiopogonis, Radix Asparagi, Radix Rehmanniae and Radix Rehmanniae Preparata nourish *yin* and moisten the lung; Radix Stemonae, Jecur Lutrae and Bulbus Fritillaria Cirrhosae moisten the lung, check cough and kill tubercle bacillus; Colla Corii Asini and Radix Notoginseng regulate *ying* (the nutrient system) and check bleeding; and Poria and Rhizoma Dioscoreae invigorate the spleen and replenish *qi*.

If *qi* deficiency is more pronounced, modified Powder of Ginseng, Poria and Atractylodis Macrocephalae (190) is prescribed. In this recipe, Radix Ginseng, Rhizoma Atractylodis Macrocephalae,

Poria and Rhizoma Dioscoreae invigorate the spleen and replenish *qi*; and Semen Lablab Album, Semen Coicis, Fructus Amomi and Pericarpium Citri Reticulatae invigorate the spleen and check diarrhea. Rhizoma Polygonati Odorati, Bulbus Lilii and Herba Dendrobii can be added to nourish lung *yin*. Radix Astragali is used to constrict the body surface and check spontaneous sweating.

3. Deficiency of *Yin* and Hyperactivity of Fire

Clinical manifestations: Hectic fever, night sweating, insomnia, dream-disturbed sleep, restlessness, hot sensations in the palms, soles and chest, irritability, choking cough with little sputum or yellow and thick sputum, spitting of profuse and bright red blood, pain in the chest and hypochondrium, nocturnal emission, amenorrhea, a crimson tongue, and a thready and rapid pulse.

Analysis: Deficiency of lung *yin* implies the failure of metal to produce water, resulting in deficiency of kidney *yin*. This in turn deprives the lung of nourishment, making lung *yin* even more deficient. *Yin* deficiency produces fire, which forces body fluids to go outward, causing night sweating and hectic fever. Deficiency of kidney *yin* deprives the liver of nourishment, thus the hyperactivity of liver fire results along with irritability. Liver fire stirs heart fire, and restlessness, hot sensations in the palms, soles and chest, insomnia or dream-disturbed sleep will follow. Dryness of the lung and hyperactive fire due to the *yin* deficiency cause bright red blood and pain in the chest and hypochondrium. Deficiency of kidney *yin* leads to hyperactivity of ministerial fire, which disturbs the residence of essence and causes nocturnal emission. Excessive internal phlegm-fire causes yellow and thick sputum. A crimson tongue and a thready and rapid pulse are signs of hyperactive fire due to the *yin* deficiency.

Treatment: To nourish *yin* and reduce fire.

Prescription: Modified Powder of Gentianae Macrophyllae and Carapax Trionycis (221). Carapax Trionycis and Rhizoma Anemarrhenae nourish *yin* and disperse heat; Radix Angelicae Sinensis enriches and harmonizes the blood; Radix Gentianae Macrophyllae, Radix Bupleuri, Cortex Lycii and Herba Artemisiae Annuae disperse heat and reduce fire; and Fructus Mume consolidates *yin* and checks sweating.

If night sweating is severe, Fructus Tritici Levis (light), Fructus Schisandrae and Concha Ostreae are added to nourish *yin* and check sweating. In cases of nocturnal emission, Carapax et Plastrum Testudinis, Fructus Corni, Semen Euryales and Fructus Rosae Laevigatae are added to nourish the kidneys and consolidate the essence. In cases of restlessness and insomnia, Fructus Gardeniae, Plumula Nelumbinis, Semen Ziziphi Spinosae and Caulis Polygoni Multiflori are added to disperse heat and calm the mind. If the sputum is yellow and sticky, powdered Concha Meretricis seu Cyclinae, Radix Scutellariae, Cortex Mori, Fructus Trichosanthis, and Succus Bambusae are added to disperse heat and resolve phlegm. In cases of persistent hemoptysis, Powder of Ten Drugs' Ashes (6) is added to cool blood and stop bleeding. If *yin* deficiency is more pronounced than fire hyperactivity, Pill for Replenishing *Yin* (22) is prescribed with additional drugs. Here, Radix Rehmanniae Preparata and Carapax et Plastrum Testudinis nourish *yin* and subdue hyperactive *yang*; pig's spinal cord replenishes marrow; and Cortex Phellodendri and Rhizoma Anemarrhenae disperse heat and subdue ministerial fire to protect the kidney *yin*.

4. Deficiency of Both *Yin* and *Yang*

Clinical manifestations: Choking cough, hemoptysis, hectic fever, night sweating, nocturnal emission, dysphonia, emaciation, aversion to wind, spontaneous sweating, dyspnea, shortness of breath, edema of the face and limbs, poor appetite, loose stool, a red and glossy tongue with little moisture, or a pale and swollen tongue with tooth prints, and a feeble and thready pulse.

Analysis: Protracted pulmonary tuberculosis causes *yin* deficiency which affects *yang*, and finally the deficiency of both *yin* and *yang* results, along with the malfunction of the lung, spleen and kidneys. Cough and hemoptysis consume lung *yin* and deprive the vocal cord of nourishment, resulting in dysphonia. Consumption of lung *qi* results in the weakness of defensive *yang*, which causes dyspnea, shortness of breath, spontaneous sweating and aversion to wind. Hectic fever and night sweating consume body fluids, while nocturnal emission consumes essence and blood, resulting in emaciation. Poor appetite and loose stool result from the damage of spleen *yang*; the malfunction of the spleen deprives the body of nourishment, thus the patient will lose weight gradually, and edema of the face and limbs will occur. At this stage, the deficiency of *qi* and nutrient system is so severe, making the recovery almost impossible. A dry and red tongue indicates the exhaustion of *yin*, while a pale and swollen tongue with tooth prints is the result of *yang* deficiency. A feeble and weak pulse is a sign of deficiency of both *yin* and *yang*.

Treatment: To reinforce essence and blood, and to warm and replenish the spleen and kidneys.

Prescription: Modified Decoction for Deficiency Syndrome (217). Radix Astragali, Radix Codonopsis, Poria, Rhizoma Atractylodis Macrocephalae, Radix Glycyrrhizae Preparata and Pericarpium Citri Reticulatae replenish *yang* and *qi*, and invigorate the spleen and stomach; Radix Ophiopogonis, Radix Asparagi, Radix Rehmanniae, Radix Rehmanniae Preparata, Radix Angelicae Sinensis, Radix Paeoniae Alba and Fructus Schisandrae replenish *yin* and reinforce essence and blood; and Radix Bupleuri, Cortex Lycii, Cortex Phellodendri, Rhizoma Anemarrhenae and Plumula Nelumbinis nourish *yin* and subdue fever.

If the deficiency of essence and blood is pronounced, a proper amount of Placenta Hominis, Colla Carapax et Plastri Testudinis, Colla Cornus Cervi and Cordyceps, or Extractum of Anas Domesticus (101) and Pill for Replenishing Marrow (159) are administered in addition. White duck in the former prescription, and Gallus Domesticus in the latter fortify congenital essence. In cases with cold limbs and a deep, slow pulse, drugs that disperse heat such as Cortex Phellodendri, Rhizoma Anemarrhenae and Plumula Nelumbinis are removed, and Cortex Cinnamomi is added to warm and consolidate kidney *yang*. In cases with morning diarrhea, Semen Myristicae, Fructus Evodiae and Fructus Psoraleae are added to warm and fortify the spleen and kidneys, consolidate the large intestine and check diarrhea.

Remarks

In addition to the medical treatment, dietary and physical therapy should be adopted in order to maintain health. The patient should avoid alcohol and sexual activity, cultivate a good lifestyle, refrain from emotional upset, and take care not to be exposed to cold or heat.

Prognosis of pulmonary tuberculosis depends on when the treatment is applied. All mild cases can expect complete recovery if treatment is given in time. However, in severe cases, if treatment has not been applied promptly, the patient's condition will go from bad to worse. Protracted illness, emaciation, scaly skin, dysphonia, uncontrollable diarrhea, a feeble and swift pulse, persistent fever, profuse sweating, dyspnea, shortness of breath, and edema of the face and foot all suggest poor prognosis.

Case Studies

Name: Peng XX; Sex: Female; Age: 25.

Clinical manifestations: Cough with sticky sputum, dyspnea, hectic fever, night sweating, dry throat, emaciation, hunger with no desire to eat, malar flush in the afternoon, pale complexion, a weak voice, shortness of breath, dislike of speaking, amenorrhea, a thready and rapid irregular pulse, and a crimson tongue with little coating. She had been confined to bed for six months and menstruation did not come.

Diagnosis: Blood loss and amenorrhea resulting from weak constitution complicated by excessive child birth and abortion. The disorder in the lower part of the body then affected the upper part. Hyperactivity of internal heat caused pulmonary tuberculosis.

Treatment: To disperse heat in the lung and moisten the lung.
Prescription: Powder for Expelling Lung-Heat (174) with additional drugs:

Cortex Mori	12 g;
Cortex Lycii	9 g;
Bulbus Fritillariae Cirrhosae	6 g;
Radix Glehniae	9 g;
Radix Asparagi	9 g;
Fructus Arctii	6 g;
Radix Stemonae	9 g;
Rhizoma Anemarrhenae	9 g;
Rhizoma Cynanchi Stauntonii	6 g;
Radix Glycyrrhizae	3 g.

Cough was slightly improved after six doses. Powder for Relieving Deficiency-Heat Syndrome (282) was then prescribed with some modifications:

Carapax Trionycis Preparata	24 g;
Rhizoma Anemarrhenae	9 g;
Radix Stellariae	9 g;
Herba Artemisiae Annuae	9 g;
Cortex Lycii	9 g;
Radix Gentianae Macrophyllae	6 g;
Radix Rehmanniae	15 g;
Cortex Mori	9 g;
Bulbus Fritillariae Cirrhosae	6 g;
Semen Armeniacae Amarum	6 g;
Radix Glycyrrhizae	3 g.

Cough, hectic fever, and night sweating improved after six doses. Treatment was changed to nourish *yin*, moisten the lung and check cough. Decoction of Glycyrrhizae Preparata (186) was prescribed with modifications:

Radix Glycyrrhizae Preparata	12 g;
Radix Glehniae	12 g;
Radix Ophiopogonis	9 g;
Radix Rehmanniae	15 g;
Fructus Cannabis	12 g;
Rhizoma Anemarrhenae	9 g;
Bulbus Fritillariae Cirrhosae	6 g;
Fructus Jujubae	4 pieces;
Colla Corii Asini	12 g.

After eight doses, cough, dyspnea and night sweating considerably improved, but hectic fever recurred, and a rapid feeble pulse and a crimson tongue still presented. The same treatment was adopted, though some of the ingredients were changed:

Radix Glycyrrhizae Preparata	12 g;
Radix Glehniae	9 g;

Radix Ophiopogonis	6 g;
Radix Rehmanniae	9 g;
Rhizoma Anemarrhenae	9 g;
Radix Stellariae	9 g;
Herba Artemisiae Annuae	9 g;
Radix Asteris	9 g;
Radix Stemonae	9 g;
Colla Corii Asini	12 g.

After another eight doses, all symptoms improved, the pulse slowed down, and appetite improved. Then the method of nourishing the lung and replenishing nutrient *qi* was adopted:

Radix Glycyrrhizae Preparata	12 g;
Radix Glehniae	24 g;
Radix Asparagi	6 g;
Radix Rehmanniae	15 g;
Radix Asteris	9 g;
Radix Stellariae	9 g;
Radix Ophiopogonis	9 g;
Semen Platycladi	9 g;
Radix Angelicae Sinensis	12 g;
Cortex Lycii	9 g;
Colla Corii Asini	12 g.

The symptoms improved further. The tongue became moist. The new prescription was based on Decoction for Benefiting *Yin*:

Radix Rehmanniae	15 g;
Radix Rehmanniae Preparata	15 g;
Radix Asparagi	9 g;
Rhizoma Polygonati Odorati	9 g;
Carapax Trionycis Preparata	12 g;
Herba Artemisiae Annuae	6 g;
Cortex Lycii	9 g;
Radix Paeoniae Alba (prepared with wine)	6 g;
Radix Asteris	9 g;
Colla Corii Asini	18 g;
Semen Juglandis	12 g.

After four doses, cough and dyspnea calmed down, and both appetite and sleep became normal, but the patient still had occasional hectic fever and spontaneous sweating. The pulse was weak, and the tongue was crimson and thinly coated. All this showed that *yin* had not yet recovered. The prescription was then based on Decoction of Astragali and Carapax Trionycis (268):

Radix Astragali	15 g;
Carapax Trionycis Preparata	12 g;
Cortex Lycii	9 g;
Radix Gentianae Macrophyllae	4.5 g;

Fructus Tritici Levis (light)	18 g;
Rhizoma Dioscoreae	12 g;
Poria	9 g;
Radix Rehmanniae	12 g;
Radix Stellariae	9 g;
Rhizoma Anemarrhenae	9 g;
Radix Paeoniae Alba	9 g.

After six doses, fever subsided and sweating stopped. The patient showed a slightly red tongue with thin and white coating and a soft feeble pulse. This implied that the invading pathogenic factors had been eliminated, although the body resistance was weak. Eight Precious Ingredients Decoction (13) was prescribed to consolidate both *qi* and blood:

Radix Codonopsis	12 g;
Rhizoma Atractylodis Macrocephalae	9 g;
Poria	9 g;
Radix Rehmanniae Preparata	12 g;
Radix Angelicae Sinensis	9 g;
Rhizoma Chuanxiong	6 g;
Radix Paeoniae Alba	9 g;
Colla Corii Asini	12 g;
Cordyceps	9 g;
Radix Glycyrrhizae Preparata	6 g.

After twenty doses, all symptoms disappeared except for listlessness. Decoction of Angelicae Sinensis and Astragali for Reinforcing Middle *Jiao* was then prescribed:

Radix Astragali	18 g;
Paeoniae Alba	18 g;
Ramulus Cinnamomi	6 g;
Radix Angelicae Sinensis	9 g;
Radix Glycyrrhizae Preparata	6 g;
Fructus Jujubae	4 pieces;
Rhizoma Zingiberis Recens	9 g.

The decoction was taken warm with 60 g of Saccharum Granorum. Twenty doses were administered in succession. These drugs did not help a lot, because the disease had a long duration, and the deficient state was extremely severe. Then large doses of Decoction for Invigorating Spleen and Nourishing Heart (110) and Powder for Restoring Pulse (96) were prescribed as a tonic to the heart and spleen. After twenty doses, appetite improved, body weight increased, and she was more vigorous. Menstruation returned six months later.

Explanation: Splenic deficiency causes emaciation, and renal deficiency gives rise to the fire of the deficiency type, causing cough and hectic fever. At the beginning, treatment for temporary relief was applied by dispersing heat and moistening the lung. Then the treatment for permanent cure was given by nourishing *yin*, moistening the lung, benefiting *qi* and harmonizing *ying* (the nutrient system). Finally, the method of replenishing both *qi* and blood, benefiting *qi* and *yin*, and invigorating the heart and spleen was adopted. To nourish *yin* was the main focus of the overall treatment, but meanwhile, care should be taken not to damage the spleen and lung. Thus water ascends while the fire descends, and the spleen and lung develop healthily, enabling a complete recovery from pulmonary tuberculosis.

Name: Xian XX; Sex: Male; Age: 45.

The patient suffered pulmonary tuberculosis from 1967, and began to cough blood intermittently since 1970. He was admitted to the hospital on May 22, 1973 due to severe hemoptysis for five days. The examination showed body temperature was 36.8°C and blood pressure 100/70 mm Hg. He had lassitude, shortness of breath, weak constitution and a pale complexion. X-rays revealed infiltrative pulmonary tuberculosis. Over the 40 days since admission, he had severe hemoptysis 20 times, losing blood ranging from 100 to 300ml each time. He lost consciousness once during hemoptysis and was rescued by first aid. He received blood transfusion for three times, and was given various Chinese and Western drugs, including hemostatics, which only proved temporary relief.

On July 8, the patient began to take Pill for Replenishing *Yin* (22) with additional ingredients. At that time, he presented pale complexion, debility, shortness of breath, a hot sensation in the chest, restlessness, irritability, insomnia, a pale tongue with scanty coating and light purple color on the border, and a thready and rapid pulse. Although the color of the tongue indicated blood loss, other symptoms suggested disturbance of the lung by flaring fire of the deficiency type. Treatment should aim at nourishing water, checking fire and sending fire back to its origin. In view of the previous drugs mainly based on the Decoction of Lilii for Strengthening Lung (116), although they were in accord with the principle, they proved more effective in moistening the lung than reducing fire. The new prescription, based on Pill for Replenishing *Yin* (22), proved effective after a single dosage. It included the following ingredients:

Radix Rehmanniae	12 g;
Radix Rehmanniae Preparata	12 g;
Fructus Gardeniae (charred)	9 g;
Rhizoma Anemarrhenae	9 g;
Carapax et Plastrum Testudinis (decocted first)	30 g;
Radix Ophiopogonis	15 g;
Radix Achyranthis Bidentatae	9 g;
Folium Eriobotryae	9 g;
Cacumen Platycladi	30 g;
Herba Ecliptae	30 g.

The amount of blood expectorated considerably decreased, and the stuffiness and hot sensation in the chest disappeared. Another two doses proved complete relief of hemoptysis. After 12 dosages, the patient felt refreshed and vigorous. In the following 46 days, hemoptysis did not occur again till the patient left hospital.

Name: Zhou XX; Sex: Female; Age: 24; Occupation: Worker.

Case history: The patient had X-ray check due to long-standing cough in 1964, and pulmonary tuberculosis was detected with a cavity in the right middle lung. A recent X-ray revealed that the cavity had already closed, since she began taking medication two years ago.

First visit: April 23, 1966. The patient reported repeated hemoptysis over recent months. Although the blood spat was scanty, it continued for a long time. The color of the expectoration was pinkish or brown sometimes, and blood traces appeared occasionally. Recently, she presented pale complexion, mild cough, lumbago during menstruation, a pale blue tongue with sticky coating, a thready pulse, and normal appetite. The diagnosis was deficiency of *yin* blood, complicated by blood stagnation in the collaterals. Therefore the treatment aimed at nourishing blood and removing blood stasis, assisted by checking hemoptysis. The following herbs were prescribed:

Radix Angelicae Sinensis	9 g;
Radix Salviae Miltiorrhizae	9 g;
Radix Paeoniae Rubra	9 g;
Radix Glycyrrhizae	3 g;
Radix Asparagi	9 g;
Cacumen Platycladi (charred)	9 g;
Radix Rubiae	9 g;
Pollen Typhae (stir-baked and wrapped)	4.5 g;
Nodus Nelumbinis Rhizomatis	5 pieces.

Hemoptysis improved after four doses and ceased within the recent week after another eight dosage. To consolidate the therapeutic results, another five doses were administered.

Explanation: Hemoptysis is the chief symptom in the above two cases. The causes of hemoptysis include hyperactivity of internal fire-heat, which causes reckless blood movement; internal heat produced by *yin* deficiency which forces blood to move outward; blockage of vessels by blood stasis which prevents blood from circulating normally; failure of *qi* to control blood, causing blood to move outside the vessels. The second case presents hyperactivity of fire due to the *yin* deficiency, which compels blood to move outward. Treatment thus aims to nourish *yin* and reduce fire. The third one exhibits *yin* blood-deficiency complicated by blood stasis. Treatment thus focuses on activating blood circulation and removing blood stasis, assisted by nourishing *yin* and checking bleeding.

Name: Wang XX; Sex: Male; Age: 51; Occupation: Worker.

In the winter of 1966, the patient had X-ray check due to persistent cough and fever, and pulmonary tuberculosis with cavitation of the right lung was detected. He came to seek medical treatment because the long term application of tuberculostatic agents proved invalid. The recent X-ray check revealed increased markings on both sides, infiltrative caseous focus and a cavity of 2-3 cm in diameter in the upper middle part of the right lung. He also had a history of bronchitis.

First visit (February 23, 1972): The clinical manifestations included fever, cough with yellow and thick sputum, chest pain, shortness of breath on exertion, dry mouth, a slightly red tongue with yellow and sticky coating, and a smooth and rapid pulse. Diagnosis of Western medicine was infiltrative pulmonary tuberculosis at the stage of dissolution and dissemination. Traditional Chinese medicine diagnosis was retention of heat and phlegm in the lung. Treatment was to disperse heat in the lung, check cough, and resolve phlegm. The following herbs were prescribed:

Radi Stemonae	18 g;
Radix Scutellariae	9 g;
Radix Salviae Miltiorrhizae	9 g;
Rhizoma Corydalis	15 g;
Rhizoma Pinelliae	9 g;
Pericarpium Citri Reticulatae	4.5 g;
Radix Asteris Preparata	9 g;
Radix Ranunculi Ternati	30 g.

Seven doses were prescribed.

Second visit (March 2): Fever subsided and chest pain improved. Another seven doses were administered.

Third visit (March 16): Fever completely subsided, and chest pain disappeared; but cough with profuse sputum and shortness of breath remained unchanged. The following herbs were prescribed then:

Radix Stemonae	18 g;
Radix Scutellariae	9 g;
Radix Salviae Miltiorrhizae	9 g;
Pericarpium Citri Reticulatae	9 g;
Rhizoma Pinelliae (prepared with ginger)	9 g;
Semen Cuscutae	9 g;
Semen Armeniacae Amarum	9 g;
Radix Platycodi	9 g;
Rhizoma Corydalis	15 g.

Seven doses were prescribed.

Fourth visit (March 23): Cough improved. A smooth pulse and a thin and white-yellowish tongue coating were present. 30 g of Herba Houttuyniae, 18 g of Pumex, and 3 g of Rhizoma Pinelliae prepared with Pericarpium Citri Reticulatae and Bulbus Fritillariae Cirrhosae (to be taken in the form of infusion) were added to the prescription.

This prescription continued for three months. X-ray check three months later showed improvement of infiltrative focus of the right lung and reduction of the cavity to 1×1 cm. But shortness of breath still occurred occasionally. Treatment was continued by administering Tablet for Protecting Lung, which consisted of Fructus Psoraleae, Radix Dipsaci, Radix Angelicae Sinensis, Semen Juglandis, Semen Cuscutae, Fructus Ligustri Lucidi, Radix Rehmanniae Preparata, Fructus Rubi, and Radix Glycyrrhizae.

Explanation: Deficiency of *yin* is a common pathogenesis of pulmonary tuberculosis. Therefore, the therapeutic principle is to nourish *yin* with sweet and cold herbs. But some cases of TB present an excess of pathogenic factors, like the fourth case. Since this case was marked by the retention of phlegm-heat in the lung, treatment aimed at dispersing heat, resolving phlegm and checking cough. Satisfactory results were achieved after a short-term treatment.

VII. Retention of Phlegm and Fluid

Retention of phlegm and fluid refers to pathological changes caused by excessive water in a certain part of the body, which results from the disorder of body transportation, transformation and distribution.

The Inner Canon of the Yellow Emperor states that the main pathogenesis of accumulated fluid is excessive water and dampness due to the malfunction of spleen *yang*. On this basis, Zhang Zhongjing of the Eastern Han Dynasty initiated the discussion of phlegm and fluid retention in his work *Synopsis of Prescriptions of the Golden Chamber*. There was no descriptive difference between phlegm and retained fluid before the end of Sui and Tang dynasties. Medical scholars then thought that the phlegm and retained fluid were of the same origin, holding that the latter was the initial form of phlegm, while phlegm was the further development of retained fluid. It was since the Song Dynasty that phlegm and retained fluid had been differentiated. After that, physicians usually apply this idea in their practice, believing phlegm is thick and turbid, resulting from fire-dryness, while retained fluid caused by cold-dampness is clear and thin. There are similarities as well as differences between the two, therefore care should be taken to distinguish them. In the treatment of phlegm and fluid retention, Zhang Zhongjing initiated the method of mediation with warm herbs. His detailed explanation of the cause and treatment proved very helpful to the later generations, who make diagnosis based on his theory.

The following diseases at certain stages can be differentiated and treated according to the corresponding descriptions given below: chronic bronchitis, bronchial asthma, exudative pleurisy, chronic heart failure caused by pulmonary heart disease, functional disturbance of the stomach and intestines, incomplete pyloric obstruction, and intestinal obstruction.

Etiology and Pathogenesis

There are internal and external causes of phlegm and fluid retention. External causes include invasion by cold-dampness and improper diet, both of which impair the transformative function of the spleen. The internal cause refers to *yang-qi* deficiency, which means weakness in transporting and transforming the body fluid. As a result, water accumulates at a certain part of the body. The external and internal causes often influence each other.

1. Invasion by Cold-Dampness

Abnormal weather changes, such as high humidity, or frequent contact with cold-dampness, like being caught in the rain, wading in rivers and dwelling in damp places, allows cold-dampness to invade the body surface and the spleen. The spleen *yang* is therefore hindered and splenic function impaired. As a result, the clear *qi* fails to be sent upward, and the turbid fails to be sent downward, causing phlegm and fluid retention.

2. Improper Diet

Drinking large quantities of water, or drinking excessive cold drinks in summer while feeling tired, or drinking cold water or eating cold food after alcohol, may abruptly hinder spleen *yang* and impair splenic function, resulting in phlegm and fluid retention.

3. Deficiency of *Yang-Qi*

The body fluid, belonging to *yin* in nature, depends on the body's *yang-qi* for transport and transformation. Splenic and renal *yang*-deficiency due to poor recuperation from a protracted illness, or weak *qi* of old patients prevents the normal transportation and transformation. When this is complicated by pathogenic cold-dampness or improper diet, retention of phlegm and fluid is more likely to occur.

Normally, fluid transport, transformation, and excretion are accomplished by the coordination of the spleen, lung and kidneys. The lung dominates *qi*, regulates water passage, and transmits the waste fluid to the urinary bladder. The spleen distributes fluid throughout the body, and the kidneys dominate water metabolism and urination. With normal functioning, the essence of food and drink is well distributed to nourish various parts of the body, and the waste fluid is excreted as sweat or urine. The spleen is the most important of the three organs in relation to the production of phlegm and retained fluid. Deficiency of spleen *yang* means insufficient production of essence, which will deprive the lung of nourishment on the one hand, and impair the renal function on the other.

Body fluid circulates through *sanjiao*, which connects the surface with the *zang-fu* organs and communicates with the interior, exterior, upper and lower parts of the body. It is through *sanjiao* that the essence produced by the spleen and stomach is distributed. Therefore, the obstruction of *sanjiao* is another cause of phlegm and fluid retention.

Differential Diagnosis

Both retention and edema result from abnormal fluid transportation, transformation and distribution, but there is a difference between them. Retention refers to a local accumulation of excessive fluid. Edema refers to a condition of which excessive fluid overflows throughout the body with swelling as its main syndrome.

Distinction and Treatment

Retention is marked by *yang* deficiency and *yin* excess, weak resistance and hyperactive pathogenic factors. If *yin* excess predominates, pathogenic phlegm and retained fluid are eliminated with purgatives, diuretics, or diaphoretics according to where they are retained. If *yang* deficiency is more pronounced, treatment should focus on invigorating the spleen and warming the kidneys. When *yang-qi* is invigorated, pathogenic phlegm and retained fluid will be resolved spontaneously. Phlegm and retained fluid are *yin* pathogenic factors, which coagulate with cold and circulate with warmth; thus warm herbs should be used in the treatment. Commonly-used herbs include Ramulus Cinnamomi, Poria and Rhizoma Zingiberis Recens, all of which are warm and mild in nature. Herbs that are extremely acrid and hot, such as Radix Aconiti Lateralis Preparata, and herbs that are cold, such as Rhizoma Anemarrhenae and Rhizoma Coptidis, are not used. The three warm and mild herbs are applied throughout the whole course of treatment, in order to achieve the purpose of warming *yang*, resolving dampness, circulating *qi*, eliminating phlegm, promoting diuresis and purging retained fluid. When most phlegm and retained fluid have been eliminated, herbs that invigorate the spleen and warm the kidneys are then used to consolidate the therapeutic results.

In addition, in cases of protracted retention, or retention complicated by wind-heat, the treatment is to warm the kidneys, while using herbs warm or cool in nature at the same time.

1. Excess Syndromes
(1) Retention in the intestines and stomach

Clinical manifestations: Fullness and pain in the epigastrium and abdomen, a splashing sound in the stomach or intestines, a deep, taut and forceful pulse, or diarrhea which does not relieve fullness, a white and sticky or slightly yellow tongue coating, constipation, absence of flatus, dry mouth and tongue, a yellow and thick tongue coating.

Analysis: Retention in the stomach and intestines gives rise to a splashing sound, fullness and pain in severe cases. A taut and deep pulse suggests retention inside the body. Diarrhea which does not relieve the feeling of fullness shows excessive fluid retention. A white and sticky or a slightly yellow tongue coating indicates that the fluid has not turned to heat yet, or heat is not pronounced. Constipation, absence of flatus, dry mouth and tongue, and a yellow and thick tongue coating are all signs of heat, which mixes with the turbid *qi*, blocking the large intestines.

Treatment: To eliminate retained fluid with purgatives.

Prescription: In cases of fluid retention in the stomach with no apparent heat signs, Decoction of Kansui and Pinelliae (86) can be prescribed to eliminate pathogenic factors and protect resistance at the same time. Rhizoma Pinelliae and Radix Kansui function to relieve stagnation, conduct the unhealthy *qi* downward, and purge fluid; while the Radix Kansui and Radix Glycyrrhizae function to the contrary. The combination strengthens drug potency for the complete purgation of fluid. Radix Paeoniae Alba and Mel, sweet and sour in nature, is added to protect the middle *jiao* and prevent damage to the resistance.

In case of fluid retention in the intestines, such as the constipation, Pill of Stephaniae Tetrandrae, Zanthoxyli, Lepidii seu Descurainiae and Rhei (31) can be prescribed. In the prescription, Semen Lepidii seu Descurainiae and Radix et Rhizoma Rhei function to disperse heat and promote bowel movement; and Radix Stephaniae Tetrandrae and Pericarpium Zanthoxyli promote diuresis. In this way, retained fluid and heat in the intestines are dispelled through defecation and urination.

(2) Retention in the chest and hypochondrium

Clinical manifestations: A distending pain in the chest and hypochondrium, which is aggravated by cough, movement of the body, and respiration, shortness of breath, palpitation, a thin and white tongue coating, and a deep and taut pulse.

Analysis: The chest and the hypochondrium serve as a channel through which *qi* could ascend or descend. Retention in the chest and hypochondrium causes retardation of *qi* with symptoms of distending pain in the chest and hypochondrium, which are aggravated by cough, movement of the body and respiration. If the retained fluid impairs the heart and lung, then pulmonary function will be affected and heart *yang* hindered; thus symptoms of shortness of breath and palpitation occur. A thin and white tongue coating and a deep and taut pulse are signs of fluid retention in the chest and hypochondrium.

Treatment: To eliminate retained fluid with purgatives.

Prescription: Decoction of Jujubae (7) or Decoction of Lepidii seu Descurainiae and Jujubae for Purging Lung-Heat (294). In the former, Radix Kansui, Flos Genkwa and Radix Euphorbiae Pekinensis are ground into powder, serving as drastic purgatives; Fructus Jujubae strengthens the resistance, invigorates the spleen and reduces the poisonous effects of the herbs. Attention should be paid to the constitution of the patient. If the patient is too weak to take drastic herbs, the latter prescription is recommended. If the case is complicated by the exterior-syndrome, these two prescriptions are not used until the exterior-syndrome is relieved.

(3) Retention in the chest and lung

Clinical manifestations: Cough, dyspnea, fullness in the chest, orthopnea in severe cases, expectoration of profuse, white and frothy sputum, edema of the face and eyelids following long-standing cough, a white and sticky tongue coating, and a taut and tense pulse. The illness is persistent and likely to recur when contacting cold, accompanied by chilliness, fever and general ache.

Analysis: Located in the upper *jiao*, the lung dominates respiration. If retained fluid invades the heart and lung, preventing the lung *qi* from circulation, this will result in cough, fullness in the chest, dyspnea, and orthopnea in severe cases. Retained fluid belongs to *yin* and was cold in nature, therefore expectoration of profuse, white and frothy sputum appears. Long-standing cough does not allow *qi* to transform water; the upward flow of water and fluid leads to edema of the face and eyelids. A white and sticky tongue coating, and a taut and tense pulse are signs of excessive fluid retention. Retention is likely to be stirred by external pathogenic cold, therefore the illness lasts for years. The external pathogenic cold stirs up the retained fluid, causing the syndromes of wind-cold.

Treatment: To warm the lung and resolve phlegm.

Prescription: Small Blue Dragon Decoction (33) is the main one. Herba Ephedrae and Ramulus Cinnamomi, ingredients of the prescription, disperse wind-cold, promote the lung's dispersive function and relieve dyspnea; Radix Paeoniae Alba, and Ramulus Cinnamomi combine to regulate nutrient and defensive *qi*; Rhizoma Zingiberis, Herba Asari and Rhizoma Pinelliae warm the lung, resolve retained fluid, disperse cold and conduct the unhealthy *qi* downward; Fructus Schisandrae, an astringent, protects lung *qi* from excessive dispersion; and Radix Glycyrrhizae regulates the middle *jiao*. This prescription is recommended in cases of retention induced by the external cold.

If there is profuse phlegm accompanied by cough, dyspnea and a suffocating sensation in the chest, Decoction of Lepidii seu Descurainiae and Jujubae for Purging Lung-Heat (294) should be described. If retained fluid has turned to heat with symptoms of fullness and stuffiness in the chest, distress in the abdomen, restlessness, thirst, and a yellow and sticky tongue coating, modified Decoction of Cocculi Trilobi (43) is recommended to promote diuresis, disperse heat, benefit *qi*, and dispel masses. If the above symptoms still exist, remove Gypsum Fibrosum and add in Poria and Natrii Sulfas to eliminate water through purgation and do away with stagnation. If there is dizziness and a falling sensation, Decoction of Alismatis (169) is used in combination. If fullness in the abdomen and constipation are present, Decoction of Magnoliae Officinalis and Rhei (209) is used. If nausea and vomiting appear without thirst, add in Rhizoma Pinelliae, Rhizoma Zingiberis Recens and Poria.

(4) Fluid retention in the four extremities

Clinical manifestations: Heaviness or even edema in the four limbs, absence of sweating, chilliness, general ache, absence of thirst, cough with profuse, white and frothy sputum, or dyspnea, a white and sticky tongue coating, and a taut and tense pulse.

Analysis: Overflow of water and fluid to the surface leads to the heaviness or even edema in the four limbs. Invasion of cold complicated by internal fluid retention explains absence of sweating, chilliness, general ache, cough with profuse, white and frothy sputum. Disturbance of the lung by phlegm and retained fluid causes dyspnea. A white and sticky tongue coating, a taut and tense pulse, and absence of thirst all suggest cold both on the exterior and in the interior of the body.

Treatment: To resolve retained fluid by warming and dispersing.

Prescription: Small Blue Dragon Decoction (33) is the main prescription. If there is invasion by the external cold, and retained fluid has turned to heat, with symptoms of fever, restlessness and a white-yellowish tongue coating, Great Blue Dragon Decoction (23) is recommended. In the prescription, Herba Ephedrae, Ramulus Cinnamomi, Semen Armeniacae Amarum, Radix Glycyrrhizae, Rhizoma Zingiberis Recens and Fructus Jujubae cause sweating, disperse retained fluid and regulate nutrient and defensive *qi*; and Gypsum Fibrosum disperses heat and relieves restlessness.

If there is subjective throbbing in the lower abdomen, spitting of fluid, dizziness and blurring of vision, Powder of Five Drugs Containing Poria (51) is recommended. Here Ramulus Cinnamomi invigorates *yang* and conducts the unhealthy *qi* downward; Poria, Polyporus and Rhizoma Alismatis promote diuresis; and Rhizoma Atractylodis Macrocephalae invigorates the spleen and promotes diuresis. When water runs downward, all the symptoms will disappear.

2. Deficiency Syndromes

These syndromes are marked by spleen and kidney *yang*-deficiency complicated by invasion of pathogenic dampness or improper diet. In these conditions, manifestations of deficiency syndrome are more pronounced than those due to the fluid retention. If retained fluid in cases of excess syndrome has been basically eliminated and weak resistance becomes more pronounced, the following methods can also be adopted.

(1) Deficiency of spleen and stomach *yang*

Clinical manifestations: A distended and full sensation in the chest and hypochondrium, preference for warmth and pressure in the epigastric and abdominal region, a splashing sound in the stomach, a cold sensation on the back, preference for a small quantity of warm drinks, lack of desire to drink, or vomiting soon after drinking, nausea, vomiting of clear fluid, palpitation, shortness of breath, dizziness, blurring of vision, a white and slippery tongue coating, and a taut, thready and smooth pulse.

Analysis: Deficiency of the spleen and stomach *yang* leads to the preference for warmth and pressure in the epigastrium and abdomen. Retention of fluid in the stomach explains a splashing sound there, lack of desire to drink, or vomiting soon after drinking, nausea, and vomiting of clear fluid. Internal fluid retention prevents *yang-qi* from reaching the back thus a cold sensation is present. Inability to send the clear *yang* upward causes dizziness and blurring of vision. Invasion of the heart and lung by water and fluid produces a distend and full sensation in the chest and hypochondrium, palpitation and shortness of breath. A white and slippery tongue coating and a taut, thready and smooth pulse are signs of *yang* deficiency complicated by fluid retention.

Treatment: To warm the spleen and resolve retained fluid.

Prescription: Decoction of Poria, Cinnamomi, Atractylodis Macrocephalae and Glycyrrhizae (170) is the main one. Poria invigorates the spleen and promotes diuresis; Ramulus Cinnamomi warms *yang* and produces *qi*; Rhizoma Atractylodis Macrocephalae invigorates splenic function and dries up dampness; and Radix Glycyrrhizae regulates the spleen and stomach. In cases of vomiting, add Rhizoma Pinelliae, Rhizoma Zingiberis Recens and Poria to pacify the stomach and conduct the unhealthy *qi* downward. In cases of dizziness and blurring of vision, the main prescription is combined with Decoction of Alismatis (169) to eliminate dampness and send the clear *qi* upward.

(2) Deficiency of kidney *yang*

Clinical manifestations: Aversion to cold, cold limbs, muscular stiffness and subjective throbbing in the lower abdomen, shortness of breath, dysuria, or spitting of fluid accompanied by dizziness and blurring of vision, a swollen tongue with white and sticky, or gray and sticky coating, and a deep, thready and smooth pulse.

Analysis: Protracted fluid retention enables the splenic deficiency to affect the kidneys. Since elderly people with fluid retention lack kidney *yang*, which deprives the body of warmth, thereby the following syndromes: aversion to cold, cold limbs and muscular stiffness in the lower abdomen occur. As the renal function is impaired, dysuria occurs. Movement of water gives rise to subjective throbbing in the lower abdomen. Upward disturbance of water leads to the spitting of fluid, dizziness and blurred vision. Renal dysfunction in receiving *qi* causes shortness of breath. A swollen tongue with white and sticky coating and a deep, thready and smooth pulse are all due to *yang* deficiency and fluid retention.

Treatment: To warm the kidneys and resolve retained fluid.

Prescription: Pill for Invigorating Kidney *Qi* (182) is the main one. Pill of Six Drugs Containing Rehmanniae Preparata (56) replenishes kidney *yin*; and Cortex Cinnamomi and Radix Aconiti Lateralis Preparata replenish kidney *yang*. The drugs should be administered continuously, then therapeutic results will be seen. Modified *Zhenwu* Decoction (223) is also recommended, and when the condition improves, Pill for Invigorating Kidney *Qi* (182) could be prescribed.

Case Studies

Miss Zhang, age 20, complained of cough, dyspnea, chest pain, afternoon fever, and expectoration of sticky and thick sputum for over ten days. The body temperature remained between 38°C and 39°C, and chest X-ray showed exudative pleurisy. Hydrothorax was not reduced following twice thoracentesis. That was why she was referred to the Department of TCM for further consultation. The pulse was smooth and forceful. Diagnosis was retention of fluid in the chest and hypochondrium. Treatment aimed to eliminate retained fluid with purgatives by prescribing Decoction of Jujubae (7).

After the first dose, the patient discharged two spittoons of water through defecation, cough and dyspnea improved, body temperature dropped, and appetite improved. She took another dose three days later, and again discharged a large amount of water. All the symptoms disappeared soon.

Discussion: Since the patient was still young, the disease lasted only ten days. Since her pulse was smooth and forceful, indicating the body resistance was not weakened, Decoction of Jujubae (7) was therefore prescribed to purge retained fluid. However, the decoction was not administered every day for fear of damaging her body resistance, and the second packet was taken three days later.

VIII. Spontaneous Sweating and Night Sweating

Both spontaneous sweating and night sweating result from the weakness of the body surface and imbalance of *yin-yang*. Frequent sweating in daytime, exacerbated by slight exertion but not affected by environmental conditions, is known as spontaneous sweating. Sweating that occurs during sleep and stops upon wakening is referred to as night sweating.

The recognition of sweating can be traced back to *The Inner Canon of the Yellow Emperor*, which says, "Sweat is transformed from blood. Acted upon by *yang-qi*, *yin* fluid transforms into sweat. Therefore, sweat stems from *yin* and originates from *yang*." The book also states that the body adjusts its temperature by regulating the amount of sweat in order to adapt to the environmental temperature. *A Guide to Clinical Practice with Case Records* says, "Spontaneous sweating due to *yang* deficiency is treated by invigorating *qi* and strengthening body surface, and night sweating due to *yin* deficiency is treated by replenishing *yin* and nourishing the interior of the body." It is generally acknowledged that spontaneous sweating is caused by *yang* deficiency, and night sweating by *yin* deficiency. But there are exceptions, for instance, *Correction of Medical Classics* says, "There are cases of spontaneous and night sweating which become worse when invigorating *qi* and consolidating body surface, or nourishing *yin* and subduing fire. This is because blood stagnation can also cause spontaneous sweating and night sweating. In these cases, Decoction for Removing Blood Stasis in the Chest (135) should be used."

Abnormal sweating in vegetative nerves causes functional disturbance, tuberculosis, shock, rheumatic fever, hyperthyroidism, transient hypoglycemia, and some infectious diseases, which can be differentiated and treated according to the following descriptions.

Etiology and Pathogenesis
Sweating is a physiological phenomenon which plays an important role in eliminating pathogenic factors and adjusting body temperature. Normally, the amount of sweat increases in summer, after drinking hot beverages, heavy physical exertion, or diaphoretics. Since sweat is the fluid of the heart, and transforms from the body's essential *qi*, it is not advisable to sweat excessively.

1. Weakness of the Lung and Body Surface
Lung *qi* is consumed, especially with patients of weak constitution, or after a protracted illness, prolonged cough and dyspnea. The deficiency of lung *qi* weakens the body surface and loosens the skin and muscles. As a result, their function of protecting body fluid and controlling the pores is impaired, and sweating occurs.

2. Disharmony of Nutrient *Qi* and Defensive *Qi*
This condition follows the imbalance of *yin-yang*, or an exterior syndrome of the deficiency type complicated by exposure to external wind. Disharmony of nutrient *qi* and defensive *qi* weakens the body surface, as a result, it could no longer prevent body fluid from being excreted.

3. Deficiency of *Yin* and Hyperactivity of Fire
This is the consequence of strain and stress, loss of blood and essence, or consumption of *yin* by pathogenic heat. Deficiency of *yin* essence produces internal heat of the deficiency type, which in turn disturbs *yin* essence and dispels it as sweat.

4. Hyperactivity of Pathogenic Heat

This results from emotional upset, leading to stagnation of liver *qi* and consequently hyperactivity of liver fire, or from overeating acrid and highly flavored food, or from excessive body dampness-heat. Either hyperactive liver fire or retained excess dampness-heat inside the body can cause body fluid to be excreted as sweat.

Differential Diagnosis
1. Sweating in Shock

This occurs in severe or critical conditions, manifested as continuous profuse sweating, short and feeble breath, lassitude, cold limbs, a feeble and fading pulse or a large and weak pulse. It is due to the exhaustion of body anti-pathogenic *qi* after a serious disease marked by failure of *yang* to preserve *yin*.

2. Sweating with Shivering

This type of sweating follows fever, thirst, restlessness and chills in an acute febrile disease. Sweating is a manifestation of the struggle between the body anti-pathogenic *qi* and pathogenic factors. If the anti-pathogenic *qi* wins, the patient's condition improves after sweating. If sweating does not occur after shivering when the anti-pathogenic *qi* is deficient, the pathogenic factors tend to penetrate into the body. If the anti-pathogenic *qi* dissipates along with sweating, the case becomes critical. Therefore, it is necessary to carefully observe the patient who sweats after shivering. If fever subsides and the pulse becomes calm after sweating, the prognosis is favorable, for it suggests the strengthening of anti-pathogenic *qi* and elimination of pathogenic factors. But if sweating is followed by cold limbs, restlessness and an irregular pulse, it indicates that the case has deteriorated because the anti-pathogenic *qi* fails to win over pathogenic factors and prostration tends to occur.

3. Yellow Sweat

Yellow sweat stains the clothes, as yellow as the juice of Cortex Phellodendri. It is often accompanied by "edema, fever, thirst and deep pulse," as described in *Synopsis of Prescriptions of the Golden Chamber*.

Distinction and Treatment

The dialectical relationship of spontaneous sweating and night sweating should be classified as *yin*, *yang*, deficiency and excess. Generally, deficiency syndromes are more common than excess syndromes, but there are cases which present a heat syndrome of the excess type, or a syndrome with both deficiency and excess. For instance, spontaneous sweating and night sweating due to hyperactivity of liver fire or excess dampness-heat are of the excess type. A complicated condition occurs in a protracted or severe case. Long-standing spontaneous sweating may damage *yin*, while long-standing night sweating may impair *yang*; thus a syndrome of both *qi* and *yin* deficiency, or both *yin* and *yang* deficiency is produced. Excess pathogenic heat consumes *yin* in a protracted illness, presenting a syndrome of both deficiency and excess.

The general principle of treatment is to replenish *qi*, nourish *yin*, consolidate the body surface and check sweating for deficiency syndromes; to disperse heat in the liver, resolve dampness and harmonize nutrient *qi* for excess syndromes; as for cases with both deficiency and excess, the treatment should take both the deficiency and excess into consideration, paying special attention to which one predominates. Astringents which arrest sweating may be used in combination, such as Radix Ephedrae, Fructus Tritici Levis (light), Radix Oryzae Glutinosae, Fructus Schisandrae, and Concha Ostreae Usta.

1. Weakness of the Lung and Body Surface

Clinical manifestations: Sweating which is worse on slight exertion, aversion to wind, susceptibility to cold, lassitude, pale complexion, a thready and weak pulse, and a thin and white tongue coating.

Analysis: Protracted illness damages lung *qi* and weakens the body surface; this explains sweating, aversion to wind and susceptibility to cold. Exertion consumes *qi*, preventing it from controlling sweating, and thus making sweating even worse. Lassitude, pale complexion, and a thready and weak pulse are signs of *qi* deficiency.

Treatment: To replenish *qi* and consolidate the body surface.

Prescription: Jade Screen Powder (73) with additional drugs. Radix Astragali is used in large doses to replenish *qi* and consolidate body surface; Rhizoma Atractylodis Macrocephalae invigorates the spleen and strengthens the source of *qi* and blood; and Radix Ledebouriellae acts on the body surface and assists Radix Astragali. The combination of Radix Astragali and Radix Ledebouriellae makes it possible to eliminate external pathogenic factors while reinforcing body resistance. In cases of profuse sweating, Fructus Tritici Levis (light), Radix Oryzae Glutinosae and Concha Ostreae Usta are added to consolidate body surface and check sweating. If *qi* deficiency is pronounced, Radix Codonopsis and Radix Polygonati are added to replenish *qi* and promote astringency. If signs of *yin* deficiency are present, such as a red tongue and a thready and rapid pulse, Radix Ophiopogonis and Fructus Schisandrae are added to nourish *yin* and check sweating.

2. Disharmony Between Nutrient *Qi* and Defensive *Qi*

Clinical manifestations: Sweating, aversion to wind, general ache, alternate chills and fever, a retarded pulse, and a thin and white tongue coating.

Analysis: This results from an exterior syndrome of the deficiency type complicated by exposure to pathogenic wind, or from the weak constitution after childbirth. Disharmony of the nutrient *qi* and defensive *qi* loosens the skin and muscles, resulting in sweating and aversion to wind. Alternate chills and fever, general ache, a retarded pulse and a thin and white tongue coating are all signs of disharmony between nutrient *qi* and defensive *qi*.

Treatment: To harmonize nutrient *qi* and defensive *qi*.

Prescription: Decoction of Cinnamomi (224) with additional drugs. Here, Ramulus Cinnamomi warms the meridians, disperses cold and relieves exterior syndrome; Radix Paeoniae Alba harmonizes nutrient *qi* and consolidates *yin*; the combination of these two herbs promotes dispersion and astringency at the same time, thus creating a harmonious state between nutrient *qi* and defensive *qi*; Rhizoma Zingiberis Recens and Fructus Jujubae assist the two previous herbs; and Radix Glycyrrhizae regulates the effects of other drugs in the prescription. To strengthen the effect of checking sweating, Os Draconis and Concha Ostreae are added. In cases of *qi* deficiency, Radix Astragali is added to replenish *qi* and consolidate the body surface. If palpitation and insomnia are also present, Semen Ziziphi Spinosae and Fructus Tritici Levis are added to nourish the heart and calm the mind.

3. Deficiency of *Yin* and Hyperactivity of Fire

Clinical manifestations: Night sweating, or spontaneous sweating, restlessness, a hot sensation in the palms, soles and chest, afternoon fever, malar flush, thirst, lassitude, a red tongue with scanty coating, and a thready and rapid pulse.

Analysis: Deficiency of *yin* essence produces fire of the deficiency type, which causes body fluid to be excreted, resulting in night sweating or spontaneous sweating. Fire of the deficiency type leads to the restlessness, a hot sensation in the palms, soles and chest, afternoon fever and malar flush. Hyperactivity of fire consumes body fluid, which causes thirst. A red tongue with scanty coating and a thready and rapid pulse are signs of *yin* deficiency with hyperactivity of fire.

Treatment: To nourish *yin* and subdue fire.

Prescription: Modified Decoction of Angelicae Sinensis and Six Ingredients (129). Here, Radix Angelicae Sinensis, Radix Rehmanniae and Radix Rehmanniae Preparata nourish *yin*, replenish the blood and strengthen kidney fluid so as to check fire; Radix Scutellariae, Rhizoma Coptidis and Cortex Phellodendri disperse heat and subdue fire to consolidate *yin*; and Radix Astragali replenishes *qi* and consolidates body surface. In cases of profuse sweating, Concha Ostreae, Fructus Tritici Levis (light) and Radix Oryzae Glutinosae are added. If afternoon fever is pronounced, Radix Stellarial, Cortex Lycii, Radix Gentianae Macrophyllae and Radix Cynanchi Atrati are added to disperse heat of the deficiency type. In cases with insomnia and palpitation, Semen Ziziphi Spinosae and Fructus Schisandrae are added to nourish the heart, calm the mind and check sweating. If *yin* deficiency is more pronounced than hyperactivity of fire, Pill of Ophiopogonis, Schisandrae and Rehmanniae Preparata (141) is used to nourish *yin* and disperse heat.

4. Hyperactivity of Pathogenic Heat

Clinical manifestations: Persistent perspiration with sticky or yellow-stained sweat, flushed face with a hot sensation, restlessness, irritability, a bitter taste in the mouth, yellow urine, a thin and yellow tongue coating, and a taut and rapid pulse.

Analysis: Hyperactivity of liver fire or retention of excessive dampness-heat leads to flushed face, restlessness, irritability, a bitter taste in the mouth and yellow urine. Heat causes fluid excretion and results in persistent perspiration. Dampness-heat affects the liver and gallbladder, causing bile to flow out with sweating, which explains yellow sweat. A thin and yellow tongue coating and a taut and rapid pulse are signs of heat retention.

Treatment: To disperse heat in the liver, resolve dampness and harmonize nutrient *qi*.

Prescription: Modified Decoction of Gentianae for Purging Liver-Fire (78). In this prescription, Radix Gentianae, Radix Scutellariae, Fructus Gardeniae and Radix Bupleuri disperse heat in the liver; Rhizoma Alismatis, Caulis Aristolochiae Manshuriensis and Semen Plantaginis disperse heat and eliminate dampness; Radix Angelicae Sinensis and Radix Rehmanniae nourish *yin*, replenish the blood and harmonize nutrient *qi*; and Radix Glycyrrhizae regulates the effects of all the other ingredients in the prescription, disperses heat and reduces fire.

If retention of dampness-heat is not accompanied by pronounced heat syndrome, Pill of Four Wonderful Ingredients (89) is prescribed. Here, Rhizoma Atractylodis, Cortex Phellodendri and Semen Coicis disperse heat and eliminate dampness; and Radix Achyranthis Bidentatae benefits the tendons and collaterals.

Simplified prescription:

(1) Spontaneous sweating due to *qi* deficiency

Radix Astragali	15 g;
Fructus Jujubae	5 pieces;
Fructus Tritici Levis (light)	15 g.

(2) Night sweating due to *yin* deficiency

Fructus Mume	10 pieces;
Fructus Tritici Levis (light)	15 g;
Fructus Jujubae	5 pieces.

(3) Night sweating

Fructus Persicae	15 pieces;
Fructus Jujubae	10 pieces.

(4) Night sweating

A proper amount of powder of Galla Chinensis is mixed with warm water and applied to the umbilicus externally.

Since sweat stems from the body's essential *qi*, excessive sweating inevitably damages the body's anti-pathogenic *qi*. Spontaneous sweating or night sweating without any accompanying symptoms generally has a good prognosis. If they are present in other diseases, however, the pathological conditions are often serious. The primary disease should then be treated first.

Since the skin is loose and the pores are open during sweating, care should be taken not to catch cold. The body should be dried soon after sweating, and wet underclothes should be taken off to prevent attack by cold-dampness.

Case Studies

Name: Yu XX; Sex: Female; Age: 72.

First visit (June 9, 1964): The patient complained of a hot sensation in the stomach, which traveled outward and caused sweating several times a day, especially on wakening. Following sweating were aversion to cold, thirst but with no desire to drink and mild cough. Her appetite, urination and defecation were normal. The illness occurred after a bout of pneumonia in the middle of May. X-ray check was normal. The patient had taken Radix Codonopsis, Radix Ophiopogonis, Fructus Schisandrae, Os Draconis, Concha Ostreae and Jade Screen Powder (73), but without effect. The pulse was deep and thready at *cun* and *chi* positions, and bounding and rapid at the *guan* position on both sides. The tongue was red with yellow and sticky coating. All this was due to the accumulation of residual dampness-heat in the lung and stomach. Treatment aimed to clear away dampness-heat. The following drugs were prescribed:

Semen Benincasae	10 g;
Semen Coicis	12 g;
Semen Armeniacae Amarum	6 g;
Rhizoma Phragmitis	18 g;
Herba Lophatheri	6 g;
Gypsum Fibrosum	9 g;
Folium Eriobotryae	6 g;
Folium Nelumbinis	6 g;
Fructus Oryzae Sativae	12 g.

Second visit (June 12, 1964): After four doses, the patient felt the hot sensation traveling downward to the lower legs like a crawling ant. Sweating was reduced, and no profuse sweating occurred on wakening. There was dryness and a sweet taste in the mouth, mild stuffiness in the chest, a red tongue with yellow and sticky coating, and a taut and smooth pulse with missed beats. All this suggested downward movement of dampness-heat and retention of residual heat in the lung and stomach. The same treatment was adopted:

Semen Benincasae	9 g;
Semen Coicis	12 g;
Semen Armeniacae Amarum	9 g;
Rhizoma Phragmitis	12 g;
Herba Lophatheri	6 g;
Gypsum Fibrosum	9 g;
Herba Artemisiae Scopariae	6 g;
Semen Sojae Germinatum	9 g;

Radix Stephaniae Tetrandrae	4.5 g;
Rhizoma Curcumae Longae	4.5 g;
Medulla Tetrapanacis	3 g.

Three doses were prescribed.

Third visit (June 15, 1964): The hot sensation and sweating were both relieved. Thirst also improved. The pulse was taut, rapid and forceful on the left side, and slightly retarded on the right. The tongue was slightly red with thin, yellow and sticky coating. All this showed the presence of residual heat. Treatment aimed to harmonize the lung and stomach, and clear away dampness-heat.

Poria	9 g;
Semen Armeniacae Amarum	6 g;
Cortex Mori	6 g;
Semen Sojae Germinatum	9 g;
Radix Scutellariae	3 g;
Herba Artemisiae Scopariae	9 g;
Rhizoma Curcumae Longae	3 g;
Talcum	9 g;
Medulla Tetrapanacis	3 g;
Semen Coicis	12 g.

All symptoms disappeared after three doses.

Explanation: Sweating several times a day followed by aversion to cold, which occurred after pneumonia, is a sign of weak defensive *yang*. A hot sensation in the stomach, a red tongue with yellow and sticky coating, and a bounding and rapid pulse at the *guan* position on both sides all suggest retention of excessive dampness-heat in the stomach and lung. Thus White Tiger Decoction was prescribed to disperse heat in the stomach, and Decoction of Phragmitis (30) and Decoction of Three Kinds of Seed were used to disperse heat and resolve dampness. Elimination of dampness-heat harmonized the stomach, consolidated the lung, and thus relieved sweating.

IX. Hemorrhagic Syndrome

Hemorrhagic syndrome is a general term for hemoptysis, epistaxis, hematemesis, hemafecia and hematuria.

The description of hemorrhagic syndrome first appeared in *The Inner Canon of the Yellow Emperor*. For instance, it says, "The middle *jiao* receives food essence, then produces a kind of red fluid, which is blood", therefore, "Blood is food essence produced by the spleen." After its formation, blood is propelled by the heart and circulates in the vessels throughout the body, hence there is a saying"the heart dominates blood." Blood circulates on exertion and flows back to the liver during sleep, therefore "the liver stores blood." With the assistance of the spleen, blood circulates inside the vessels, and no blood extravasation occurs, therefore "the spleen controls blood." The kidneys store the essence of the five *zang* organs, which is transformed into blood. *Qi* and blood rely on each other and circulate throughout the body endlessly. They jointly nourish the body, carry on metabolism, promote growth and development, and perform various physiological activities. As a result, disharmony between *qi* and blood will produce various diseases.

The Inner Canon of the Yellow Emperor holds that the cause of hemorrhagic syndrome is the excess *yin* or *yang* inside the body. It says, "Voracious eating, irregular life style, or over-exertion may damage vessels. If *yang* (superficial and ascending) vessels are damaged, extravasated blood will flow upwards, and epistaxis will occur. If *yin* (deep and descending) vessels are damaged, extravasated blood will flow downwards, and hemafecia and hematuria will ensue." *Synopsis of Prescriptions of the Golden Chamber* dedicated a whole chapter to the description of hemorrhagic syndrome. It holds that excess of fire-heat, *yang* deficiency and heart *qi*-deficiency can lead to hemorrhagic syndrome. The major focus of *Prescriptions for Life Saving* is on heat: "Reckless movement of blood is caused by heat. Acted upon by heat, blood follows *qi* in its upward movement and causes epistaxis." *Danxi's Experience on Medicine* explains the cause of hemoptysis and hematemesis as "excess of *yang* and deficiency of *yin* prevent blood from moving downward, and cause fire to flare up, resulting in hematemesis." The book also says, "Epistaxis is mostly due to the blood deficiency," and "hematuria is due to heat." *A Complete Collection of Jingyue's Treatise* believes that "bleeding involves fire and *qi*, therefore attention should be paid to the presence of fire and *qi* in analyzing the cause." *Diseases of Blood* of the Qing Dynasty, explicitly describes the relation between *qi* and blood, pathogenesis and treatment of hemorrhagic syndrome. These descriptions provide valuable experience to physicians of the later generations. It points out that extravasated blood include those fresh in color as well as those black, "Pure and fresh extravasated blood is also referred to as stagnant blood." As to the treatment of hemorrhagic syndrome, it says, "To stop bleeding is the first step of treatment. When bleeding ceases, blood outside the vessels is stagnant blood. Therefore, the second step is to remove blood stasis. To prevent the blood from stirring up again, drugs must be administered to calm it, therefore checking blood is the third step. Excessive blood loss inevitably leads to *yin* deficiency, thus the treatment ends by remedying deficiency. The above four steps are the main principle in the treatment of hemorrhagic syndrome."

Hemorrhagic syndrome covers a wide range, either in acute or chronic cases. This chapter will mainly discuss the hemorrhagic syndromes commonly seen in internal medicine.

Etiology and Pathogenesis

Most hemorrhagic syndrome is caused by fire or *qi*, for instance, hyperactivity of fire-heat inside the body, or the *yin* deficiency forces the blood to move irregularly, or the malfunctioning of the five *zang* organs, like the spleen's failing to control blood, the liver's failing to store blood, and the collapse of *qi* in the middle *jiao* which fails to control blood. Since fire-heat attacks the blood, the blood tends to run out of the vessels, resulting in hemorrhagic syndrome. The fire inside the *zang-fu* organs damages its collaterals, which can also cause hemorrhagic syndrome in different places. The fire can be divided into excess and deficiency type. Fire of the excess type results from the attack of the body by pathogenic factors (wind, fire and dryness), improper diet, or emotional upsets (as in the case of liver fire). Fire due to the *yin* deficiency is often present in chronic disorders. For instance, deficiency of kidney *yin* leads to hyperactivity of ministerial fire; deficiency of lung *yin* deprives the lung of nourishment and moisture, which causes the dryness and damages the vessels; deficiency of liver *yin* leads to hyperactivity of liver fire; and deficiency of heart *yin* produces hyperactivity of heart fire, which transports the heat to the small intestines.

Hemorrhagic syndrome can also result from *qi* deficiency complicated by cold. *Qi* is the commander of blood; propelled by *qi*, blood circulates normally; controlled by *qi*, it does not flow outside the vessels. Therefore,"*qi* conveys blood, and blood consolidates *qi*". The *qi* that does not control blood is the *qi* of the middle *jiao*. Since the *qi* of the middle *jiao* belongs to the spleen, thus the failure of *qi* in controlling the blood usually means splenic failure. If the spleen and stomach are deficient and affected by cold, or if the *qi* of the middle *jiao* is insufficient, either bloody stools or uterine bleeding will occur. Clinically, bleeding due to heat is more commonly seen than bleeding from *qi* deficiency complicated by cold.

Attack by external pathogenic wind, heat and dryness, or cold which then turns into heat, damages the pulmonary vessels and causes blood to run upward, resulting in hemoptysis and epistaxis.

Excessive alcohol or overeating acrid and dry food produces dryness and heat in the stomach and intestines, which then turn into fire and cause blood extravasation, leading to hematemesis, epistaxis and hemafecia.

Hyperfunction of the liver, or flaring up of liver fire due to hepatic and renal *yin*-deficiency affects the lung and results in hemoptysis and epistaxis. Either mental depression or excessive anger will damage the liver, which in turn attacks the stomach, damaging its vessels; hematemesis then occurs.

Strain and stress do harm to the spleen and impair its ability to control the blood. Upward movement of the extravasated blood leads to hematemesis and epistaxis; downward movement leads to hemafecia.

A protracted illness, febrile disease, or excessive sexual activity consumes kidney *yin* and produces hyperactivity of the ministerial fire, which then causes reckless blood movement, resulting in hematuria. Excessive worry consumes heart *yin* and causes hyperactivity of heart fire, which then draws blood down to the small intestines, resulting in hematuria.

In addition, stagnant blood blocks vessels and prevents blood from circulating normally, which also may cause bleeding. If the blood stasis is not removed, bleeding will not cease.

Distinction and Treatment
1. Hemoptysis

Hemoptysis results from damage to the pulmonary vessels, with blood brought up through the air passage. In such cases, blood mixed with sputum, sputum with blood streaks, or blood bright red with foam will appear. The causes of hemoptysis include deficiency of lung *yin* complicated by the attack of external pathogenic wind, heat and dryness, impairment of the lung's descending function following the attack of the lung by liver fire, and damage to the pulmonary vessels by hyperactive fire due to the *yin* deficiency. Therefore, treatment aims to disperse heat, moisten the lung, disperse heat in the liver, calm the vessels, nourish *yin*, subdue fire, cool blood and check bleeding. There is bleeding through the air passage without cough, which could be treated in the same way.

(1) Attack of the lung by wind-heat

Clinical manifestations: Itching of the throat, cough with blood-tinged sputum, dry mouth and nose, a red tongue with thin and yellow coating, and a superficial and rapid pulse. Before hemoptysis occurs, there often appear symptoms of fever, chilliness, sore throat and cough with difficulty in expectoration.

Analysis: Attack of the lung by external pathogenic wind-heat impairs the pulmonary descending function, and results in cough and itching of the throat. Damage to the pulmonary vessels causes hemoptysis. Dry mouth, nose, and red tongue are due to the consumption of body fluids by wind-heat. Fever, a thin and yellow tongue coating and a superficial and rapid pulse are signs of the attack by external wind-heat.

Treatment: To disperse heat, moisten the lung, calm the vessels and check bleeding.

Prescription: Modified Decoction of Mori and Armeniacae Amarum (256). Here, Folium Mori and Semen Sojae Preparatum disperse dryness and heat; Semen Armeniacae Amarum benefits lung *qi*; Bulbus Fritillariae Thunbergii checks cough and resolves phlegm; Fructus Gardeniae disperses heat and cools blood; and Radix Adenophorae and Exocarpium Pyri moisten the lung and produce body fluids. If fever is not present, Semen Sojae Praeparatum is removed from the prescription and Rhizoma Imperatae, Nodus Nelumbinis Rhizomatis, Cacumen Platycladi and Radix Rubiae are added to cool blood and check bleeding. In cases with fever, Flos Lonicerae and Fructus Forsythiae are added.

If hemoptysis is due to the damage of the lung by pathogenic dryness, Bulbus Fritillariae Cirrhosae, Fructus Trichosanthis and Radix Trichosanthis are prescribed to disperse heat, resolve phlegm, moisten the lung and check bleeding; Radix Platycodi promotes the lung's dispersive function and eases the throat; and Poria harmonizes the middle *jiao* and resolves retained fluid. If dryness and heat consume *yin*, producing a red and dry tongue or persistent hemoptysis, Radix Rehmanniae, Colla Corii Asini, Cacumen Platycladi and Folium Artemisiae Argyi are added to nourish *yin*, cool blood and check bleeding. In cases with constipation, Radix et Rhizoma Rhei is added.

(2) Attack of the lung by liver fire

Clinical manifestations: Paroxysmal cough with blood-tinged sputum or bright red blood, pain in the chest and hypochondrium during coughing, restlessness, irritability, constipation, scanty and deep yellow urine, a red tongue with thin and yellow coating, and a taut and rapid pulse.

Analysis: Attack of the lung by liver fire damages the vessels, causing paroxysmal cough with blood-tinged sputum or bright red blood in severe cases. Since the Liver Meridian passes through the hypochondriac region, cough due to liver fire causes pain there. Hyperactivity of liver fire gives rise to restlessness and irritability. Constipation, scanty and deep yellow urine, a red tongue with thin and yellow coating and a taut and rapid pulse are signs of hyperactive liver fire.

Treatment: To clear away liver fire, reduce heat in the lung, calm the vessels and check bleeding.

Prescription: Powder of Indigo Naturalis and Concha Meretricis seu Cyclinae (321), and Powder for Expelling Lung-Heat (174) added with other drugs. This prescription disperses heat in the liver and lung. Here, Cortex Mori and Cortex Lycii reduce fire in the lung; Concha Meretricis seu Cyclinae disperses heat in the lung and resolves phlegm; and Indigo Naturalis disperses heat in the liver and cools blood. If hemoptysis is persistent, along with symptoms of cough and dyspnea, Fructus Gardeniae is added to reduce liver fire; Fructus Trichosanthis and Pumex are added to disperse heat, subdue fire, moisten dryness and resolve phlegm; and Fructus Chebulae is added to consolidate the lung, check cough and relieve dyspnea. Since hemoptysis due to the attack of the lung by liver fire is often accompanied by the liver *yin*-deficiency, drugs that nourish liver *yin*, such as Radix Rehmanniae, Fructus Lycii and Herba Ecliptae, should be added.

(3) Hyperactivity of fire due to *yin* deficiency

Clinical manifestations: Cough with scanty blood-tinged sputum, afternoon fever, night sweating, malar flush, dry mouth and tongue, a red tongue, and a thready and rapid pulse.

Analysis: Lung *yin*-deficiency impairs the lung's descending function, resulting in cough with scanty sputum. Damage to the pulmonary vessels by fire causes tinged sputum with a color of bright red. Hyperactivity of fire due to *yin* deficiency causes body fluid to move outwards, and thereby night sweating, afternoon fever and malar flush occur. Failure of body fluid to ascend leads to the dry mouth and tongue. A red tongue and a thready and rapid pulse are signs of heat caused by *yin* deficiency.

Treatment: To nourish *yin*, moisten the lung, cool blood and check bleeding.

Prescription: Modified Decoction of Lilii for Strengthening Lung (116). In this prescription, Bulbus Lilii and Radix Ophiopogonis moisten the lung and produce fluid; Radix Scrophulariae, Radix Rehmanniae and Radix Rehmanniae Preparata nourish *yin* and disperse heat; Radix Angelicae Sinensis and Radix Paeoniae Alba produce moisture and nourish blood; and Radix Platycodi, Bulbus Fritillariae Cirrhosae and Radix Glycyrrhizae disperse heat in the lung and resolve phlegm. To disperse heat, Radix Scutellariae and Fructus Gardeniae are added. To cool blood and check bleeding, Rhizoma Bletillae, Rhizoma Imperatae and Nodus Nelumbinis Rhizomatis are added. In cases of persistent hemoptysis with profuse blood, Colla Corii Asini and Radix Notoginseng are added to nourish blood and check bleeding. In cases with afternoon fever and malar flush, Herba Artemisiae Annuae, Cortex Lycii and Radix Cynanchi Atrati are added to disperse heat of the deficiency type. For night sweating, Radix Oryzae Glutinosae, Testa Glycine and Concha Ostreae are added.

If deficiency of lung *yin* is complicated by that of lung *qi*, Decoction of Colla Corii Asini for Invigorating Lung (153) is prescribed with additional drugs. Here, Colla Corii Asini nourishes *yin*, fortifies the lung, replenishes blood and checks bleeding; Fructus Aristolochiae disperses heat, resolves phlegm and checks cough; Fructus Arctii promotes the lung's dispersive function, eases the diaphragm and disperses phlegm; Semen Armeniacae Amarum conducts the unhealthy *qi* downward and relieves dyspnea; and Semen Oryzae Glutinosae and Radix Glycyrrhizae invigorate the spleen and benefit the lung. To invigorate the spleen and replenish *qi*, such drugs as Radix Ginseng, Rhizoma Polygonati and Poria can be added.

In the treatment of serious cases with damage of the lung vessels, like hemoptysis of profuse bright red blood, Decoction of Cornu Rhinocerotis and Rehmanniae (306) is administered in combination with Powder of Radix Notoginseng to disperse heat, cool the blood and check bleeding. In cases with cold feet, pounded Radix Aconiti Lateralis Preparata is applied onto *Yongquan* (KI 1) soon after washing feet in hot water. This can conduct blood downward and bring fire back to its origin. If hemoptysis is often induced by cough, Pericarpium Papaveris is added for consolidating the lung and checking cough. It is not advisable to use it for a long time, or when there is attack of external pathogenic factors. If a collapse of *yin* occurs with symptoms of shortness of breath, spontaneous sweating, malar flush and a thready and rapid pulse, Powder for Restoring Pulse (96) is prescribed with Os Draconis and Concha Ostreae. When profuse bleeding occurs, the patient must keep calm and lie down quietly to prevent prostration.

2. Epistaxis

Epistaxis included bleeding in the nose, gums, ears, tongue and sweat pores without traumatic injury. The lung opens into the nose, and the Stomach Meridian goes to the gums. Excessive heat in the lung and stomach causes reckless blood movement. Retention of pathogenic heat in the interior can also lead to this. Hepatic and renal *yin*-deficiency may cause fire of the deficiency type to flare up, which damages the vessels and causes bleeding. And epistaxis can also be caused by *qi* and blood deficiency; *qi* fails to control the blood which runs upward, thus epistaxis occurs. Bleeding in the eyes is often caused by excessive fire in the liver meridian; and bleeding in the tongue is usually the consequence of hyperactive heart fire. Heat that causes epistaxis is of two types, excess and deficiency, and epistaxis can be chronic or acute. The primary principle of treatment is to nourish *yin*, disperse heat, cool blood and check bleeding.

(1) Heat in the lung

Clinical manifestations: Dryness and bleeding of the nose, dry mouth and throat, or fever and cough with scanty sputum, a red tongue with thin coating, and a rapid pulse.

Analysis: The lung opens into the nose. Attack of the lung by wind-heat or retention of heat in the lung allows pathogenic factors to move upward and causes dryness and bleeding of the nose. Attack of the lung by wind-heat also impairs the lung's dispersive function, resulting in fever and cough with scanty sputum. Dry mouth, a red tongue and a rapid pulse are signs of consumption of body fluids by heat.

Treatment: To disperse heat in the lung, cool blood and check bleeding.

Prescription: Decoction of Mori and Chrysanthemi (257) is the main one, which disperses heat in the lung. To cool blood and check bleeding, Cortex Moutan, Rhizoma Imperatae and Herba Ecliptae are added. If heat in the lung is excessive without exterior syndrome (e.g., fever), Herba Menthae and Radix Platycodi are removed from the prescription and Radix Scutellariae and Fructus Gardeniae are added to disperse heat in the lung.

If bleeding in the nose is caused by fire of the deficiency type due to deficiency of lung *yin*, with symptoms of restlessness, a hot sensation in the palms, soles and chest, scanty and sticky sputum and a red tongue, drugs that nourish *yin* and disperse heat in the lung, such as Radix Rehmanniae, Radix Ophiopogonis, Radix Scrophulariae and Radix Adenophorae, should be added.

(2) Heat in the stomach

Clinical manifestations: Bleeding in the nose or gums with bright red blood, thirst, stuffiness in the chest, foul breath, constipation, a red tongue with yellow coating, and a rapid pulse.

Analysis: The Stomach Meridian of Foot-*Yangming* originates in the nose and enters the upper gums, while the Large Intestine Meridian of Hand-*Yangming* passes by the nostril and enters the lower gums. Eating too much pungent and hot food leads to hyperactive fire-heat in the *Yangming* Meridians, which causes blood extravasation and subsequent bleeding in the nose and gums with bright red blood. Consumption of body fluids by stomach heat causes thirst and constipation. Upward flaring of stomach fire causes stuffiness in the chest and foul breath. A red tongue with yellow coating and a rapid pulse are signs of excessive heat in the stomach.

Treatment: To disperse heat and fire in the stomach, cool blood and check bleeding.

Prescription: Modified Jade Maid Decoction (71). In this prescription, Gypsum Fibrosum disperses heat in the stomach; Radix Ophiopogonis and Rhizoma Anemarrhenae nourish *yin* and disperse heat; Radix Rehmanniae cools blood and checks bleeding; and Radix Achyranthis Bidentatae conducts blood downward. To disperse heat and cool blood, Fructus Gardeniae and Cortex Moutan are added. In cases with constipation, Radix et Rhizoma Rhei is added to disperse heat in the intestines. In cases with thirst, Radix Trichosanthis, Rhizoma Imperatae and Herba Dendrobii are added to nourish *yin* and produce body fluids.

(3) Liver fire

Clinical manifestations: Bleeding in the nose or eyes, headache, dizziness, red eyes, irritability, restlessness, dry mouth with bitter taste, deep yellow urine, constipation, a red tongue with thin, sticky and yellow coating, and a taut and rapid or smooth and rapid pulse.

Analysis: Mental depression may cause liver *qi*-stagnation, which turns into fire in prolonged cases; if liver fire is constitutionally excessive, it disturbs the upper part of the body, forcing blood to run upward, resulting in bleeding in the nose or eyes. Disturbance of the upper orifices by hyperactive liver *yang* leads to headache, dizziness and red eyes. Hyperactivity of liver *qi* causes irritability and restlessness. A bitter taste in the mouth, thirst, deep yellow urine and constipation are all caused by hyperactivity of liver fire. A red tongue with thin, yellow and sticky coating, and a taut and rapid or smooth and rapid pulse are all the result of excessive liver fire in the interior.

Treatment: To disperse heat in the liver, reduce fire, cool blood and check bleeding.

Prescription: Modified Decoction of Gentianae for Purging Liver-Fire (78). In the prescription, Radix Gentianae disperses fire in the liver; Fructus Gardeniae and Radix Scutellariae, bitter and cold in nature, disperse heat and reduce fire; Radix Rehmanniae and Radix Angelicae Sinensis nourish liver blood, protecting healthy *qi* while eliminating pathogenic factors; Radix Bupleuri eases liver *qi*; Semen Plantaginis, Rhizoma Alismatis and Caulis Aristolochiae Manshuriensis disperse heat through urination; and Radix Achyranthis Bidentatae conducts heat downward. In cases of liver *yin*-deficiency, this prescription is combined with *Yiguan* Decoction (1).

Bleeding in the gums due to the fire caused by hepatic and renal *yin*-deficiency presents bleeding of light red blood, loose teeth, atrophy of gums, sore and weak the lumbus and knees, dizziness, tinnitus and lassitude. Decoction for Nourishing Fluid and Clearing Away Liver-Heat (303) and Powder of Rubiae (201) are prescribed together. The former drug emphasizes on nourishing *yin* and dispersing fire with Pill of Six Drugs Containing Rehmanniae Preparata (56) nourishing *yin* and reducing fire, and Radix Bupleuri, Cortex Moutan and Fructus Gardeniae dispersing liver fire. The latter prescription focuses on cooling blood and checking bleeding; Radix Rehmanniae Preparata, Radix Rubiae, Cacumen Platycladi and Colla Corii Asini cool blood and check bleeding, while Radix Glycyrrhizae disperses heat and regulates the middle *jiao*. This prescription can also be used in the treatment of bleeding in the ears.

(4) Pathogenic heat

Clinical manifestations: Bleeding in the nose, tongue, gums, eyes and pores, fever, restlessness, irritability, headache, or loss of consciousness and delirium in severe cases, a rapid pulse, and a crimson tongue with thorn-like coating.

Analysis: Excessive heat inside the body causes reckless blood movement and subsequent bleeding in the nose, tongue, gums, eyes and sweat pores. Attack of the pericardium by heat leads to restlessness, irritability, loss of consciousness and delirium. A rapid pulse and a crimson and thorny tongue indicate consumption of *yin* by excessive heat.

Treatment: To disperse heat in the *ying* system, eliminate toxins and protect *yin*.

Prescription: Decoction for Clearing Away Heat in the *Ying* System (283) is the main prescription. Here, Cornu Rhinocerotis and Radix Salviae Miltiorrhizae disperse heat in the *ying* system and eliminate toxins; Radix Rehmanniae, Radix Scutellariae and Radix Ophiopogonis nourish *yin* and disperse heat; and Herba Lophatheri, Flos Lonicerae, Fructus Forsythiae and Rhizoma Coptidis disperse heat and eliminate toxins. In cases with loss of consciousness and delirium, Bolus of Calculus Bovis for Resurrection (127) or Pill of Precious Drugs (124) is added to disperse heat and restore consciousness.

(5) Deficiency of *qi* and blood

Clinical manifestations: Bleeding in the nose or gums, or pores in severe cases, pale complexion, lassitude, dizziness, tinnitus, palpitation, insomnia, a pale tongue, and a thready and weak pulse.

Analysis: Deficiency of *qi* and blood means failure of *qi* to control blood which causes bleeding. Blood deficiency explains pale complexion, dizziness and palpitation. A pale tongue and a thready and weak pulse are signs of *qi* and blood deficiency.

Treatment: To replenish *qi* to control blood.

Prescription: Powerful Tonic Decoction of Ten Drugs (5) or Decoction for Invigorating Spleen and Nourishing Heart (110); both are *qi* and blood tonics. The former warmly replenishes *qi* and blood, while the latter replenishes *qi* and blood by invigorating the spleen and nourishing the heart.

Deficiency of *qi* and blood is often complicated by *yang* deficiency, *yin* deficiency, or deficiency of both *yin* and *yang*; deficiency of *yin* or *yang* can also be mixed with deficiency of *qi* and blood. Therefore, it is necessary to add *yin* or *yang* tonics in nourishing *qi* and blood. In cases of *yin* deficiency, Colla Corii Asini and Radix Polygoni Multiflori are added. In cases of *yang* deficiency, Cornu Cervi, Placenta Hominis and Herba Cistanches are added. Drugs that check bleeding include Radix Sanguisorbae, Pollen Typhae and Herba Agrimoniae.

3. Hematemesis

Hematemesis refers to bleeding in the esophagus and stomach, with blood passing through the mouth. Blood can also be brought up by vomiting while dark purple blood is mixed with food residue. In ancient times, the term "spitting of blood" was used to refer to bleeding in both respiratory and upper digestive tracts. Since the Jin and Sui dynasties, hematemesis and hemoptysis have been separated in discussion.

Hematemesis often results from the accumulated heat in the stomach, or stagnant liver *qi* that turns into heat, attacking the stomach and damaging *yang* vessels, or strain and stress, which damage stomach *qi* and prevent it from controlling blood, resulting in hematemesis and hemafecia simultaneously, or long-standing alcoholic drinking, which impairs the liver's ability to store blood. Attention should be paid to the conditions of the liver, stomach and spleen in differentiating hematemesis. Methods of treatment include conducting the unhealthy *qi* downward, dispersing fire, easing the liver, warming the middle *jiao* and promoting the circulation of blood. Three principles of treatment are described in the Ming Dynasty *Extensive Notes on Medicine*. The first is "to circulate blood instead of checking bleeding," because no blood stasis will form when blood circulates smoothly. The second is "to nourish the liver instead of reducing hyperactivity of the liver." If the liver is treated with the reducing method, it will become even more deficient, and its ability in storing blood will be further impaired. Nourishing the liver will ease liver *qi* and invite blood to return to the liver. The third is "to conduct the unhealthy *qi* downward instead of driving the fire downward." Surplus *qi* is fire, thus when *qi* descends, fire will reduce, and the blood will follow *qi* to run downward. These three principles may provide reference in clinical work.

(1) Accumulation of heat in the stomach

Clinical manifestations: Distress and distention in the epigastrium and abdomen, with pain in severe cases, hematemesis with bright red or dark purple blood, or food residue, foul breath, constipation or black stool, a red tongue with yellow and sticky coating, and a smooth and rapid pulse.

Analysis: Either excessive alcohol or overeating pungent and hot food produces heat in the stomach, which impairs the stomach's descending function, resulting in dyspepsia. This explains distress and distention in the epigastrium and abdomen, with pain in severe cases. Damage to the vessels of the stomach by heat leads to hematemesis with bright red or dark purple blood if blood stasis is formed. The stool becomes tarry if bleeding follows defecation. Dyspepsia causes vomiting of food residue. A red tongue with yellow and sticky coating and a smooth and rapid pulse are signs of accumulated heat in the stomach.

Treatment: To disperse heat in the stomach, reduce fire, remove blood stasis and check bleeding.

Prescription: Decoction for Purging Stomach-Fire (173) combined with Powder of Ten Drugs' Ashes (6). In the former, Radix et Rhizoma Rhei, Radix Scutellariae and Rhizoma Coptidis, bitter and cold in nature, disperse heat in the stomach and reduce fire. In the latter, Herba seu Radix Cirsii Japanici,

Herba Cirsii, Radix Rubiae, Cacumen Platycladi, Rhizoma Imperatae and Fructus Gardeniae cool blood and check bleeding; Vagina Trachycarpi checks bleeding; Cortex Moutan cools blood and removes blood stasis; and Folium Nelumbinis removes blood stasis and checks bleeding. Radix et Rhizoma Rhei is the key drug in the prescription for treatment of hematemesis due to excessive heat in the stomach.

(2) Attack of the stomach by liver fire

Clinical manifestations: Hematemesis with bright red or purplish blood, a bitter taste in the mouth, hypochondriac pain, irritability, insomnia with dream-disturbed sleep, restlessness, a crimson tongue, and a taut and rapid pulse.

Analysis: Excessive anger damages the liver and produces liver fire, which invades the stomach, damaging its vessels and causing hematemesis with bright red or purplish blood. Upward disturbance of liver and gallbladder fire leads to a bitter taste in the mouth, hypochondriac pain and irritability. Disturbance of the heart by liver fire results in restlessness and insomnia with dream-disturbed sleep. A crimson tongue and a taut and rapid pulse indicate consumption of *yin* fluid by liver fire.

Treatment: To reduce liver fire and disperse stomach heat.

Prescription: Modified Decoction of Gentianae for Purging Liver-Fire (78). Here, Radix Gentianae reduces excessive liver and gallbladder fire; Radix Scutellariae and Fructus Gardeniae, bitter and cold in nature, reduce fire and check bleeding; and Cortex Moutan and Radix Rehmanniae cool blood and check bleeding. Drugs that cool blood and check bleeding, such as Rhizoma Imperatae, Nodus Nelumbinis Rhizomatis and Herba Ecliptae, are added. Persistent hematemesis accompanied by fullness and distention in the chest and epigastrium, along with dry mouth with no desire to drink suggests blood stagnation, for which Powder of Ophicalcitum (166) and Powder of Radix Notoginseng are prescribed together to remove blood stasis and check bleeding. In cases of liver *yin*-deficiency, drugs that nourish the liver, such as Fructus Lycii, Fructus Ligustri Lucidi and Radix Paeoniae Alba, are added.

(3) Cold of deficiency type in the spleen and stomach

Clinical manifestations: Hematemesis, which is bright pinkish, pain in the epigastrium aggravated by cold and alleviated by warmth and pressure, pale complexion, poor appetite, cold limbs, a thin and white tongue coating, and a deep and thready pulse.

Analysis: Deficiency of the spleen leads to the impaired ability to control blood, and cold in the stomach leads to upward disturbance of stomach *qi*. In such cases, blood follows the unhealthy *qi*, causing hematemesis, which is bright pinkish. Deficiency of *yang* of the middle *jiao* causes pain in the epigastrium which is aggravated by cold and alleviated by warmth. Pale complexion, poor appetite, cold limbs, a thin and white tongue coating or a pale tongue, and a deep and thready pulse are syndromes of cold deficiency of the spleen and stomach.

Treatment: To warm the middle *jiao*, pacify the stomach, conduct the unhealthy *qi* downward and check bleeding.

Prescription: Decoction of Aconiti Lateralis Preparata for Regulating Middle *Jiao* (163) combined with Decoction of Cacumen Platycladi (195). In this prescription, Radix Aconiti Lateralis Preparata and Rhizoma Zingiberis warm the middle *jiao* and benefit *yang*; Radix Ginseng and Rhizoma Atractylodis Macrocephalae invigorate the spleen and replenish *qi*; and Cacumen Platycladi and Folium Artemisiae Argyi warm the middle *jiao* and check bleeding. To nourish blood and check bleeding, Colla Corii Asini are added. In cases of unhealthy stomach *qi* with persistent belching, Flos Inulae and Haematitum are added to conduct the unhealthy *qi* downward, and Rhizoma Pinelliae and Pericarpium Citri Reticulatae are added to pacify the stomach.

If hematemesis is severe, treatment should focus on dispersing heat and cooling blood. Decoction of Cornu Rhinocerotis and Rehmanniae (306) added with Powder of Radix Notoginseng is prescribed. If signs of prostration follow, such as pale complexion, cold limbs, sweating and feeble pulse, Decoction of Ginseng (218) should be administered without delay to replenish *qi* and prevent collapse. If hematemesis does not respond to drugs that cool the blood, it indicates that the fire of the deficiency type has run upward. Decoction of Cacumen Platycladi (195) is then prescribed to conduct the unhealthy *qi* downward and check bleeding. This prescription includes warm and cold drugs, and can be administered together with Powder of Ten Drugs' Ashes (6). If fire is caused by the *yin* deficiency, and there are symptoms of thirst with desire to drink, restlessness, a red tongue and a thready and rapid pulse, Jade Maid Decoction (71) is then recommended, which nourishes *yin* and reduces fire.

The patient should keep calm and lie in bed quietly at the moment of hematemesis. In addition to taking the drugs, the patient must pay attention to diet, avoiding voracious eating or overeating hot and pungent food. Food which can be easily digested is recommended. The patient should also maintain emotional stability and a proper lifestyle.

4. Hemafecia

Hemafecia refers to blood being produced together with stool, which occurs before or after bowel motion, or only blood being discharged. According to *A Complete Collection of Jingyue's Treatise*, "Bleeding before bowel motion comes from areas such as the rectum and the anus, while bleeding soon after bowel motion comes from more distant areas, such as the small intestines and stomach." At present, doctors determine where bleeding comes from according to the color of the blood. Generally, bright red blood in the stool comes from the rectum and anus, dark purplish blood from the large and small intestines, and tarry blood from the stomach.

Blood color also helps to differentiate syndromes. For instance, bright red blood in the stool suggests heat, dark purplish blood suggests stagnation, and tarry blood suggests deficiency. The basic principle of treatment for hematemesis is to invigorate the spleen, replenish *qi*, disperse heat and resolve dampness.

(1) Cold of deficiency type in the spleen and stomach

Clinical manifestations: Dark purplish blood in the stool or tarry blood in severe cases, dull abdominal pain, preference for warm drinks, pale complexion, lassitude, dislike of speaking, loose stool, a pale tongue, and a thready pulse.

Analysis: Cold of deficiency type in the spleen and stomach implies the spleen's inability to control blood, which causes blood extravasation in the intestinal tract and bloody stool. Cold of deficiency type in the middle *jiao* deprives the stomach and intestines of warmth, thereby hindering *qi* circulation. This explains dull abdominal pain, preference for warm drinks and loose stool. Pale complexion, lassitude, dislike of speaking, a pale tongue and a thready pulse are signs of *qi* and blood deficiency following weak spleen *yang*.

Treatment: To warm the spleen and control blood.

Prescription: Modified Decoction of Terra Flava Usta (259). Here, Terra Flava Usta warms the spleen and checks bleeding; Radix Aconiti Lateralis Preparata and Rhizoma Atractylodis Macrocephalae warm *yang* and invigorate the spleen; Radix Rehmanniae and Colla Corii Asini nourish *yin* and blood; Radix Scutellariae, bitter and cold in nature, consolidates *yin* and prevents acrid and warm drugs in the prescription from consuming and disturbing the blood; and Radix Glycyrrhizae harmonizes the middle *jiao*. Rhizoma Zingiberis (charred) is added to provide warmth and check bleeding. Powder of Rhizoma Bletillae is also added to check bleeding. When bleeding ceases, Decoction for Strengthening Middle *Jiao* and Benefiting *Qi* (154) is administered to strengthen the *qi* of the middle *jiao*; or Decoction for Invigorating Spleen and Nourishing Heart (110) is prescribed to treat both the heart and spleen.

(2) Accumulation of heat in the stomach and intestines

Clinical manifestations: Dark purplish or purplish-red blood in the stool, a burning pain in the epigastrium or abdomen, dry mouth with a bitter taste, preference for cold drinks, foul breath, restlessness, a red tongue with yellow coating and little moisture, and a taut and thready or thready and rapid pulse.

Analysis: Prolonged accumulation of heat in the stomach and intestines turns into fire, which damages blood vessels and causes bloody stool. This also leads to retarded circulation of *qi*, causing a burning pain in the epigastrium and abdomen. Excessive interior heat consumes body fluids, which causes dry mouth with a bitter taste, along with preference for cold drinks. Foul breath and restlessness are consequences of accumulation of heat in the stomach and intestines. A red tongue with yellow coating and little moisture and a taut and thready pulse or thready and rapid pulse are signs of fluid consumption by heat.

Treatment: To disperse heat, reduce fire, cool blood and check bleeding.

Prescription: Powder for Clearing Away Stomach-Heat (281) combined with Powder of Sophorae (314). In this prescription, Rhizoma Coptidis, bitter and cold in nature, reduces fire; Radix Rehmanniae and Cortex Moutan disperse heat, cool the blood and check bleeding; Radix Angelicae Sinensis nourishes and regulates the blood, and also checks bleeding; Rhizoma Cimicifugae clears away stomach fire and cools heat in the blood; Flos Sophorae and Cacumen Platycladi disperse heat in the intestines and check bleeding; Herba Schizonepetae regulates *qi* and eliminates wind; and Fructus Aurantii promotes the circulation of *qi*.

If *yin* deficiency is more pronounced than hyperactivity of fire, Decoction of Coptidis and Colla Corii Asini (261) is prescribed to nourish *yin* and reduce fire. Here, Rhizoma Coptidis and Radix Scutellariae, bitter and cold in nature, reduce fire; and Colla Corii Asini and Radix Paeoniae Alba nourish *yin*, replenish blood and check bleeding. Drugs that disperse heat and cool blood, such as Radix Sanguisorbae, Radix Rehmanniae and Cortex Moutan, can also be added.

(3) Downward movement of dampness-heat

Clinical manifestations: Bright red blood in the stool, bleeding before bowel movement, unsmooth discharge of feces, a bitter taste in the mouth, a yellow and sticky tongue coating, and a soft and rapid pulse.

Analysis: Excessive alcohol drinking or eating too much hot and pungent food produces dampness-heat, which then goes downward to the large intestine, damaging the blood vessels and causing bright red blood in the stool or bleeding before bowel movement. Retention of dampness-heat in the large intestine impairs its transmission function and results in unsmooth discharge of feces. A bitter taste in the mouth, a yellow and sticky tongue coating and a soft and rapid pulse are signs of retention of dampness-heat in the interior.

Treatment: To disperse heat, eliminate dampness, regulate *ying* and check bleeding.

Prescription: Powder of Phaseoli and Angelicae Sinensis (164) combined with Powder of Sanguisorbae (119). Radix Scutellariae, Rhizoma Coptidis and Fructus Gardeniae disperse heat; Poria and Semen Phaseoli discharge dampness and eliminate toxins; and Radix Sanguisorbae, Radix Rubiae and Radix Angelicae Sinensis check bleeding and nourish the blood.

If *ying* and *yin* have become deficient due to the excessive bleeding, but dampness-heat still remains, *Zhuju* Pill (187) is prescribed to regulate *ying*, disperse heat, and treat both deficiency and excess simultaneously.

5. Hematuria

Hematuria refers to abnormal presence of blood in the urine, which can be found by the naked eyes, or by laboratory examination. Generally, hematuria does not produce pain, although a mild distensive pain or burning pain is occasionally present. Simple hematuria is therefore different from stranguria with hematuria, which is characterized by unbearable pain and dribbling urination.

Hematuria is often caused by retention of heat in the kidneys and urinary bladder. Cardiac and hepatic fire can also move downward to the urinary bladder. Splenic and renal deficiency implies weakness in controlling blood, which is another cause of hematuria. Hematuria of the excess type is caused by excessive heat and marked by an abrupt onset with bright red blood in the urine and a hot sensation in the urethra. The deficiency type often occurs in a protracted illness with pinkish blood in the urine but without the hot sensation. If bleeding comes from the kidneys, a distant place, the color of the urine is red and well-distributed. If it comes from the urinary bladder, a nearby place, the urine is bright red in color, and bleeding often follows urination. If it comes from the urethra, the urine is also bright red in color with bleeding preceding the urination. Treatment aims to disperse heat, reduce fire, nourish *yin*, check bleeding and invigorate the spleen and kidneys.

(1) Dampness-heat in the lower *jiao*

Clinical manifestations: Abrupt onset of hematuria, a hot sensation in the urethra during urination, increased frequency of urination with bright red urine, fever and chilliness, a thin or yellow and sticky tongue coating, and a smooth and rapid or a thready and rapid pulse.

Analysis: Retention of dampness-heat in the kidneys and urinary bladder damages the blood vessels, causing hematuria. Heat produces reckless blood movement, which causes bright red blood in the urine. Dampness-heat causes a hot sensation in the urethra during urination; if the patient has contracted the external dampness-heat, which penetrates into the kidneys and urinary bladder, fever and chilliness will occur. A thin, yellow and sticky tongue coating, a smooth and rapid, or thready and rapid pulse are signs of retention of dampness-heat.

Treatment: To disperse heat, eliminate dampness, cool blood and check bleeding.

Prescription: Modified Powder for Dispersing Heat and Promoting Urination (12). In the prescription, Herba Dianthi and Herba Polygoni Avicularis disperse heat and eliminate dampness; Semen Plantaginis, Talcum, Caulis Aristolochiae Manshuriensis and Radix Glycyrrhizae disperse heat, promote diuresis and resolve dampness; and Fructus Gardeniae and Radix et Rhizoma Rhei disperse heat and reduce fire. Drugs that cool blood and check bleeding, such as Herba Cirsii, Herba Agrimoniae and Pollen Typhae are added. If exterior syndrome is present, Semen Sojae Preparatum, Herba Schizonepetae and Herba Menthae are added.

(2) Deficiency of *yin* and hyperactivity of fire

Clinical manifestations: Scanty deep yellow urine tinged with blood, dizziness, blurring of vision, tinnitus, lassitude, malar flush, hectic fever, soreness and weakness in the lumbar region and knees, a red tongue, and a thready and rapid pulse.

Analysis: Hyperactive fire due to *yin* deficiency damages the blood vessels and results in scanty deep yellow urine tinged with blood. *Yin* deficiency leads to hyperactivity of *yang*, which then disturbs the upper orifices and causes dizziness, blurring of vision, malar flush and hectic fever. Since the kidneys dominate the bones, open into the ears and reside in the lumbar region, renal deficiency will produce soreness and weakness in the lumbar region and knees, lassitude and tinnitus. A red tongue and a thready and rapid pulse are signs of hyperactivity of fire due to *yin* deficiency.

Treatment: To nourish *yin*, reduce fire, cool blood and check bleeding.

Prescription: Modified Bolus of Anemarrhenae, Phellodendri and Rehmanniae Preparata (181). In the prescription, Radix Rehmanniae Preparata, Fructus Corni and Rhizoma Dioscoreae replenish kidney *yin*; Rhizoma Anemarrhenae and Cortex Phellodendri disperse heat and reduce fire; and Cortex Moutan disperses heat and cools the blood. To cool the blood and check bleeding, Herba seu Radix Cirsii Japonici, Herba Cirsii, Nodus Nelumbinis Rhizomatis and Herba Ecliptae are added.

If renal *yin*-deficiency fails to control fire, giving rise to ministerial fire, and manifesting symptoms of hectic fever and night sweating, the prescription will be based on Pill for Replenishing *Yin* (22) to nourish *yin* and reduce fire.

(3) Hyperactivity of heart fire

Clinical manifestations: A hot sensation during urination with bright red blood, restlessness, thirst, flushed face, aphthae, insomnia, a red tongue tip, and a rapid pulse.

Analysis: Strain and stress consume heart *yin* and cause hyperactivity of cardiac heart fire. Symptoms include restlessness, thirst, flushed face and aphthae. Downward movement of heart fire to the small intestine damages the blood vessels, causing a hot sensation during urination, and urine with bright red blood. Disturbance of the heart by fire gives rise to insomnia. A red tongue tip and a rapid pulse are both signs of hyperactive heart fire.

Treatment: To disperse heat in the heart, reduce fire, cool blood and check bleeding.

Prescription: Modified Decoction of Cirsii (38). Herba Cirsii, Radix Rehmanniae, Pollen Typhae and Nodus Nelumbinis Rhizomatis cool the blood and check bleeding; Caulis Aristolochiae Manshuriensis, Herba Lophatheri and Fructus Gardeniae disperse heat and reduce fire; Talcum promotes diuresis, disperses heat and conducts heat downward; Radix Angelicae Sinensis nourishes blood; and Radix Glycyrrhizae coordinates the effects of all drugs in the prescription. To check bleeding and remove blood stasis, Succinum is added.

(4) Splenic and renal deficiency

Clinical manifestations: Frequent urination with pinkish blood in the urine, poor appetite, lassitude, sallow complexion, soreness in the lumbar region, dizziness, tinnitus, a pale tongue, and a weak and feeble pulse.

Analysis: Strain and stress or prolonged illness damages the spleen and kidneys, and gives rise to a collapse of *qi* of the middle *jiao*. Splenic deficiency means the inability to control blood, and renal deficiency results in ill controlling of urination. This explains frequent urination with pinkish blood in the urine. Impaired splenic function in transportation and transformation results in *qi* and blood deficiency. The consequences are poor appetite, lassitude and sallow complexion. Deficiency of kidney essence is the cause of soreness in the lumbar region, dizziness and tinnitus. A pale tongue and weak and feeble pulse are both signs of splenic and renal deficiency.

Treatment: To invigorate the spleen, replenish *qi*, strengthen the kidneys and promote astringency.

Prescription: Decoction for Strengthening Middle *Jiao* and Benefiting *Qi* (154) combined with Pill of Dioscoreae for Nourishing Kidney (41). The former strengthens the spleen to control blood, and the latter fortifies the kidneys to control urination. In this prescription, Radix Rehmanniae Preparata, Rhizoma Dioscoreae and Fructus Corni nourish kidney *yin*; Herba Cistanches, Semen Cuscutae, Cortex Eucommiae and Radix Morindae Officinalis warm and replenish kidney *yang*; and Halloysitum Rubrum promotes astringency. In chronic cases, Concha Ostreae Usta, Os Draconis Ustum and Fructus Rosae Laevigatae are added to strengthen the effect of checking bleeding.

Remarks

Bleeding in the same area of the body may result from disorders of different *zang-fu* organs, and disorders of the same organ may cause bleeding in different areas. *Treatise on Cold Diseases* introduces the treatment of hemorrhagic syndrome by saying, "In the treatment of epistaxis, the method of inducing perspiration should not be adopted" and "it should also be avoided in cases with severe loss of blood." This is because sweat is transformed from body fluid which is an important part of blood. Since hemorrhagic patients lack body fluid, if the method of inducing perspiration is adopted, it would further consume the body fluid, resulting in fluid and blood exhaustion.

Excessive bleeding often results in primordial *qi* deficiency with symptoms of pale complexion and a hollow pulse. Generally, bleeding with a thready, weak and slow pulse is easier to deal with than bleeding with a rapid, large and taut pulse.

Case Studies

Name: Shao XX; Sex: Male; Age: 33.

First visit: Attack of the lung by dryness and fire, which induced persistent cough, damaged the blood vessels and resulted in hemoptysis with mouthfuls of blood. Other symptoms were sore throat, hoarse voice, lassitude, a dry and crimson tongue and a thready and rapid pulse. Treatment aimed to nourish *yin* and moisten the lung. The patient was asked to rest well, and the following drugs were prescribed:

Folium Mahoniae	9 g;
Cortex Moutan	4.5 g;
Radix Adenophorae	9 g;
Bulbus Fritillariae Cirrhosae	9 g;
Radix Curcumae	4.5 g;
Haematitum	15 g;
Radix Tinosporae	4.5 g;
Cortex Eucommiae	12 g;
Semen Armeniacae Amarum	9 g;
Concha Meretricis seu Cyclinae	15 g;
Fructus Chebulae	4.5 g;
Bulbus Lilii	4.5 g.

Second visit: Both cough and sore throat improved, hemoptysis ceased, but hoarse voice remained unchanged, and the pulse was still thready, rapid and weak. Since the disease responded to the first treatment, the same method was adopted with emphasis on nourishing:

Radix Adenophorae	9 g;
Bulbus Fritillariae Cirrhosae	9 g;
Radix Asparagi	6 g;
Radix Ophiopogonis	6 g;
Cortex Moutan	6 g;
Fructus Chebulae	4.5 g;
Cortex Eucommiae	12 g;
Semen Benincasae	15 g;
Bulbus Lilii	6 g;
Semen Armeniacae Amarum	9 g;
Concha Meretricis seu Cyclinae (powder)	6 g;
Fructus Aristolochiae Preparata	6 g;
Herba Ecliptae	9 g.

Explanation: Prolonged cough with hemoptysis was due to the damage of *yang* vessels following the dryness of the lung. Radix Adenophorae, Concha Meretricis seu Cyclinae and Bulbus Fritillariae Cirrhosae nourish *yin* and moisten the lung; Bulbus Lilii, Cortex Moutan and Folium Mahoniae disperse heat and cool blood; Haematitum conducts the unhealthy *qi* downward; Fructus Chebulae consolidates lung *qi*; Cortex Eucommiae fortifies the kidneys; and Radix Curcumae activates *qi* and blood circulation. After these drugs were taken, cough improved and hemoptysis ceased, but the pulse was still thready and rapid. This suggested the deficiency of lung *yin*, therefore Decoction of Colla Corii Asini for Invigorating Lung (153) was prescribed again.

Name: Shi XX; Sex: Female; Age: 30.

First visit: Attack by the external wind-heat caused headache, fever, cough with difficulty in expectoration, dry throat and mouth. In the morning, epistaxis with profuse bright red blood occurred. The pulse was superficial and rapid, and the tongue red with yellow coating. The disease was due to heat retention in the lung. Treatment aimed to disperse heat in the lung by prescribing the following herbs:

Folium Mori	9 g;
Semen Armeniacae Amarum	9 g;
Folium Menthae (decocted later)	3 g;
Fructus Forsythiae	9 g;
Fructus Gardeniae	9 g;
Flos Chrysanthemi	4.5 g;
Rhizoma Phragmitis (fresh with nodes removed)	1/3 meter;
Radix Scutellariae	4.5 g;
Radix Peucedani Preparata	6 g;
Rhizoma Imperatae	15 g;
Bulbus Fritillariae Thunbergii	9 g.

Second visit: She took the above drugs on the previous day. Fever subsided, epistaxis ceased, and both headache and thirst disappeared. Cough remained unchanged, however, the pulse was taut and smooth, and the tongue coating was thin and yellow. Treatment aimed to disperse heat from the *qi* system and promote the lung's dispersive function with the following prescription:

Folium Mori	9 g;
Semen Armeniacae Amarum	9 g;
Caulis Bambusae in Taeniam	9 g;
Bulbus Fritillariae Cirrhosae	4.5 g;
Flos Chrysanthemi	6 g;
Radix Scutellariae	4.5 g;
Pericarpium Trichosanthis	12 g;
Radix Peucedani Preparata	6 g;
Semen Benincasae	12 g;
Rhizoma Phragmitis (fresh with nodes removed)	1/3 meter;
Folium Eriobotryae Preparata	9 g.

Discussion: The skin and hair are dominated by the lung. If wind-heat cannot be eliminated from the exterior of the body, it accumulates in the lung, which could only be dispersed through epistaxis; hence epistaxis is also referred to as red sweat. The treatment for this is to disperse heat from the lung. When wind-heat is dispersed and fever subsides, epistaxis will cease spontaneously.

Name: Duan XX; Sex: Male; Age: 28; Date: October 1, 1960.

The patient had a history of gastric ulcers with hemorrhage. The occult blood test of stool 20 days earlier was positive. He felt fatigued recently due to overwork. He was caught in a heavy rain two days earlier. To warm up, he drank a cup of grape wine, which caused sudden hematemesis. He was thus sent to the hospital, where a diagnosis of gastric bleeding was established. But hematemesis continued in spite of treatment during hospitalization. For fear that he might suffer gastric perforation, the decision of operation was made, but his family members oppose the idea. They came to Dr. Pu Fuzhou at midnight, asking for a prescription. Dr. Pu said that although hematemesis continued for two days, oral administration of Chinese herbal medicine could still help if there was no perforation of the stomach. Considering the fact that bleeding was caused by drinking grape wine following the exposure to cold, it is not advisable to cool the blood and check bleeding. Decoction of Cacumen Platycladi (195) was prescribed instead to warm spleen *yang*, remove blood stasis and check bleeding. The prescription consisted of 9 grams of Cacumen Platycladi, 6 grams of Rhizoma Zingiberis Preparata, and 6 grams of Folium Artemisiae Argyi. They were made into a highly concentrated decoction, which was then mixed with 60ml. of children's urine to be taken bit by bit at short intervals.

Dr. Pu visited the patient the next morning, and found that hematemesis had started improving. The pulse was deep, thready and unsmooth, and the tongue pale without coating. He then added 12 grams of Radix Panacis Quinquefolii to the previous prescription to replenish *qi* and control the blood, and six grams of Radix Notoginseng (powder) to be taken separately for removing blood stasis and checking bleeding. It was also taken bit by bit at short intervals.

The next morning, hematemesis ceased, and the patient wanted to sleep and began to feel hungry. Flatus occurred. The pulse was feeble at *cun* position, and deep and weak at *guan* and *chi* positions on both sides. The tongue was still pale without coating. However, the prognosis was good, because the pulse agreed with the symptoms following severe bleeding. Treatment aimed primarily to warm spleen *yang* and nourish the blood, and remove blood stasis secondarily. Decoction for Regulating Middle *Jiao* (258) added with Radix Angelicae Sinensis, Radix Paeoniae Alba and Radix Notoginseng was then prescribed.

The patient developed dizziness and tinnitus after taking these herbs, and the pulse became thready and rapid. This was caused by an upward disturbance of heat of the deficiency type. Added to the prescription were 6 grams of Cortex Lycii and 9 grams of Nodus Nelumbinis Rhizomatis. All the drugs were made into a highly concentrated decoction, mixed with 60ml. of children's urine, and were taken bit by bit at short intervals.

When the doctor visited him again, all the chief symptoms had disappeared, the pulse was smooth and appetite also improved. But the patient only had flatus without bowel movement. Consequently, the primary aim of treatment was to replenish *qi* and blood, nourish *yin* and moisten dryness, and secondarily to remove blood stasis. The prescription consisted of the following herbs:

Radix Ginseng	9 g;
Semen Platycladi	6 g;
Herba Cistanches	12 g;
Fructus Cannabis	12 g;
Radix Angelicae Sinensis	6 g;
Nodus Nelumbinis Rhizomatis	15 g;
Pericarpium Citri Reticulatae	3 g;
Fructus Crataegi	3 g.

A highly concentrated decoction was made of these drugs, together with 12 grams of Colla Corii Asini and 60ml. of children's urine, and was taken warm, 1/4 of the total each time.

After taking the decoction, the bowel began to move, and both appetite and sleep became normal. The occult blood test of stool turned negative. The patient was then advised to stop taking medicine, and eat nutritious food to help restore health.

Explanation: Since the patient had a history of stomach ulcers, he did not drink alcohol all the time. This time, he drank grape wine after exposing to cold, causing cold and heat to attack the stomach.

Since hematemesis was not caused by extreme heat, treatment aimed to warm spleen *yang* and send the unhealthy *qi* downward by prescribing Decoction of Cacumen Platycladi (195). In the prescription, Cacumen Platycladi, light in weight and fragrant and sweet in nature, disperses heat and checks bleeding; Rhizoma Zingiberis Preparata, Folium Artemisiae Argyi, acrid and warm in nature, and children's urine, salty and cold, are combined to provide warmth, disperse heat, conduct the unhealthy *qi* downward and remove blood stasis at the same time. As a result, the syndromes of bleeding started to improve after treatment.

The addition of Radix Notoginseng and Radix Panacis Quinquefolii in the second prescription replenishes *qi*, removes blood stasis and checks bleeding. Thus hematemesis completely ceased, and no operation was needed.

The aim to warm the spleen *yang*, nourish the blood and remove blood stasis was then accomplished by prescribing Decoction for Regulating Middle *Jiao* (258). Mild dizziness and tinnitus occurred after taking these drugs, which were due to an upward disturbance of deficiency heat. So Cortex Lycii was added to cool the blood without producing stasis; Nodus Nelumbinis Rhizomatis was added to remove vascular obstruction and blood stasis; and children's urine acted to reduce fire. All the symptoms disappeared, the pulse became smooth, and sleep became sound after treatment. Finally, the treatment ended by replenishing *qi* and blood.

Since this case of hematemesis was not caused by reckless blood movement following pathogenic heat, it was not advisable to cool the blood and check bleeding. Erroneous administration of cold and cool drugs would have caused *qi* and blood stagnation, thus making the disease critical.

Name: Miao XX; Sex: Female; Age: 58.

The patient complained of severe bleeding through the anus after bowel movement or without movement at all, 1-2 tea cups of fresh blood each time, 2-3 times a day, for more than 20 days. The other symptoms included a dull pain in the lower abdomen, dizziness, palpitation, shortness of breath, spontaneous sweating, facial puffiness, a deep and rapid pulse, and a slightly pale tongue with no coating. The appetite was moderate. She often had insomnia and painful joints. It had been two years after her menopause.

The disease was due to an accumulation of *yin-qi*, which blocked blood circulation and allowed downward movement of blood to the intestines. Treatment was to warm and nourish the spleen and kidneys by prescribing Decoction of Terra Flava Usta (259) with some modifications:

Radix Rehmanniae Preparata	30 g;
Rhizoma Atractylodis Macrocephalae	9 g;
Radix Glycyrrhizae Preparata	9 g;
Radix Aconiti Lateralis Preparata	9 g;
Radix Scutellariae	6 g;
Colla Corii Asini	15 g;
Cacumen Platycladi	9 g;
Terra Flava Usta	60 g.

Mix Terra Flava Usta with boiling water, let it settle down and take the clear supernatant fluid to decoct with the other ingredients.

Second visit: After two doses, symptoms improved. She had three bowel movements on the previous day, and bleeding occurred only once. She had bleeding again following defecation on the second day. Dizziness, spontaneous sweating and insomnia all disappeared. She still had palpitation, shortness of breath, a tongue with no coating, and a deep and rapid pulse.

Another three doses were prescribed.

Third visit: Very little blood in the stool. Both palpitation and shortness of breath improved. The tongue coating was thin and slightly yellow. The pulse remained unchanged, which was due to the excessive blood loss and damage to *qi* of the middle *jiao*. Treatment aimed to replenish *qi*, nourish *yin* and replenish blood:

Radix Astragali	15 g;
Radix Angelicae Sinensis	6 g;
Radix Rehmanniae	12 g;
Colla Corii Asini	9 g;
Radix Glycyrrhizae	6 g;
Radix Sanguisorbae	6 g;
Cacumen Platycladi (stir-baked)	6 g;
Radix Scutellariae	4.5 g;
Flos Sophorae (stir-baked)	6 g;
Cortex Lycii	6 g.

Five doses were prescribed.

A follow-up visit three months later showed no relapse of bloody stool, and palpitation and shortness of breath had improved.

Explanation: According to *Synopsis of Prescriptions of the Golden Chamber*, if bleeding occurs after bowel movement, blood should have come from distant areas; Decoction of Terra Flava Usta (259) is then prescribed. Terra Flava Usta is warm in nature, therefore when combined with Rhizoma Atractylodis Macrocephalae and Radix Aconiti Lateralis Preparata, it invigorates the spleen and promotes smooth *qi* and blood circulation. Colla Corii Asini, Radix Rehmanniae and Radix Glycyrrhizae nourish the kidneys and replenish blood. To prevent acrid and warm drugs from causing bleeding, Radix Scutellariae is added. Cacumen Platycladi strengthens the hemostatic effect.

X. Palpitation

Being mild or severe, palpitation is a sensation of involuntary bounding or unduly rapid heart beat. It often occurs paroxysmally, induced by emotional fluctuation or stain and stress. Common accompanying symptoms include insomnia, poor memory, dizziness and tinnitus. Palpitation linked with various heart diseases or functional disturbances of the vegetative nervous system in Western medicine can be differentiated and treated according to the following descriptions.

Etiology and Pathogenesis
1. Timidity due to Heart Deficiency

If a constitutionally diffident person is suddenly overwhelmed by fear and fright, uncontrollable palpitation will occur. Anger damages the liver and causes unhealthy *qi*; fright damages the kidneys and consumes essence. In either case, *yin* deficiency in the lower part of the body produces hyperactive fire in the upper part, which then disturbs the heart and gives rise to palpitation. Retention of phlegm-heat in the interior complicated by mental depression or excessive anger may also cause phlegm-fire to disturb the heart and mind, resulting in palpitation.

2. Deficiency of Blood in the Heart

This is often found in patients after a protracted illness with consumption of *yin* blood, or in patients with excessive blood loss, or with impaired splenic function in producing blood due to overthinking or strain and stress. If the heart fails to be nourished, its ability to house the mind will be impaired, and palpitation then occurs.

3. Deficiency of *Yin* and Hyperactivity of Fire

Protracted illnesses, excessive sexual activity, or febrile diseases can all consume *yin*, especially the kidney *yin*. Deficiency of kidney *yin* can also be the result of constitutional weakness. In either case, kidney water will fail to coordinate with fire. The disturbance of the heart by such deficiency fire leads to palpitation.

4. Deficiency of Heart *Yang*

This often follows a severe or protracted illness. Since *yang-qi* is deficient, it is unable to warm and nourish the heart, resulting in palpitation.

5. Attack of the Heart by Retained Fluid

Deficient splenic and renal *yang* fails to transform body fluid, thus the retained fluid moves upward and hinders heart *yang*.

6. Stagnation of Blood in the Heart

Heart *yang*-deficiency implies retarded blood circulation. Palpitation can also be the further development of *bi*-syndrome. When pathogenic wind-cold affects the heart, its vessels are blocked. Retarded blood circulation leads to palpitation.

Differential Diagnosis
Attention should be paid to the similarities and differences between mild and severe palpitation.

The differences between the two lie in the etiological factors and severity of pathological conditions. Severe palpitation is often caused by internal factors and induced by slight exertion. Although it develops gradually, the general condition of the patient is poor, and the symptoms are severe. Mild palpitation is often caused by external factors such as fear, fright and anger. Although the onset is rapid, the general condition of the patient is still good, and the symptoms are mild. However, the two types of palpitation are closely related. Mild palpitation can develop into severe one if it lasts long. The patient with severe palpitation is more likely to be affected by external stimuli, thus making the pathological condition even worse.

Distinction and Treatment

The following three points should be carefully considered. First, it is necessary to make sure that the patient has the characteristic symptoms. Second, it is necessary to determine the nature of palpitation according to the pathological conditions. For instance, it is necessary to determine whether palpitation is of the excess or the deficiency type, whether it is caused by heart *yang*-deficiency or heart *yin*-deficiency, and whether it is complicated by phlegm or blood stagnation. Finally, it is necessary to differentiate mild and severe palpitation. Mild palpitation is mostly of the excess type, mixed with deficiency in some cases. Severe palpitation is mostly of the deficiency type, presenting frequent fits of involuntary bounding of the heart, stuffiness in the chest, and possibly intermittent cardiac pain. Some cases of severe palpitation manifest deficiency syndrome complicated by the excesses.

As for cases complicated by deficiency syndrome, the method of nourishing blood and calming the mind is adopted. For instance, replenishing heart *qi*, warming and invigorating heart *yang* are used for heart *yang*-deficiency, or *yang* deficiency complicated by retained fluid. In the treatment of cases with excess syndrome, the method of activating blood circulation and removing blood stasis is used in cases of blood stagnation; and the method of dispersing heat and resolving phlegm is employed in cases of phlegm-heat. In the treatment of cases with both deficiency and excess syndromes, both causative and symptomatic treatment should be employed to eliminate pathogenic factors and restore resistance simultaneously.

1. Timidity due to Heart Deficiency

Clinical manifestations: Palpitation, fear and fright, restlessness, insomnia, dream-disturbed sleep, a thin and white tongue coating, and a tremulous and rapid or taut and feeble pulse.

Analysis: Fright deranges *qi*, thus the heart could not house the mind as usual, resulting in palpitation. As consequences, fear and fright, restlessness, insomnia and dream-disturbed sleep will occur. A tremulous and rapid pulse or a taut and feeble pulse suggests derangement of *qi* and blood circulation. The mild cases are characterized by intermittent attacks, while the severe ones by uncontrollable palpitations.

Treatment: To relieve timidity, nourish the heart and calm the mind.

Prescription: Pill for Tranquilizing (128) combined with Succinum, Magnetitum and Cinnabaris. In this recipe, Dens Draconis, Succinum and Magnetitum relieve timidity and soothe the heart; and Lignum Pini Poriaferum, Rhizoma Acori Tatarinowii and Radix Polygalae calm and tranquilize the mind.

In cases of heart deficiency accompanied by diffidence, Radix Glycyrrhizae Preparata is added to replenish heart *qi*. If heart *yin* is insufficient, Semen Platycladi, Fructus Schisandrae and Semen Ziziphi Spinosae are added to nourish the heart, calm the mind and astringe heart *qi*.

If palpitation is accompanied by restlessness, frequent fright, profuse sputum, poor appetite, nausea, a yellow and sticky tongue coating, and a smooth and rapid pulse, it is due to the disturbance of the heart by phlegm-heat. Thus the Decoction of Coptidis for Clearing Away Gallbladder-Heat (264) is prescribed to disperse phlegm-heat and arrest palpitation. To calm the mind and nourish the heart, Radix Polygalae and Semen Ziziphi Spinosae are added.

2. Deficiency of Blood in the Heart

Clinical manifestations: Palpitation, dizziness, pale complexion, lassitude, a slightly red tongue, and a thready and weak pulse.

Analysis: Since the heart dominates the blood and vessels, and manifests in the complexion, deficiency of heart blood leads to pale complexion. Deficiency of blood in the heart also deprives the heart of nourishment, so palpitation occurs. If the brain receives no nourishment, dizziness follows. Blood deficiency also means *qi* deficiency, which causes lassitude. Since the tongue is the mirror of the heart, heart blood-deficiency gives rise to a slightly red tongue and a thready and weak pulse.

Treatment: To replenish blood, nourish the heart, benefit *qi* and calm the mind.

Prescription: Modified Decoction for Invigorating Spleen and Nourishing Heart (110). Radix Angelicae Sinensis and Arillus Longan replenish heart blood; Radix Ginseng, Radix Astragali, Rhizoma Atractylodis Macrocephalae and Radix Glycyrrhizae Preparata benefit *qi* and invigorate the spleen to strengthen the source of blood; Semen Ziziphi Spinosae, Lignum Pini Poriaferum and Radix Polygalae calm the mind and tranquilize emotions and Radix Aucklandiae circulates *qi* to prevent the stagnation that may possibly result from tonics.

If palpitation is accompanied by a pulse with missed beats, this is due to the *qi* and blood deficiency which deprives the heart of nourishment. Decoction of Glycyrrhizae Preparata (186) is then prescribed to benefit *qi* and blood, nourish *yin* and restore normal pulse. In the prescription, Radix Glycyrrhizae Preparata, sweet and warm in nature, restores normal pulse and benefits heart *qi*; Radix Ginseng and Fructus Jujubae replenish *qi* and invigorate the stomach; Ramulus Cinnamomi and Rhizoma Zingiberis Recens, acrid and warm in nature, invigorate *yang*; and Radix Rehmanniae, Colla Corii Asini, Radix Ophiopogonis and Fructus Cannabis nourish heart *yin* and blood.

If palpitation results from deficiency of heart *yin* at the later stage of a febrile disease, Powder for Restoring Pulse (96) is prescribed to replenish *qi* and nourish *yin*. In the prescription, Radix Ginseng strengthens primordial *qi* of the body; Radix Ophiopogonis nourishes *yin*; and Fructus Schisandrae consolidates heart *qi*.

3. Deficiency of *Yin* and Hyperactivity of Fire

Clinical manifestations: Palpitation, restlessness, insomnia, dizziness, blurring of vision, a hot sensation in the palms and soles, tinnitus, lumbago, a red tongue with scanty or no coating, and a thready and rapid pulse.

Analysis: Deficiency of kidney *yin* means lack of coordination between water and fire; hyperactive heart fire thus produced causes palpitation, restlessness and insomnia. Kidney *yin*-deficiency also gives rise to lumbago. Hyperactive *yang* causes dizziness, tinnitus and the hot sensation in the palms and soles. A red tongue and a thready and rapid pulse are signs of hyperactivity of fire due to the *yin* deficiency.

Treatment: To replenish *yin*, clear away fire, nourish the heart and calm the mind.

Prescription: King of Heaven Tonic Pill for Mental Discomfort (39) or Pill of Cinnabaris for Tranquilizing (134). In cases of *yin* deficiency without hyperactivity of fire, King of Heaven Tonic Pill for Mental Discomfort (39) is used with modifications. In the recipe, Radix Rehmanniae, Radix Scrophulariae, Radix Ophiopogonis and Radix Asparagi nourish *yin* and disperse heat; Radix Angelicae Sinensis and Radix Salviae Miltiorrhizae replenish blood and nourish the heart; Radix Ginseng replenishes heart *qi*; Cinnabaris, Poria, Radix Polygalae, Semen Ziziphi Spinosae and Semen Platycladi calm the mind and nourish the heart; Fructus Schisandrae consolidates heart *qi*; and Radix Platycodi conducts the action of drugs upward to circulate heart *qi*.

If heat signs, such as restlessness, dry mouth and throat, and a bitter taste in the mouth are pronounced, Pill of Cinnabaris for Tranquilizing (134) is applied. In this prescription, Cinnabaris calms the mind; Radix Angelicae Sinensis and Radix Rehmanniae nourish *yin* and blood; and Rhizoma Coptidis disperses heat and reduces fire. The combination of all these drugs reduces heart fire, nourishes heart *yin*, replenishes heart blood and calms the mind. It is commonly used for palpitation marked by restlessness and irritability.

If symptoms of a hot sensation in the palms, soles and chest, nocturnal emission and lumbago are present, this suggests a disturbance of ministerial fire. Bolus of Anemarrhenae, Phellodendri and Rehmanniae Preparata (181) is then prescribed with modifications to nourish *yin* and reduce fire.

4. Deficiency of Heart *Yang*

Clinical manifestations: Palpitation, restlessness, stuffiness in the chest, shortness of breath, pale complexion, cold limbs, a pale tongue, a weak pulse or a deep, thready and rapid pulse.

Analysis: Deficiency of heart *yang* after a protracted illness deprives the heart of warmth and nourishment, and thereby causes palpitation and restlessness. Insufficient *yang-qi* in the chest causes stuffiness and shortness of breath. Heart *yang*-deficiency results in slow blood circulation; the consequences are cold limbs and a pale complexion. A pale tongue and a weak or deep, thready and rapid pulse are signs of heart *yang*-deficiency.

Treatment: To warm and replenish heart *yang*, calm the mind and relieve palpitation.

Prescription: Decoction of Cinnamomi, Glycyrrhizae, Os Draconis and Concha Ostreae (225) with additional drugs. In this recipe, Ramulus Cinnamomi and Radix Glycyrrhizae warm and replenish heart *yang*; and Os Draconis and Concha Ostreae calm the mind and relieve palpitation. To warm *yang* and benefit *qi*, Radix Ginseng and Radix Aconiti Lateralis Preparata are added.

In severe cases with sweating, cold limbs, cyanosis and orthopnea, Radix Ginseng and Radix Aconiti Lateralis Preparata are prescribed in large doses, and Pill of Stannum Nigrum (300) is added to restore *yang* and prevent collapse.

5. Attack of the Heart by Retained Fluid

Clinical manifestations: Palpitation, dizziness, fullness in the chest and epigastrium, cold limbs, scanty urine, edema of the lower limbs, thirst with no desire to drink, nausea, retching, a white and slippery tongue coating, and a taut and smooth pulse.

Analysis: Fluid, a *yin* pathogenic factor, is resolved by *yang-qi*. *Yang* deficiency implies inability to resolve fluid, which then retains in the body and attacks the heart, resulting in palpitation. Inability of *yang-qi* to reach the four limbs causes cold limbs. Retained fluid in the middle *jiao* hinders the clear *yang* from ascending, thus causing dizziness. Retarded *qi* circulation produces fullness in the chest and epigastrium. Fluid retention leads to dry mouth with no desire to drink, scanty urine and edema of the lower limbs. Upward disturbance of retained fluid gives rise to nausea and retching. A white and slippery tongue coating and a taut and smooth pulse are signs of fluid retention.

Treatment: To invigorate heart *yang*, produce *qi* and resolve fluid.

Prescription: Modified Decoction of Poria, Cinnamomi, Atractylodis Macrocephalae and Glycyrrhizae (170). In the recipe, Poria, bland in nature, promotes diuresis; Ramulus Cinnamomi and Radix Glycyrrhizae invigorate *yang* and produce *qi*; and Rhizoma Atractylodis Macrocephalae invigorates the spleen and eliminates dampness. In cases of upward disturbance of retained fluid with symptoms of nausea and vomiting, Rhizoma Pinelliae, Pericarpium Citri Reticulatae and Rhizoma Zingiberis Recens are added to regulate the stomach and conduct the unhealthy *qi* downward.

If kidney *yang* is too deficient to control water, the fluid will attack the heart. Clinical manifestations are palpitation, cough, orthopnea, dysuria and edema. *Zhenwu* Decoction (223) is prescribed with modifications to warm kidney *yang* and resolve fluid.

6. Stagnation of Blood in the Heart

Clinical manifestations: Palpitation, restlessness, stuffiness in the chest, occasional cardiac pain, cyanosis of the lips and nails, a dark purple tongue or a tongue with petechiae, and an unsmooth pulse or a pulse with knotted and intermittent beats.

Analysis: The heart dominates the blood and vessels. Blockage of heart vessels deprives the heart of nourishment, causing palpitation and restlessness. Stagnation of *qi* and blood hinders heart *yang* and gives rise to stuffiness in the chest. Contraction of the heart collaterals causes cardiac pain. Stagnation of heart blood produces cyanosis of the lips and nails. A dark purple tongue or a tongue with petechiae, an unsmooth pulse or a pulse with knotted and intermittent beats are signs of blood stagnation which hinders heart *yang*.

Treatment: To activate blood circulation, remove blood stasis, regulate *qi* and reopen the collaterals.

Prescription: Modified Decoction of Persicae and Carthami (233). In the recipe, Semen Persicae, Flos Carthami, Radix Paeoniae Rubra and Rhizoma Chuanxiong activate blood circulation and remove stasis; Rhizoma Corydalis, Rhizoma Cyperi and Pericarpium Citri Reticulatae Viride regulate *qi* and remove obstruction in the vessels; and Radix Rehmanniae and Radix Angelicae Sinensis nourish and regulate the blood. To invigorate *yang-qi*, Ramulus Cinnamomi and Radix Glycyrrhizae are added. To calm the mind, Os Draconis and Concha Ostreae are added.

Remarks

Palpitation at the initial stage can be easily treated. Delayed or improper treatment may aggravate the disease, causing the excess type to develop into the deficient. As for elderly and weak patients, palpitation tends to be very stubborn, because the kidneys have been affected and the anti-pathogenic *qi* is weak. During treatment, the patient should maintain emotional stability, rest well in a quiet environment, and avoid hot and pungent food.

Case Studies

Name: Kong XX; Sex: Male; Occupation: Office worker.

First visit (February 6, 1975): The patient complained of intermittent attacks of palpitation for two years. The accompanying symptoms included stuffiness in the chest, sighing, shortness of breath, constipation, a slightly red tongue with thin coating, and a slightly taut pulse with knotted and intermittent beats. An ECG in 1972 showed premature ventricular beats. The disease was due to *qi* and blood deficiency, which deprived the heart of nourishment and gave rise to heart *yang*-deficiency and retarded *qi* and blood circulation. Treatment aimed primarily to replenish heart *qi*, nourish *yin* blood and invigorate heart *yang*; secondarily to regulate *qi* and activate blood circulation. The following drugs were prescribed:

Radix Codonopsis	12 g;
Radix Glycyrrhizae Preparata	9 g;
Ramulus Cinnamomi	6 g;
Radix Paeoniae Rubra	12 g;
Radix Angelicae Sinensis	12 g;
Fructus Tritici Levis	30 g;
Fructus Citri Sarcodactylis	4.5 g;
Radix Curcumae	12 g;
Fructus Citri	9 g;
Radix Camelliae	30 g;
Fructus Jujubae	5 pieces.

Seven doses were prescribed.

Second visit (April 7, 1975): All symptoms disappeared. Appetite was good. Pulse with knotted and intermittent beats was not found. Another seven doses were prescribed to consolidate the results.

Explanation: The palpitation of this case is due to *qi* and blood deficiency along with heart *yang*-deficiency. Due to heart *yang*-deficiency, blood fails to circulate; and *qi* and blood deficiency deprives the heart of nourishment, resulting in palpitation. The prescription was based on Decoction of Glycyrrhizae Preparata (186) and Decoction of Glycyrrhizae, Tritici Levis and Jujubae (84). The sticky tonics, such as Radix Rehmanniae and Colla Corii Asini, were removed from the prescription, and drugs that regulate *qi* and blood were added. When heart *qi* circulates smoothly and heart *yang* is restored, a pulse with knotted and intermittent beats will disappear. Drugs that nourish the blood in the heart are prescribed to replenish the vessels with sufficient blood, thus preventing *yang-qi* from floating away. Attention should be paid that stuffiness in the chest and sighing in this case are due to heart *qi*-deficiency, not *qi* stagnation and dampness retention.

XI. Chest *Bi*-Syndrome

Chest *bi*-syndrome presents a feeling of suffocation in mild cases, and chest pain penetrating to the back, shortness of breath, dyspnea, or even orthopnea in severe cases.

The earliest description of chest *bi*-syndromes can be found in *The Inner Canon of the Yellow Emperor*, which also introduced the acupuncture treatment of the disease. The term "chest *bi*-syndrome" first appeared in *Synopsis of Prescriptions of the Golden Chamber* by Zhang Zhongjing, who initiated the method of removing obstructions in *qi* and blood circulation, and invigorating *yang*. Nowadays, his prescriptions are still used by physicians as guidelines.

Etiology and Pathogenesis

The causes of this disease include the attack by external pathogenic cold, improper diet, emotional upsets, and weak constitution of elderly people. There are two types of syndromes —deficiency and excess. Excess syndrome results from obstruction of *yang-qi* in the chest and blockage of heart vessels due to the attack by cold, stagnation of *qi*, stagnation of blood and retention of phlegm. Deficiency syndrome is caused by cardiac, splenic, hepatic and renal deficiency and malfunctioning. When the disease develops, the excess syndrome often precedes the deficiency one, but there are some exceptions. Nevertheless, clinical manifestations are often the combination of excess and deficiency.

1. Attack by Pathogenic Cold

Constitutional *yang* deficiency causes deficiency of chest *yang*, which enables external pathogenic cold to invade. Retention of cold and stagnation of *qi* in the chest lead to chest *bi*-syndrome.

2. Improper Diet

This refers to eating too much greasy, sweet, or cold food, or excessive drinking, which damages the spleen and stomach and impairs their transportation and transformation functions. The dampness and phlegm thus produced block the channels and collaterals, causing *qi* and blood stagnation and hindering the normal distribution of chest *yang*.

3. Emotional Upsets

Excessive worry damages the spleen and causes *qi* stagnation, which blocks the fluid distribution, resulting in phlegm. Mental depression or anger damages the liver and causes liver *qi*-stagnation. In severe cases, stagnant liver *qi* turns into fire, which condenses fluid into phlegm. Both stagnation of *qi* and retention of phlegm may cause blood stagnation, which hinders the circulation of heart *yang* and blocks the heart vessels, producing pain in the chest.

4. Weak Constitution of Elderly People

This occurs in middle-aged or elderly patients with weak kidney *qi*. If there is kidney *yang*-deficiency, heart *qi*- or heart *yang*-deficiency will result. Deficiency of kidney *yin* causes deficiency of heart *yin*. Deficiency of either kidney *yin* or kidney *yang* blocks the *qi* and blood circulation, thus creating complicated syndromes of both the deficiency type and the excess type.

Differential Diagnosis

Distinction of chest *bi*-syndrome with fluid retention in the hypochondrium, epigastric pain and cardiac pain.

1. Retention of Fluid in the Hypochondrium

Chest pain due to fluid retention in the hypochondrium is similar to chest *bi*-syndrome. But in the chest *bi*-syndrome, the pain is accompanied by a feeling of suffocation at the anterior part of the chest. This pain can extend to the shoulder and back on the left side, or to the left inner upper arm. It occurs suddenly but does not last long. The inducing factors include strain and stress, voracious eating, exposure to cold, and emotional irritation. Rest and proper medication can alleviate the pain.

Chest pain due to fluid retention in the hypochondrium is located in the costal and hypochondriac regions, and lasts long, accompanied by cough, sleeplessness, pain during respiration, productive cough and fullness in the costal region.

2. Epigastric Pain

Some chest *bi*-syndromes are not so typical, which may appear in the epigastric region. This makes it easy to confuse chest *bi*-syndrome with epigastric pain. But epigastric pain is often accompanied by belching, hiccup and acid regurgitation or vomiting of clear fluid.

3. Cardiac Pain

Real cardiac pain is the further development of chest *bi*-syndrome. It is much more severe and lasts for a long time. Other accompanying symptoms include sweating, cold limbs, pale complexion, cyanosis of the lips and nails, a feeble and thready pulse, or a pulse with knotted and intermittent beats, which indicates a critical condition.

Distinction and Treatment

This disease is marked by a feeling of suffocation and chest pain. In severe cases, chest pain may penetrate to the back, accompanied by shortness of breath, dyspnea and orthopnea. The illness mainly locates in heart, with the spleen and kidneys involved.

Chest *bi*-syndrome is a disorder of both the deficiency and the excess. To treat the root cause first then the symptoms is the general principle, although in some cases both are treated at the same time. To treat the root cause is often by activating blood circulation and removing blood stasis, invigorating *yang* with acrid and warm drugs, and eliminating turbid phlegm. While to treat the symptoms is often by warming *yang* and replenishing *qi*, benefiting *qi*, nourishing *yin* and strengthening the kidneys.

1. Stagnation of Blood in the Heart

Clinical manifestations: Fixed stabbing pain in the chest, which is more severe at night, occasional palpitation, restlessness, a dark purple tongue, and a deep and unsmooth pulse.

Analysis: Prolonged *qi* stagnation leads to blood stagnation in the vessels, resulting in the stabbing pain in the chest; since blood is stagnated, the pain remains in the same place. Blood belongs to *yin*, and so does the night, therefore the pain becomes acute during the evening. Blood stagnation in the vessels deprives the heart of nourishment, resulting in palpitation and restlessness. A dark purple tongue, and a deep and unsmooth pulse are signs of blood stagnation.

Treatment: To activate blood circulation, remove blood stasis in the vessels and relieve pain.

Prescription: Modified Decoction for Removing Blood Stasis in the Chest (135). In the recipe, Radix Angelicae Sinensis, Radix Paeoniae Rubra, Rhizoma Chuanxiong, Semen Persicae and Flos Carthami activate blood circulation and remove blood stasis; Radix Bupleuri soothes the liver; and Fructus Aurantii regulates *qi*. When *qi* circulates well, blood circulates smoothly. If chest pain is severe, a proper amount of Ligni Dalbergiae Odoriferae, Radix Curcumae and Rhizoma Corydalis is added to activate blood circulation, regulate *qi* and relieve pain.

If blood stagnation is not severe, Decoction of Salviae Miltiorrhizae (62) is used instead. In the recipe, Radix Salviae Miltiorrhizae activates blood circulation, removes stasis and relieves pain; Lignum Santali Albi warms the middle *jiao*, regulates *qi*, relieves cardiac and abdominal pain as well. Fructus

Amomi warms the stomach and removes obstruction in the middle *jiao*, relieving the feeling of suffocation in the chest.

2. Retention of Turbid Phlegm

Clinical manifestations: Chest pain extending to the shoulders and back, a feeling of suffocation, shortness of breath, sluggishness of the limbs and body, obesity, profuse sputum, a turbid and sticky tongue coating, and a smooth pulse.

Analysis: Retention of turbid phlegm hinders chest *yang*, causing suffocation and pain in the chest. Blockage of the vessels causes pain penetrating to the shoulders and back. Retarded circulation of *qi* leads to the shortness of breath. Since the spleen dominates the four limbs, and retention of turbid phlegm in the spleen impairs its function of transportation and transformation, sluggishness of the body and limbs will ensue. Obesity, profuse sputum, a turbid and sticky tongue coating and a smooth pulse are signs of turbid phlegm retention.

Treatment: To invigorate *yang* and eliminate turbid phlegm.

Prescription: Decoction of Trichosanthis, Allii Macrostemi and Pinelliae (236) with additional drugs. In this recipe, Fructus Trichosanthis disperses phlegm in the chest; Rhizoma Pinelliae resolves phlegm and conducts the unhealthy *qi* downward; and Bulbus Allii Macrostemi invigorates *yang* with its acrid and warm nature, eliminates phlegm and conducts the unhealthy *qi* downward. To achieve even better results in invigorating *yang*, eliminating phlegm, warming the middle *jiao* and regulating *qi*, Rhizoma Zingiberis, Pericarpium Citri Reticulatae and Semen Amomi Rotundus are added.

Clinically, retention of turbid phlegm and stagnation of blood often appear at the same time. Thus the method of invigorating *yang* and eliminating phlegm is often combined with activating blood circulation and removing blood stasis. The treatment should be given according to dominant factor.

3. Stagnation of *Yin* Cold

Clinical manifestations: Chest pain penetrating to the back, which becomes acute when exposed to cold, a feeling of suffocation, shortness of breath, palpitation, dyspnea or even orthopnea in severe cases, pale complexion, cold limbs, a white tongue coating, and a deep and thready pulse.

Analysis: *Yang-qi* normally accumulates in the chest and then flows to the back. Attack by pathogenic cold hinders the circulation of *yang-qi*, resulting in chest pain which penetrates to the back and acute pain when exposed to cold. Deficiency of chest *yang* leads to *qi* obstruction, consequently, a feeling of suffocation, shortness of breath, palpitation, dyspnea or even orthopnea in severe cases will occur. *Yang-qi* deficiency results in pale complexion and cold limbs. A white tongue coating and a deep and thready pulse are signs of *yin* cold and *yang-qi* stagnation.

Treatment: To invigorate *yang* with acrid and warm drugs and disperse cold.

Prescription: Decoction of Trichosanthis, Allii Macrostemi and Wine (237) combined with Fructus Aurantii Immaturus, Ramulus Cinnamomi, Radix Aconiti Lateralis Preparata, Radix Salviae Miltiorrhizae and Lignum Santali Albi. In the recipe, Ramulus Cinnamomi, Radix Aconiti Lateralis Preparata, and Bulbus Allii Macrostemi, acrid and warm in nature, invigorate *yang* and disperse cold; Fructus Trichosanthis and Fructus Aurantii Immaturus resolve phlegm, disperse masses, relieve the feeling of fullness and conduct the unhealthy *qi* downward; Lignum Santali Albi regulates *qi* and warms the middle *jiao*; and Radix Salviae Miltiorrhizae activates blood circulation and removes obstruction in the vessels. If chest *bi*-syndrome is accompanied by productive cough due to the retention of phlegm-dampness, Rhizoma Zingiberis Recens, Pericarpium Citri Reticulatae, Poria and Semen Armeniacae Amarum are added to circulate *qi* and resolve phlegm.

Incessant and severe cardiac pain spreading to the back, cold limbs and body, orthopnea and a deep and tense pulse all indicate a chest *bi*-syndrome due to severe *yin* cold. Pill of Aconiti Preparata and Halloysitum Rubrum (65) combined with Bolus of Styrax (143) is the proper prescription. In the recipe, Pericarpium Zanthoxyli and Rhizoma Zingiberis warm the middle *jiao* and disperse cold; Radix Aconiti Lateralis Preparata and Radix Aconiti Preparata relieve cardiac pain and cold limbs; Halloysitum Rubrum nourishes heart *qi*; and the combination of Halloysitum Rubrum and Bolus of Styrax warms chest *yin* and relieves pain. Radix Aconiti Lateralis Preparata and Radix Aconiti Preparata are rarely used at the same time. For better results, Cortex Cinnamomi is adopted instead of Radix Aconiti Preparata. Bolus of Styrax for Coronary Heart Disease, frequently used nowadays, is produced on the basis of Bolus of Styrax (143).

4. Cardiac and Renal *Yin*-Deficiency

Clinical manifestations: A feeling of suffocation and pain in the chest, palpitation, night sweating, restlessness, insomnia, soreness of the lumbar region and weak knees, tinnitus, dizziness, a red tongue or a tongue with petechiae, a thready and slightly rapid, or a thready and unsmooth pulse.

Analysis: Retarded *qi* and blood circulation for a long time due to the protracted illness causes stagnation in the chest. As consequences, a feeling of suffocation and pain occurs. Deficiency of heart *yin* causes palpitation, night sweating, restlessness and insomnia. Renal *yin*-deficiency results in tinnitus, soreness of the lumbar region and weak knees. If water is unable to nourish wood, liver *yang* becomes hyperactive, causing dizziness, a red tongue, or a tongue with petechiae. A thready and slightly rapid, or a thready and unsmooth pulse indicates *yin* blood-deficiency and vascular obstruction.

Treatment: To nourish *yin* and benefit the kidneys, nourish the heart and calm the mind.

Prescription: Modified *Zuogui* Decoction (80). In the recipe, Radix Rehmanniae Preparata, Fructus Corni and Fructus Lycii nourish *yin* and benefit the kidneys; and Rhizoma Dioscoreae, Poria and Radix Glycyrrhizae invigorate the spleen to strengthen the source of *qi* and blood. In cases of cardiac *yin*-deficiency with symptoms of palpitation, night sweating, restlessness and insomnia, Radix Ophiopogonis, Fructus Schisandrae, Semen Platycladi and Semen Ziziphi Spinosae are added to nourish the heart and calm the mind, and Radix Ophiopogonis can be applied in a large dose. If a feeling of suffocation is accompanied by pain, Radix Angelicae Sinensis, Radix Salviae Miltiorrhizae, Rhizoma Chuanxiong and Radix Curcumae are added to nourish blood and remove vascular obstruction. If *yin* deficiency leads to hyperactive *yang* with symptoms of dizziness, blurring of vision, numb tongue and limbs, and a hot sensation in the face, a proper amount of Radix Polygoni Multiflori Preparata, Fructus Ligustri Lucidi, Ramulus Uncariae cum Uncis, Concha Haliotidis, Concha Ostreae and Carapax Trionycis is added to nourish *yin* and subdue hyperactive *yang*.

5. Deficiency of Both *Qi* and *Yin*

Clinical manifestations: A feeling of suffocation and intermittent dull pain in the chest, palpitation, shortness of breath, lassitude, dislike of speaking, pale complexion, dizziness and blurring of vision which become worse on exertion, a red tongue or a tongue with tooth prints, and a thready and weak pulse, or a pulse with knotted and intermittent beats.

Analysis: Protracted chest *bi*-syndrome results in the deficiency of both *qi* and *yin*. Deficiency of *qi* prevents blood from normal circulation; and *yin* deficiency leads to vascular disorders, resulting in blood stagnation. As a result of stagnation of *qi* and blood, intermittent feeling of suffocation and dull pain in the chest appears. Malnutrition of the heart produces palpitation. Deficiency of *qi* explains the shortness of breath, lassitude, dislike of speaking and pale complexion. Hyperactivity of *yang* due to the *yin* deficiency causes dizziness and blurred vision, which become more serious on exertion. A red tongue or a tongue with tooth prints, and a thready and weak pulse or a pulse with knotted and intermittent beats are signs of deficiency of both *qi* and *yin*.

Treatment: To benefit *qi* and nourish *yin*.

Prescription: Powder for Restoring Pulse (96) combined with Decoction of Ginseng for Nourishing *Qi* and *Ying* (11). In the recipe, Radix Ginseng, Radix Astragali, Rhizoma Atractylodis Macrocephale,

Poria and Radix Glycyrrhizae invigorate the spleen and benefit *qi* to strengthen the source of *qi* and blood; Radix Ophiopogonis, Radix Rehmanniae, Radix Angelicae Sinensis and Radix Paeoniae Alba nourish *yin* blood; and Radix Polygalae and Fructus Schisandrae nourish the heart and calm the mind. To relieve the feeling of suffocation and pain in the chest, Radix Salviae Miltiorrhizae, Radix Notoginseng, Herba Leonuri, Radix Curcumae and Faeces Trogopterori are added to activate blood circulation and remove vascular obstruction. A pulse with knotted and intermittent beats is the result of *qi* and blood deficiency which deprives the heart of nourishment. Decoction of Glycyrrhizae Preparata (186) can be used to replenish *qi*, nourish blood and *yin*, and restore normal pulse.

6. Deficiency of *Yang-Qi*

Clinical manifestations: A feeling of suffocation in the chest, shortness of breath, chest pain extending to the back in severe cases, palpitation, sweating, aversion to cold, cold limbs, lumbar soreness, lassitude, pale complexion, pale or dark purple lips and nails, a pale or dark purple tongue, and a deep and thready, or deep, feeble and fading pulse.

Analysis: Deficiency of *yang-qi* results in *qi* and blood stagnation, therefore suffocation, shortness of breath, and chest pain spreading to the back in severe cases occur. Heart *yang*-deficiency causes palpitation and sweating; kidney *yang*-deficiency produces aversion to cold, cold limbs, lumbar soreness, pale complexion and pale or dark purple lips and nails. A pale or dark purple tongue, and a deep and thready, or deep, feeble and fading pulse indicate *yang-qi* deficiency and blood stagnation.

Treatment: To benefit *qi* and warm *yang*.

Prescription: Decoction of Ginseng and Aconiti Lateralis Preparata (188) combined with *Yougui* Decoction (83). In this recipe, Radix Ginseng replenishes the body's primordial *qi*; Radix Aconiti Lateralis Preparata and Cortex Cinnamomi warm and invigorate kidney *yang*; and Radix Rehmanniae Preparata, Fructus Corni, Fructus Lycii and Cortex Eucommiae replenish kidney essence. In cases of cardiac *yang* collapse with symptoms such as cyanosis of the face and lips, profuse sweating, cold limbs and a deep, feeble and fading pulse, Radix Ginseng and Radix Aconiti Lateralis Preparata should be prescribed in large doses, and Os Draconis and Concha Ostreae are also used to restore *yang* and prevent collapse. If *yang* deficiency affects *yin* and causes deficiency of both *yin* and *yang*, Radix Ophiopogonis and Fructus Schisandrae are added. In cases of renal *yang*-deficiency complicated by the attack of the heart due to retained fluid with symptoms such as palpitation, shortness of breath, orthopnea, scanty urine and edema of the limbs and body, *Zhenwu* Decoction (223) is prescribed with Radix Stephaniae Tetrandrae, Polyporus and Semen Plantaginis to warm *yang* and eliminate retained fluid.

The commonly used Chinese medicines for chest *bi*-syndromes are as follows:

(1) Bolus of Styrax for Coronary Heart Disease

When the pain is acute, administer one bolus once or one bolus twice or three times a day. It consists of Oleum Styrax, Lignum Santali Albi, Cinnabaris, Borneolum Syntheticum, Radix Aristolochiae and Olibanum.

(2) Injection of Salviae Miltiorrhizae Co

2ml each time, intramuscular injection once or twice a day. Or 2ml mixed with 20ml of 50% glucose intravenously, or 4-8ml mixed with 250ml of 5% glucose by intravenous drips. Each ml contains 2 g of Radix Salviae Miltiorrhizae and Ligni Dalbergiae Odoriferae respectively.

(3) Injection of Ilicis Pubescentis

One ampoule each time, once or twice a day. Each ampoule contains 8 g of Radix Ricis Pubescentis.

(4) Pill of Styrax and Borneolum Syntheticum

Two to three pills each time, twice a day.

(5) Tablet of Trichosanthis

Four tablets each time, three times a day.

Case Studies

Name: Wu XX; Sex: Female; Age: 73.

First visit (April 20, 1974): The patient had a history of coronary heart disease with frequent attacks of suffocation and pain in the left chest. On the morning of that day, severe pain occurred again in the left chest. Other symptoms included aversion to cold, cold limbs, sweating, palpitation, shortness of breath, orthopnea, a pulse with knotted and intermittent beats, and a pale tongue with white coating. Diagnosis in Western medicine was coronary heart disease, angina pectoris and auricular fibrillation. The pathogenesis of traditional Chinese medicine was heart *yang*-deficiency complicated by retention of turbid phlegm. The following herbs were prescribed to relieve acute symptoms:

Radix Aconiti Lateralis Preparata (decocted first)	12 g;
Ramulus Cinnamomi	6 g;
Radix Codonopsis	18 g;
Radix Salviae Miltiorrhizae	18 g;
Radix Angelicae Sinensis	12 g;
Rhizoma Chuanxiong	6 g;
Bulbus Allii Macrostemi	6 g;
Fructus Trichosanthis	12 g;
Rhizoma Pinelliae Preparata	9 g;
Ligni Dalbergiae Odoriferae	4.5 g.

Two doses were prescribed.

Second visit (April 22, 1974): Suffocation, pain in the left chest and palpitation improved, and shortness of breath and orthopnea disappeared, although there were mild dizziness and dry stool. The pulse became thready and even, and the tongue coating thin. These symptoms showed the gradual improvement of heart *yang*, and the dry stool was due to the dryness in the intestines. Radix Codonopsis was removed from the prescription, and 12 g of Fructus Cannabis were added. Three doses were prescribed.

Third visit (April 25, 1974): Suffocation, pain in the left chest, palpitation, and dry stool all disappeared. The pulse was slightly taut, and the tongue coating thin. The heart *yang* was gradually restored, but phlegm-dampness was not completely resolved. Treatment aimed to invigorate *yang*, activate blood circulation, and promote the circulation of *qi*. The following herbs were prescribed:

Ramulus Cinnamomi	6 g;
Bulbus Allii Macrostemi	6 g;
Fructus Trichosanthis	12 g;
Rhizoma Pinelliae Preparata	9 g;
Poria	12 g;
Radix Salviae Miltiorrhizae	15 g;
Radix Angelicae Sinensis	9 g;
Flos Carthami	6 g;
Ligni Salbergiae Odoriferae (decocted later)	4.5 g.

Seven doses were prescribed.

Explanation: When the acute attack of coronary heart disease with angina pectoris occurs, the major focus in the treatment should be relieving pain. For this reason, the method of invigorating *yang*, eliminating turbid phlegm, removing blood stasis and regulating *qi* was adopted to treat the symptoms. When *qi* and blood circulate smoothly, pain is relieved. Although there is a saying "tonics should not be used to relieve the severe pain," it is not applicable in such a case. Because cardiac pain is due to the heart *yang*-deficiency complicated by retention of turbid phlegm. If heart *yang* is not invigorated, turbid phlegm will keep on causing pain in the chest. Therefore, the drugs that warm *yang* and benefit *qi*, such as Radix Aconiti Lateralis Preparata and Radix Codonopsis, are prescribed with drugs that relieve pain for the treatment of the acute symptoms.

Name: Wang XX; Sex: Female; Age: 48; Date of Admission: February 17, 1975.

Chief complaint: Severe pain in the left chest, palpitation and profuse sweating for four hours due to overwork.

Examination: The body temperature was 36°C, pulse rate 96/min. and blood pressure 160/90mm Hg. Respiratory sound was clear. The heart was slightly enlarged towards the left side. Premature beats were occasionally present. Systolic blowing murmur of Grade II was heard in cardiac apex. ECG showed acute inferior myocardial infarction and occasional premature beats.

Diagnosis: Coronary heart disease, acute inferior myocardial infarction.

First visit: Clinical manifestations included severe pain in the left precordial region, which was colicky and persistent, radiating to the left shoulder and arm, shortness of breath, dizziness, lassitude, palpitation, profuse sweating, cold limbs, a pale tongue with thin and white coating, and a deep, thready and taut pulse. The pathogenesis was *qi* and blood stagnation in the heart vessels complicated by *yang* deficiency. Treatment aimed to warm *yang*, benefit *qi*, activate blood circulation, remove stasis and relieve pain. The following drugs were prescribed:

Radix Aconiti Lateralis Preparata	9 g;
Cortex Cinnamomi	6 g;
Radix Ginseng (decocted and taken separately)	9 g;
Semen Persicae	9 g;
Radix Salviae Miltiorrhizae	9 g;
Bolus of Styrax (143) (to be taken separately with warm boiled water)	one.

Second visit: Chest pain greatly improved after three doses, but a feeling of suffocation still existed. She complained of a bitter taste in the mouth, deep yellow urine, a red tongue and a taut pulse. The symptoms indicate retention of phlegm-heat and blood stagnation in the heart vessels. Treatment aimed to disperse heat, resolve phlegm, activate blood circulation and remove blood stasis. The following drugs were prescribed:

Rhizoma Pinelliae	9 g;
Radix Sophorae Flavescentis	9 g;
Fructus Trichosanthis	18 g;
Semen Persicae	9 g;
Flos Carthami	9 g;
Pollen Typhae	9 g;
Faeces Trogopterori	9 g.

Third visit: Both the feeling of suffocation and pain in the chest slightly improved after ten doses. The patient complained of shortness of breath and profuse sweating on exertion. The tongue became pale, and the pulse was deep, taut and weak. Treatment aimed to warm *yang*, activate blood circulation and remove blood stasis. The following drugs were prescribed:

Radix Aconiti Lateralis Preparata	3 g;
Cortex Cinnamomi	3 g;
Radix Ginseng (decocted and taken separately)	9 g;
Semen Persicae	9 g;
Radix Salviae Miltiorrhizae	9 g;
Radix Astragali	15 g.

ECG revealed a remote inferior myocardial infarction, and almost all symptoms disappeared after administering the above drugs for one and a half months. The patient was then discharged.

Explanation: The pathogenesis of this case is heart *yang*-deficiency and blood stagnation in the heart vessels. Radix Ginseng, Radix Aconiti Lateralis Preparata and Cortex Cinnamomi restore *yang* and prevent collapse. Radix Salviae Miltiorrhizae and Semen Persicae activate blood circulation and remove stasis. Bolus of Styrax warms *yang*, promotes resuscitation and relieves pain. Red tongue, a bitter taste in the mouth, and yellow urine were found on the second visit, which indicated that the retained phlegm had turned into heat. Thus Radix Sophorae Flavescentis, Fructus Trichosanthis and Rhizoma Pinelliae were prescribed to disperse heat and resolve phlegm; and Powder for Dissipating Blood Stasis (98), Semen Persicae and Flos Carthami were used to activate blood circulation and remove stasis. On the third visit, the tongue became pale, heat signs subsided, and the pulse was taut and thready. Thus the method of warming *yang*, benefiting *qi*, activating blood circulation and removing stasis was still adopted, with which almost all the symptoms disappeared.

XII. Insomnia

Insomnia means the inability to have a normal sleep. Mild insomnia includes the difficulty in falling asleep, shallow sleep, difficulty to resume sleep once waking up, and sometimes asleep, sometimes awake. Severe insomnia refers to the inability to fall asleep for the whole night.

As early as in *Basic Questions*, it says, "Disharmony of the stomach leads to insomnia." In the *Synopsis of Prescriptions of the Golden Chamber*, it explains that insomnia is due to the deficiency caused by overwork or anxiety. *A Complete Collection of Jingyue's Treatise* elaborates the causes of insomnia.

Insomnia may appear alone or in combination with other symptoms, such as headache, dizziness, palpitation and poor memory. It is commonly seen as neurosis and climacteric syndromes in modern medicine.

Etiology and Pathogenesis
1. Damage of the Heart and Spleen due to Strain and Stress

Damage of the heart causes the consumption of *yin* blood, resulting in wandering of the mind. Damage of the spleen affects the appetite, therefore, the heart is deprived of nourishment, and insomnia ensues.

2. Disharmony Between the Heart and Kidneys due to the Imbalance of *Yin* and *Yang*

With people congenitally weak and those after a protracted illness, their kidney *yin* is too deficient to nourish the heart. Therefore, the heart fire or heart *yang* becomes hyperactive. Emotional upsets directly lead to hyperactivity of heart fire, which cannot coordinate with kidney water. Hyperactive heart fire caused by the disharmony between the heart and kidneys interferes with the mind, resulting in insomnia.

3. Disturbance of Liver *Yang* and Fire due to *Yin* Deficiency

Emotional upsets impair the renal function and cause liver *qi*-stagnation, which then turns into fire. Deficiency of *yin* leads to hyperactivity of *yang*, which interferes with the mind, resulting in insomnia.

4. Timidity due to Heart Deficiency

Being timid, indecisive, and easily frightened can all lead to insomnia. In addition, nervousness caused by sudden fright can also gradually develop into insomnia.

5. Disturbance of Stomach *Qi*

Improper diet damages the intestines and stomach, and causes retention of food, which produces phlegm-heat. Retained phlegm-heat in the middle *jiao* disturbs stomach *qi*, resulting in insomnia.

There are many causes of insomnia, but most of them are related to the heart, spleen, liver, kidneys, and *yin* blood-deficiency. The pathogenesis is the disharmony between hyperactive *yang* and insufficient *yin*.

Distinction and Treatment

Insomnia is of two types, the deficiency and excess. Deficiency syndromes result from *yin* blood-deficiency, for which the heart, spleen, liver and kidneys are responsible. The treatment for this is benefiting *qi*, nourishing blood and strengthening the liver and kidneys. Excess syndromes are caused by liver *qi*-stagnation which turns into fire, and food retention which results in turbid phlegm. They are dealt with by promoting digestion, harmonizing the middle *jiao*, dispersing heat in the heart and resolving phlegm. Protracted excess syndromes may change into the deficiency syndromes. When treating cases complicated by both the deficiency and excess, the method of strengthening the body resistance and eliminating pathogenic factors should be used in combination.

1. Excess Syndromes

(1) Liver *qi*-stagnation turning into fire

Clinical manifestations: Insomnia, irritability, poor appetite, thirst, red eyes, a bitter taste in the mouth, deep yellow urine, constipation, a red tongue with yellow coating, and a taut and rapid pulse.

Analysis: Anger damages the liver and causes liver *qi*-stagnation, which then turns into fire disturbing the heart and mind, and insomnia ensues. If the stomach is attacked by liver *qi*, poor appetite will follow. Stagnation of liver *qi* turns into fire, which attacks the stomach, resulting in thirst with a desire to drink. Hyperactive liver fire causes irritability. Upward disturbance of fire and heat causes red eyes and bitter taste in the mouth. Deep yellow urine, constipation, a red tongue with yellow coating and a taut and thready pulse all indicate heat syndrome.

Treatment: To soothe the liver, disperse heat and calm the mind.

Prescription: Decoction of Gentianae for Purging Liver-Fire (78) with additional drugs. In the recipe, Radix Gentianae, Radix Scutellariae and Fructus Gardeniae disperse heat in the liver and reduce fire; Rhizoma Alismatis, Caulis Aristolochiae Manshuriensis and Semen Plantaginis clear away dampness-heat in the Liver Meridian; Radix Angelicae Sinensis and Radix Rehmanniae nourish blood and the liver; Radix Bupleuri regulates the liver and gallbladder *qi*; and Radix Glycyrrhizae harmonizes the middle *jiao*. To soothe the heart and calm the mind, Lignum Pini Poriaferum and Os Draconis are added. In cases with stuffiness in the chest, hypochondriac distention and sighing, Radix Curcumae and Rhizoma Cyperi are added to soothe the liver and relieve stagnation.

(2) Internal disturbance of phlegm-heat

Clinical manifestations: Insomnia, a heavy sensation in the head, profuse sputum, stuffiness in the chest, anorexia, belching, acid regurgitation, nausea, restlessness, a bitter taste in the mouth, blurred vision, a sticky and yellow tongue coating and a smooth and rapid pulse.

Analysis: Phlegm-dampness caused by retention of food produces heat which disturbs upward, resulting in restlessness and insomnia. Retention of phlegm-dampness in the middle *jiao* causes stuffiness in the chest. Hindrance of clear *yang* leads to a heavy sensation in the head and blurred vision. Retention of food blocks *qi* circulation and impairs the function of stomach, and anorexia, belching and nausea ensue. A sticky and yellow tongue coating, and a smooth and rapid pulse are signs of phlegm-heat and retention of phlegm-heat.

Treatment: To resolve phlegm, disperse heat, harmonize the middle *jiao* and calm the mind.

Prescription: Decoction for Clearing Away Gallbladder-Heat (302) with Rhizoma Coptidis and Fructus Gardeniae. In this recipe, Rhizoma Pinelliae, Pericarpium Citri Reticulatae, Caulis Bambusae in Taeniam and Fructus Aurantii Immaturus regulate *qi*, resolve phlegm, harmonize the stomach and conduct the unhealthy *qi* downward; Rhizoma Coptidis and Fructus Gardeniae disperse heat in the heart and reduce fire; and Poria soothes the heart and calms the mind. In cases of palpitation and restlessness, Concha Margaritifera Usta and Cinnabaris are added to soothe the heart and calm the mind. In cases of stomach disharmony due to food and phlegm retention, Decoction of Pinelliae and Panicum (108) is prescribed with Massa Medicata Fermentata, Fructus Crataegi and Semen Raphani. As for phlegm-heat with constipation, which is a severe case, Pill of Lapis Chloriti Usta for Expelling Phlegm (323) is prescribed to reduce fire, disperse heat, eliminate phlegm and calm the mind.

2. Deficiency Syndromes

(1) Hyperactivity of fire due to *yin* deficiency

Clinical manifestations: Insomnia, restlessness, palpitation, dizziness, tinnitus, poor memory, lumbar soreness, nocturnal emission, a hot sensation in the palms, soles and chest, thirst, lack of saliva, a red tongue, and a thready and rapid pulse.

Analysis: Kidney *yin*-deficiency leads to hyperactivity of heart and liver fire, which disturbs the mind and results in insomnia, restlessness and palpitation. Consumption of renal essence leads to the empty sea of marrow, therefore, dizziness, tinnitus and poor memory appear. Lack of nourishment in the lumbar region explains the soreness. The disharmony between the heart and kidneys weakens the gate of essence, resulting in nocturnal emission. Thirst, lack of saliva, a hot sensation in the palms, soles and chest, a red tongue and a thready and rapid pulse all indicate hyperactivity of fire due to the *yin* deficiency.

Treatment: To replenish *yin*, reduce fire, nourish the heart and calm the mind.

Prescription: Both Decoction of Coptidis and Colla Corii Asini (261) and Pill of Cinnabaris for Tranquilizing (134) are prescribed to disperse heat and calm the mind. The former nourishes *yin* and reduces fire, and is applied to cases of insomnia caused by restlessness. If *yang* increases, causing a hot sensation in the face, dizziness and tinnitus, Concha Ostreae, Carapax et Plastrum Testudinis and Magnetitum are added to suppress hyperactive *yang*. When *yang* and *yin* are balanced, the patient may have normal sleep. The latter prescription, which also selects Rhizoma Coptidis as the main ingredient, is similar to the former in terms of the principle. Being pills, it is more convenient for administration. To replenish *yin*, reduce fire, nourish the heart and calm the mind, Semen Platycladi and Semen Ziziphi Spinosae could be added.

(2) Cardiac and splenic deficiency

Clinical manifestations: Dream-disturbed sleep, shallow sleep, palpitation, poor memory, dizziness, blurred vision, lassitude, lack of taste, pale complexion, a pale tongue with thin coating, and a thready and weak pulse.

Analysis: Deficiency of both the heart and spleen deprives the heart of nourishment, and causes wandering mind. As a result, dream-disturbed sleep, shallow sleep, poor memory and palpitation appear. *Qi* and blood deficiency deprives the brain of nourishment, thus dizziness and blurred vision ensue. Blood deficiency leads to pale complexion and a pale tongue. The spleen's failing to transport results in the lack of taste. Lack of blood and *qi* causes lassitude and a thready and weak pulse.

Treatment: To fortify the heart and spleen, and produce *qi* and blood.

Prescription: Decoction for Invigorating Spleen and Nourishing Heart (110) is the main prescription. In the recipe, Radix Ginseng, Rhizoma Atractylodis Macrocephalae, Radix Astragali and Radix Glycyrrhizae replenish *qi* and invigorate the spleen; Radix Polygalae, Semen Ziziphi Spinosae, Lignum Pini Poriaferum and Arillus Longan invigorate the heart and spleen and calm the mind; Radix Angelicae Sinensis nourishes *yin* and replenishes blood; and Radix Aucklandiae eases the circulation of *qi* and the spleen, nourishing it without causing stagnation. In case of cardiac blood deficiency, Radix Rehmanniae Preparata, Radix Paeoniae Alba and Colla Corii Asini are added. If insomnia is severe, a proper amount of Fructus Schisandrae and Semen Platycladi could be added to nourish the heart and calm the mind; or Flos Albiziae, Caulis Polygoni Multiflori, Os Draconis and Concha Ostreae are added to calm the mind. If epigastric discomfort, poor appetite, a slippery and sticky tongue present, Rhizoma Pinelliae, Pericarpium Citri Reticulatae, Poria and Cortex Magnoliae Officinalis are added to invigorate the spleen, regulate *qi* and resolve phlegm.

Another effective method is to combine Decoction for Invigorating Spleen and Nourishing Heart (110) with Decoction for Nourishing Heart (208).

(3) *Qi* deficiency of the heart and gallbladder

Clinical manifestations: Insomnia, dream-disturbed sleep, shallow sleep, timidity, palpitation, being easily to be caught in a fright, shortness of breath, lassitude, profuse clear urine, pale tongue, and a taut and thready pulse.

Analysis: Cardiac deficiency leads to restlessness, while gallbladder deficiency makes one easily to be frightened. As the results, dream-disturbed sleep, shallow sleep, palpitation, and being easily to be caught in a fright appear. Shortness of breath, lassitude and profuse clear urine all indicate *qi* deficiency. A pale tongue and a taut and thready pulse are due to the *qi* and blood deficiency.

Treatment: To benefit *qi*, soothe the heart, calm the mind and tranquilize emotions.

Prescription: Pill for Tranquilizing (128) is the main prescription. In the recipe, Radix Ginseng benefits *qi*; Dens Draconis soothes the heart; Poria, Lignum Pini Poriaferum and Rhizoma Acori Tatarinowii replenish *qi*, benefit the gallbladder and calm the mind. In cases of floating *yang* and blood deficiency with symptoms of restlessness and insomnia, Decoction of Ziziphi Spinosae (315) is recommended. In this prescription, Semen Ziziphi Spinosae calms the mind and nourishes the liver; Rhizoma Chuanxiong regulates blood and assists Semen Ziziphi Spinosae to nourish the heart; Poria resolves phlegm and soothes the heart, helping Semen Ziziphi Spinosae to calm the mind; and Rhizoma Anemarrhenae disperses heat in the gallbladder and calms the mind.

These two prescriptions can be used in combination to treat severe cases of insomnia.

If after illness, insomnia is accompanied by emaciation, pale complexion, lassitude, a pale tongue, and a thready and weak pulse, or elderly people wake up too early in the morning, it indicates *qi* and blood deficiency. Decoction for Invigorating Spleen and Nourishing Heart (110) should be prescribed.

If insomnia is due to blood deficiency and heat in the liver, Pill of Succinum for Relieving Insomnia (292) should be applied.

In cases of disharmony between the heart and kidneys, and upward disturbance of *yang* of the deficiency type, Pill of Coptidis and Cinnamomi (126) is recommended. In the recipe, Rhizoma Coptidis, the main ingredient, clears away fire; and Cortex Cinnamomi warms the heart and kidneys and conducts fire back to its origin.

Remarks

In the treatment of insomnia, medication should be combined with psychotherapy. The patient is asked to keep calm, avoid excitement and anxiety, and do some labor work and exercises, such as *qigong*. It is not advisable for the patient to smoke, drink alcohol or strong tea before sleep.

Case Studies

Name: Zheng XX; Sex: Female; Age: 58; Occupation: Housewife.

First visit (October 17, 1976): The patient complained of insomnia accompanied by restlessness for years. In severe cases, insomnia lasted two or three days. Other symptoms included aversion to heat and cold, numb lips and limbs, headache on the right side, a thin white and slippery tongue coating, and a taut and thready pulse. The disease was due to disharmony between the heart and kidneys. Treatment aimed to harmonize the heart and kidneys by replenishing kidney *yin* and reducing heart fire. The following drugs were prescribed:

Radix Salviae Miltiorrhizae	9 g;
Semen Platycladi	12 g;
Fructus Tritici Levis	30 g;
Fructus Forsythiae (Cinnabaris coated)	9 g;

Fluoritum (decocted first)	30 g;
Rhizoma Chuanxiong	6 g;
Folium Ilicis Cornutae	9 g;
Bulbus Lilii	9 g;
Rhizoma Alismatis	12 g;
Fructus Toosendan	9 g;
Rhizoma Acori Tatarinowii	9 g;
Herba Taxilli	9 g;
Rhizoma Coptidis	1 g;
Cortex Cinnamomi	1 g.

Rhizoma Coptidis and Cortex Cinnamomi were ground to powder to be taken before sleep. Seven doses were prescribed.

Second visit (November 7, 1976): Sleep improved and headache disappeared, but there was a dull pain in the chest. The disease was due to the imbalance between water and fire. The method of nourishing the blood and soothing the heart was adopted. The following drugs were prescribed:

Radix Salviae Miltiorrhizae	9 g;
Fluoritum (decocted first)	30 g;
Fructus Tritici Levis	30 g;
Radix Glycyrrhizae Preparata	6 g;
Semen Platycladi	9 g;
Bulbus Lilii	9 g;
Rhizoma Alismatis	9 g;
Fructus Forsythiae (Cinnabaris coated)	9 g;
Folium Ilicis Cornutae	9 g;
Herba Taxilli	9 g;
Rhizoma Corydalis	9 g;
Lignum Sappan	9 g;
Rhizoma Coptidis	1 g;
Cortex Cinnamomi	1 g.

Rhizoma Coptidis and Cortex Cinnamomi were ground to powder to be taken before sleep. Ten doses were prescribed.

Third visit (November 28, 1976): The patient could calmly go to sleep. Although there was a hot sensation on the right scalp, the dull pain on the right scalp was relieved. The tongue coating was smooth, and the pulse was taut and thready, which was due to the *qi* and *yin* deficiency. Deficiency of both the heart and kidneys resulted in the imbalance of water and fire, therefore, liver *yang* disturbed upward. Treatment aimed to nourish the blood, soothe the heart, and replenish water to strengthen wood by prescribing the following drugs:

Radix Changii	12 g;
Radix Salviae Miltiorrhizae	9 g;
Fluoritum (decocted first)	30 g;
Fructus Tritici Levis	30 g;
Radix Glycyrrhizae Preparata	6 g;
Semen Platycladi	9 g;
Radix Ophiopogonis	9 g;
Radix Paeoniae Alba	12 g;

Flos Chrysanthemi	9 g;
Stigma Maydis	30 g;
Herba Taxilli	12 g;
Fructus Forsythiae (Cinnabaris coated)	9 g;
Fructus Crataegi	12 g;
Rhizoma Coptidis	1 g;
Cortex Cinnamomi	1 g.

Rhizoma Coptidis and Cortex Cinnamomi were ground to powder to be taken before sleep. Ten doses were prescribed.

Explanation: This is a typical case of insomnia due to the disharmony between the heart and kidneys. The principle of treatment is to reduce heart fire and replenish kidney fluid. When the fluid and fire are well coordinated, the patient can sleep soundly.

XIII. *Jue*-Syndrome (Syncope)

Jue-syndrome is marked by sudden collapse, loss of consciousness, and occasional cold limbs. The patient can gradually recover consciousness soon after the outbreak, without the sequelae of hemiplegia, dysphasia and deviation of the mouth and eyes. But severe cases may lead to death.

The earliest description of *jue*-syndrome can be found in *The Inner Canon of the Yellow Emperor*. It mentions two conditions: one is the sudden collapse and loss of consciousness, and the other is cold limbs and body. *Jue*-syndrome may manifest cold limbs, but the converse theorem is not necessarily true. Based on the experiences of predecessors, later medical workers give different names to the causes of *jue*-syndrome, among them are *jue*-syndrome due to *qi* disorder, blood disorder, phlegm, voracious eating, attack by summer heat, round worms, epilepsy, and alcoholic drinking.

According to clinical manifestations, doctors may consult the following descriptions to treat symptoms of syncope and shock in Western medicine, such as serious hypertension, hypoglycemic coma, cardiogenic shock, infectious-toxic shock, hysterical syncope, and sunstroke.

Etiology and Pathogenesis

The etiological factors for *jue*-syndrome include emotional upset, improper diet, and the attack by pathogenic summer heat, among which emotional upset is the main cause. The pathogenesis is the sudden derangement of *qi* leading to abnormal movement of *qi* and blood. Derangement of *qi* can be divided into two types, namely, the deficiency and excess. Excess *qi* causes unhealthy *qi* which carries blood along, thus phlegm and retained food block the clear cavity and *jue*-syndrome ensues. Deficient *qi* prevents clear *yang* (including blood) from ascending. As the spleen *qi* sinks, blood cannot reach the upper part of the body, thus the brain is deprived of nourishment, and *jue*-syndrome occurs. These two conditions are different in nature, so attention should be paid in differentiating them.

1. *Jue*-Syndrome due to *Qi* Disorder

There are two causes of this illness, namely, the excess and deficiency. The excess case results from emotional upsets, such as anger and fright, which cause derangement of *qi* in the heart and chest, thus the clear cavity is blocked and the *jue*-syndrome ensues. The deficiency case is caused by weak primordial *qi* complicated by grief, fear or fatigue. Consequently, the spleen *qi* sinks, preventing clear *yang* from ascending, and *jue*-syndrome ensues.

2. *Jue*-Syndrome due to Blood Disorder

There are two causes of the illness, the deficiency and excess. The excess case results from constitutional hyperactivity of liver *yang* complicated by fury. Consequently, blood follows the unhealthy *qi*, blocking the clear cavity and causing *jue*-syndrome. The deficiency case is caused by loss of blood, such as severe hemorrhage after childbirth, haematemesis and others. The prostration of *qi* after great loss of blood will cause *jue*-syndrome.

3. *Jue*-Syndrome due to Phlegm

This illness is often found in obese patients with weak *qi*. Overeating greasy and sweet food damages the spleen and stomach, causing retained dampness and phlegm. It can also be found in patients who always have excessive dampness and phlegm inside. For both conditions, if induced by irritation, phlegm blocks *qi*, resulting in *qi* derangement. Phlegm goes upward together with *qi* and blocks the clear cavity, resulting in *jue*-syndrome.

4. *Jue*-Syndrome due to Voracious Eating

Voracious eating causes food retention in the stomach, thus preventing stomach *qi* from descending. The upward disturbance of *qi* blocks the clear cavity, causing syncope. Although this illness is often found in children, adults also suffer from *jue*-syndrome if they fly into a fury after voracious eating.

5. *Jue*-Syndrome due to Summer Heat

This often occurs in summer if exposing to the blazing sun or working in poorly ventilated places. Attacked by the summer heat, *qi* will run upward and block the clear cavity, resulting in *jue*-syndrome. Retained summer heat inside the body forces fluid to go outward, and *qi* will prostrate together with sweat, which also causes *jue*-syndrome.

Differential Diagnosis

1. Coma

Coma usually lasts long with severe pathological manifestations. After recovery of consciousness, he still suffers from the primary disease.

2. Wind Stroke

Loss of consciousness of the *zang-fu* organs usually lasts long with severe pathological manifestations, such as deviation of mouth and eyes, and hemiparalysis. After recovery of consciousness, there often exists sequelae.

3. Epilepsy

Epilepsy manifests sudden loss of consciousness, falling down in a fit, screaming with foam on the lips, eyes staring upward, transient systemic convulsions, and incontinence of urine and feces. If the tongue is bitten, the foam spat out will be bloody. When convulsions stop, the patient will fall asleep deeply; after regaining consciousness, he will feel tired. Each epileptic seizure lasts for a short period of time with similar symptoms.

Distinction and Treatment

Sudden collapse and loss of consciousness are the main symptoms of *jue*-syndrome. Before the outbreak of *jue*-syndrome, the etiological factors are easily found. For instance, a *jue*-syndrome of the deficiency type due to *qi* disorder is often found in patients with weak constitution, if induced by fatigue, insufficient sleep, hunger or cold. A syndrome of the deficiency type due to blood disorder often results from blood loss, such as severe hemorrhage, menorrhagia, and childbirth. A syndrome of the excess type due to *qi* and blood disorder is often found in patients with strong constitution, if induced by emotional irritation. *Jue*-syndrome due to phlegm is likely to be found in patients with excessive phlegm-dampness. *Jue*-syndrome due to voracious eating often occurs after overeating and drinking. And *jue*-syndrome due to summer heat is characterized by the season, which is induced by overexposure to blazing sun or working in poorly ventilated places.

In the treatment of *jue*-syndrome, the first step is to distinguish whether it is an excess type or a deficient one. If the patient has coarse breathing, rigidity of the limbs, lockjaw, and a deep and taut, or deep and hidden pulse, usually, Powder for Causing Sneezing (310) is prescribed first. If the drugs are not effective, Bolus of Styrax (143) or *Yushu* Pill (72) is administered to restore consciousness. If syncope is due to the pathogenic factors inside the pericardium, with symptoms of high fever and restlessness, Bolus of Calculus Bovis for Resurrection (127), Pill of Precious Drugs (124), or Purple-Snow Pellet (299) is used to disperse heat and restore consciousness. In cases of feeble breathing with open mouth, sweating, cold limbs and skin, and a deep, feeble and thready pulse, Decoction of Ginseng and Aconiti Lateralis Preparata (188) is prescribed to restore *yang* and prevent collapse. In cases of red tongue, thready and rapid pulse, sweating and fever, Powder for Restoring Pulse (96) is recommended to fortify *qi* and rescue *yin*. To help regain mental clarity, acupoints *Renzhong* (DU 26) and *Yongquan* (KI 1) could be needled, and if necessary, Chinese and Western medicine can both be adopted. After recovery of consciousness, treatment is then based on the distinction of syndromes.

1. *Jue*-Syndrome due to *Qi* Disorder

(1) Excess syndrome

Clinical manifestations: Falling down in a fit, loss of consciousness, lockjaw, clenched fists, coarse breathing, cold limbs, a thin and white tongue coating, and a hidden, or a deep and taut pulse.

Analysis: Emotional irritation is an inducing factor of the illness. Disturbance of the heart and chest by liver *qi* blocks the clear cavity, therefore falling down in a fit, loss of consciousness, lockjaw and clenched fists occur. Upward movement of liver *qi* impairs the lung's dispersive function, resulting in coarse breathing. Inability of *yang-qi* to reach the exterior of the body causes cold limbs. Hindrance of *qi* in the interior produces a hidden pulse, and stagnation of liver *qi* leads to the deep and taut pulse.

Treatment: To promote circulation of *qi* and relieve stagnation.

Prescription: Modified Decoction of Six Ground Ingredients (57). In this prescription, Lignum Aquilariae Resinatum and Radix Linderae conduct the unhealthy *qi* downward and relieve stagnation; and Semen Arecae, Fructus Aurantii Immaturus and Radix Aucklandiae circulate *qi* and relieve stagnation. This prescription is recommended for patients with strong constitution. If the patient is weak, Radix Codonopsis could be added. In cases of hyperactive liver *yang* with symptoms of dizziness, headache, and flushed face, Ramulus Uncariae cum Uncis, Concha Haliotidis and Spica Prunellae are added to clarify liver. In cases of profuse sputum obstructing the air passage, Arisaema cum Bile, Bulbus Fritillariae Cirrhosae and Succus Bambusae are added to eliminate phlegm and disperse heat. If after recovering oneself, the following symptoms appear, such as weeping and wailing, capricious weeping and laughing, and insomnia, Decoction of Glycyrrhizae, Tritici Levis and Jujubae (84) added with Radix Polygalae, Semen Ziziphi Spinosae, Rhizoma Acori Tatarinowii, Radix Curcumae and Radix Salviae Miltiorrhizae is prescribed to nourish the heart, calm the mind and stabilize emotions.

Since mental irritation may cause the illness to recur, *Xiaoyao* Powder (250) should be administered in daily life to regulate *qi*, relieve stagnation and harmonize the liver and spleen.

(2) Deficiency syndrome

Clinical manifestations: Dizziness, syncope, pale complexion, feeble breathing, sweating, cold limbs, a pale tongue, and a deep and weak pulse.

Analysis: Since the patient congenitally lacks *qi*, added by grief, fear or fatigue, which leads to the sinking of *qi* of the middle *jiao* and prevents the clear *yang* from ascending, he is likely to suffer from dizziness, syncope, pale complexion and feeble breathing. Deficiency of *yang-qi* causes cold limbs. Unconsolidated defensive energy explains sweating. This syndrome often occurs in the morning, or when the stomach is empty, or when changing the body posture suddenly. A pale tongue, and a deep and weak pulse are signs of weak constitution.

Treatment: To replenish *qi* and restore *yang*.

Prescription: Modified Decoction of Four Ingredients for Recapturing *Yang* (92). In the recipe, Radix Ginseng replenishes *qi*; Radix Aconiti Lateralis Preparata and Rhizoma Zingiberis (stir-baked) restore *yang*; and Radix Glycyrrhizae harmonizes the middle *jiao*. In cases of exterior syndrome of the deficiency type with spontaneous sweating, Radix Astragali and Rhizoma Atractylodis Macrocephalae are added to replenish *qi* and constrict the body surface. If sweating is persistent, Os Draconis and Concha Ostreae are added to stop sweating. If palpitation and restlessness occur, Radix Salviae Miltiorrhizae, Semen Platycladi and Semen Ziziphi Spinosae are added to nourish the heart and calm the mind. In cases of suffocation and pain in the cardiac region, Bolus of Styrax should be administered immediately to promote *qi* circulation and restore consciousness. If the tongue is red due to the *yin* deficiency, Radix Ophiopogonis and Fructus Schisandrae are added.

Since this illness is likely to recur, Pill of Six Mild Drugs with Aucklandiae and Amomi (211) or Decoction of Astragali for Strengthening Middle *Jiao* (267) is recommended for daily administration to invigorate the spleen, benefit *qi* and harmonize the middle *jiao*.

2. *Jue*-Syndrome due to Blood Disorder

(1) Excess syndrome

Clinical manifestations: Sudden falling down, loss of consciousness, lockjaw, flushed face, purple lips, a red or dark purple tongue, and a deep and taut, or an unsmooth pulse.

Analysis: If the patient congenitally has hyperactive liver *yang-qi*, he is likely to get excited. When in a fury, liver *qi* disturbs upward, bringing blood along with it. This blocks the clear cavity and causes sudden falling down, loss of consciousness, and lockjaw. A flushed face, purple lips, a red or dark purple tongue, and a deep and taut, or unsmooth pulse, are signs of *qi* derangement and blood stagnation.

Treatment: To activate blood and *qi* circulation.

Prescription: The main description is Decoction for Removing Blood Stasis (254). In the recipe, Radix Angelicae Sinensis (terminal part), Flos Carthami and Fructus Crataegi activate blood circulation and remove stasis; Radix Linderae, Pericarpium Citri Reticulatae Viride, Radix Aucklandiae and Rhizoma Cyperi promote *qi* circulation and relieve stagnation. In cases with irritation, insomnia and dream-disturbed sleep, Ramulus Uncariae cum Uncis, Concha Haliotidis, Radix Gentianae and Cortex Moutan are added to subdue hyperactive liver *yang* and disperse heat in the liver. If hyperactive liver *yang* is persistent, Fructus Ligustri Lucidi, Fructus Lycii and Concha Margaritifera Usta could be added to nourish *yin* and subdue hyperactive *yang*. If sputum is profuse, Succus Bambusae and Arisaema cum Bile are added. If unconsciousness remains, Pill of Precious Drugs (124) should be administered immediately to restore consciousness.

(2) Deficiency syndrome

Clinical manifestations: Sudden loss of consciousness, pale complexion, pale lips, tremor of the four limbs, sinking of the eyes, open mouth, spontaneous sweating, cold skin, feeble breathing, a pale tongue, and a thready and weak pulse.

Analysis: Excessive blood loss prevents the blood from nourishing the upper part of the body, which causes sudden loss of consciousness, pale complexion, and pale lips. The inability of blood to reach four limbs deprives the tendons of nourishment and produces internal wind, resulting in tremor. Deficiency of *yin* blood and weakness of *qi* lead to the sinking of the eyes, open mouth, sweating, cold skin and feeble breathing. A pale tongue and a thready and weak pulse are signs of *qi* and blood deficiency due to excessive blood loss.

Treatment: To replenish *qi* and blood.

Prescription: Decoction of Ginseng (218) is given immediately, followed by Decoction of Ginseng for Nourishing *Qi* and *Ying* (11). The former replenishes *qi* to control blood. In the latter, Radix Ginseng and Radix Astragali, the main ingredients, replenish *qi* to produce blood; Radix Angelicae Sinensis and Radix Rehmanniae Preparata nourish blood; and Radix Paeoniae Alba and Fructus Schisandrae astringe *yin*. If bleeding is persistent, Colla Corii Asini, Herba Agrimoniae and Cacumen Platycladi are added to check bleeding. In cases of sweating, cold limbs and feeble breathing, Radix Aconiti Lateralis Preparata and Rhizoma Zingiberis are added to warm *yang*. In cases of palpitation and insomnia, Radix Polygalae, Arillus Longan and Semen Ziziphi Spinosae are added to nourish the heart and calm the mind.

3. *Jue*-Syndrome due to Phlegm

Clinical manifestations: Sudden loss of consciousness, gurgling in the throat or vomiting of sputum-like substance, coarse breathing, a white and sticky tongue coating, and a deep and smooth pulse.

Analysis: This illness is likely to be found in patients with retention of phlegm-dampness. Either induced by excessive anger, *qi* goes upward, bringing phlegm along or attack of the body by external pathogenic factors stirs up retained phlegm, which blocks the clear cavity may cause sudden loss of consciousness, gurgling in the throat or vomiting of sputum-like substance. Blockage of the air passage by phlegm leads to coarse breathing. A white and sticky tongue coating and a deep and smooth pulse are signs of internal retention of phlegm-dampness.

Treatment: To circulate *qi* and resolve phlegm.

Prescription: Decoction for Eliminating Phlegm (138) is the main prescription. In the recipe, Pericarpium Citri Reticulatae and Fructus Aurantii Immaturus regulate *qi* and conduct the unhealthy *qi* downward; Rhizoma Pinelliae, Arisaema cum Bile and Poria dry up dampness and eliminate phlegm. In cases of excessive phlegm and *qi*, Fructus Perillae and Semen Sinapis Albae are added to conduct the *qi* downward and resolve phlegm. In cases with yellow and sticky sputum, thirst, constipation, a yellow and sticky tongue coating and a smooth and rapid pulse, Radix Scutellariae, Herba Houttuyniae and Succus Bambusae are added to disperse heat and resolve phlegm. For constipation, Radix et Rhizoma Rhei and Natrii Sulfas Exsiccatus are added, or Pill of Lapis Chloriti Usta for Expelling Phlegm (323) is prescribed to disperse heat, resolve phlegm and reduce fire. To promote restoration of consciousness, Radix Polygalae, Rhizoma Acori Tatarinowii and Radix Curcumae are added.

4. *Jue*-Syndrome due to Voracious Eating

Clinical manifestations: After voracious eating or drinking alcohol, if induced by emotional irritation, the following symptoms will appear, such as sudden loss of consciousness, a feeling of suffocation in the chest, distention and fullness in the epigastrium and abdomen, a thick and sticky tongue coating, and a smooth and forceful pulse.

Analysis: Voracious eating, overdrinking alcohol, and emotional irritation combine to cause food retention in the stomach, which causes stomach *qi* to disturb upward, blocking the clear cavity and thus resulting in loss of consciousness. The unhealthy stomach *qi* disturbs the chest and affects the lung *qi*, therefore, there is a feeling of suffocation in the chest. Retention of food leads to distention and fullness in the epigastrium and abdomen. A thick and sticky tongue coating, and a smooth and forceful pulse indicate food retention and retained turbid *qi*.

Treatment: To harmonize the middle *jiao* and promote digestion.

Prescription: If syncope occurs soon after eating, the method of inducing vomiting could be adopted first to get rid of retained food. Then Magic Powder (210) and Pill for Promoting Digestion (216) are prescribed. In the recipe, Fructus Crataegi, Massa Medicata Fermentata and Semen Raphani digest food; Herba Agastaches, Rhizoma Atractylodis, Cortex Magnoliae Officinalis and Fructus Amomi regulate *qi* and resolve the turbid; and Rhizoma Pinelliae, Pericarpium Citri Reticulatae and Poria harmonize the stomach and resolve dampness. In cases of abdominal distension and constipation, Decoction for Mild Purgation (35) is used to relieve stagnation by inducing defecation. In cases with a white and slippery tongue coating and cold limbs, Radix Aconiti Lateralis Preparata and Rhizoma Zingiberis are added to warm *yang* and disperse cold.

5. *Jue*-Syndrome due to Summer Heat

Clinical manifestations: Before fainting the patient usually complains of dizziness, headache, a feeling of suffocation, feverishness, impeded sweating and flushed face, then he falls down unconsciously, with possible delirium in severe cases. The tongue is red and dry, and the pulse bounding rapidly, or feeble, taut and rapid.

Analysis: Attack of the head by pathogenic summer heat leads to dizziness and headache. Retained summer heat causes a feeling of suffocation, feverishness, impeded sweating and flushed face. Attack of the heart by pathogenic summer heat blocks the clear cavity, thus leading to the sudden loss of consciousness and even delirium. A red and dry tongue and a bounding and rapid pulse indicate the impairment of *yin* by summer heat.

Treatment: To clear away summer heat, benefit *qi*, disperse heat in the heart and restore consciousness.

Prescription: In cases of fainting, Bolus of Calculus Bovis for Clearing Heart-Heat (67) or Purple-Snow Pellet (299) should be taken immediately with cool boiled water to disperse heat in the heart and restore consciousness. Then, White Tiger Decoction with Ginseng (103) or Decoction for Clearing Away Summer-Heat and Benefiting *Qi* (286) is administered to clear away summer heat, reduce fever, benefit *qi* and produce body fluid. In this prescription, Gypsum Fibrosum, Rhizoma Anemarrhenae, Rhizoma Coptidis, Herba Lophatheri, Petiolus Nelumbinis and Exocarpium Citrulli clear away summer heat; and Radix Panacis Quinquefolii, Radix Ophiopogonis, Herba Dendrobii, Fructus Oryzae Sativae and Radix Glycyrrhizae benefit *qi* and produce fluid. Since this illness is often caused by overexposure to the blazing sun in summer, the patient should be moved to a cool and well ventilated place immediately. If fever is severe, well water or ice water could be applied to his body, or an ice bag could be put on his head. If necessary, acupuncture can be used to assist treatment.

In cases of attack by pathogenic summer heat, which causes sweating and prostration of *qi*, with symptoms of dizziness, palpitation, weak limbs, pale complexion, excessive sweating, cold limbs, sudden loss of consciousness, and a soft and rapid pulse, the treatment should focus on benefiting *qi* and checking sweating by administering Decoction of Ginseng, Aconiti Lateralis Preparata, Os Draconis and Concha Ostreae (193). In the recipe, Radix Ginseng replenishes *qi*; Radix Aconiti Lateralis Preparata restores *yang*; and Os Draconis and Concha Ostreae check sweating.

If summer heat damages *yin*, stirring up liver wind, with symptoms of convulsion of the limbs, profuse sweating, thirst, dizziness, nausea and a taut and rapid pulse, the treatment aims to calm liver wind, nourish *yin* and clear away summer heat. Therefore, modified Decoction of Cornu Saigae Tataricae and Ramulus Uncariae cum Uncis (278) is prescribed. In the recipe, Cornu Saigae Tataricae and Ramulus Uncariae cum Uncis, Folium Mori and Flos Chrysanthemi disperse heat, calm liver wind and arrest convulsion; and Radix Rehmanniae, Radix Paeoniae Alba and Radix Glycyrrhizae cool the blood and nourish the liver. To disperse summer heat, Exocarpium Citrulli, Folium Nelumbinis and Gemma Bambusae are added.

Case Studies

Name: Chen Maochu; Sex: Male.

He was caught in a sudden pain in the chest and diaphragm after breakfast. After several cries, he fell down and blacked out. Although his limbs were cold, his body was warm. The pulse on the *chi* position was not palpable, but the pulse on the *cun* and *guan* positions was still strong. The facial color was normal, and there was no gurgling sound in the throat. Apparently the disease was not caused by the attack of wind and cold, or disorder of *qi*. Since the severe pain occurred soon after breakfast, the pathogenesis was retention of food in the cardiac region which prevented *yang-qi* from moving downward. That was why the pulse on *chi* position was not palpable. The treatment was to induce vomiting by drinking a bowl of salty water, which contained 30 g of salt. Large amounts of sputum and food were soon brought up, and the patient regained consciousness.

Explanation: This is a case of *jue*-syndrome due to voracious eating. Retained food in the stomach impairs its function of transportation and transformation, resulting in *qi* blockage and further the *jue*-syndrome. Consciousness can be restored by inducing vomiting.

Name: Chen XX; Sex: Male; Age: 92.

One day, the patient was repairing a pail, squatting. He fell down suddenly when standing up. His son nearby helped him sit on a chair and fed him with salty water. Soon vomiting of sputum-like substance and incontinence of feces occurred at the same time, indicating a critical condition. The patient was sent to hospital immediately.

On his first visit, the clinical manifestations were cyanosis of lips, pale complexion, a slightly red tongue, shortness of breath, incontinence, feeble pulse on the right side and feeble, thready and interrupted pulse on the left side, cold limbs and nose. Only the forehead was warm.

Due to old age, yang-qi was insufficient already, if added by overwork, the primordial qi would sink, resulting in the collapse of kidney yang. Fortunately, there was no sweat on his head. Treatment aimed to consolidate kidney yang with large doses of Aconiti Lateralis Preparata and Cinnamomi Decoction, which regulates the middle jiao:

Radix Codonopsis	15 g;
Rhizoma Atractylodis Macrocephalae Preparata	9 g;
Rhizoma Zingiberis Preparata	9 g;
Radix Glycyrrhizae Preparata	4.5 g;
Radix Aconiti Lateralis Preparata	9 g;
Cortex Cinnamomi	3 g;
Rhizoma Zingiberis Recens	3 g;
Fructus Jujubae	5 pieces.

The drugs were taken every two hours, and three times a day.

Second visit: On the next morning, the pulse became smooth, long and forceful in all positions. The hands and feet became warm, and the bowel movements were under control. The patient was calm, and could manage to sit and eat a little. Drugs for invigorating the stomach were then prescribed:

Radix Codonopsis	9 g;
Rhizoma Atractylodis Macrocephalae	9 g;
Rhizoma Zingiberis Preparata	6 g;
Radix Glycyrrhizae Preparata	3 g;
Rhizoma Dioscoreae Preparata	15 g;
Rhizoma Zingiberis Recens	3 g;
Fructus Jujubae	3 pieces.

These drugs were taken three times a day.

Explanation: Due to the qi deficiency of elderly people and overwork, the disorder of qi occurs, causing the sinking of primordial qi, preventing the clear yang from being distributed. Consequently, the wandering of the mind occurs, which results in prostration. If classified according to the jue-syndrome, this case is a jue-syndrome of the deficiency type. If the patient had been allowed to lie down and rest quietly soon after fainting, and treated with warming and tonic drugs, he would have recovered consciousness. However, he was made to sit in a chair and vomit. This further damaged the body's anti-pathogenic qi, making the condition even more critical. With such an illness, attention must be paid to adopt the proper treatment.

XIV. Stagnation Syndrome

Stagnation syndrome refers to pathological conditions resulting from emotional upsets and *qi* stagnation. The main clinical manifestations include mental depression, restlessness, distention and pain in the costal and hypochondriac region, proneness to anger and cry, feeling of a foreign body in the throat, and insomnia.

According to *Danxi's Experience on Medicine*, no disease occurs if *qi* and blood are in harmony. But if one is perplexed by emotional upsets, various diseases will occur. Thus almost all diseases result from stagnation due to emotional upsets. There are six kinds of stagnation syndrome: *qi*, blood, dampness, phlegm, heat and food stagnation, with *qi* stagnation being the inducing factor. This chapter will mainly discuss the stagnation syndrome caused by emotional upsets, as well as the cause and treatment of *qi* stagnation.

Neurasthenia, hysteria and climacteric syndrome in Western medicine belong to this category of stagnation syndrome.

Etiology and Pathogenesis

Emotional upsets and liver *qi*-stagnation lead to the disharmony of *qi* in the five *zang* organs, resulting in stagnation syndrome. However, the main cause is the disharmony of *qi* and blood caused by the impairment of the liver, spleen, and heart.

Mental depression or anger impairs the function of the liver in regulating the flow of *qi*, and thus liver *qi*-stagnation occurs. Stagnant liver *qi* gradually turns into fire, or causes blood stagnation. If the spleen is affected by the liver *qi*-stagnation, added by anxiety or strain and stress, it cannot transport normally, thus producing dampness and phlegm. Retained dampness, food, and heat transformed from damp phlegm can all develop into dampness, food, and heat stagnation.

Stagnant liver *qi* due to emotional upsets consumes heart *qi* and blood, and thereby the heart is deprived of nourishment and fails to house the mind. When the spleen is affected by liver *qi*, appetite will be poor, resulting in *qi* and blood deficiency and further the deficiency of both the heart and spleen. Stagnant liver *qi* gradually turns into fire, which consumes *yin* blood and affects the kidneys, resulting in hyperactivity of fire due to *yin* deficiency. Consequently, various consumptive symptoms will occur.

Stagnation syndrome at the early stage, which is usually caused by stagnation of *qi* complicated by retention of damp phlegm, food and heat, is mostly of the excess type. But chronic cases change from the excess to the deficiency type, such as the malfunctioning of the heart, deficiency of both the heart and spleen, and hyperactivity of fire due to *yin* deficiency.

Distinction and Treatment

In the early stage of stagnation syndrome, with manifestations of mental depression, listlessness, stuffiness in the chest, hypochondriac pain, sighing and poor appetite, the treatment concentrates on soothing the liver and regulating *qi*. This method bears important meaning in preventing the illness from deterioration. If the proper treatment has not been applied in time, and the five *zang* organs are affected, the therapy can only be decided after analyzing the stagnation syndrome together with other accompanied symptoms. The analysis should focus on whether the illness belongs to *qi* or blood, cold or heat, deficiency or excess type, as well as to which organ the illness relate.

1. Excess Syndromes

(1) Stagnation of liver *qi*

Clinical manifestations: Mental depression, restlessness, sighing, distention and wandering pain in the costal and hypochondriac region, distress in the epigastrium, abdominal distention, poor appetite, or vomiting, irregular bowel movements, amenorrhea, a thin and sticky tongue coating, and a taut pulse.

Analysis: Emotional upsets impair the liver's function of regulating the flow of *qi*, resulting in mental depression and restlessness. Since the Liver Meridian passes through the lower abdomen, stomach, costal and hypochondriac region, stagnation of liver *qi* and blood produces abdominal distention, stuffiness in the chest, hypochondriac pain and amenorrhea. Invasion of the stomach by liver *qi* results in the disturbance of its descending function, therefore the distress in the epigastrium, poor appetite and vomiting occur. Invasion of the spleen by liver *qi* explains abdominal distention and irregular bowel movements. A thin and sticky tongue coating and a taut pulse indicate the disharmony between the liver and stomach.

Treatment: To soothe the liver, regulate *qi* and relieve stagnation.

Prescription: Modified Powder of Bupleuri for Releasing Stagnant Liver-*Qi* (239). In the recipe, Radix Bupleuri, Fructus Aurantii and Rhizoma Cyperi release the liver, promote *qi* circulation and relieve stagnation; Pericarpium Citri Reticulatae regulates *qi* flow and harmonizes the middle *jiao*; and Rhizoma Chuanxiong, Radix Paeoniae Alba and Radix Glycyrrhizae activate blood circulation, remove blood stasis and relieve pain. Radix Curcumae and Pericarpium Citri Reticulatae Viride are added to help relieve stagnation. Since liver *qi*-stagnation is the root cause of other five kinds of stagnation, *Yueju* Pill (Additional Formulae) is administered along with the above prescription. *Qi* circulation leads blood to circulate, and also resolves phlegm, heat, dampness and retained food. In cases of frequent belching and a distressed sensation in the chest and hypochondrium, Flos Inulae, Haematitum and Pericarpium Citri Reticulatae are added to calm the liver and conduct the unhealthy *qi* downward. In cases of food retention complicated by abdominal distention, Massa Medicata Fermentata, Fructus Crataegi and Endothelium Corneum Gigeriae Galli are added to digest food and relieve stagnation. In cases of *qi* and blood stagnation with a fixed pain in the costal and hypochondriac region, amenorrhea and a taut and unsmooth pulse, Radix Angelicae Sinensis, Radix Salviae Miltiorrhizae, Semen Persicae and Flos Carthami are added to activate blood circulation and remove stasis.

(2) Stagnation of *qi* turning into fire

Clinical manifestations: Irritability, stuffiness in the chest, hypochondriac distention, an uncomfortable and empty sensation in the stomach, acid regurgitation, dry and bitter mouth, constipation, or headache, red eyes, tinnitus, a red tongue with yellow coating, and a taut and rapid pulse.

Analysis: Stagnant *qi* turns into fire, which moves upward along the Liver Meridian, thus headache, red eyes, and tinnitus occur. Invasion of the stomach by liver fire leads to dry and bitter mouth, constipation and irritability. A red tongue with yellow coating, and a taut and rapid pulse are signs of hyperactivity of the liver fire.

Treatment: To disperse heat in the liver, reduce fire, relieve stagnation and harmonize the stomach.

Prescription: *Xiaoyao* Powder with Moutan and Gardeniae (63) combined with *Zuojin* Pill (81). The former soothes the liver, relieves stagnation and disperses heat, while the latter reduces fire in the liver and harmonizes the stomach. In cases of a bitter taste in the mouth, a yellow tongue coating and constipation, Radix Gentianae and Radix et Rhizoma Rhei are added to reduce fire and relieve constipation.

(3) Stagnation of *qi* complicated by retention of phlegm

Clinical manifestations: Feeling a foreign body in the throat, which cannot be relieved by spitting or swallowing, suffocation in the chest, or hypochondriac pain, a white and sticky tongue coating, and a taut and smooth pulse.

Analysis: Invasion of the spleen by liver qi impairs the splenic function in transportation and transformation, and thus produces dampness and phlegm. Retention of phlegm and qi in the upper chest causes the feeling of a foreign body in the throat, which is also called "plum-stone qi." Hindrance of qi causes a feeling of suffocation in the chest. Since the Liver Meridian passes through the hypochondrium, liver qi-stagnation results in hypochondriac pain. A white and sticky tongue coating and a taut and smooth pulse are signs of liver qi-stagnation complicated by retention of damp phlegm.

Treatment: To resolve phlegm, benefit qi and relieve stagnation.

Prescription: Modified Decoction of Pinelliae and Magnoliae Officinalis (107). In the recipe, Rhizoma Pinelliae, Cortex Magnoliae Officinalis and Poria conduct the unhealthy qi downward and resolve phlegm; Folium Perillae and Rhizoma Zingiberis Recens benefit qi and disperse stagnation. To strengthen these effects, a proper amount of Rhizoma Cyperi Preparata, Fructus Aurantii, Fructus Citri Sarcodactylis, Flos Inulae and Haematitum is added. In cases of phlegm-heat retention with symptoms of nausea, vomiting, a bitter taste in the mouth, and a yellow and sticky tongue coating, Decoction for Clearing Away Gallbladder-Heat (302) is prescribed along with Radix Scutellariae, Bulbus Fritillariae Cirrhosae, and Pericarpium Trichosanthis to resolve phlegm, disperse heat and benefit qi.

2. Deficiency Syndromes

(1) Damage of the mind due to melancholia

Clinical manifestations: Absent-mindedness, restlessness, grief, proneness to weeping, frequent yawning, a pale tongue with thin and white coating, and a taut and thready pulse.

Analysis: Persistent melancholia consumes heart qi and nutrient blood, and thus the heart and mind are deprived of nourishment, resulting in absent-mindedness and restlessness. This is called hysteria in *Synopsis of Prescriptions of the Golden Chamber*, and often found in women. A pale tongue with thin and white coating, and a taut and thready pulse are signs of blood deficiency and qi stagnation.

Treatment: To nourish the heart and calm the mind.

Prescription: Decoction of Glycyrrhizae, Tritici Levis and Jujubae (84) with additional drugs. In the recipe, Radix Glycyrrhizae and Fructus Jujubae relieve acute symptoms; Fructus Tritici Levis nourishes heart qi and calms the mind. The additional Semen Platycladi, Semen Ziziphi Spinosae, Lignum Pini Poriaferum and Flos Albiziae strengthen potency.

(2) Deficiency of heart and spleen

Clinical manifestations: Anxiety and worry, palpitation, timidity, insomnia, poor memory, pale complexion, dizziness, lassitude, poor appetite, a pale tongue, and a thready and weak pulse.

Analysis: Deficiency of both the heart and spleen due to excessive worry leads to cardiac malnutrition, thus palpitation, timidity, insomnia and poor memory occur. Since the spleen and stomach are the source of qi and blood, splenic deficiency causes pale complexion, dizziness, lassitude, a pale tongue and a thready and weak pulse.

Treatment: To invigorate the spleen, nourish the heart, and replenish qi and blood.

Prescription: Modified Decoction for Invigorating Spleen and Nourishing Heart (110). This prescription is a combination of Decoction of Four Mild Drugs (91) and Decoction of Angelicae Sinensis for Enriching Blood (131) with some other drugs. The former replenishes qi and invigorates the spleen. When the spleen and stomach function well, qi and blood will be sufficient. The latter consists of Radix Angelicae Sinensis and Radix Astragali, which are effective in replenishing qi and producing blood. Semen Ziziphi Spinosae, Radix Polygalae and Arillus Longan nourish the heart and spleen, calm the mind and stabilize emotions. Radix Aucklandiae regulates qi flow and strengthens the spleen, nourishing it without causing stagnation. A proper amount of Radix Curcumae and Flos Albiziae is added to relieve stagnation and calm the mind. Since *yin* develops as *yang* grows, and blood flourishes if *qi* is sufficient, the heart will eventually receive sufficient nourishment.

(3) Deficiency of *yin* and hyperactivity of fire

Clinical manifestations: Dizziness, palpitation, insomnia, restlessness, irritability, or nocturnal emission, lumbar soreness, irregular menstruation, a red tongue, and a taut, thready and rapid pulse.

Analysis: Deficiency of *yin* leads to the upward floating of *yang* in deficiency, with symptoms of dizziness and irritability. Consumption of *yin* blood deprives the heart of nourishment, resulting in heat produced by *yin* deficiency. The heat disturbs the mind and causes palpitation, insomnia and restlessness. Renal *yin*-deficiency deprives the lumbar region of nourishment, thus causes lumbar soreness. Hyperactivity of fire due to *yin* deficiency disturbs the residence of essence, and thus nocturnal emission occurs. Malnutrition of the liver and kidneys impairs the function of the *Chong* and *Ren* meridians (vessels), thus causing irregular menstruation. A red tongue, and a taut, thready and rapid pulse all indicate fire caused by *yin* deficiency.

Treatment: To nourish *yin*, disperse heat, soothe the heart and calm the mind.

Prescription: Modified Decoction for Nourishing Fluid and Clearing Away Liver-Heat (303). In the recipe, Pill of Six Drugs Containing Rehmanniae Preparata (56) replenishes *yin*, nourishes the kidneys, and strengthens fluid to control fire; Radix Bupleuri, Fructus Gardeniae and Cortex Moutan reduce fire in the liver. The addition of Concha Margaritifera Usta, Magnetitum and Iron Scale soothes the heart and calms the mind. In cases of lumbar soreness, nocturnal emission and lassitude, Carapax et Plastrum Testudinis, Rhizoma Anemarrhenae, Cortex Eucommiae and Concha Ostreae are added to strengthen the kidneys and consolidate essence. In cases of irregular menstruation, Rhizoma Cyperi and Herba Leonuri are added to regulate *qi*, relieve stagnation and normalize menstruation.

Remarks

Drugs that regulate *qi* should be used with caution in treating chronic cases with consumption of *yin* blood, because most of these drugs are dry and aromatic in nature. Since Fructus Citri and Fructus Citri Sarcodactylis are mild in nature, regulating the flow of *qi* without consuming *yin*, they can be used for either acute or protracted illness.

It is very important to apply psychotherapy while using medicine. If the patient can do some physical exercises, such as *qigong* and *taijiquan*, the therapeutic effect will be even better.

Case Studies

Name: Li XX; Sex: Female; Age: 48; Occupation: Worker.

First visit (May 17, 1975): During recent years, the patient suffered persistent headache, with nausea in severe cases. Other manifestations included mental depression, irritability, suspiciousness, trance, auditory hallucination, grief, weeping, insomnia, nightmare, tinnitus, dizziness, lumbar soreness, profuse leucorrhea, lassitude, pale complexion, a thin and sticky tongue coating, and a thready and rapid pulse. She had taken sedatives for a long time without conspicuous effect. The above symptoms were caused by the consumption of heart *qi* due to anxiety and worry, added by liver *qi*-stagnation and upward disturbance of liver wind and *yang*. Treatment aimed to nourish the heart and calm the mind, soothe the liver and relieve stagnation:

Radix Glycyrrhizae Preparata	9 g;
Fructus Tritici Levis	30 g;
Fructus Jujubae	5 pieces;

Radix Curcumae	9 g;
Rhizoma Acori Tatarinowii	9 g;
Arisaema cum Bile	9 g;
Iron Scale (decocted first)	60 g;
Caulis Polygoni Multiflori	30 g;
Tablet of Scorpio and Scolopendra (three tablets each time; swallow with water)	6 tablets.

Seven doses were prescribed.

Second visit (May 24, 1975): Menstruation arrived with less severe headache and auditory hallucination. Other symptoms remained the same, and she was still impetuous. She suffered frequent, urgent and painful urination. Urinalysis showed white blood cells full of visual field. Since Furadantin caused discomfort in her stomach, she had stopped taking it. The new prescription was based on the previous one, with Fructus Jujubae and Rhizoma Acori Tatarinowii removed from it and 12 g of Radix Scutellariae and 12 g of Rhizoma Anemarrhenae added. Another seven doses were prescribed.

Third visit (May 31, 1975): Recently, headache did not appear in the morning, and was mild in the afternoon. The condition of insomnia and irritability improved and the frequency of urination had reduced. However, the auditory hallucination still existed. The same treatment was adopted:

Radix Glycyrrhizae Preparata	9 g;
Fructus Tritici Levis	30 g;
Fructus Jujubae	5 pieces;
Radix Curcumae	9 g;
Radix Salviae Miltiorrhizae	9 g;
Rhizoma Anemarrhenae	15 g;
Iron Scale (decocted first)	60 g;
Caulis Polygoni Multiflori	30 g;
Tablet of Scorpio and Scolopendra (three tablets each time; swallow with water)	6 tablets.

Seven doses were prescribed.

Fourth visit (June 7, 1975): Menstruation arrived with mild headache in the afternoon. She had sound sleep at night, and an one-hour sleep at noon. The state of auditory hallucination improved. The tongue coating was thin and sticky and the pulse was thready. The same treatment continued:

Radix Glycyrrhizae Preparata	9 g;
Fructus Tritici Levis	30 g;
Fructus Jujubae	5 pieces;
Radix Curcumae	9 g;
Rhizoma Acori Tatarinowii	9 g;
Iron Scale (decocted first)	60 g;
Radix Salviae Miltiorrhizae	9 g;
Caulis Polygoni Multiflori	30 g.

Seven doses were prescribed.

In addition, 100 tablets of Angelicae Dahuricae Tablet were also prescribed (five tablets each time, three times a day, and swallow with water). Each tablet contains 0.3 g of powdered Radix Angelicae Dahuricae.

Fifth visit (June 14, 1975): The patient could sleep well but had dreams. A mild headache occurred when feeling fatigue. Other symptoms were pale complexion, thready pulse, and red tongue. The same drugs were prescribed with Rhizoma Acori Tatarinowii removed from it, and 9 g of Radix Paeoniae Alba added. Seven doses were prescribed.

Sixth visit (June 21, 1975): In the recent week, mild headache only occurred on the previous day. The patient could sleep well for more than nine hours at noon and night. The symptoms of irritability and dreams lessened. Auditory hallucination only occurred when it was quiet and she was cheerful. Other symptoms were thready pulse and thin and sticky tongue coating. Drugs that replenish *qi* and blood were added to the prescription:

Radix Glycyrrhizae Preparata	9 g;
Fructus Tritici Levis	30 g;
Fructus Jujubae	5 pieces;
Radix Codonopsis	9 g;
Rhizoma Atractylodis Macrocephalae	9 g;
Radix Paeoniae Alba	9 g;
Radix Salviae Miltiorrhizae	9 g;
Radix Polygalae Preparata	4.5 g.

Seven doses were prescribed.

Explanation: This case was diagnosed as schizophrenia in another hospital, but the sedatives proved invalid. According to traditional Chinese medicine, this is a case of "hysteria". Mental depression and excessive worry consume heart *qi* and cause *yin* deficiency of the *zang* organs. Therefore, Fructus Tritici Levis is used to nourish heart *qi*. Radix Glycyrrhizae and Fructus Jujubae relieve acute symptoms with their sweet nature. Caulis Polygoni Multiflori, Arisaema cum Bile, Rhizoma Acori Tatarinowii and Radix Curcumae calm the mind, restore consciousness and relieve stagnation. Iron Scale and Tablet of Scorpio and Scolopendra calm liver wind and relieve pain. The addition of Radix Scutellariae and Rhizoma Anemarrhenae in the second prescription disperses heat and resolves dampness, treating urinary infection. All symptoms remarkably improved after a month of treatment.

XV. Manic-Depressive Syndrome

Psychosis in traditional Chinese medicine includes manic and depressive syndromes. The depressive syndrome is characterized by reticence, mental dullness, incoherent speech, silent and happy; while the manic is characterized by shouting, restlessness, irritability, and violent behavior. Since the two syndromes cannot be separated clearly, and they may transform into one another, they are usually called manic-depressive syndrome, which is often found in young and middle-aged people.

As early as in *The Inner Canon of the Yellow Emperor*, there is systematic description of the etiology, pathogenesis and treatment of manic-depressive syndrome. For instance, it says, "Various kinds of irritability and insanity belong to fire." Also in this book, the Yellow Emperor asked, "What causes insanity?" Qi Bo replied, "It is caused by disorders of *yang*." The Yellow Emperor asked, "How to treat it?" Qi Bo replied, "It can be treated simply by stopping eating. Let the patient take Decoction of Iron Scale."

Liu Hejian, a physician of the Jin and Yuan dynasties, held that "Hyperactivity of heart fire and deficiency of kidney *yang* destroy emotional stability and thus cause insanity." According to *Danxi's Experience on Medicine*, the depressive state belongs to *yin*, while the manic state belongs to *yang*; usually the two syndromes are caused by retention of phlegm in the chest and heart. It put forward a theory that the manic-depressive syndrome is related with phlegm, which greatly influenced physicians at that time, and established a theoretical basis for the therapy of inducing vomiting to treat manic-depressive syndrome, greatly benefiting the later generations.

Wang Qingren of the Qing Dynasty initiated the theory of stagnant blood. He said, "Manic-depressive syndrome manifesting as persistent weeping, laughing, scolding and singing ... is due to *qi* and blood stagnation, which prevents the *qi* in the brain from linking with the *qi* of the *zang-fu* organs. Thus the patient behaves as if he were in a dream." Since it is caused by *qi* and blood stagnation, the treatment aims to promote blood flow and eliminate blood stasis.

Psychosis in Western medicine, such as schizophrenia, symptomatic psychosis and reactive psychosis, can be differentiated and treated according to the following descriptions.

Etiology and Pathogenesis
1. Emotional Upsets

This is the main cause of manic-depressive syndrome. Failing to realize personal ambition and anxiety can all damage the heart and spleen. Cardiac deficiency prevents the heart from housing the mind, and splenic deficiency influences its function of producing *qi* and blood, which deprives the heart of nourishment, resulting in the wandering of the mind. Upward movement of stagnant liver *qi* due to mental depression disturbs the mind, resulting in depressive syndrome which belongs to *yin* in nature and is characterized by quietness. Excessive anger, on the other hand, damages the liver and turns stagnant liver *qi* into fire, thus causing the hyperactivity of liver and gallbladder fire. Changeable moods consume heart *yin* and thereby cause abrupt hyperactivity of heart fire. Fire of both the liver and heart may disturb the mind, causing the manic state which belongs to *yang* and is characterized by violent behavior.

2. Upward Disturbance of Phlegm-Fire

Attack of the spleen by stagnant liver *qi* impairs its function of transportation and transformation, and thus producing turbid phlegm. Stagnant liver *qi* brings phlegm along and disturbs the mind, blocking the clear cavity of the heart. Stagnant liver *qi* can also turn into fire, attacking the stomach. Heated by the fire, stomach fluid is condensed into phlegm-fire, which goes upward and disturbs the mind, resulting in confusion of the mind and further the manic-depressive syndrome.

3. Stagnation of *Qi* and Blood

Qi and blood stagnation blocks the meridians and collaterals, and prevents *qi* in the brain from connecting with *qi* of the *zang-fu* organs, resulting in manic-depressive syndrome.

Generally speaking, manic-depressive syndrome is caused by emotional upsets, the upward disturbance of phlegm, and the stagnation of *qi* and blood. These factors are inter-related, for instance, the combination of phlegm and stagnant liver *qi* forms phlegm *qi*; phlegm and fire of both the liver and gallbladder form phlegm-fire; excessive worry damages the heart and spleen, thus producing turbid phlegm; long-standing *qi* stagnation leads to blood stagnation. Long-standing excessive fire consumes *qi* and *yin*, resulting in weak body-resistance.

Heredity and constitution also play an important role in the manic-depressive syndrome.

Differential Diagnosis

Manic-depressive syndrome should be differentiated from epilepsy.

Epilepsy is a paroxysmal mental disorder characterized by falling down in a fit, loss of consciousness, convulsion, staring upward, and screaming like animals, while the patient behaves normally after the seizure.

Manic-depressive syndrome refers to mental disorders, manifesting as either reticence, dullness and incoherent speech, or irritability, restlessness and violent behavior.

Distinction and Treatment

The causes of manic-depressive syndrome are stagnation of *qi*, phlegm-heat, and the imbalance between the *yin* and *yang*; the diseased organs are the liver, gallbladder, heart and spleen. Clinically, attention should be paid first to the distinction of manic and depressive states. The depressive syndrome is treated by soothing the liver, regulating *qi*, resolving phlegm, restoring consciousness, nourishing blood, calming the mind and replenishing the heart and spleen. While the manic syndrome is treated by soothing the heart, eliminating phlegm and reducing liver fire, or nourishing *yin*, reducing fire and calming the mind. Although the two syndromes are clinically different, they are interchangeable. Manic-depressive syndrome at the initial stage usually belongs to the excess type, and is treated by dispersing heat, eliminating phlegm, soothing the liver, regulating *qi* and calming the mind. In protracted cases, since the body-resistance is weak, the treatment should base on the different state of *qi*, blood, *yin*, and *yang* deficiency, invigorating the spleen, benefiting *qi*, nourishing *yin* and replenishing blood. If there is blood stagnation, treatment aims to activate blood circulation and remove blood stasis.

1. Depressive State

(1) Stagnation of phlegm *qi*

Clinical manifestations: Mental depression, indifference, dullness, incoherent speech or muttering to oneself, changeable moods, poor appetite, a sticky tongue coating, and a taut and smooth pulse.

Analysis: Excess worry or failing to achieve personal ambition leads to liver *qi*-stagnation and prevents spleen *qi* from ascending. Consequently, the stagnant phlegm *qi* blocks the mind, manifesting as indifference and dullness. Retention of turbid phlegm in the middle *jiao* leads to poor appetite, a sticky tongue coating, and a taut and smooth pulse.

Treatment: To regulate *qi*, relieve stagnation, resolve phlegm and restore consciousness.

Prescription: Decoction for Promoting Smooth Circulation of *Qi* and Eliminating Phlegm (214) with Radix Polygalae, Radix Curcumae and Rhizoma Acori Tatarinowii. In the recipe, Rhizoma Pinelliae, Pericarpium Citri Reticulatae, Arisaema cum Bile and Poria benefit *qi* and resolve phlegm; Rhizoma Cyperi, Radix Aucklandiae and Rhizoma Acori Tatarinowii relieve stagnation and restore consciousness. Pill for Treating Phlegm-Syndrome (270) can be used in severe cases to eliminate turbid phlegm in the chest and diaphragm. For patients with strong constitution, who manifest symptoms such as excessive turbid phlegm, fullness in the chest and diaphragm, profuse phlegm-fluid, and a smooth, large and forceful pulse, Powder of Three Holy Ingredients (17) can be administered temporarily to purge phlegm-fluid by vomiting. Since the property of the drug is rather strong, it should be used with caution. After vomiting, the patient will be very tired, nutritious diet is recommended for his recuperation. The following symptoms, mental perplexity and dullness, incoherent speech, staring upward and a white and sticky tongue coating, indicate the mental confusion caused by phlegm. The treatment aims to eliminate phlegm, restore consciousness, regulate *qi* and disperse masses. Bolus of Styrax (143), aromatic in nature, can be administered first to restore consciousness; then Decoction of Magnoliae Officinalis and Pinelliae (88) added with Arisaema cum Bile, Radix Curcumae, Rhizoma Acori Tatarinowii and Radix Polygalae can be administered to resolve phlegm and circulate *qi*. Symptoms such as insomnia, susceptibility to fright, restlessness, a red tongue with yellow coating, and a smooth and rapid pulse are caused by the upward disturbance of phlegm and heat. Therefore, Decoction for Clearing Away Gallbladder-Heat (302) with Rhizoma Coptidis, and Pill of Alumen and Curcumae (102) are recommended to disperse heat and resolve phlegm. In cases with mental confusion, Pill of Precious Drugs (124) is prescribed to disperse cardiac heat and restore consciousness. If the patient starts shouting and smashing, that indicates the depressive syndrome characterized by hyperactivity of fire.

(2) Heart and spleen deficiency

Clinical manifestations: Absent-mindedness, dream-disturbed sleep, palpitation, fright, grief, weeping, lassitude, poor appetite, a pale tongue, and a thready and weak pulse.

Analysis: Prolonged depressive state consumes heart blood and deprives the heart of nourishment, resulting in palpitation, fright, absent-mindedness, grief and weeping. Splenic deficiency impairs its function of transportation and transformation, poor appetite and lassitude thus appear. A pale tongue and a thready and weak pulse are signs of *qi* and blood deficiency due to the deficiency of the heart and spleen.

Treatment: To invigorate the spleen, nourish the heart, replenish *qi* and calm the mind.

Prescription: The prescription is based on Decoction for Nourishing Heart (208) and Decoction of Glycyrrhizae, Tritici Levis and Jujubae (84). In the recipe, Radix Ginseng, Radix Astragali, Radix Glycyrrhizae and Fructus Jujubae replenish spleen *qi*; Rhizoma Chuanxiong and Radix Angelicae Sinensis nourish heart blood; Poria, Radix Polygalae, Semen Platycladi, Semen Ziziphi Spinosae, Fructus Schisandrae and Fructus Tritici Levis nourish the heart and calm the mind; and Cortex Cinnamomi conducts the efficacy of drugs to the heart to nourish it and calm the mind.

2. Manic State

(1) Upward disturbance of phlegm-fire

Clinical manifestations: The illness suddenly occurs with symptoms like irritability, headache, insomnia, staring angrily, flushed face and red eyes. Then violent behavior will follow, such as climbing over walls and houses, shouting, smashing, hitting people, refusing to eat and sleep. The tongue of the patient is crimson with yellow and sticky coating, and the pulse is taut, large, smooth and rapid.

Analysis: Excess anger damages the liver and causes abrupt hyperactivity of liver fire; liver fire agitates phlegm-heat in the *Yangming* meridians, going upward and disturbing the mind. Consequently, irritability, headache, insomnia and violent behavior will follow. As the limbs are related to *yang*, sufficient *yang* would strengthen limbs, thus the patient is strong and could climb over walls and houses. Disturbance of the head by hyperactive liver fire leads to headache, flushed face and red eyes. A crimson tongue with yellow coating and a taut, large, smooth and rapid pulse are signs of excessive phlegm-fire and *yang-qi*. Fire belongs to *yang* and *yang* influences human behavior, thus the illness is acute and the patient behaves violently.

Treatment: To soothe the heart, eliminate phlegm, reduce fire and disperse heat in the liver.

Prescription: Decoction of Iron Scale (97) is the main prescription. In the recipe, Iron Scale soothes the heart and conducts the fire downward; Arisaema cum Bile, Bulbus Fritillariae Cirrhosae and Exocarpium Citri Rubrum disperse heat and eliminate phlegm; Rhizoma Acori Tatarinowii, Radix Polygalae, Lignum Pini Poriaferum and Cinnabaris restore consciousness and calm the mind; and Radix Asparagi and Radix Ophiopogonis, Radix Scrophulariae and Fructus Forsythiae nourish *yin* and disperse heat. In cases with excessive phlegm-fire, extremely yellow and sticky tongue coating, the above formula should be combined with Pill of Lapis Chloriti Usta for Expelling Phlegm (323) to reduce fire and eliminate phlegm; then Bolus of Calculus Bovis for Resurrection (127) could be used to disperse heat in the heart and promote the restoration of consciousness. In cases of hyperactive liver and gallbladder fire with a taut and forceful pulse, Pill of Angelicae Sinensis, Gentianae and Aloe (130) is prescribed.

In cases of excessive *Yangming* fire with symptoms of constipation, a yellow and coarse tongue coating, and a large and forceful pulse, Decoction for Purgation with Modification (113) is prescribed to reduce fire of the excess type in the stomach and intestines. To relieve restlessness and thirst, Gypsum Fibrosum and Rhizoma Anemarrhenae are added to disperse heat. In severe cases, a proper amount of *Longhu* Pill (77) is prescribed to remove phlegm-fire. Since the drugs may cause vomiting and diarrhea, it is not advisable to take large dosages for a long time for fear of damaging the stomach and intestines. If the mind is clear, but phlegm-heat, restlessness and insomnia still exist, Decoction for Clearing Away Gallbladder-Heat (302) and Pill of Cinnabaris for Tranquilizing (134) are prescribed at the same time to resolve phlegm and calm the mind. If the fire is getting weaker but turbid phlegm remains, manifesting a depressive state characterized by mental confusion, the treatment should focus on the depressive syndrome.

(2) Consumption of *yin* by hyperactive fire

Clinical manifestations: The manic state will gradually lessen, followed by lassitude, garrulousness, susceptibility to fright, occasional irritability, emaciation, flushed face, a red tongue, and a thready and rapid pulse.

Analysis: Prolonged manic state consumes *yin* and *qi*. The patient fatigues easily due to the *qi* deficiency; *yin* deficiency produces fire, causing restlessness, irritability, emaciation, flushed face and a red tongue. If malnutrition of the heart is added by disturbance of deficiency fire, then garrulousness and fragility to fright will follow. A thready and rapid pulse also indicates heat produced by *yin* deficiency.

Treatment: To nourish *yin*, reduce fire, calm the mind and stabilize emotion.

Prescription: *Eryin* Decoction (4). In the recipe, Radix Rehmanniae, Radix Ophiopogonis and Radix Scrophulariae nourish *yin* and disperse heat; Rhizoma Coptidis, Caulis Aristolochiae Manshuriensis, Herba Lophatheri and Medulla Junci disperse heat in the heart and calm the mind; and Lignum Pini Poriaferum, Semen Ziziphi Spinosae and Radix Glycyrrhizae nourish the heart and calm the mind. Pill for Stabilizing Emotion (177) can be used in combination.

In cases of manic-depressive syndrome, there often exists blood stagnation, accompanied by sallow complexion, dark purple tongue, purple sublingual veins and a deep and unsmooth pulse. For such cases, treatment should focus on activating blood circulation and removing blood stasis by using Decoction for Removing Blood Stasis in the Chest (135) or modified Decoction for Relieving Manic-Depressive Syndromes (326). Recommended drugs include Radix Angelicae Sinensis, Radix Paeoniae Rubra, Semen Persicae, Flos Carthami, Rhizoma Chuanxiong and Radix Bupleuri.

Remarks

Besides taking medicine, the patient should live a regular life, and pay attention to diet; if necessary, psychotherapy or safety attendance should be applied to avoid emergency.

Case Studies

Name: Liu XX; Sex: Male; Age: 54; Occupation: Worker.

First visit (October 28, 1963): The diagnosis of psychosis was established six months ago. The symptoms included mental depression, insomnia, uncontrollable delusion, palpitation, persistent restlessness, dullness, muttering to himself, and no response to inquiries.

Upon arrival at the hospital, the patient kept complaining of family trivia in a confusing manner. Other symptoms included mild shortness of breath, constipation (having bowel movement every three to four days), scanty urine, a red tongue tip with thick, white and sticky coating, and a smooth, thready and rapid pulse.

The disease was due to *qi* and phlegm stagnation, which blocks the clear cavity. Treatment aimed to relieve stagnation, resolve phlegm, restore consciousness and calm the mind. The following herbs were prescribed:

Exocarpium Citri Rubrum	6 g;
Rhizoma Pinelliae Preparata	9 g;
Poria	12 g;
Radix Glycyrrhizae	3 g;
Caulis Bambusae in Taeniam	9 g;
Fructus Aurantii	6 g;
Fructus Oryzae Glutinosae	15 g;
Radix Curcumae	6 g;
Fructus Trichosanthis	3 g.

Two doses were prescribed, added with two pills of Bolus of Styrax (one bolus each time).

Second visit (November 1, 1963): Mental dullness disappeared after taking the medicine. The patient was calm, and could sleep well. He started conversation himself. The bowel movement was normal. Other symptoms were slightly red tongue with white and thin coating, and deep, thready and smooth pulse. Three grams of Rhizoma Coptidis were added to the previous prescription. Twelve doses were prescribed.

Third visit: The symptoms were normal mental state, slightly dry stool, white, thick and slightly yellowish tongue coating, smooth and rapid pulse. All symptoms suggested that dampness-heat remained at *Yangming* meridians. To prevent relapse, the following drugs were prescribed to relieve dampness:

Fructus Aurantii Immaturus	9 g;
Cortex Magnoliae Officinalis	6 g;
Radix et Rhizoma Rhei	4.5 g;
Rhizoma Coptidis	3 g;

Radix Scutellariae	6 g;
Rhizoma Pinelliae	6 g;
Rhizoma Zingiberis	3 g;
Fructus Trichosanthis	24 g;
Radix Curcumae	6 g;
Rhizoma Acori Tatarinowii	6 g.

Twelve doses were prescribed.

The check after two months showed further improvement. To consolidate the effects, he was asked to stop taking decoction and start administering pills and powder. The powder was composed of 12 g of Radix Curcumae, 6 g of Alumen, and 3 g of Cinnabaris. One-tenth of the powder was administered each time at night. Six grams of Pill of Lapis Chloriti Usta for Expelling Phlegm (323) was taken each time in the morning for ten days.

A follow-up survey after ten months showed no relapse.

Explanation: In this case, the depressive state was effectively treated by Decoction for Clearing Away Gallbladder-Heat and Bolus of Styrax; this is because the main pathogenesis was *qi* and phlegm stagnation. The symptoms (such as a yellow tongue coating and a smooth and rapid pulse) appeared when the disease was getting better, indicating that the *yin* syndrome was changing into *yang* syndrome, which was a good sign. Therefore, the method of purgation and dispersing fire in the heart was adopted to eliminate dampness-heat at the *Yangming* meridians, getting rid of the root cause thoroughly. When all symptoms were relieved, pills, powder and Pill of Lapis Chloriti Usta for Expelling Phlegm (323) were prescribed to consolidate the results and prevent relapse.

Name: Bao XX; Sex: Female; Age: 53; Occupation: Housewife.

First visit (July 16, 1963): For years, the patient was mentally depressed, narrow-minded and suspicious. Ten days ago, mental disorder suddenly occurred following a breakout of anger. Other symptoms included intermittent weeping and laughing, garrulousness, insomnia, visual and auditory hallucination, occasional fear and fright, and occasional violence, such as smashing doors and windows, which could not be stopped for her strong constitution, a burning sensation in the chest, stickiness in the mouth, refusal to eat, and constipation. The diagnosis was senile psychosis by another hospital.

Presently, the symptoms were nervousness, clear speech, inability to answer inquiries correctly, crimson and cracked tongue with yellow and dry coating at the root, thready, smooth and rapid pulse.

The pathogenesis was stagnant liver *qi*, which was caused by mental depression and had turned into phlegm fire, blocking the clear cavity. Treatment aimed to relieve stagnation, reduce fire, eliminate phlegm and restore consciousness:

Concha Margaritifera Usta	24 g;
Radix Salviae Miltiorrhizae	9 g;
Radix Scrophulariae	9 g;
Radix Ophiopogonis (Cinnabaris coated)	9 g;
Lignum Pini Poriaferum (Cinnabaris coated)	9 g;
Radix Paeoniae Alba	12 g;
Caulis Polygoni Multiflori	15 g;
Cortex Albiziae	9 g;
Fructus Gardeniae (stir-baked)	6 g;
Rhizoma Coptidis	3 g;
Semen Ziziphi Spinosae (stir-baked)	15 g;

Radix Polygalae	9 g;
Rhizoma Acori Tatarinowii	6 g;
Concretio Silicae Bambusae	9 g;
Pulvis Succinum (to be taken separately)	1.2 g.

Three doses were prescribed.

Second visit (July 19, 1963): The patient calmed down after taking the medicine. Fear, fright and violent behavior disappeared. Other symptoms were inadequate sleep, occasional auditory hallucination, less drinking of water, nausea or vomiting if taking food compulsively, normal bowel movement, less yellow and dry tongue coating, red and cracked tongue, and smooth and rapid pulse. The same treatment was adopted. Semen Ziziphi Spinosae and Concretio Silicae Bambusae were removed from the previous prescription, and 12 g of Colla Corii Asini and 9 g of Radix Astragali were added. Another six doses were prescribed.

Third visit (July 31, 1963): Clinical manifestations were normal mental state, sound sleep, less obvious auditory hallucination. Nausea and vomiting disappeared, but anorexia still existed. The tongue was slightly red and cracked and the pulse was thready and retarded.

These symptoms showed that fire had been reduced and phlegm eliminated. But due to the damage of stomach *yin*, stomach *qi* had not yet recovered. Thus drugs that nourish *yin* and improve appetite were prescribed:

Radix Rehmanniae	15 g;
Radix Ophiopogonis	9 g;
Herba Dendrobii	9 g;
Pericarpium Citri Reticulatae	6 g;
Rhizoma Pinelliae Preparata	9 g;
Caulis Bambusae in Taeniam	9 g;
Fructus Aurantii	6 g;
Fructus Oryzae Glutinosae	15 g;
Radix Paeoniae Alba	12 g;
Semen Ziziphi Spinosae (stir-baked)	15 g;
Radix Polygalae	9 g;
Rhizoma Acori Tatarinowii	6 g;
Cortex Albiziae	9 g;
Caulis Polygoni Multiflori	9 g.

Six doses were prescribed.

Fourth visit (August 9, 1963): Appetite improved after taking the medicine. Although sometimes the patient was suspicious, she presented a normal mental state and could do housework on her own. Her tongue was slightly red with scanty coating and her pulse was deep and thready. The treatment aimed to nourish the heart and calm the mind. Pericarpium Citri Reticulatae, Rhizoma Pinelliae and Caulis Bambusae in Taeniam were removed from the previous prescription. Radix Rehmanniae Preparata, Radix Scrophulariae, Fructus Schisandrae and Radix Glycyrrhizae were added. Ten doses were prescribed.

Fifth visit (August 31, 1963): The patient was in normal mental state. Suspiciousness did not present for quite a few days. She could do heavy housework.

A follow-up survey after one year showed that psychosis never appeared. She was advised not to eat cold, raw and oily food, so as to further strengthen the results.

Explanation: According to clinical manifestations, this case belonged to the manic syndrome. The cause was phlegm-fire which went upward, disturbing the mind and blocking the clear cavity. Thus treatment aimed to relieve stagnation, reduce fire, resolve phlegm and restore consciousness. In the first prescription, Concha Margaritifera Usta and Succinum calm the mind; Radix Salviae Miltiorrhizae and Radix Scrophulariae replenish fluid to control fire; Radix Ophiopogonis and Lignum Pini Poriaferum (both were coated with Cinnabaris), and Semen Ziziphi Spinosae reduce fire, nourish the heart and calm the mind; Radix Paeoniae Alba and Cortex Albiziae relieve stagnation and nourish the liver; Fructus Gardeniae and Rhizoma Coptidis disperse fire in the heart; Radix Polygalae and Rhizoma Acori Tatarinowii harmonize the heart and kidneys to promote the restoration of consciousness; and Concretio Silicae Bambusae disperses heat and eliminates phlegm. Other symptoms, such as the disappearance of violent behavior, normal mental state, poor appetite with nausea and vomiting if eating compulsively, thready and retarded pulse, showed that although the fire was reduced, the stomach *yin* and *qi* had not recovered yet. Thus drugs that nourish stomach *yin* and regulate stomach *qi* were prescribed. Consequently, the appetite improved, enabling her to do labor work again. Finally, the drugs that nourish the heart and calm the mind were prescribed.

XVI. Epilepsy

Epilepsy is a paroxysmal mental disorder that manifests as episodic loss of consciousness, spitting foam, staring upward, convulsions of the limbs and screaming like a pig or goat. Consciousness recovers very soon, and the patient behaves like ordinary people.

Medical classics hold that the depressive syndrome and epilepsy are the same, therefore, they are often mentioned together. Later medical workers notice that the two illness are entirely different, although there are similarities between them.

Both primary and secondary epilepsy in Western medicine can be differentiated and treated according to the following descriptions.

Etiology and Pathogenesis

Causes of epilepsy include congenital factors, emotional upsets, improper diet, strain and stress, head trauma and other diseases. These pathogenies impair the functions of the *zang-fu* organs, producing turbid phlegm which disturbs the flow of *qi*, and causes wind and hyperactive *yang* inside the body. Phlegm is the most important pathogenic factor.

1. Congenital Factors

If epilepsy syndrome appears in one's childhood, it is often congenital. According to ancient medical workers, the infant is likely to suffer from epilepsy if his mother has been frightened during pregnancy. This is because fear and fright derange *qi* and consume kidney essence. Consumption of essential *qi* of the mother will lead to the dysplasia of the fetus, and future epilepsy syndrome.

2. Emotional Upsets

This is usually caused by fear and fright. In the book *Basic Questions*, it says, "Fear causes *qi* to decline, and fright deranges *qi*." Drastic fear and fright not only cause disorders of *qi* but also damage the *zang-fu* organs. Damage of the liver and kidneys prevents *yin* from keeping *yang*, thus producing heat and wind. Splenic and gastric damage produces turbid phlegm, which, if affected by deranged *qi*, fire, or wind, will block the clear cavity and cause epilepsy.

3. Head Trauma

Trauma on the head may result from contusions or forceps delivery. Such injuries cause mental disturbance, loss of consciousness, *qi* and blood stagnation. Thus the obstruction in meridians and collaterals will follow, which causes convulsion and further epilepsy.

In addition, invasion by external pathogenic factors, improper diet, and other diseases can all damage the *zang-fu* organs and produce phlegm. If complicated by strain and stress or irregular lifestyle, the retained phlegm will disturb the upper part of the body and block the clear cavity, meridians and collaterals, therefore, epilepsy occurs.

Prolonged epileptic seizures inevitably make the *zang-fu* organs deficient, resulting in the accumulation of turbid phlegm, which will cause the relapse of epilepsy.

Differential Diagnosis

Epilepsy, wind stroke and *jue*-syndromes are all characterized by falling down suddenly and loss of consciousness. But epilepsy is often accompanied by spitting foam, staring upward, convulsions of the limbs and screaming like a pig or goat.

Distinction and Treatment

Although epilepsy has typical symptoms, its pathological conditions vary. For instance, the duration of a seizure ranges from several seconds or minutes to hours; they may occur once a day, several times a day, once a few days, or once a few years. The severity of epileptic seizures also differs. Mild cases present mental dullness, indifference, reticence, pale complexion, absence of convulsions, stopping activities abruptly, dropping things suddenly, sudden forward bending of the neck, transient staring upward. All these symptoms may last only for a few seconds or minutes. When consciousness returns, the patient knows nothing of the seizure. Severe cases manifest as falling down suddenly, loss of consciousness, screams, convulsions and spitting foam. After the seizure, the patient knows nothing of the illness, feels dizzy and tired, and has no recall. Generally, the severity of the illness is related to the condition of turbid phlegm and body resistance. At the initial stage, the syndromes are mild, the duration is short, and the intervals are long, because the body resistance is still strong and turbid phlegm is not severe. Recurrent epileptic seizures weaken the body resistance and aggravate turbid phlegm, making the pathological conditions even worse. If an epileptic seizure lasts for a long time, it indicates a critical condition.

In treatment, the cause and symptoms, and the excess and deficiency should be clarified first. During the seizure, the method of needling *Renzhong* (DU 26) could be adopted to restore consciousness; if the illness occurs regularly, medicine could be taken before the onset of epilepsy. The method of eliminating phlegm and circulating *qi*, calming wind and restoring consciousness is adopted during seizures. At ordinary times, the treatment aiming at curing the root cause is recommended, including invigorating the spleen, resolving phlegm, nourishing the liver, kidneys and heart and calming the mind.

1. Blockage by Wind and Phlegm

Clinical manifestations: Dizziness, stuffiness in the chest, and lassitude before the breakout, falling down suddenly, loss of consciousness, convulsions, spitting foam, screams and incontinence of urine and feces during seizures, possible transient loss of consciousness or trance without convulsions, white and sticky tongue coating, and taut and smooth pulse.

Analysis: Dizziness, stuffiness in the chest, and lassitude indicate the upward disturbance of wind-phlegm. Liver wind brings phlegm along, disturbing the mind and causing epilepsy with spitting of foam. A white and sticky tongue coating, and a taut and smooth pulse all indicate liver wind along with turbid phlegm.

Treatment: To eliminate phlegm, calm wind, restore consciousness, and arrest epileptic seizures.

Prescription: Pill for Relieving Epilepsy (178). In this recipe, Succus Bambusae, Radix Acori Tatarinowii, Arisaema cum Bile and Rhizoma Pinelliae eliminate phlegm and restore consciousness; Rhizoma Gastrodiae, Scorpio and Bombyx Batryticatus calm liver wind and arrest convulsion; and Succinum, Cinnabaris, Lignum Pini Poriaferum and Radix Polygalae soothe the heart and calm the mind. In cases of *qi* stagnation with profuse sputum, Pill of Alumen and Curcumae (102) is prescribed.

2. Excess Internal Phlegm-Fire

Clinical manifestations: Falling down suddenly, loss of consciousness, convulsion, spitting foam, and possibly screams, irritability, restlessness, insomnia, difficult expectoration of sputum, dry and bitter mouth, constipation, a red tongue with yellow and sticky coating, and a taut, smooth and rapid pulse at ordinary times.

Analysis: Hyperactive liver fire produces wind, which brings phlegm along, blocking the mind and causing the sudden falling-down, loss of consciousness, convulsion and spitting foam. Stagnant liver *qi* leads to irritability. Disturbance of the mind by liver fire results in restlessness and insomnia. A red tongue with yellow coating and a taut, smooth and rapid pulse indicate excess liver-fire and phlegm-heat.

Treatment: To disperse heat in the liver, reduce fire, resolve phlegm and restore consciousness.

Prescription: Decoction of Gentianae for Purging Liver-Fire (78) combined with Decoction for Cleansing Phlegm (243). In this formula, Radix Gentianae, Radix Scutellariae, Fructus Gardeniae and Caulis Aristolochiae Manshuriensis disperse heat in the liver and reduce fire; and Rhizoma Pinelliae, Exocarpium Citri Rubrum, Arisaema cum Bile and Rhizoma Acori Tatarinowii resolve phlegm and restore consciousness. To disperse heat, calm wind, resolve phlegm, remove obstructions in the meridians and relieve convulsion, Concha Haliotidis, Ramulus Uncariae cum Uncis, Succus Bambusae (fresh) and Lumbricus are added. In cases of excess phlegm-fire with constipation, Pill of Succus Bambusae for Eliminating Phlegm (133) is prescribed to eliminate phlegm, reduce fire and relieve constipation.

3. Hepatic and Renal *Yin*-Deficiency

Clinical manifestations: Protracted illness, dizziness, insomnia, poor memory, soreness and weakness in the lumbar region and knees, possible constipation, a red tongue with scanty coating, and a thready and rapid pulse.

Analysis: Prolonged epileptic seizures disturb liver wind and *yang*, and consume hepatic and renal *yin*. Consequently, *yin* fails to keep *yang*, resulting in fire of the deficiency type, which disturbs the mind and causes insomnia. Renal deficiency and consumption of essence lead to the soreness and weakness of the lumbar region and knees. Deficiency of renal essence deprives the brain of nourishment, causing dizziness and poor memory. Deficiency of *yin* fluid fails to moisten the large intestines, thus constipation ensues. A red tongue with scanty coating and a thready and rapid pulse indicate internal heat due to *yin* deficiency.

Treatment: To nourish the liver and kidneys, suppress hyperactive *yang* and calm the mind.

Prescription: Modified *Zuogui* Pill (79). In the recipe, Radix Rehmanniae Preparata, Rhizoma Dioscoreae, Fructus Corni, Fructus Lycii and Carapax et Plastrum Testudinis nourish the liver and kidneys. To replenish *yin* and suppress hyperactive *yang*, Concha Ostreae and Carapax Trionycis are added. To soothe the heart and calm the mind, Semen Platycladi, Magnetitum and Cinnabaris are added. To disperse heat and eliminate phlegm, Bulbus Fritillariae Cirrhosae, Concretio Silicae Bambusae and Caulis Bambusae in Taeniam are added. In cases with dry stool, Radix Scrophulariae and Fructus Cannabis are added. In a prolonged case due to deficiency of *yin*, essence, *qi* and blood with symptoms of lassitude and pale complexion, Bolus of Placenta Hominis (172) could be administered regularly to nurture essence and blood. With prolonged cases manifesting trance, fear, worry and anxiety, Decoction of Glycyrrhizae, Tritici Levis and Jujubae (84) is prescribed together to nourish the heart and moisten dryness.

4. Splenic and Gastric Weakness

Clinical manifestations: Protracted illness, lassitude, dizziness, poor appetite, pale complexion, loose stool, possible nausea and vomiting, a pale tongue, and a soft and weak pulse.

Analysis: Weakness of the spleen and stomach impairs their function of producing *qi* and blood, resulting in pale complexion and lassitude. Impaired splenic function to transport and transform causes loose stool. Phlegm-dampness blocks *yang-qi* and gives rise to dizziness. Deficiency of stomach *qi* leads to poor appetite, nausea and vomiting. A pale tongue and a soft and weak pulse indicate weakness of the spleen and stomach.

Treatment: To invigorate the spleen, benefit *qi*, harmonize the stomach and resolve the turbid.

Prescription: Modified Decoction of Six Mild Drugs (55). In this formula, Radix Codonopsis, Poria, Rhizoma Atractylodis Macrocephalae and Radix Glycyrrhizae invigorate the spleen and benefit *qi*; and Rhizoma Pinelliae and Pericarpium Citri Reticulatae harmonize the stomach and resolve the turbid. To eliminate turbid phlegm and calm the mind, Rhizoma Acori Tatarinowii, Radix Polygalae, Arisaema cum Bile and Bombyx Batryticatus are added.

In order to calm wind, relieve convulsion, and enhance the therapeutic results, Scorpio and Scolopendra are added to all the above prescriptions. Scorpio and Scolopendra are pounded into powder to be taken separately twice a day, 1.0-1.5 g or taken together 0.5-1.0 g each time. Epilepsy is often related to *qi* and blood stagnation, especially when caused by trauma. In such cases, medicines that activate blood circulation and remove stasis, such as Radix Salviae Miltiorrhizae, Flos Carthami, Semen Persicae and Rhizoma Chuanxiong are added.

Remarks

A regular lifestyle plays an important role in the treatment of epilepsy. The patient must try to avoid emotional irritation, strain and stress. It is not advisable for him to drive car, or work high above the ground or in water. When epileptic seizures take place, false teeth should be removed in order to protect the tongue. If the patient remains unconscious for a long time, special attention should be paid to oral hygiene and sputum elimination.

Case Studies

Name: Li XX; Sex: Female; Age: 26.

First visit (July 31, 1976): The patient experienced two epileptic seizures that month. The recent one manifested syncope, convulsion, spitting white foam, dark blue complexion, dizziness, lassitude, palpitation, a thin and sticky tongue coating, and a thready and taut pulse. All this suggested the blockage of the pericardium and disturbance of the mind by turbid phlegm due to blood deficiency and hyperactive liver fire. Treatment aimed to nourish the blood, calm the liver, disperse heat in the heart and eliminate phlegm:

Dens Draconis	30 g;
Os Draconis	30 g;
Radix Paeoniae Alba	15 g;
Haematitum	30 g;
Radix Salviae Miltiorrhizae	12 g;
Concretio Silicae Bambusae	4.5 g;
Arisaema cum Bile	9 g;
Rhizoma Acori Tatarinowii	9 g;
Radix Polygalae (coated with Cinnabaris)	4.5 g;
Fructus Tritici Levis	30 g;
Semen Ziziphi Spinosae (stir-baked)	9 g;
Semen Platycladi	9 g;
Plumula Nelumbinis	3 g;
Pill of Alumen and Curcumae (to be taken separately, 4.5 g each time)	9 g.

Seven doses were prescribed.

Second visit (August 5, 1976): Epileptic seizures did not occur. Dizziness, palpitation, and dark blue complexion improved. The tongue was slightly red with thin coating. The pulse was thready and taut. The same treatment was adopted:

Cornu Bubali (decocted first)	30 g;
Cortex Moutan	9 g;
Radix Salviae Miltiorrhizae	12 g;
Haematitum	30 g;
Os Draconis (decocted first)	30 g;
Concretio Silicae Bambusae	4.5 g;
Arisaema cum Bile	9 g;
Rhizoma Acori Tatarinowii	9 g;
Radix Polygalae (coated with Cinnabaris)	4.5 g;
Fructus Tritici Levis	30 g;
Semen Ziziphi Spinosae (stir-baked)	9 g;
Semen Platycladi	9 g;
Plumula Nelumbinis	3 g;
Pill of Alumen and Curcumae (to be taken separately, 4.5 g each time)	9 g.

Seven doses were prescribed.

Discussion: Since this case was at the early stage of epilepsy, treatment emphasized on soothing the liver, reducing fire in the heart, eliminating phlegm and dispersing heat. The patient paid ten visits before her condition became stable. Thirty grams of Caulis Vitis Romanetii were added at her fifth visit, which proved effective. The special effect of Caulis Vitis Romanetii needs further study.

XVII. Epigastric Pain

Epigastric pain is also called stomach-ache. In Western medicine, acute and chronic gastritis, gastric and duodenal ulcers, gastric cancer, gastric neurosis, certain types of pancreatitis and disorders in the biliary tract with symptom of epigastric pain can all be differentiated and treated according to the following descriptions.

Etiology and Pathogenesis
1. Attack of the Stomach by Pathogenic Factors

Attack of the stomach by external pathogenic cold or cold in the middle *jiao* due to overeating raw and cold food may lead to epigastric pain. Constitutional *yang* deficiency of the spleen and stomach makes the spleen easier to be affected by pathogenic cold, which will result in epigastric pain. Improper diet, such as overeating greasy and sweet food, produces dampness-heat or causes retention of food in the stomach, resulting epigastric pain.

2. Invasion of the Stomach by Liver *Qi*

Stagnant liver *qi* due to mental depression or anger affects the stomach and blocks *qi*, thereby causing epigastric pain. Stagnant liver *qi* may turn into fire, which consumes stomach *yin* and aggravates epigastric pain. Long-standing *qi* stagnation leads to blood stagnation, making epigastric pain even more difficult to be cured.

3. Splenic and Gastric Weakness

Constitutional weakness of the spleen and stomach, strain and stress, or long-standing illness, can all cause cold in the middle *jiao* and further gastric pain. Spleen *yang*-deficiency produces internal cold that deprives the stomach collaterals of warmth, resulting in epigastric pain due to deficiency and cold. The combination of external and internal cold produces epigastric pain due to cold accumulation. Damage of stomach *yin* deprives the stomach of nourishment, thus causing epigastric pain due to *yin* deficiency.

In cases with epigastric pain, the stomach is affected. Since the spleen and stomach are interior-exteriorly related, and the liver regulates the flow of *qi*, epigastric pain directly influences the spleen and liver. Although there are many causes of epigastric pain, "obstruction causes pain" is the common pathogenesis.

Differential Diagnosis
The following is the distinction of epigastric pain, cardiac pain and abdominal pain.
1. Cardiac Pain

Medical classics used to confuse epigastric pain with cardiac pain. As a matter of fact, these two diseases are different in location, nature and prognosis.

Cardiac pain is located in the precordial (left thoracic) region, while epigastric pain is in the upper abdominal region close to the heart.

Epigastric pain is usually dull and insidious. Although occasionally there is a sharp stab of pain, it is less intense than cardiac pain. The latter is characterized by a sudden onset of cramping, intolerable or suffocating pain, which goes up to the left shoulder and back or down the left arm. The patient experiences palpitation, a feeling of suffocation and impending death during the seizure of cardiac pain.

The prognosis of epigastric pain is favorable, but that of cardiac pain is ominous. Persistent cardiac pain often results in death in the evening if it occurs in the morning, or death in the next morning if it occurs at night. In a severe case, it may lead to immediate death.

2. Abdominal Pain

The difference between abdominal and epigastric pain lies in the location. Epigastrium locates between the cardia and pylorus, and the pain in this area is called epigastric pain, while abdominal pain is found below the epigastrium.

Distinction and Treatment

In the distinction of epigastric pain, the following points must be clarified: Is the pain caused by stagnant pathogenic factors (cold, heat, food retention) or by dysfunction of the *zang-fu* organs (stagnation of liver *qi*, weak spleen and stomach)? Which organ is diseased, the liver, or the spleen and stomach? Is it of the excess type (stagnation of pathogenic factors, liver *qi*-stagnation, liver fire) or of the deficiency type (splenic and renal *yang*-deficiency, stomach *yin*-deficiency)? Is it caused by *qi* stagnation or blood stasis?

The principle of treatment for epigastric pain is to regulate *qi* and relieve pain. Different methods are used according to the syndromes. For instance, the method of eliminating pathogenic factors may vary since the nature of these factors are different. In cases of liver *qi*-stagnation, the method of soothing the liver and regulating *qi* is adopted, while the method of warming the middle *jiao* and dispersing cold is employed in cases of splenic and gastric deficiency with stagnant cold. In cases of long-standing epigastric pain due to fire, consumption of *yin* or blood stagnation, the method of reducing fire, nourishing *yin* and removing blood stasis is used respectively.

1. Attack of the Stomach by Pathogenic Cold

Clinical manifestations: Abrupt onset of epigastric pain which could be alleviated by hot compression, aversion to cold and preference for warmth, absence of thirst or preference for warm drinks, a white tongue coating, a taut and tense, or a taut and slow pulse.

Analysis: Accumulation of cold in the middle *jiao* due to external cold or overeating raw and cold food hinders *yang-qi*, and thus causes epigastric pain. White tongue coating and tense or slow pulse all suggest cold stagnation, which causes epigastric pain.

Treatment: To warm the stomach, disperse cold, circulate *qi* and relieve pain.

Prescription: In a mild case of epigastric pain, local hot compression or warm ginger soup can relieve the pain. In a severe case, Pill of Alpiniae Officinarum and Cyperi (151) is prescribed. In the recipe, Rhizoma Alpiniae Officinarum warms the stomach and disperses cold; and Rhizoma Cyperi circulates *qi* and relieves pain. If cold is intense, Rhizoma Zingiberis, Fructus Evodiae, Fructus Piperis Longi, Cortex Cinnamomi, Fructus Litseae and Pericarpium Citri Reticulatae are added to help dispersing cold and relieving pain. If there is vomiting of clear fluid, Rhizoma Zingiberis Recens is added; Rhizoma Pinelliae could be used if vomit is severe. If there are also abdominal pain and diarrhea, Rhizoma Zingiberis (roasted) and Fructus Crataegi (charred) are added. In cases of distress in the chest and epigastrium, anorexia and belching, medicines that eliminate wind, disperse cold and relieve pain are added. In cases of food retention, Fructus Aurantii Immaturus, Massa Medicata Fermentata and Endothelium Corneum Gigeriae Galli are added to promote digestion.

2. Retention of Food

Clinical manifestations: Fullness and distention, or pain in the epigastrium, belching, acid regurgitation, vomiting of undigested food, alleviation of pain after vomiting, difficult bowel movements, a thick and sticky, or dirty and sticky tongue coating, and a smooth pulse.

Analysis: Overeating causes food retention and upward disturbance of turbid *qi*, resulting in fullness, distention and pain in the epigastric region, belching, acid regurgitation, and vomiting of undigested food. Vomiting relieves food retention, thus alleviates epigastric pain. Difficult bowel movements, a thick and sticky, or a dirty and sticky tongue coating, and a smooth pulse all indicate food retention.

Treatment: To promote digestion, eliminate stagnation, harmonize the stomach and relieve pain.

Prescription: Modified Pill for Promoting Digestion (216). In this formula, Fructus Crataegi, Massa Medicata Fermentata and Semen Raphani digest food; Rhizoma Pinelliae, Pericarpium Citri Reticulatae and Poria harmonize the stomach and eliminate dampness; and Fructus Forsythiae disperses stagnation and heat. A proper amount of Fructus Aurantii Immaturus, Fructus Amomi, and Semen Arecae can be added to the prescription. If the prescription is not effective, Decoction for Mild Purgation (35) added with Radix Aucklandiae, and Rhizoma Cyperi could be used. If retained food produces heat with symptoms of burning epigastric pain, uncomfortable and empty sensation in the stomach, vomiting of yellow fluid, restlessness, a bitter taste or dryness of the mouth with no desire to drink, constipation or difficult bowel movement, a red tongue with yellow and sticky coating, Pill of Aurantii Immaturus for Relieving Stagnation (196) is prescribed. If damage of the stomach is due to overeating meat, Endothelium Corneum Gigeriae Galli and a large dosage of Fructus Crataegi (charred) are added. If the damage is due to eating too much rice and flour, Fructus Hordei Germinatus (charred) and Massa Medicata Fermentata (charred) are prescribed; if the damage is caused by eating fish and crabs, Folium Perillae is added. If the pain is caused by administering Radix Ginseng, which produces *qi* stagnation with symptoms of fullness, distention and pain in the epigastrium, a large dosage of Semen Raphani is used.

3. Attack of the Stomach by Liver *Qi*

Clinical manifestations: Epigastric pain which penetrates to the hypochondrium on both sides, frequent hiccups, difficult bowel movement, fullness and distention in the epigastrium caused by emotional upsets, thin and white tongue coating, and a taut pulse.

Analysis: Stagnant liver *qi* due to mental depression affects the stomach, causing epigastric pain. Since the Liver Meridian passes through the hypochondrium, epigastric pain caused by liver *qi* will reach there. Failure of stomach *qi* to descend causes epigastric fullness and distention, belching and difficult bowel movements. A taut pulse suggests liver disorders and pain.

Treatment: To soothe the liver, regulate *qi*, harmonize the stomach and ease the middle *jiao*.

Prescription: Modified Powder of Bupleuri for Releasing Stagnant Liver-*Qi* (239). In the recipe, Radix Bupleuri, Rhizoma Cyperi, Fructus Aurantii, Radix Paeoniae Alba and Rhizoma Chuanxiong calm the liver and relieve stagnation; and Pericarpium Citri Reticulatae and Radix Glycyrrhizae regulate *qi* and harmonize the middle *jiao* to relieve pain. In order to strengthen these effects, Fructus Citri, Fructus Citri Sarcodactylis, Flos Mume, Flos Rosae Rugosae and Radix Curcumae are added.

4. Retention of Heat in the Liver and Stomach

Clinical manifestations: Burning epigastric pain, irritability, acid regurgitation, uncomfortable and empty sensation in the stomach, a bitter taste and dryness of the mouth, red tongue with yellow coating, and a taut or rapid pulse.

Analysis: Stagnant liver *qi* turns into fire, which affects the stomach and causes the burning pain in the epigastrium, irritability, acid regurgitation and an uncomfortable and empty sensation in the stomach. Since the liver and gallbladder are exterior-interiorly related, heat in the liver helps gallbladder fire to disturb upward, resulting in a bitter taste and dryness of the mouth. Yellow tongue coating, and a taut or rapid pulse indicate heat in the stomach and liver.

Treatment: To disperse heat in the liver, reduce fire, harmonize the stomach and relieve pain.

Prescription: Decoction for Clearing Liver-Heat (59) is the main formula. Pericarpium Citri Reticulatae and Pericarpium Citri Reticulatae Viride regulate *qi*; Radix Paeoniae Alba constricts the liver; and Cortex Moutan and Fructus Gardeniae disperse heat in the liver. *Zuojin* Pill (81) can be added, with Rhizoma Coptidis reducing fire with its bitter and cold nature and Fructus Evodiae dispersing stagnation to reduce fire. *Xiaoyao* Powder with Moutan and Gardeniae (63) can also be used.

5. *Yin* Deficiency

Clinical manifestations: Dull epigastric pain, dry mouth and throat with a desire to drink, constipation, red tongue with little moisture, and a thready and taut pulse.

Analysis: Constitutional stomach *yin*-deficiency or consumption of *yin* by fire due to long-standing illness deprives the stomach collaterals of nourishment and moisture, resulting in a dull gastric pain. *Yin* deficiency results in the lack of fluid, and thus dry mouth and throat appear. Deficiency of *yin* fluid deprives the intestines of moisture, which causes constipation. Red tongue with little moisture, and a thready and taut pulse are signs of *yin* deficiency.

Treatment: To nourish *yin*, benefit the stomach and relieve acute pain.

Prescription: Decoction for Nourishing Stomach (207) combined with Decoction of Paeoniae Alba and Glycyrrhizae (122). In the recipe, Radix Adenophorae, Radix Ophiopogonis, Radix Trichosanthis, Rhizoma Polygonati Odorati and Herba Dendrobii nourish *yin* and benefit the stomach; Semen Lablab Album, combined with *yin* tonics, help invigorate the spleen and stomach; Fructus Toosendan soothes the liver, regulates *qi* and disperses heat; and Radix Paeoniae Alba and Radix Glycyrrhizae relieve acute pain. In cases of burning epigastric pain, nausea, an uncomfortable and empty sensation in the stomach, *Zuojin* Pill (81) is added to eliminate stagnation and disperse heat. In cases of poor appetite, Radix Ophiopogonis and Rhizoma Polygonati Odorati are removed from the formula and Rhizoma Dioscoreae and Rhizoma Atractylodis Macrocephalae are added. In cases of *yin* blood-deficiency and dry stool, Radix Polygoni Multiflori, Semen Platycladi and Fructus Cannabis are added to nourish the blood and moisten the large intestines. In severe cases, a proper amount of Fructus Mume and Fructus Chaenomelis is added to appease the liver and activate the stomach. In cases of emaciation, lassitude and loose stool due to splenic and gastric deficiency and consumption of *yin* fluid, Radix Ophiopogonis, Rhizoma Polygonati Odorati and Radix Trichosanthis are removed from the formula, and Radix Ginseng, Pericarpium Citri Reticulatae and Fructus Citri Sarcodactylis are added to regulate *qi* and improve appetite.

This syndrome can also be treated by *Yiguan* Decoction (1) or Decoction for Nourishing Fluid and Clearing Away Liver-Heat (303).

6. Deficiency Cold in the Spleen and Stomach

Clinical manifestations: Dull epigastric pain, vomiting of clear fluid, preference for warmth and massage in certain parts, poor appetite, lassitude, cold limbs, pale complexion, loose stool, pale tongue with white coating, and a deep, thready, slow and weak pulse.

Analysis: Deficiency cold in the spleen and stomach indicates *yang-qi* deficiency and sluggish transportation. This results in fluid retention in the stomach, producing cold from the inside, with symptoms of dull epigastric pain, preference for warmth and pressure, vomiting of clear fluid and poor appetite. Deficiency of *yang* causes cold limbs, lassitude, loose stool and pale complexion. Pale tongue with white coating and a thready and weak pulse are signs of deficiency in the middle *jiao* with stagnant cold.

Treatment: To warm the middle *jiao*, invigorate the spleen and relieve acute pain.

Prescription: Modified Decoction of Astragali for Strengthening Middle *Jiao* (267). In cases with serious blood deficiency, Decoction of Angelicae Sinensis for Strengthening Middle *Jiao* is prescribed. In cases with both *qi* and blood deficiency, Decoction of Angelicae Sinensis and Astragali for Strengthening Middle *Jiao* is used. In these formulae, Radix Astragali fortifies the middle *jiao* and benefits *qi*; Saccharum Granorum, sweet and warm in nature, enters the spleen to warm the middle *jiao*, replenish deficiency, harmonize the interior and relieve acute pain; Ramulus Cinnamomi warms *yang-qi*; Radix

Paeoniae Alba replenishes *yin* blood and relieves acute pain when combined with Radix Glycyrrhizae Preparata; Rhizoma Zingiberis Recens, acrid and warm in nature, and Radix Glycyrrhizae Preparata and Fructus Jujubae, sweet and warm in nature, are combined to warm the middle *jiao* and remedy the deficiency. In cases of acid regurgitation, Saccharum Granorum can be removed or reduced in amount, while Rhizoma Coptidis and Fructus Evodiae, stir-baked with ginger juice, or Concha Arcae Usta is added. If vomiting of clear fluid is serious, Rhizoma Pinelliae, Pericarpium Citri Reticulatae and Poria are added to resolve retained fluid and conduct the unhealthy *qi* downward. In cases with poor appetite, belching and a thick and sticky tongue coating, Fructus Aurantii Immaturus, Cortex Magnoliae Officinalis, Massa Medicata Fermentata and Fructus Hordei Germinatus are added to promote digestion and relieve stagnation. In cases of black stool due to bleeding, Decoction of Terra Flava Usta (259) is prescribed to warm the middle *jiao* and check bleeding. Pill of Alpiniae Officinarum and Cyperi (151) could be used to warm the middle *jiao*, regulate *qi* and relieve pain. If the cold is intense, with symptoms of severe epigastric pain and cold limbs, Decoction for Potently Warming Middle *Jiao* (25) is prescribed to boost *yang-qi* and disperse *yin* cold. In cases of loose stool, Bolus of Aconiti Lateralis Preparata for Regulating Middle *Jiao* (163) is prescribed with some modifications. When the pain is relieved, Pill of Six Mild Drugs with Aucklandiae and Amomi (211) can be used to promote recuperation.

7. Stagnation of Blood

Clinical manifestations: Piercing epigastric pain with a fixed location, vomiting of dark purple blood, tarry stool, blue-purplish tongue, and a thready and unsmooth pulse.

Analysis: Chronic epigastric pain damages the vessels and produces blood stagnation as the saying goes "Prolonged illness affects blood" and "Long-standing pain damages the vessels." It can also be caused by stagnation of *qi* or retention of excessive cold. Since stagnant blood is substantial, the pain has a fixed location. Damage to the vessels leads to the piercing pain, vomiting of blood, or tarry stool. Blood stagnation also causes purple tongue and an unsmooth pulse.

Treatment: To activate blood circulation, remove blood stasis, regulate *qi* and relieve pain.

Prescription: Powder for Dissipating Blood Stasis (98) combined with Decoction of Salviae Miltiorrhizae (62). In the formula, Pollen Typhae, Faeces Trogopterori and Radix Salviae Miltiorrhizae activate blood circulation, remove blood stasis and relieve pain; and Lignum Santali Albi and Fructus Amomi regulate *qi*, harmonize the stomach and relieve pain. In cases of hematemesis and hemafecia, Radix Notoginseng and Radix Sanguisorbae are added to remove blood stasis and check bleeding.

This syndrome can also be treated by modified Decoction for Removing Blood Stasis Under Diaphragm (318).

Remarks

The above seven syndromes of epigastric pain are interrelated. Epigastric pain due to stagnant pathogenic factors is often acute; while the pain resulting from stagnant liver *qi* or spleen and stomach deficiency and cold is often chronic. Acute epigastric pain responds to the treatment quickly, however, it may turn into chronic with improper diet and lifestyle, emotional upsets, and incomplete treatment. Persistent epigastric pain may cause blood stagnation. In general, the above syndromes do not exist alone; they can be complicated by both excess and deficiency, and both cold and heat.

The principle of treatment for epigastric pain is to regulate *qi* and relieve pain. Since drugs that regulate *qi* are mostly aromatic and dry, they should be used with caution if there is hepatic hyperfunction or *yin* deficiency, for the consumption of stomach *yin* may cause long-standing epigastric pain.

Epigastric pain is often related with emotional upsets or improper diet. Therefore, the patient must maintain emotional stability and take proper diet.

Appendix I   Acid Regurgitation

Acid regurgitation often accompanies epigastric pain, although sometimes it appears alone. It results from disharmony of stomach *qi* due to retained liver fire or deficiency cold in the spleen and stomach. Acid regurgitation can be found in cases of gastric ulcer, duodenal ulcer, chronic gastritis and dyspepsia in Western medicine.

The stagnation of liver fire manifests acid regurgitation accompanied by restlessness, dryness and a bitter taste in the mouth, red tongue tip, thin and yellow tongue coating, and a taut or rapid pulse. Treatment aims to disperse heat in the liver and reduce fire by prescribing *Zuojin* Pill (81) added with Concha Bellamyae Quadratae and Concha Arcae, which check acid secretion and harmonize the stomach.

Deficiency cold in the spleen and stomach manifests acid regurgitation accompanied by distention and distress in the chest and epigastrium, preference for warmth and pressure, belching, white tongue coating, and a taut and thready pulse. Treatment aims to warm the middle *jiao* and regulate *qi* by prescribing Pill of Six Mild Drugs with Aucklandiae and Amomi (211). To disperse cold and conduct the unhealthy *qi* downward, Fructus Evodiae and Rhizoma Zingiberis Recens are added. In cases with acid regurgitation after eating, poor appetite and sticky tongue coating, Massa Medicata Fermentata, Fructus Setariae Germinatus and Fructus Hordei Germinatus are added to promote digestion and harmonize the stomach. In cases of retained turbid dampness with sticky tongue coating, Rhizoma Atractylodis, Cortex Magnoliae Officinalis, Herba Agastaches and Herba Eupatorii are added to disperse dampness by their aromatic nature.

Appendix II   Gastric Upset

Gastric upset manifests an empty feeling in the stomach like a feeling of hunger, heat or pain. It often appears at the same time with epigastric pain and acid regurgitation, although sometimes alone. The causes are as follows:

Heat in the stomach: An empty and uncomfortable feeling in the stomach accompanied by hunger, thirst with a desire for cold drinks, foul breath, restlessness, yellow tongue coating, and possibly rapid pulse. Treatment aims to harmonize the middle *jiao* and disperse heat by prescribing Decoction for Clearing Away Gallbladder-Heat (302). If the heat is intense, Rhizoma Coptidis and Fructus Gardeniae are added to strengthen the above effects.

Gastric deficiency: Lack of taste, epigastric distention after eating, pale tongue, and feeble pulse. Treatment aims to invigorate the spleen and harmonize the stomach by prescribing Decoction of Four Mild Drugs (91) with Rhizoma Dioscoreae and Semen Lablab Album. If the syndrome is accompanied by *qi* stagnation, Radix Aucklandiae and Fructus Amomi are added to regulate *qi* and harmonize the middle *jiao*. In cases with obvious gastric cold, Rhizoma Zingiberis is added to warm the stomach and disperse cold.

Blood deficiency: Pale complexion, tongue and lips, palpitation, dizziness, and thready pulse. Treatment aims to nourish the heart and spleen by prescribing Decoction for Invigorating Spleen and Nourishing Heart (110).

Case Studies

Name: Liang XX; Sex: Male; Age: 42; Occupation: Doctor.
First visit: December 24, 1974.
Chief complaint: Epigastric pain for 15 years.
Examination: Barium meal fluoroscopy in 1964 showed ulcer of the lesser curvature of the stom-

ach. Another examination this year revealed a peanut-sized ulcer.

The patient received treatment of Western medicine for three months. Epigastric pain had not been completely relieved when he was discharged. Recently, clinical manifestations included an empty feeling in the stomach, acid regurgitation, belching, a burning sensation in the epigastrium, aversion to cold which was even worse at night, preference for hot drinks, thin and sticky tongue coating, taut and smooth pulse.

Pathogenesis: *Qi* stagnation due to splenic and gastric deficiency and cold stagnation.

Treatment: To warm the middle *jiao*, relieve pain, soothe the liver and harmonize the stomach.

Prescription:

Rhizoma Cyperi Preparata	9 g;
Radix Aucklandiae	9 g;
Fructus Piperis Longi	4.5 g;
Rhizoma Pinelliae	9 g;
Fructus Toosendan	9 g;
Radix Paeoniae Alba	9 g;
Radix Codonopsis	9 g;
Pericarpium Citri Reticulatae	9 g;
Concha Arcae Usta	30 g.

Six doses were prescribed.

Second visit: January 21, 1975.

Epigastric pain was completely relieved after 21 doses, but belching and nausea still presented when getting up in the morning. Other symptoms included normal appetite, stickiness in the mouth, thin tongue coating, taut and smooth pulse. The same prescription was used with 6 g of Cortex Magnoliae Officinalis added. Another six doses were prescribed.

Third visit: February 20, 1975.

After 14 doses, the burning sensation disappeared. When getting up in the morning, he still had belching and mild nausea. The pulse was taut, and tongue coating was thin and sticky. Treatment aimed to replenish *qi*, harmonize the stomach and conduct the unhealthy *qi* downward.

Prescription:

Radix Codonopsis	9 g;
Rhizoma Atractylodis Macrocephalae	9 g;
Radix Paeoniae Alba	9 g;
Pericarpium Citri Reticulatae	9 g;
Caulis Bambusae in Taeniam (ginger treated)	6 g;
Rhizoma Cyperi Preparata	9 g;
Radix Aucklandiae	6 g;
Cortex Magnoliae Officinalis	6 g;
Concha Arcae Usta	30 g.

Six doses were prescribed.

Explanation: It is rather confusing when making diagnosis of this illness, for the patient had an aversion to cold drinks although he suffered a burning gastric pain. Gastric pain with a burning sensation does not necessarily indicate heat syndrome, for excessive gastric acid due to *qi* stagnation can also produce it. In this case, Radix Paeoniae Alba was adopted to soothe the liver and Concha Arcae to check acid secretion. Retention of cold in the stomach was treated by Fructus Piperis Longi, Rhizoma Cyperi and Radix Aucklandiae. If epigastric pain was accompanied by a burning sensation, restlessness, irritability, dry mouth, red tongue with yellow coating, and a taut pulse, the treatment should aim to soothe the liver, harmonize the stomach, and disperse heat. To achieve better effects, attention should be paid to the distinction of cold and heat syndromes.

Name: Wang XX; Sex: Male; Age: 38.
First visit: December 11, 1965.
Chief complaint: Irregular pain in the upper abdomen for 15 years, accompanied by diarrhea.
Case history: The irregular pain in the upper abdominal region began in 1949, and had nothing to do with eating. Other symptoms included poor appetite, nausea and belching. In 1953, diarrhea occurred and he was hospitalized twice. Gastroscopy showed smoothening and thinning of the rugae of gastric mucosa. Gastric juice analysis revealed lack of free acid, which did not increase with injection of histamine.
Diagnosis: Chronic atrophic gastritis (diarrhea type).
Clinical manifestations: Epigastric pain, poor appetite, occasional nausea, frequently belching, loose stool, emaciation, taut pulse, thin and sticky tongue coating.
Pathogenesis: Attack of the stomach by liver *qi* made stomach *qi* ascend, thus impairing the splenic function of transportation and transformation.
Treatment: To soothe the liver and harmonize the stomach in order to conduct the unhealthy *qi* downward, and to invigorate the spleen and replenish *qi* to check diarrhea.
Prescription:

Radix Codonopsis	9 g;
Rhizoma Atractylodis Macrocephalae (charred)	9 g;
Rhizoma Pinelliae Preparata	9 g;
Pericarpium Citri Reticulatae	6 g;
Fructus Amomi (decocted later)	3 g;
Fructus Amomi Rotundus (decocted later)	3 g;
Radix Aucklandiae	4.5 g;
Poria	9 g;
Radix Glycyrrhizae Preparata	3 g;
Flos Inulae (wrapped)	6 g;
Haematitum (decocted first)	18 g;
Radix Paeoniae Rubra (stir-baked)	9 g;
Caulis Spatholobi	12 g.

Three doses were prescribed.
Second visit: December 14, 1965.
Both epigastric pain and diarrhea improved, and the same prescription was adopted with Flos Inulae and Haematitum removed and 18 g of Concha Arcae Usta (decocted first) added. Nine grams of Os Sepiae (powder) were taken twice. Another four doses were prescribed.
Therapeutic results: After over 50 decoctions, the patient became more vigorous with sanguine complexion and normal appetite. He had gained weight and diarrhea stopped. A blood test showed a considerable increase of hemochrome and red blood cells.
Explanation: Atrophic gastritis is marked by hypohydrochloria, and is treated with drugs that assist secretion of acid, such as Fructus Schisandrae, Fructus Mume, or diluted hydrochloric acid. Con-

cha Arcae and Os Sepiae (powder), which check secretion of acid, were used in this case. Ideal therapeutic results were achieved through the treatment contrary to the routine prescription. Drugs that activate blood circulation, such as Caulis Spatholobi and Radix Paeoniae Rubra, were also used although blood stagnation did not occur. This is to save blood vessels from being affected by long-standing illness. Concha Arcae is thought to be effective in relieving epigastric pain caused by blood stagnation.

Name: Fu XX; Sex: Male; Age: 37; Occupation: Worker.
First visit: March 20, 1975.
Severe epigastric pain occurred last November, which did not respond to Western medication. The diagnosis of antral gastritis was established through barium meal fluoroscopy.

Clinical manifestations: epigastric pain located slightly toward the right side, a feeling of something pushing in the epigastrium, dry stool discharged once a day, absence of belching and acid regurgitation, red tongue, thready and taut pulse.

The disease was due to *qi* stagnation complicated by blood stagnation. Treatment aimed to regulate *qi* and remove blood stasis. The following drugs were prescribed:

Radix Aucklandiae	6 g;
Rhizoma Cyperi Preparata	9 g;
Rhizoma Corydalis	9 g;
Radix Angelicae Sinensis	9 g;
Radix Paeoniae Rubra	9 g;
Radix Paeoniae Alba	9 g;
Radix Glycyrrhizae Preparata	4.5 g;
Fructus Toosendan	9 g;
Pericarpium Citri Reticulatae Viride	6 g;
Pericarpium Citri Reticulatae	6 g.

Seven doses were prescribed.
Second visit: March 27, 1975.
Epigastric pain was relieved, and the stool became moist, but the same feeling of something pushing in the stomach still existed. The tongue was red, and the pulse thready and taut. The same treatment continued with 4.5 g of Flos Carthami added to the prescription. Another seven doses were prescribed.

Third visit: April 3, 1975.
Epigastric pain disappeared, and the feeling of something pushing in the stomach lessened. The stool became normal with more flatus. The patient could sleep well, feeling more comfortable than before. The tongue was still red, and the pulse thready and slightly taut. Twelve grams of Radix Salviae Miltiorrhizae was added. Another seven doses were prescribed.

Fourth visit: April 10, 1975.
Epigastric pain did not relapse and the feeling of something pushing in the stomach further lessened. The tongue was red and the pulse thready and slightly taut. The patient was satisfied with the rapid improvement. To consolidate the results, the following drugs were prescribed:

Radix Aucklandiae	6 g;
Rhizoma Cyperi Preparata	9 g;
Caulis Inulae	9 g;
Radix Angelicae Sinensis	9 g;
Radix Paeoniae Rubra	9 g;

Radix Paeoniae Alba	9 g;
Radix Glycyrrhizae Preparata	4.5 g;
Radix Salviae Miltiorrhizae	12 g;
Pericarpium Citri Reticulatae	9 g;
Pericarpium Citri Reticulatae Viride	9 g;
Endothelium Corneum Gigeriae Galli	9 g.

Another seven doses were prescribed.

Explanation: Antral gastritis confirms the diagnosis of epigastric pain in traditional Chinese medicine. This case was caused by *qi* and blood stagnation in the collaterals of the stomach. In the book, *A Guide to Clinical Practice with Case Records*, it says, "At the early stage, the illness affects the meridians; it enters the collaterals (vessels) in a prolonged case. The meridians dominate *qi* and the collaterals (vessels) dominate blood.... Drugs acrid and aromatic in nature are prescribed to regulate *qi*, and drugs acrid and warm in nature are used to regulate blood." In this case, Radix Aucklandiae, Rhizoma Cyperi and Pericarpium Citri Reticulatae, acrid and aromatic in nature, regulate *qi*, while Radix Angelicae Sinensis and Flos Carthami, acrid and warm in nature, regulate blood. Once *qi* circulates smoothly and blood stasis is removed, epigastric pain and the accompanying symptoms will disappear. The pain was relieved after 21 decoctions. Upon his last visit, the patient was advised to wear clothes according to the changing of temperature, and take proper diet.

XVIII. Dysphagia

Dysphagia is called "*yege*" in Chinese language, with "*ye*" referring to the difficulty in swallowing and "*ge*" the refusal to swallow or vomit soon after eating. "*Ye*" may occur alone or as a prodromal symptom of "*ge*".

Emotional upsets cause dysphagia. *Basic Questions* states, "Dysphagia is the blockage between the upper and lower parts of the body and is caused by excessive worry." *Prescriptions for Life Saving* holds that dysphagia is related with improper diet. *A Complete Collection of Jingyue's Treatise* says that dysphagia is caused by indulgence in alcohol and sex, and rarely found in young people.

Dysphagia found with esophageal cancer, cancer of the cardia, cardiac spasm, esophageal diverticulum, esophageal neurosis and esophagitis in Western medicine can be differentiated and treated according to the following descriptions.

Etiology and Pathogenesis
1. Worry, Over-Thinking, Mental Depression and Anger

Worry and over-thinking damage the spleen, thus causing *qi* stagnation. Body fluid turns into phlegm since it cannot spread within the body as usual. Stagnant *qi* and phlegm combine to block the esophagus, making it difficult to swallow. Then food with saliva goes upward.

Mental depression and anger damage the liver, causing the overactivity of wood on earth. Body fluid therefore accumulates and turns into phlegm. Blockage of the esophagus by stagnant *qi* and phlegm gives rise to dysphagia.

Prolonged *qi* stagnation will affect blood, causing phlegm retention and blood stagnation.

2. Improper Diet

Improper diet damages the spleen and stomach, and subsequently causes dysphagia. For example, overeating pungent and dry food consumes body fluid and dries blood, causing dryness in the esophagus with difficulty in swallowing. Indulgence in alcohol, drinking too much hot alcohol, or overeating greasy, sweet and highly flavored food may produce heat of deficiency type, which consumes fluid and causes phlegm. Consequently, phlegm blocks the esophagus, resulting in difficult swallowing.

3. Attack by Cold or Heat

Attack by cold or heat damages the spleen and stomach, thus causing difficulty in swallowing. For example, attack of the chest and diaphragm by cold blocks food passage. Consequently, the spleen and stomach fail to transport and transform, preventing the body from taking in food. Retention of heat in the spleen and stomach consumes body fluid and dries the blood. Abnormal receptive and digestive function blocks the esophagus and causes a reflux of food after eating in a prolonged illness.

4. Excessive Sex

Excessive sex consumes essence and blood, affecting the internal organs. Renal essence-deficiency affects the spleen and stomach and exhausts the source of health. Consumption of *yin* and body fluid dries the esophagus, making it difficult to swallow. When *yin* deficiency affects *yang*, decline of the fire from the vital gate will follow, depriving the spleen and stomach of warmth. As a result, the *qi* of the middle *jiao* will be too weak to promote transportation and transformation. Blockage of the food passage by phlegm and stagnant blood results in difficult swallowing.

Dysphagia is a disorder in esophagus. Ye Tianshi, a famous physician of the Qing Dynasty, once said, "Dysphagia is caused by stricture of the esophagus." Generally, the pathogenesis of mild dysphagia is esophageal blockage by phlegm and stagnant *qi* due to hepatic and splenic *qi*-stagnation, and esophageal dryness due to the consumption of stomach fluid. The pathogenesis of severe dysphagia is esophageal blockage by phlegm and stagnant blood resulting from the combination of phlegm and stagnant *qi*, or renal *yin*-deficiency caused by consumption of stomach fluid. Clinical manifestations of severe dysphagia include pain when swallowing food, vomiting soon after eating, and difficulty in drinking. The following symptoms, such as *yin* deficiency turning into *yang* deficiency, the exhaustion of essential renal *qi*, and splenic inability to transport and transform, withered skin, emaciation, or edema of the limbs and body indicate that the condition becomes worse.

Differential Diagnosis
1. Plum-Stone *Qi*

Plum-stone *qi* is marked by the sensation of a foreign body in the throat, which cannot be relieved by spitting or swallowing. There is no difficulty in swallowing, however.

2. Reflux of Food from the Stomach

This is caused by food retention in the stomach due to poor digestion. The food taken in the morning is brought up in the evening, and vice versa.

3. Vomiting

Vomiting is often the result of the upward movement of stomach *qi*. There is no difficulty in swallowing.

4. Hiccup

Hiccup is due to the upward movement of *qi*, and is marked by involuntary sound in the throat, which is continuous, short and frequent.

Distinction and Treatment

The initial stage of dysphagia is marked by difficulty in swallowing food, especially solid food. When the condition becomes worse, pain in the chest and diaphragm gradually develops, and vomiting occurs soon after eating. Vomit in a severe case looks like red bean juice. Emaciation, withered skin and weariness are accompanying symptoms.

The resistance and the pathogenic factor should be carefully examined. The pathogenic factor predominates at the initial stage, presenting blockage of the esophagus by stagnant *qi*, phlegm and blood. Deficient resistance predominates at the later stage, manifesting exhaustion of fluid and blood, and *yin* deficiency leading to *yang* deficiency. Severe dysphagia often exhibits complicated syndromes of weak resistance and excessive pathogen.

1. Blockage by Phlegm and Stagnant *Qi*

Clinical manifestations: Difficulty in swallowing, fullness or dull pain in the chest and diaphragm, which becomes less severe if the patient is in better spirit, dry mouth and throat, red tongue, and taut and smooth pulse.

Analysis: Esophageal blockage leads to swallowing difficulty, and fullness and a dull pain at the chest and diaphragm. *Qi* circulates more smoothly when one is in better spirit, which explains the alleviation of symptoms. Stagnant *qi* produces heat, which consumes fluid and prevents it from going upward to provide nourishment; the consequence is dry mouth and throat. A red tongue and a taut and smooth pulse are signs of *qi* stagnation and phlegm retention complicated by consumption of body fluid by heat.

Treatment: To relieve stagnation, moisten dryness and resolve phlegm.

Prescription: Powder for Easing Diaphragm (152). In the recipe, Radix Salviae Miltiorrhizae, Radix Curcumae and Fructus Amomi remove blood stasis and benefit *qi* to relieve stagnation; Radix Adenophorae, Bulbus Fritillariae Cirrhosae and Poria moisten dryness and resolve phlegm to disperse stagnation; and Petiolus Nelumbinis and Testa Oryzae Sativae resolve the turbid and harmonize the stomach to conduct the unhealthy *qi* downward. Meanwhile, Caulis Aristolochiae Manshuriensis, Radix Asparagi and Fructus Trichosanthis are added to strengthen these effects.

2. Consumption of Fluid and Retention of Heat

Clinical manifestation: Difficulty and pain in swallowing, especially with solid food. Other symptoms include emaciation, dry mouth and throat, constipation, restlessness and a hot sensation in the palms, soles and chest, red and dry tongue with cracks, and taut, thready and rapid pulse.

Analysis: Consumption of stomach fluid deprives the esophagus of moisture, thus leading to difficulty and pain in swallowing, especially with solid food. Consumption of gastric and intestinal fluid and retention of heat cause dry mouth and throat and constipation. Stomach fluid-consumption also causes renal *yin*-deficiency and produces internal heat with symptoms of restlessness, a hot sensation in the palms, soles and chest as well as emaciation. Red and dry tongue with cracks and taut, thready and rapid pulse are signs of fluid consumption and heat retention.

Treatment: To nourish body fluid.

Prescription: Decoction of Five Kinds of Juice for Relieving Dysphagia (49). In the recipe, Succus Pyri, Succus Nelumbinis Rhizomatis and Lactis Bovis nourish the stomach and produce fluid; Succus Zingiberis Recens harmonizes the stomach and conducts the unhealthy *qi* downward; and Succus Allii Tuberosi Herbae activates blood circulation and removes stasis. Meanwhile, Radix Adenophorae, Herba Dendrobii, Radix Rehmanniae and Radix Scrophulariae are added to nourish the stomach and kidneys. The drugs are advised to be taken bit by bit at short intervals. In cases of constipation with dry stool, a proper amount of Radix et Rhizoma Rhei is added.

3. Retention of Stagnant Blood

Clinical manifestations: Fixed pain in the chest and diaphragm, inability to swallow food and fluid, hard and scanty stool, vomit like red bean juice, emaciation, dry skin, purplish tongue with little moisture, and thready and unsmooth pulse.

Analysis: Blockage of the esophagus by stagnant blood leads to pain with a fixed location, dysphagia, and even difficulty in swallowing fluid. Consumption of *yin* and blood in a chronic case dries up the intestinal tract, causing hard and scanty stool. Damage to the vessels results in bleeding, which explains vomit like red bean juice. Inability to eat exhausts the source of nutrients, resulting in emaciation, dry skin and purplish tongue with little moisture. Purplish tongue and thready and unsmooth pulse are signs of *yin* and blood consumption, and retention of stagnant blood.

Treatment: To nourish *yin* and blood, and remove blood stasis.

Prescription: Decoction for Relieving Stagnation (251). In this formula, Radix Rehmanniae and Radix Angelicae Sinensis nourish *yin* and blood; Semen Persicae and Flos Carthami remove blood stasis; and Radix Glycyrrhizae relieves the acute symptoms and moistens dryness. To remove stasis in the vessels, Radix Notoginseng, Radix Salviae Miltiorrhizae, Radix Paeoniae Rubra and Catharsius Molossus are added. To soften hard masses and resolve phlegm, Sargassum, Thallus Laminariae seu Eckloniae and Bulbus Fritillariae Cirrhosae are added. If vomiting occurs when drinking the decoction, *Yushu* Pill (72) is administered first to ease the diaphragm and conduct the unhealthy *qi* downward. This enables the patient to swallow the decoction.

4. *Qi* Deficiency and *Yang* Weakness

Clinical manifestations: Inability to swallow for a long time, pale complexion, listlessness, shortness of breath, vomiting of clear fluid, facial puffiness, edema of the feet, abdominal distention, pale tongue with white coating, and thready and weak, or deep and thready pulse.

Analysis: *yin* deficiency develops into *yang* deficiency when the illness aggravates. Splenic and gastric *yang-qi* deficiency causes the inability to receive, transport and transform food, resulting in inability to swallow, vomiting of clear fluid and listlessness. It also results in the inability to transform body fluid, with facial puffiness, edema of the feet and abdominal distention as its manifestations. Renal *yang*-deficiency presents pale complexion, shortness of breath, pale tongue with white coating, and thready and weak or deep and thready pulse.

Treatment: To warm and nourish the spleen and kidneys.

Prescription: To warm the spleen, apply Decoction for Replenishing *Qi* and Invigorating Spleen (155); to warm the kidneys, use *Yougui* Pill (82). In the former, Radix Ginseng, Radix Astragali seu, and Poria replenish *qi* and invigorate the spleen; and Rhizoma Pinelliae, Pericarpium Citri Reticulatae and Rhizoma Zingiberis Recens, as secondary ingredients, harmonize the stomach and conduct the unhealthy *qi* downward. Meanwhile, Flos Inulae and Haematitum are added to check vomiting. In the latter formula, Radix Rehmanniae Preparata, Fructus Corni and Fructus Lycii nourish kidney *yin*; and Colla Cornu Cervi, Cortex Cinnamomi, Radix Aconiti Lateralis Preparata and Cortex Eucommiae warm kidney *yang*. Both the spleen and kidneys are in extreme deficiency at this stage of the disease. Generally, drugs that warm the spleen and replenish *qi* are administered first to rescue the source of health. When the patient can swallow thin and liquid food, drugs that fortify the spleen and warm the kidneys are taken. Decoction and pills are taken at the same time or alternately.

Remarks

To avoid the illness, the patient should alternate work with rest, strengthen the body, avoid mental stress, refrain from excessive alcohol or too much pungent food, and take care not to be exposed to external pathogenic factors. During treatment, the patient must rest well, keep calm, avoid highly-flavored food, fragrant food which is dry in nature, refrain from anger, and avoid sexual life.

Case Studies

Name: Chen XX; Sex: Male; Age: 31.

The patient suffered difficulty in swallowing food for two years. The disease became worse over the last month. He complained of epigastric fullness and distention after eating, vomiting of a large amount of mucus and clear fluid soon after eating, insomnia, dizziness and sore limbs. In the early spring two years ago, he developed a difficulty in swallowing after eating cold rice. He also had an uncomfortable feeling in his chest and diaphragm, and intermittent vomiting of large amounts of mucus. The barium meal fluoroscopy showed a 6cm-long stricture of the lower end of the esophagus. The impression was cardiac spasm.

The patient now manifested sallow complexion, emaciation, soft abdomen, normal epigastrium, constipation, hot and deep yellow urine, a red tongue with slightly slippery and sticky coating, and a taut, thready and smooth pulse.

The disease was due to the transformation of cold into fire complicated by phlegm and stagnant *qi*. Treatment aimed at conducting the unhealthy *qi* downward, eliminating phlegm, relieving stagnation, and moistening dryness. The following drugs were prescribed:

Radix Pseudostellariae	9 g;
Flos Inulae	9 g;
Haematitum	18 g;

Rhizoma Pinelliae Preparata	9 g;
Radix Angelicae Sinensis	6 g;
Radix Asparagi	9 g;
Rhizoma Anemarrhenae	6 g;
Poria	9 g;
Radix et Rhizoma Rhei (charred)	4.5 g;
Fructus Liquidambaris	9 g.

All symptoms considerably improved after six doses. He had taken 16 doses of the prescription altogether. After that, his complexion became rosy and moist, and he could eat normally.

Explanation: Decoction of Ginseng and Haematitum for Nourishing *Qi* is recommended in the treatment of dysphagia according to *Records of Traditional Chinese Medicine in Combination with Western Medicine*. In the recipe, Haematitum, used in large dosage, promotes gastric activity, arrests spasm, and relieves constipation; Radix Ginseng, used in small dosage, replenishes *qi*; and Rhizoma Pinelliae Preparata, Radix Angelicae Sinensis, Radix Asparagi and Rhizoma Anemarrhenae conduct the stomach *qi* to descend, eliminate phlegm, moisten dryness and produce fluid. Fructus Liquidambaris and Flos Inulae are added to relieve stagnation.

Name: Chen XX; Sex: Male; Age: 44.

The patient felt blockage in the throat for two months. He took barium meal fluoroscopy three times, which showed a focus of 0.8cm-wide and 9cm-long at the lower 1/3 of the esophagus. This established the diagnosis of esophageal cancer.

Clinical manifestations now included emaciation, blockage of the esophagus which became worse when lying down, constipation with dry stool, and a taut and rapid pulse.

The esophagus connects with the stomach, and thus belongs to the Stomach Meridian of Foot-*Yangming*. Thus the method of nourishing *yin* and benefiting the stomach was adopted. Drugs that soften hard masses were added to drugs that produce fluid and moisten dryness. The following were prescribed:

Radix Adenophorae	15 g;
Rhizoma Polygonati Odorati	15 g;
Radix Ophiopogonis	9 g;
Rhizoma Dioscoreae	24 g;
Flos Inulae (wrapped)	9 g;
Rhizoma Imperatae	60 g;
Herba Hedyotis Diffusae	60 g;
Mel (to be added to the prepared decoction)	120 g.

In addition, the patient was asked to drink the blood of a white goose every five or seven days, eat meat cooked over slow fire and take the oil gland of a goose in form of fine powder mixed in rice soup or porridge. If a white goose is unavailable, a white duck also works.

The symptoms considerably improved after three months of treatment. The barium meal fluoroscopy then showed an expanded lower part of the esophagus. Treatment continued. A follow-up survey after seven years showed that he was strong and healthy, and could do heavy manual work.

Explanation: This case was caused by *yin* deficiency, dryness in the stomach, and blockage of the esophagus by stagnant blood. Thus a version of Decoction of Adenophorae and Ophiopogonis was prescribed to nourish *yin* and benefit the stomach; and the blood of a white goose was also administered to remove stasis and soften the hard masses. Herba Hedyotis Diffusae was used in large dosage to treat the cancer and eliminate toxins. In recent years, there have been reports about successful treatment of dysphagia and esophageal cancer with the blood of white geese. This method is also described in *Zhang's Medical Treatise*. Clinical practice has shown that goose blood can eliminate stagnation without damaging the stomach.

XIX. Vomiting

Vomiting forces the contents of the stomach or phlegm to go out of the mouth. It is caused by the adverse movement of stomach *qi*. In Chinese, it is called "*outu*". According to medical classics, "*ou*" refers to forcing out the contents of the stomach with sounds, "*tu*" refers to soundless regurgitation, and dry "*ou*" (retching) refers to a vehement attempt to vomit without bringing anything up. As a matter of fact, it is difficult to separate "*ou*" and "*tu*" for they often occur at the same time. There is a difference between vomiting and retching, but their distinction and treatment are almost the same.

The earliest description of vomiting can be found in *The Inner Canon of the Yellow Emperor*, according to which the causes of vomiting include attack of the stomach and intestines by pathogenic cold, consumption of stomach *yin* by hyperactive fire and heat, and attack of the spleen by dampness accompanied by impaired transportation and transformation. *Synopsis of Prescriptions of the Golden Chamber* not only recommends effective prescriptions that are still used today, but also recognizes vomiting as a protective reaction to harmful substances in the stomach, which should not be checked in such cases. *A Complete Collection of Jingyue's Treatise* classifies vomiting into two types, deficiency and excess, and recommends different methods of treatment.

Vomiting occurs in many diseases, e.g., acute gastritis, cardiac spasm, pyloric spasm, hepatitis, pancreatitis, cholecystitis, certain acute infectious diseases, and some craniocerebral diseases. If it appears as a main symptom, the following descriptions could be used for distinction and treatment. Vomiting may also be found with intestinal obstruction, tumor in the digestive tract, and uremia. In such cases, the chapters discussing vomiting, regurgitation of food from the stomach, dysuria and constipation with incessant vomiting, and retention of urine could be used as reference.

Etiology and Pathogenesis
The stomach is in charge of receiving and digesting food. When stomach *qi* descends, the stomach functions well. The inability of stomach *qi* to descend due to the attack of the stomach by pathogenic factors or gastric deficiency causes vomiting.

1. Attack by External Pathogenic Factors
External pathogenic factors include wind, cold, summer-heat, dampness and pestilential factors. Their attack of the stomach causes an upward movement of stomach *qi* which results in vomiting.

2. Improper Diet
Overeating raw, cold, greasy, or unclean food impairs the stomach's receptive function, and the spleen's ability to transport and transform, thereby causing the upward flow of stomach *qi*.

3. Emotional Upsets
Anger damages the liver and leads to the attack of the stomach by liver *qi*, resulting in the upward movement of stomach *qi*. Worry and over-thinking damage the spleen and impair its function, and further lead to the failure of stomach *qi* to descend.

4. Deficiency of the Spleen and Stomach
Splenic deficiency due to strain and stress or deficiency of *yang-qi* of the middle *jiao* in a prolonged illness impairs the spleen's function of transportation and transformation. In addition, retention of cold and phlegm-fluid in the stomach also causes vomiting. Another cause of vomiting is consump-

tion of fluid in the stomach following a febrile disease, or by fire due to *qi* stagnation, which deprives the stomach of moisture and thus impairs its descending function.

Vomiting is divided into two types, deficiency and excess. The excess syndrome is caused by pathogenic factors, while the deficiency syndrome results from gastric deficiency that prevents *qi* from descending; such deficiency may involve either *yin* or *yang*. Although vomiting is primarily a stomach problem, its pathogenesis is closely related to the liver and spleen.

Differential Diagnosis
1. Regurgitation

Regurgitation is marked by distention and fullness at the epigastrium and abdomen after eating, poor digestion, vomiting in the evening what was taken in the morning, and vice versa. Its accompanying symptoms include emaciation, pale complexion, and lassitude. This disease often develops gradually, and is very hard to be cured.

Vomiting of the excess type develops rapidly and occurs soon after eating or without eating. The deficiency type occurs intermittently and has no definite pattern; retching and nausea may be the symptoms. In either case, food taken in the same day is brought up.

2. Dysphagia

In a mild case, the patient can swallow a small quantity of food; in a severe one, he can only swallow fluid; and in an extremely severe case, both food and fluid are resisted. The symptoms accompanying dysphagia include emaciation, sallow complexion and constipation with dry stool. Vomiting involves the stomach, while dysphagia involves the esophagus and cardia. There is also difference in prognosis: the prognosis of vomiting is favorable, while that of dysphagia is ominous.

3. Cholera

Clinical manifestations of cholera include an abrupt onset of severe vomiting and diarrhea, abdominal pain, stool that resembles rice water, severe weight loss, cold limbs, and deep and faint pulse. Usually vomiting appears without diarrhea, and shows no critical signs except in incessant and severe cases, which indicate the exhaustion of *yin* fluid and collapse of *yang-qi*.

Distinction and Treatment

Efforts should be made to differentiate excess and deficiency. The former has an acute onset and a short duration; the latter is characterized by a slow onset and a long duration.

1. Excess Syndromes

(1) Attack of the stomach by external pathogenic factors

Clinical manifestations: A sudden onset of vomiting, fever, chilliness, headache, fullness in the epigastrium and stuffiness at the chest, a thin and white tongue coating, and a superficial, smooth and rapid pulse.

Analysis: Attack of the stomach by pathogenic wind-cold, summer-heat, dampness, or pestilential factors leads to upward movement of turbid *qi*; this explains the abrupt onset of vomiting. Attack of the body surface by pathogenic factors causes disharmony between the nutrient *qi* and defensive *qi*, thereby resulting in fever, chilliness and headache. Retention of dampness in the middle *jiao* produces disorders of *qi* with symptoms of fullness and stuffiness. A thin and white tongue coating and a superficial, smooth and rapid pulse are signs of invasion by wind, cold, summer-heat and dampness.

Treatment: To eliminate external pathogenic factor, relieve exterior syndrome and resolve the turbid with aromatic drugs.

Prescription: Powder of Agastaches for Restoring Anti-Pathogenic *Qi* (322) is the main formula. In the recipe, Herba Agastaches, Folium Perillae, Cortex Magnoliae Officinalis and Radix Angelicae

Dahuricae eliminate external pathogenic factors and resolve dampness; Rhizoma Pinelliae, Pericarpium Citri Reticulatae, Poria and Pericarpium Arecae conduct the unhealthy *qi* downward and relax the middle *jiao*; and Radix Platycodi promotes the lung's dispersive function. To strengthen the effect in resolving dampness, Rhizoma Atractylodis Macrocephalae can be replaced by Rhizoma Atractylodis. Since there are fullness and stuffiness, drugs that are sweet and sticky, such as Radix Glycyrrhizae and Fructus Jujubae, are removed from the formula. To relieve food retention, Endothelium Corneum Gigeriae Galli and Massa Medicata Fermentata are added. If there are fever, chilliness, absence of sweating and general aching, Herba Schizonepetae and Radix Ledebouriellae are included to eliminate wind and relieve exterior syndrome. If vomiting is accompanied by restlessness and thirst in summer due to attack of summer-heat and dampness, drugs warm and dry in nature, such as Cortex Magnoliae Officinalis and Radix Angelicae Dahuricae, are removed, and drugs that disperse summer-heat, such as Rhizoma Coptidis, Herba Eupatorii and Folium Nelumbinis, are added instead. If there is attack by pestilential factors, one or two grams of *Yushu* Pill (72) is administered to eliminate them and check vomiting.

(2) Retention of food

Clinical manifestations: Vomiting of acid-fermented contents of the stomach, fullness and distention in the epigastrium and abdomen, belching and anorexia — all of which are aggravated by eating and alleviated by vomiting, loose and foul stool or constipation, a thick and sticky tongue coating, and a smooth and forceful pulse.

Analysis: Food retained in the middle *jiao* causes the upward flow of turbid *qi*, resulting in vomiting. Food retained in the stomach also blocks the flow of *qi*, resulting in fullness and distention in the epigastrium and abdomen, belching and anorexia, all aggravated by eating and alleviated by vomiting. When *qi* of the middle *jiao* is hindered, its function of transportation and transformation are impaired, causing abnormal bowel movements. A thick and sticky tongue coating, and a smooth and forceful pulse are signs of food retention.

Treatment: To improve digestion, relieve stagnation, harmonize the stomach, and conduct the unhealthy *qi* downward.

Prescription: Pill for Promoting Digestion (216) is the main formula. In the recipe, Massa Medicata Fermentata, Fructus Crataegi, Semen Raphani and Poria help digest and harmonize the stomach; Pericarpium Citri Reticulatae and Rhizoma Pinelliae regulate *qi* and conduct the unhealthy *qi* downward; and Fructus Forsythiae disperses retained heat. If food retention is severe and accompanied by abdominal fullness and constipation, Radix et Rhizoma Rhei and Fructus Aurantii Immaturus are added. When turbid *qi* goes downward, vomiting will cease spontaneously.

(3) Internal retention of phlegm-fluid

Clinical manifestations: Vomiting of clear fluid and sputum-like substance, epigastric discomfort, poor appetite, dizziness, blurring of vision, palpitation, a white and sticky tongue coating, and a smooth pulse.

Analysis: Impaired splenic and gastric ability to transport and transform results in internal retention of phlegm-fluid and prevents stomach *qi* from descending. Subsequently, vomiting of clear fluid and sputum-like substance, epigastric discomfort and poor appetite occur. Too much water and fluid inhibit the flow of clear *yang-qi*; thus dizziness and palpitation ensue. Retention of phlegm-fluid gives rise to a white and sticky tongue coating and a smooth pulse.

Treatment: To warm and resolve phlegm-fluid, harmonize the stomach and conduct the unhealthy *qi* downward.

Prescription: Modified Small Dose of Pinelliae Decoction (32) and Decoction of Poria, Cinnamomi, Atractylodis Macrocephalae and Glycyrrhizae (170). In the former, Rhizoma Pinelliae and Rhizoma Zingiberis Recens harmonize the stomach and conduct the unhealthy *qi* downward. In the latter, Poria,

Rhizoma Atractylodis Macrocephalae and Radix Glycyrrhizae invigorate the spleen and resolve dampness; and Ramulus Cinnamomi resolves phlegm-fluid with warmth. If retention of phlegm turns into heat and prevents stomach *qi* from descending, with symptoms of dizziness, palpitation, insomnia, nausea and vomiting, Decoction for Clearing Away Gallbladder-Heat (302) is prescribed to resolve phlegm, harmonize the stomach and check vomiting.

(4) Attack of the stomach by liver *qi*

Clinical manifestations: Vomiting, acid regurgitation, belching, fullness and pain in the costal and hypochondriac region, a tongue with red border and thin and sticky coating, and a taut pulse.

Analysis: Attack of the stomach by liver *qi* impairs the stomach's ability to send things down, giving rise to vomiting, acid regurgitation and frequent belching. Liver *qi*-stagnation causes fullness and pain in the costal and hypochondriac region. A tongue with red border and thin and sticky coating, and a taut pulse are signs of *qi* stagnation and hepatic hyperfunction.

Treatment: To soothe the liver, harmonize the stomach, and conduct the unhealthy *qi* downward.

Prescription: Modified Decoction of Pinelliae and Magnoliae Officinalis (107) and modified *Zuojin* Pill (81). In the former, Cortex Magnoliae Officinalis and Folium Perillae regulate *qi* flow and relieve the middle *jiao*; and Rhizoma Pinelliae, Rhizoma Zingiberis Recens and Poria conduct the unhealthy *qi* downward, harmonize the stomach and check vomiting. In the latter, Rhizoma Coptidis and Fructus Evodiae check vomiting with their acrid and bitter nature. If a bitter taste in the mouth, an empty and uncomfortable sensation in the stomach and constipation are present, a small amount of Radix et Rhizoma Rhei, Fructus Aurantii Immaturus and Caulis Bambusae in Taeniam is added to disperse heat and send the turbid downward.

2. Deficiency Syndromes

(1) Stagnant deficiency-cold in the spleen and stomach

Clinical manifestations: Nausea and vomiting after eating, lassitude, dizziness and vomiting after too much work. Other symptoms include dry mouth with no desire to drink, preference for warmth, aversion to cold, pale complexion, cold limbs in severe cases, loose stool, a pale tongue, and a soft and weak pulse.

Analysis: Stagnant deficiency-cold in the spleen and stomach indicates *yang* deficiency of the middle *jiao* and impairs digestive function; thus nausea and vomiting appear after eating. The patient with splenic deficiency cannot shoulder hard work, resulting in lassitude, dizziness and vomiting follow strain and stress. *Yang* deficiency produces cold; here, the head, face, limbs and body are deprived of warmth, accounting for pale complexion, preference for warmth, aversion to cold and cold limbs. Deficiency of the middle *jiao* prevents *qi* from transforming body fluid; since body fluid cannot nourish the upper part of the body, dry mouth with no desire to drink results. Impaired splenic function causes loose stool. Deficiency of spleen *yang* leads to a pale tongue and a soft and weak pulse.

Treatment: To warm the middle *jiao*, invigorate the spleen, harmonize the stomach and conduct the unhealthy *qi* downward.

Prescription: Bolus for Regulating Middle *Jiao* (258) is the main formula. In the recipe, Radix Ginseng, Rhizoma Atractylodis Macrocephalae, Rhizoma Zingiberis and Radix Glycyrrhizae warm the middle *jiao*, disperse cold, invigorate the spleen and check vomiting. To harmonize the stomach and conduct the unhealthy *qi* downward, Fructus Amomi, Rhizoma Pinelliae and Pericarpium Citri Reticulatae are added. In cases with persistent vomiting of clear fluid, Fructus Evodiae is added to warm the middle *jiao*, conduct the unhealthy *qi* downward and check vomiting.

(2) Deficiency of stomach *yin*

Clinical manifestations: Repeated attacks of vomiting or retching, dry mouth and throat, an empty and uncomfortable sensation in the stomach, anorexia, red tongue with little moisture, and a thready, or thready and rapid pulse, vomiting when smelling greasy odor.

Analysis: When the stomach is deprived of moisture, and stomach *qi* does not descend following a febrile disease or due to *yin* deficiency, or consumption of body fluid by fire originating from stagnant *qi*, there occur repeated attacks of vomiting or retching, along with dry mouth and throat. Failure of stomach *qi* to descend due to gastric *yin*-deficiency causes an empty and uncomfortable feeling in the stomach and anorexia. For the same reason, vomiting may be induced by greasy smells. Red tongue with little moisture and a thready or thready and rapid pulse are signs of heat of the deficiency type due to fluid consumption.

Treatment: To nourish stomach *yin*, conduct the unhealthy *qi* downward and check vomiting.

Prescription: Decoction of Ophiopogonis (140) is the main formula. In the recipe, Radix Ophiopogonis, Radix Ginseng (or Radix Adenophorae), Fructus Oryzae Sativae and Radix Glycyrrhizae nourish stomach *yin*; and Rhizoma Pinelliae conducts the unhealthy *qi* downward and checks vomiting. To promote the generation of body fluid and nourish the stomach, Herba Dendrobii, Radix Trichosanthis and Caulis Bambusae in Taeniam are added. In cases of constipation with dry stool, Fructus Cannabis and Mel are added to moisten the intestines and promote bowel movement.

Vomiting has different manifestations due to different causes. For instance, vomiting due to the attack by external pathogenic factors is marked by an abrupt and serious onset. Vomiting due to emotional upsets is accompanied by nausea and alleviated by belching. Vomiting due to deficiency of stomach *yin* is accompanied by an empty and uncomfortable sensation in the stomach and dry mouth, and sometimes manifests as retching. Finally, vomiting due to cold of the deficiency type in the spleen and stomach occurs intermittently and brings up clear fluid and sputum-like substance. Recognition of these characteristics is conducive to distinction and treatment.

Since vomiting damages stomach *qi* and impairs the source of *qi* and blood, it should be treated promptly. Drugs that harmonize the stomach and conduct the unhealthy *qi* downward are used in combination, no matter what principle is observed in treatment; this is because the stomach functions well when stomach *qi* descends. Medical workers share the opinion that Rhizoma Pinelliae and Haematitum are the most effective of all drugs in conducting the unhealthy *qi* downward and checking vomiting. There is also a method of applying acrid and bitter drugs to treat vomiting; the representative drugs are Rhizoma Zingiberis Recens, acrid in nature, and Rhizoma Coptidis, bitter in nature. Both can help improve the function of the stomach in sending *qi* downward.

Incorrect treatment of vomiting may change an excess syndrome into a deficiency one, and, if so, the pathological conditions will deteriorate. Extreme spleen and stomach deficiency will possibly become the consequence.

As the popular saying goes, "Diseases enter the body via the mouth." Therefore, attention should be paid to dietary hygiene. To protect stomach *qi*, one should take care to avoid external pathogenic factors.

Appendix   Regurgitation

Regurgitation is characterized by vomiting of food in the evening of what was taken in the morning, and vice versa, and is often accompanied by epigastric and abdominal distention and dyspepsia. Its causes include improper diet, indulgence in alcohol, excess sexual life and emotional stress. *Qi* stagnation, blood stagnation and phlegm retention due to spleen and stomach dysfunction are the main pathogenesis.

Regurgitation found with gastric and duodenal ulcer, the diverticulum of the stomach and duodenum, acute and chronic gastritis, prolapse of gastric mucosa, duodenal stasis and gastric tumors characterized by difficulty in emptying the stomach due to pyloric spasm, edema and stricture, is differentiated and treated in the following ways.

Improper diet, overeating raw and cold food, or excessive worry and thinking produces deficiency of the middle *jiao* with stagnation of cold. Consequently, food retention causes regurgitation. Prolonged regurgitation leads to renal *yang*-deficiency, which decreases the fire of the lower *jiao*. In this case, digestion becomes even poorer, and pathological conditions more severe.

Clinical manifestations: Distention and fullness in the epigastrium and abdomen after eating, which are alleviated by regurgitation, vomiting of undigested food in the evening of what is taken in the morning, and vice versa, lassitude, pale complexion, a pale tongue with thin coating, and a thready, slow and weak pulse.

Analysis: Deficiency of the middle *jiao* with stagnation of cold causes food retention, along with distention and fullness in the epigastrium and abdomen which are alleviated by regurgitation. Prolonged regurgitation damages *qi*, which fails to transform food to essence; this explains lassitude and pale complexion. A pale tongue with thin coating and a thready, retarded and weak pulse reflect cold of the deficiency type in the spleen and stomach.

Treatment: To warm the middle *jiao*, invigorate the spleen, conduct the unhealthy *qi* downward, and harmonize the stomach.

Prescription: Modified Powder of Caryophylli for Relieving Regurgitation (8). In the recipe, Radix Ginseng, Rhizoma Atractylodis Macrocephalae and Radix Aucklandiae warm the middle *jiao* and invigorate the spleen; and Fructus Amomi, Flos Caryophylli, Fructus Amomi Rotundus, Massa Medicata Fermentata and Fructus Hordei Germinatus conduct the unhealthy *qi* downward and harmonize the stomach. The addition of Flos Inulae and Haematitum suppresses the unhealthy *qi* and checks regurgitation.

In a chronic case marked by renal *yang*-deficiency with symptoms of pale complexion, cold limbs, a pale tongue with white coating and a deep and thready pulse, Fructus Evodiae, Flos Caryophylli and Cortex Cinnamomi are added to Bolus of Aconiti Lateralis Preparata for Regulating Middle *Jiao* (163) to reinforce the source of fire in order to warm splenic *yang*.

In cases with dry lips and mouth, constipation with dry stool, a red tongue, and a thready pulse caused by insufficient stomach fluid and deficiency of both *qi* and *yin*, Decoction of Ophiopogonis (140) is prescribed with additional drugs to replenish *qi*, promote the generation of body fluid, conduct the unhealthy *qi* downward and check regurgitation.

In summary, failure of stomach *qi* to descend is the common pathogenesis of vomiting and regurgitation, but regurgitation usually results from deficiency cold in the spleen and stomach. Vomiting is due to the upward movement of stomach *qi* caused by either attack of pathogenic factors or gastric deficiency.

Case Studies

Name: Wang XX; Sex: Male; Age: 34.

The patient complained of nausea, vomiting, belching, acid regurgitation and dizziness for two months. Other symptoms were shortness of breath, poor appetite, lack of taste, and dislike of greasy food. Sleep was basically good, and both defecation and urination were normal. Barium meal fluoroscopy and X-rays of the brain showed nothing abnormal. The diagnosis of Western medicine was neurogenic vomiting. The illness did not respond to Western treatment. The patient looked healthy when he did not vomit. The pulse was slightly taut and smooth, the tongue coating was sticky, and blood pressure was 115/74 mm Hg.

The disease was due to retention of dampness in the middle *jiao*, causing upward movement of stomach *qi*. Treatment aimed to resolve the turbid with aromatic drugs, harmonize the stomach and conduct the unhealthy *qi* downward. The following were prescribed:

Rhizoma Atractylodis	6 g;
Cortex Magnoliae Officinalis	6 g;
Pericarpium Citri Reticulatae	6 g;
Herba Agastaches	9 g;
Herba Eupatorii	9 g;
Poria	9 g;
Rhizoma Pinelliae	9 g;
Fructus Aurantii	3 g;
Caulis Bambusae in Taeniam	9 g;
Rhizoma Zingiberis Recens	6 g;
Radix Glycyrrhizae	3 g.

Second visit: After two doses, vomiting stopped; nausea and shortness of breath improved. Other symptoms were loose stool once a day, yellow urine, and a yellow tongue coating at the root. Three grams of Radix Scutellariae and 2.4 grams of Fructus Amomi were added to the above prescription. Another three doses were prescribed. All the symptoms were then relieved.

Explanation: Vomiting and acid regurgitation were caused by the attack of the stomach by liver *qi*. Lack of taste and dislike of greasy food were signs of retention of dampness in the middle *jiao*. Thus bitter and cold drugs should not be used. Decoction for Clearing Away Gallbladder-Heat (302) was prescribed to soothe the liver and conduct the unhealthy *qi* downward. The addition of Rhizoma Atractylodis, Cortex Magnoliae Officinalis, Herba Agastaches and Herba Eupatorii resolved dampness. When dampness was resolved and stomach *qi* descended, vomiting would stop.

Name: Wang XX; Sex: Female; Age: 18; Occupation: Student.

First visit (March 5, 1974): The patient had regurgitation for over a year. Her stomach felt uncomfortable after eating. The undigested food brought up had no acid smell. She felt more comfortable after regurgitating but without the feeling of hunger. If she tried to swallow a bit of food then, she would regurgitate again. Other symptoms were emaciation, constipation, thirst, red tongue and a thready and weak pulse. X-rays showed nothing abnormal in the stomach and intestines.

All this was due to mental irritation and improper diet. Incessant regurgitation caused deficiency of both *qi* and *yin*. Treatment aimed to soothe the liver, nourish the stomach, and conduct the unhealthy *qi* downward. The following drugs were prescribed:

Flos Inulae	9 g;
Haematitum Usta	12 g;
Radix Glehniae	9 g;
Radix Ophiopogonis	9 g;
Fructus Toosendan	9 g;
Rhizoma Pinelliae	9 g;
Pericarpium Citri Reticulatae	6 g;
Caulis Bambusae in Taeniam (ginger prepared)	9 g;
Fructus Setariae Germinatus	12 g;
Fructus Aurantii	4.5 g.

Three doses were prescribed.

Second visit (March 8, 1974): Regurgitation slightly improved. The empty and uncomfortable feeling in the stomach remained unchanged. One and a half grams of Rhizoma Coptidis were added. Seven doses were prescribed.

Third visit (March 15, 1974): Regurgitation further improved. Another seven doses were prescribed.

Fourth visit (March 23, 1974): Regurgitation stopped. Bowel movements were normal. The patient began to eat soybean juice, rice porridge, and then soft rice, and felt comfortable after eating; but she still had lassitude, red tongue with no coating and a thready pulse. All this showed damage to the spleen and stomach and deficiency of both qi and yin. Treatment then aimed at replenishing qi, promoting the generation of body fluid, invigorating the spleen and harmonize the stomach. Decoction of Ophiopogonis (140) was prescribed with some modifications:

Radix Ophiopogonis	9 g;
Rhizoma Pinelliae	4.5 g;
Radix Codonopsis	9 g;
Radix Glycyrrhizae	3 g;
Pericarpium Citri Reticulatae	4.5 g;
Fructus Setariae Germinatus	12 g;
Fructus Hordei Germinatus	12 g.

Ten doses were prescribed. The patient was advised not to eat too much.

Explanation: On the one hand, this patient exhibited deficiency cold in the spleen and stomach with regurgitation. On the other, she experienced consumption of stomach yin by heat with symptoms of red tongue, dry mouth, and an empty and uncomfortable feeling in the stomach. Thus drugs that nourish stomach yin and stomach qi were prescribed primarily to conduct the unhealthy qi downward, and aromatic and dry drugs were avoided. The prescription combined Decoction of Inulae and Haematitum (275), Decoction of Ophiopogonis (140) and Decoction of Coptidis for Clearing Away Gallbladder-Heat. According to Zhu Danxi's statement, "Unhealthy qi originates from the liver," Fructus Toosendan was added to soothe the liver and regulate qi. This case is complicated with cold and heat, exhibiting excess first and deficiency later. It was advisable to harmonize the stomach and conduct the unhealthy qi downward at the beginning of treatment, because incessant regurgitation prevents the patient from taking the medicinal decoction. When the effects of the drugs reach the stomach and qi circulation becomes smooth, regurgitation will cease.

Name: Yang XX; Sex: Female; Age: 45.

First visit (January 18, 1975): The patient had a long history of stomach problem. Over the past ten days, she developed vomiting after eating, acid regurgitation, a cold feeling at the epigastrium, dizziness, aversion to cold, a dark red tongue with thin coating, and a slightly taut pulse. All this was due to turbid phlegm retention which causes upward movement of stomach qi. Decoction of Inulae and Haematitum (275) and *Zuojin* Pill (81) were prescribed to harmonize the stomach, conduct the unhealthy qi downward, resolve phlegm and disperse cold:

Flos Inulae (wrapped)	12 g;
Haematitum	30 g;
Rhizoma Zingiberis Recens	6 g;
Rhizoma Pinelliae	6 g;
Radix Codonopsis	9 g;

Radix Glycyrrhizae Preparata	3 g;
Pericarpium Citri Reticulatae	6 g;
Caulis Bambusae in Taeniam (ginger prepared)	9 g;
Radix Aucklandiae	1.8 g;
Zuojin Pill (to be swallowed separately)	1.8 g.

Second visit (January 21, 1975): Both vomiting and nausea disappeared; but she still complained of dizziness, blurred vision, aversion to cold, belching and absence of bowel movements for three days. The pulse was slightly taut and smooth, and the tongue coating was white. All this was due to the attack of the stomach by liver *qi*, complicated by the failure of turbid *qi* to descend. Drugs that drain the intestines and conduct the turbid *qi* downward were added to Decoction of Pericarpium Citri Reticulatae and Caulis Bambusae in Taeniam:

Radix Codonopsis	9 g;
Pericarpium Citri Reticulatae	9 g;
Rhizoma Zingiberis Recens	2 pieces;
Rhizoma Pinelliae	6 g;
Poria	9 g;
Caulis Bambusae in Taeniam (ginger prepared)	9 g;
Fructus Citri	9 g;
Massa Medicata Fermentata	9 g;
Radix et Rhizoma Rhei Preparata	9 g.

Explanation: This patient had gastric deficiency which prevented stomach *qi* from descending. Attack of the stomach by liver *qi* resulted in vomiting. In the prescription, Flos Inulae and Haematitum conduct the unhealthy *qi* downward; and Rhizoma Zingiberis Recens and Rhizoma Pinelliae harmonize the stomach, conduct the *qi* to go downward and check vomiting. *Zuojin* Pill treats both the liver and stomach. Decoction of Inulae and Haematitum is also effective in the treatment of vomiting due to gastric deficiency and upwardly moving stomach *qi*. Decoction of Pericarpium Citri Reticulatae and Caulis Bambusae in Taeniam remedies the deficiency, harmonizes the stomach, and conducts the unhealthy *qi* downward. Dizziness and blurred vision are caused by constipation, which prevents turbid *qi* from moving downward and clear *qi* from going upward. Radix et Rhizoma Rhei sends the turbid *qi* downward.

XX. Hiccup

Hiccup refers to an involuntary spasmodic contraction of the diaphragm followed by sudden closure of the glottis due to upward disturbance of *qi*. It may occur alone or as a symptom of other diseases. Hiccup of the excess type is caused by invasion by pathogenic cold, stomach fire, stagnation of *qi*, or retention of food. Hiccup of the deficiency type results from deficiency of the middle *jiao* with stagnation of cold, deficiency of the kidneys, or weakness of body constitution after a severe illness.

The Inner Canon of the Yellow Emperor relates hiccup to the disorders of the upper and middle *jiao*, holding that the cause of hiccup is the disharmony of stomach *qi* and failure of lung *qi* to descend. This book also recommends simple methods of stopping hiccup. For instance, stimulation of the nose with certain herbs to cause sneezing, holding breath with closed mouth and nose, and sudden fright all stop hiccup. *Synopsis of Prescriptions of the Golden Chamber* classifies hiccup into three categories: hiccup due to cold with the symptoms of retching and cold limbs to be treated with Decoction of Pericarpium Citri Reticulatae, hiccup due to heat of the deficiency type to be treated with Decoction of Pericarpium Citri Reticulatae and Caulis Bambusae in Taeniam, and hiccup due to heat of the excess type accompanied by fullness and distention of the abdomen to be treated by promoting diuresis or relieving constipation. This classification of hiccup laid down a foundation of distinction and treatment for medical workers of later generations.

Western medicine holds that spasm of the diaphragm is the cause of hiccup. Hiccup found with gastrointestinal neurosis, gastritis, gastric dilatation, hepatic cirrhosis at the later stage, cerebrovascular diseases, uremia etc. is differentiated and treated according to the following descriptions.

Etiology and Pathogenesis
1. Improper Diet

Eating too fast or too much, or excess eating of raw and cold food, or excess administration of herbs cold and cool in nature, may all accumulate cold in the stomach. Invasion of the lung by cold in the stomach along the Meridian of Hand-*Taiyin* causes stomach and lung *qi* to ascend with the symptom of hiccup. Excess eating of fried food pungent and hot in nature, or excess administration of herbs warm and dry in nature produces dryness and heat in the intestines. Failure of *qi* in the intestines to descend disturbs the diaphragm and causes hiccup.

2. Emotional Upsets

Both anger and mental depression impair the liver's function in promoting flow of *qi*. Malfunction of *qi* influences distribution of body fluid, and thus produces phlegm. Invasion of the lung and stomach by liver *qi* and phlegm disturbs the diaphragm, and subsequently causes hiccup.

3. Deficiency of Spleen and Kidney *Yang*

This may result from weakness of body constitution, old age, long-standing diarrhea and dysentery, a severe illness, strain and stress, or administration by mistake of herbs that eliminate pathogenic factors for deficiency syndrome. Deficiency of *yang-qi* of the spleen and kidneys causes stomach *qi* to decline, and prevents clear *qi* from ascending and turbid *qi* from descending. Unhealthy *qi* disturbs the diaphragm, and causes hiccup. Hiccup found in old patients, patients suffering from deficiency syndrome, women at the postpartum stage, and patients at the later stage of a severe illness suggests aggravation of pathological conditions.

4. Deficiency of Stomach *Yin*

A febrile disease consumes stomach *yin*. Severe sweating, vomiting, or diarrhea consumes *yin* fluid of the stomach, and subsequently gives rise to fire of the deficiency type. Failure of stomach *qi* to descend leads to hiccup.

To conclude, hiccup is usually the result of disturbance of the diaphragm by stomach *qi* in its upward movement. Unsmooth circulation of lung *qi* can also produce the same problem. This is because the Lung Meridian goes along the upper orifice of the stomach and passes through the diaphragm. The lung and stomach promote each other physiologically and affect each other pathologically. The diaphragm is located between the lung and stomach. Invasion of the lung by pathogenic factors hinders *qi* between the lung and stomach, and causes upward disturbance of stomach *qi* with the symptom of hiccup.

Sneezing caused by the stimulation of the nose with certain herbs circulates *qi* between the lung and stomach, and thus assists descending of stomach *qi*. That is why the method recommended in *The Inner Canon of the Yellow Emperor* checks hiccup.

Differential Diagnosis
1. Retching

Retching and hiccup are two different diseases. But they were thought to be the same disease at the Jin and Yuan dynasties by some medical workers. Retching presents with a strong attempt to vomit without bringing anything up, while hiccup is marked by continuous involuntary production of sounds at short intervals.

2. Belching

Belching means sending out stagnant *qi* of the body, and sometimes is accompanied by acid fermented smell. Since belching makes *qi* of the middle *jiao* circulate more smoothly, the patient feels more comfortable after belching. This act is due to stagnation of *qi* of the middle *jiao* with the symptoms of fullness and distention at the chest and diaphragm.

Distinction and Treatment

It is necessary to clarify whether hiccup is caused by transient disturbance of *qi* or by dysfunction of *zang-fu* organs. Generally, hiccup at the initial stage presenting loud and strong sounds in a continuous manner is of the excess type. Intermittent occurrence of hiccup with low and long sounds and lassitude is of the deficiency type. Hiccup of the cold type manifests deep and slow sounds, blue complexion, cold limbs and loose stool. Hiccup of the heat type exhibits loud and short sounds, red face, hot limbs, irritability, thirst, and constipation. Hiccup appearing at the later stage of an acute and severe illness or in senile patients with weak constitution, incessant low and feeble sounds, difficulty in swallowing, and a deep, thready and hidden pulse, are critical signs indicating the decline of primordial *qi* of the body. In this case, special attention should be paid to the development of pathological conditions.

Mild hiccup can be relieved without any treatment. But if hiccup occurs repeatedly or the spleen and kidney are affected, different methods should be adopted according to the causes of the disease. These methods include eliminating cold, dispersing heat, relieving stagnation, resolving phlegm, warming and tonifying the spleen and kidneys to nourish *yin* fluid. Herbs that harmonize the stomach, conduct the unhealthy *qi* downward, and stop hiccup could be added in treating the illness. To stop hiccup, Flos Caryophylli and Calyx Kaki are commonly used.

1. Excess Syndrome

(1) Retention of cold in the stomach

Clinical manifestations: Hiccup with deep and slow sounds, discomfort at the chest, diaphragm and epigastrium, which is alleviated by warmth and aggravated by cold, poor appetite, absence of thirst, white and moist tongue coating, and slow pulse.

Analysis: Invasion by cold prevents *qi* of the lung and stomach from descending; this explains discomfort at the chest, diaphragm and epigastrium. Retention of cold in the stomach leads to upward disturbance of stomach *qi*; the result is hiccup with deep and slow sounds. *Qi* circulates more smoothly when it is warm, thus symptoms are alleviated. Exposure to cold makes the illness worse because cold aggravates stagnation. Absence of thirst, poor appetite, white and moist tongue coating and slow pulse are signs of retention of cold in the stomach.

Treatment: To warm the middle *jiao*, eliminate cold and check hiccup.

Prescription: Powder of Caryophylli (9) is the main formula, in which, Flos Caryophylli, Calyx Kaki check hiccup, and Rhizoma Alpiniae Officinarum and Radix Glycyrrhizae Preparata warm the middle *jiao* and eliminate cold. If cold is severe, add Fructus Evodiae and Cortex Cinnamomi to warm *yang*, disperse cold and conduct the unhealthy *qi* downward. In case of retention of phlegm with the symptoms of stuffiness in the chest and foul belching, add Cortex Magnolicae Officinalis, Fructus Aurantii Immaturus, Fructus Hordei Germinatus and Pericarpium Citri Reticulatae to circulate *qi*, resolve phlegm and relieve stagnation.

(2) Upward disturbance of stomach fire

Clinical manifestations: Hiccup with loud and strong sounds, foul breath, irritability, thirst, preference for cold drinks, scanty and deep yellow urine, constipation, yellow tongue coating, and smooth and rapid pulse.

Analysis: Overeating fried pungent food, or excess administration of tonics which are warm in nature, may accumulate heat and fire in the stomach and intestines. Disturbance of the diaphragm by stomach fire gives rise to hiccup with loud and strong sounds. Heat in the stomach consumes body fluid, which is the cause of foul breath, irritability, thirst, preference for cold drinks, scanty, deep yellow urine, and constipation. A yellow tongue coating and a smooth and rapid pulse are signs of retention of heat in the stomach.

Treatment: To clear heat, relieve constipation and check hiccup.

Prescription: Decoction for Mild Purgation (35) added with Calyx Kaki is prescribed. In this prescription, Radix et Rhizoma Rhei, Fructus Aurantii Immaturus and Cortex Magnolicae Officinalis clear heat, relieve constipation, relax the middle *jiao* and send *qi* downward; and Calyx Kaki checks hiccup. If there is no constipation, although stomach-heat is severe, Decoction of Lophatheri and Gypsum Fibrosum (132) added with Calyx Kaki is prescribed. In this case, Radix Ginseng can be replaced by Radix Adenophorae. This prescription nourishes the stomach, produces body fluid, conducts the unhealthy *qi* downward and checks hiccup.

(3) Blockage by stagnant *qi* and phlegm

Clinical manifestations: Hiccup in a continuous manner, stuffiness in the chest, distention in the hypochondrium induced by mental depression or anger, and alleviated when the patient is in a happy mood, nausea, poor appetite, dizziness and blurring of vision, sticky tongue coating, and taut and smooth pulse.

Analysis: Mental depression or anger causes liver *qi* to invade the stomach and lung. Upward disturbance of *qi* of the stomach results in hiccup in a continuous manner. Invasion of the lung by liver *qi* along the Liver Meridian is the cause of stuffiness in the chest and distention in the hypochondrium. Since the liver's function is closely related to emotions, hiccup of this kind is induced or alleviated by emotional changes. Nausea, poor appetite, dizziness and blurring of vision are due to the disharmony of stomach *qi* complicated with turbid phlegm in the middle *jiao*, preventing lucid *yang-qi* from ascending. Sticky tongue coating, and taut and smooth pulse are signs of stagnant liver *qi* complicated with phlegm-dampness.

Treatment: Decoction of Inulae and Haematitum (275) is the main formula, in which Flos Inulae and Haematitum send the unhealthy *qi* of the liver and lung downward, and Rhizoma Zingiberis Recens and Rhizoma Pinelliae harmonize the stomach, resolve phlegm and check hiccup, and Fructus Toosendan and Radix Curcumae relieve stagnation of liver *qi*. If body resistance is not weakened, Radix Ginseng and Radix Glycyrrhizae are removed from the formula to prevent stagnation of *qi*.

2. Deficiency Syndrome

(1) Deficiency of *yang* of the spleen and stomach

Clinical manifestations: Hiccup with low, deep and weak sounds, shortness of breath, pale complexion, cold limbs, poor appetite, lassitude, pale tongue with white coating, and a thready and weak pulse.

Analysis: Deficiency of the spleen and stomach with stagnation of cold causes upward disturbance of stomach *qi* with the result of hiccup in a low, deep and weak voice. Deficiency of *yang-qi* impairs the function of transportation and transformation and exhausts the source of *qi* and blood. This explains shortness of breath, pale complexion, cold limbs, poor appetite and lassitude. Pale tongue with white coating and thready and weak pulse are signs of *yang-qi* deficiency.

Treatment: To warm and tonify the spleen and stomach, harmonize the middle *jiao* and check hiccup.

Prescription: Decoction for Regulating Middle *Jiao* (258) added with Fructus Evodiae and Flos Caryophylli is prescribed. In this prescription, Radix Ginseng, Rhizoma Atractylodis Macrocephalae, and Radix Glycyrrhizae, sweet and warm in nature, tonify *qi*; Rhizoma Zingiberis warms the middle *jiao* and assists the spleen; and Fructus Evodiae and Flos Caryophylli warm the stomach and diaphragm to check hiccup. In case of deficiency of kidney *yang* with the symptoms of cold limbs, soreness and weakness of the lumbus and knees, pale and swollen tongue and deep and slow pulse, add Radix Aconiti Lateralis Preparata and Cortex Cinnamomi to warm the kidneys and assist *yang*.

(2) Deficiency of stomach *yin*

Clinical manifestations: Hiccup in a rapid manner, dry mouth and tongue, irritability, restlessness, red and dry tongue or tongue with cracks, and thready and rapid pulse.

Analysis: Consumption of stomach *yin* in a febrile disease causes lack of moisture in the stomach. This prevents stomach *qi* from descending, and thus produces hiccup in a rapid manner. Dry mouth and tongue, irritability and restlessness are consequences of consumption of body fluid and disturbance by heat of the deficiency type. Red and dry or cracked tongue and thready and rapid pulse are signs of consumption of body fluid.

Treatment: To produce body fluid, nourish the stomach and check hiccup.

Prescription: Decoction for Benefiting Stomach (246) added with Herba Dendrobii, Folium Eriobotryae, Calyx Kaki and Semen Canavaliae is prescribed. In this prescription, Radix Adenophorae, Radix Ophiopogonis, Radix Rehmanniae, Rhizoma Polygonati Odorati, Herba Dendrobii and crystal sugar nourish fluid of the stomach. This method is known as producing body fluid with sweet herbs cold in nature. Folium Eriobotryae, Calyx Kaki and Semen Canavaliae send *qi* of the stomach and lung downward to check hiccup.

Case Studies

Name: Xu XX; Sex: Female; Age: 34.

First visit (April 8, 1975): The patient had hiccup for three weeks. The accompanying symptoms included aversion to cold, an uncomfortable sensation in the throat and epigastrium, stuffiness in the chest, abdominal distention, borborygmus, difficult bowel movement, thin and sticky tongue coating, and thready and taut pulse.

The disease was due to the invasion by pathogenic cold, which prevented stomach *qi* from descending. The method of warming the middle *jiao*, eliminating cold, harmonizing the stomach and conducting the unhealthy *qi* downward was adopted in the treatment. The following herbs were prescribed:

Radix Aconiti Lateralis Preparata	4.5 g;
Rhizoma Zingiberis	2.4 g;
Flos Caryophylli	1.5 g;
Calyx Kaki	9 g;
Caulis Bambusae in Taeniam	6 g;
Rhizoma Pinelliae	4.5 g
Pericarpium Citri Reticulatae	9 g;
Magnetitum	30 g;
Flos Inulae (wrapped)	9 g;
Ramulus Uncariae cum Uncis	9 g;
Haematitum	18 g;
Radix Glycyrrhizae Preparata	9 g.

Second visit (April 12, 1975): Hiccup improved after taking four doses of the above prescription. Aversion to cold and an uncomfortable sensation in the throat remained unchanged. The patient did not have bowel movement for two days. The tongue coating was thin, and the pulse was thready. All this suggested remnant pathogenic factors and disharmony of stomach *qi*. The method of warming the middle *jiao*, regulating *qi*, harmonizing the stomach, and conducting the unhealthy *qi* downward was adopted. The following herbs were prescribed:

Radix Aconiti Lateralis Preparata	4.5 g;
Rhizoma Zingiberis	2.4 g;
Flos Caryophylli	15 g;
Calyx Kaki	9 g;
Rhizoma Coptidis	2.4 g;
Pericarpium Trichosanthis	15 g;
Magnetitum	30 g;
Flos Inulae (wrapped)	9 g;
Haematitum	18 g;
Caulis Akebiae	9 g;
Radix Glycyrrhizae Preparata	9 g.

Explanation: Hiccup can also be caused by spasm of the stomach. This case results from cold blockage, which prevents stomach *qi* from descending. Flos Caryophylli and Calyx Kaki harmonize the stomach and conduct the unhealthy *qi* downward. Caulis Bambusae in Taeniam, Rhizoma Pinelliae, Pericarpium Citri Reticulatae, Flos Inulae and Haematitum are combined to conduct the unhealthy *qi* downward. Ramulus Uncariae cum Uncis and Magnetitum relieve gastric spasm, and Radix Glycyrrhizae harmonizes the middle *jiao*. Hiccup stopped after ten doses were taken.

Hiccup is often complicated with cold and heat, deficiency and excess. Although there are different treatment of hiccup, the method of harmonizing the stomach and conducting the unhealthy *qi* downward is considered the basic one.

XXI. Diarrhea

Diarrhea refers to the frequent passage of loose stools, possibly containing undigested food, or watery stools in severe cases. Its main cause is the retention of excess dampness and impaired splenic and gastric functions. Here the clear and turbid *qi* is not divided, and water and food mix together on their way to the large intestine. Although diarrhea may occur during all four seasons, it is more common in the summer and the autumn.

Detailed descriptions concerning diarrhea can be found in medical classics of all ages. *The Inner Canon of the Yellow Emperor* says, "The descent of clear splenic *qi* gives rise to diarrhea with undigested food in the stools. Retained dampness causes watery diarrhea." *A Complete Collection of Jingyue's Treatise* states, "Diarrhea is the result of an improper diet, seasonal pathogenic factors and retained cold after eating raw or cold food." *Zhang Yuqing's Medical Records* points out that when stagnant *qi* of the Liver Meridian of Foot-*Jueyin* invades the spleen and stomach, this may cause the upward movement of liver and stomach *qi* which produces symptoms such as belching and sighing, and the descent of spleen *qi* resulting in diarrhea.

An Essential Medical Manual recommends nine methods of treating diarrhea: promoting diuresis with sweet and wild herbs, sending fresh air upwards, dissipating heat with cool herbs, soothing the liver and eliminating dampness, relieving acute symptoms with sweet herbs, restraining excretion with sour herbs, drying dampness, warming the kidneys, and promoting astringency.

Diarrhea due to functional and organic disorders of the digestive organs, such as acute and chronic enteritis, intestinal tuberculosis, intestinal problems or an irritable colon, can be differentiated and treated according to the following descriptions.

Etiology and Pathogenesis
1. Pathogenic Factors

External factors which cause diarrhea include heat in the summer, dampness and cold. Of these, dampness is the most common. The spleen dislikes dampness, and prefers dryness. External pathogenic dampness is likely to affect the spleen and impair its ability to transport and transform. As a result, water and food descend together, causing diarrhea. Hence there are the sayings: "excess dampness causes five types of diarrhea" and "diarrhea is impossible without dampness". The other factors invade the lungs and body surface first, and then penetrate the spleen and stomach, impairing their ability to ascend and descend. These can also damage the spleen and stomach directly, impairing their ability to divide the clear and the turbid *qi*, thus causing diarrhea. In either case, external factors causing diarrhea are often associated with pathogenic dampness.

2. Improper Diet

Overeating, especially greasy, raw, cold or unclean food, damages the spleen and stomach and impairs their ability to transport, transform, ascend and descend, thus causing diarrhea. *A Complete Collection of Jingyue's Treatise* describes the etiology as follows, "An improper diet or lifestyle damages the spleen and the stomach so that water and food are unable to be transformed into essence and turbid dampness and retained food are produced. The vital energy cannot be distributed throughout the body, so it descends along with dampness, thus produces diarrhea."

3. Emotional Trauma

When a patient who always suffers from splenic and gastric deficiency is perplexed by mental depression or anger, stagnant liver *qi* invades the spleen and impairs its ability, thus causing diarrhea.

4. Spleen and Stomach Deficiencies

These may come from improper diet, stress or prolonged illness. In these cases, the stomach is unable to receive food and water and the spleen cannot transport or transform the essence of food, and diarrhea occurs. In cases where the spleen *yang* is inadequate, too much pathogenic cold is produced and normal functions are impaired.

5. Kidney *Yang*-Deficiency

Kidney *yang* helps the spleen, stomach and intestines digest food and absorb the essence of food because fire usually promotes earth. A deficiency of renal *yang* may be the result of prolonged illness or of a weak constitution in an elderly patient. *A Complete Collection of Jingyue's Treatise* says, "As the gate to the stomach, the kidneys control the two private parts (urethra and anus), dominating urination and defecation. A deficiency of kidney *yang-qi* leads to the declining of fire from the life gate... and an excess of *yin-qi* causes incessant diarrhea."

Overdrinking is another cause of diarrhea, since water may be retained in the large intestine. In a prolonged case of retained cold, heat and dampness in the intestines, blood is liable to become stagnant and diarrhea will occur.

To conclude, pathogenic dampness is the most important pathogenic factor, and splenic deficiency the main internal cause of diarrhea. Diarrhea due to hepatic or renal disorders is also induced by splenic deficiency, namely, the dysfunction of the spleen and stomach produces dampness, which in turn further impairs their functions.

Differentiation

1. Dysentery

In diarrhea, there is neither mucus nor blood in the stools. Tenesumus does not occur and abdominal pain is not a recessary symptom. However, dysentery manifests these symptoms.

2. Cholera

Cholera is marked by an abrupt onset of abdominal pain, severe vomiting and diarrhea. The vomit contains mostly of undigested food with a sour, fermented, foul smell. The stool is yellow and watery, or like rice water. The accompanying symptoms include aversion to cold, fever, emaciation in a short period of time, and abdominal cramps. Severe vomiting and diarrhea in cholera may cause a pale complexion, sunken eyes, sweating and cold limbs, all of which are signs of dehydration and *yang* exhaustion.

Treatment

The first step is to clarify acute and chronic conditions. Acute diarrhea is often accompanied by pathogenic factors, while chronic diarrhea is marked by weak resistance. And the next step is to distinguish cold, heat, deficiency and excess. Generally speaking, diarrhea with clear and diluted stool and undigested food manifests a cold syndrome. Rapid diarrhea with yellow, brown and foul stool and a burning sensation of the anus suggests a heat syndrome. Diarrhea with acute abdominal pain aggravated by pressure is of the excess type; and diarrhea with mild pain in the lower abdomen which can be alleviated by warmth and pressure is of the deficiency type. Clinically, complicated conditions of deficiency and cold, cold and heat are often seen.

1. Acute Diarrhea

(1) Cold-dampness or wind-cold

Clinical manifestations: Diarrhea with clear and diluted stool or watery stool in severe cases, abdominal pain, borborygmus, possible aversion to cold, fever, nasal stuffiness, headache, general aching, thin or sticky white tongue coating, and a weak pulse.

Analysis: Invasion of the stomach and intestines by external pathogenic cold-dampness impairs the ability of the spleen and stomach to ascend and descend, preventing food from being transformed into essence. Instead of being divided and moving in different directions, the clear and turbid *qi* mix together, and move downwards to the large intestine; this explains the occurence of diarrhea with clear and diluted stool. Excess cold-dampness in the middle *jiao* causes disorders of gastric and intestinal *qi*, thus leading to abdominal pain and borborygmus. Aversion to cold, fever, nasal stuffiness, headache and general aching are signs of wind-cold invasion. A white or sticky tongue coating and a weak pulse are signs of cold-dampness.

Treatment: To relieve symptoms, disperse cold, and resolve the turbid *qi* with aromatic herbs.

Prescription: Powder of Agastaches for Restoring Anti-Pathogenic *Qi* (322) is the main formula. Herba Agastaches disperses cold with its acrid warmth, and resolves the turbid *qi* with its aromatic smell; Rhizoma Atractylodis Macrocephalae and Poria invigorate the spleen and remove dampness; Cortex Magnoliae Officinalis and Pericarpium Arecae dry dampness, regulate *qi* and relieve fullness; and Folium Perillae and Radix Angelicae Dahuricae relieve exterior symptoms and disperse cold. This formula not only eliminates wind-cold, but also invigorates the spleen, eliminates dampness, regulates *qi* and relieves fullness. When wind-cold is eliminated and the functions of the spleen and stomach are restored, diarrhea ceases.

If exterior symptoms are severe, add Herba Schizonepetae and Radix Ledebouriellae to further ensure that wind-cold is eliminated. In cases of excessive pathogenic dampness with the symptoms of stuffiness in the chest, poor appetite, general lassitude and a sticky or white tongue coating, *Weiling Decoction* (204) is prescribed to invigorate the spleen, dry dampness and promote diuresis.

(2) Dampness-heat or summer-heat

Clinical manifestations: Rapid or intermittent diarrhea, abdominal pain, foul, yellow-brown stools, a burning sensation in the anus, restlessness, thirst, small amounts of deep yellow urine, a sticky yellow tongue coating, and a weak, fast pulse or a smooth, fast pulse.

Analysis: Invasion of the stomach and intestines by dampness-heat or summer-heat impairs their ability to transport and transform, thus producing diarrhea. Retention of heat in the intestines leads to rapid diarrhea, while retention of dampness-heat blocks *qi* circulation and thus gives rise to intermittent diarrhea. The downward movement of dampness-heat to the large intestine causes a burning sensation in the anus, foul, yellow-brown stools, and small amounts of deep yellow urine. Restlessness, thirst, a sticky yellow tongue coating and a fast, weak pulse or a smooth, fast pulse are signs of retained dampness-heat.

Treatment: To clear heat and resolve dampness.

Prescription: Decoction of Puerariae, Scutellariae and Coptidis (293) with additional drugs. In the formula, Radix Puerariae relieves exterior symptoms, clears heat, sends the clear *qi* upward and checks diarrhea. Radix Scutellariae and Rhizoma Coptidis, bitter and cold in nature, disperse the heat and dry dampness. To further disperse heat, add Flos Lonicerae; to further eliminate dampness, add Poria, Caulis Aristolochiae Manshuriensis and Semen Plantaginis. When dampness-heat is eliminated through urination, diarrhea ceases.

In cases of excessive pathogenic dampness with symptoms of stuffiness in the chest and a feeling of fullness in the abdomen, absence of thirst or thirst with no desire to drink, a slightly yellow, thick and sticky tongue coating, and a soft, slow pulse, add Rhizoma Atractylodis and Cortex Magnoliae Officinalis, which are bitter and warm. They dry dampness, helping the *qi* to circulate and the middle *jiao* to relax. If food has retained, add Massa Medicata Fermentata, Fructus Hordei Germinatus and Fructus Crataegi to promote digestion.

If diarrhea is due to invasion of summer-heat, add Six-to- One Powder (54) and Folium Nelumbinis to clear summer-heat and eliminate dampness. Diarrhea in summer can also be caused by cold-dampness due to exposure to cold or by eating too much raw or cold food. In these cases, refer to the discussion of diarrhea due to cold-dampness.

(3) Retention of food in the stomach and intestines

Clinical manifestations: Abdominal pain alleviated after bowel movements, borborygmus, diarrhea of undigested food and with a foul smell resembling rotten eggs, fullness of the epigastrium and abdomen, foul belching, poor appetite, a sticky, dirty or a thick, sticky tongue coating, and a smooth pulse.

Analysis: Food retention in the middle *jiao* impairs transportation and transformation, thus producing abdominal pain, borborygmus and a feeling of fullness. The upward disturbance of turbid *qi* due to retained food gives rise to foul belching. Its movement downward to the large intestine causes foul stools. A dirty, sticky or a thick, sticky tongue coating and a smooth pulse are all signs of retained food.

Treatment: To promote digestion and relieve stagnation.

Prescription: Pill for Promoting Digestion (216). In the formula, Fructus Crataegi, Massa Medicata Fermentata and Semen Raphani promote digestion and relieve stagnation; Pericarpium Citri Reticulatae, Rhizoma Pinelliae and Poria harmonize the stomach and eliminate dampness; Fructus Forsythiae disperses heat and stagnation. In severe cases, when epigastric and abdominal distention, fullness and intermittent diarrhea occur, add Radix et Rhizoma Rhei, Fructus Aurantii Immaturus and Semen Arecae to eliminate stagnation. This method is contrary to routine treatment.

2. Chronic Diarrhea

(1) Invasion of the spleen by liver *qi*

Clinical manifestations: This type of diarrhea is often induced by emotional stress. Other symptoms include abdominal pain which is not alleviated by bowel movements, borborygmus, and flatus. Usually there is also stuffiness in the chest, distention of the hypochondrium, belching, poor appetite, a slightly red tongue, and a taut pulse.

Analysis: Emotional strain impairs the liver's ability to promote the flow of *qi* and causes liver *qi* to invade the spleen. Impaired splenic functions give rise to abdominal pain and diarrhea. Liver dysfunctions cause stuffiness and distention. Belching, poor appetite, a slightly red tongue and a taut pulse are signs of hyperactive liver and splenic deficiency.

Treatment: To restrain the liver and invigorate the spleen.

Prescription: Powder for Treating Diarrhea with Abdominal Pain (301) is the main formula. In the recipe, Rhizoma Atractylodis Macrocephalae invigorates the spleen and eliminates dampness; Radix Paeoniae Alba nourishes the blood and the liver; Pericarpium Citri Reticulatae regulates *qi* and harmonizes the middle *jiao*; and Radix Ledebouriellae sends the clear *qi* upwards and checks diarrhea.

(2) Weak spleen and stomach

Clinical manifestations: Loose stool or diarrhea with undigested food, increased bowel movements after eating greasy food, poor appetite, epigastric and abdominal distention, sallow complexion, lassitude, a pale tongue with white coating, and a weak pulse.

Analysis: Weak spleen and stomach indicate that their function of transportation and transformation, separating the clear *qi* from the turbid are impaired. This explains the lack of appetite, epigastric and abdominal distention, loose stool or diarrhea, and increased bowel movements after eating a small amount of greasy food. Weak spleen and stomach also imply that the sources of *qi* and blood are insufficient, which causes sallow complexion and lassitude. A pale tongue with a white coating and a weak pulse are signs of splenic and gastric weakness.

Treatment: To invigorate the spleen and smooth the flow of *qi*.

Prescription: Powder of Ginseng, Poria and Atractylodis Macrocephalae (190). The Decoction of Four Mild Drugs (91) invigorates the spleen and benefits *qi*; Rhizoma Dioscoreae, Semen Lablab Album and Semen Nelumbinis invigorate the spleen and stop diarrhea; Fructus Amomi regulates *qi* and hamonizes the stomach; and Semen Coicia invigorates the spleen and eliminates dampness through urination. Both causative and symptomatic treatment should be considered. In cases of splenic *yang*-deficiency with excessive *yin* cold, where the patient feels cold or pain in the abdomen and has cold limbs, Bolus of Aconiti Lateralis Preparata for Regulating Middle *Jiao* (163) with Cortex Cinnamomi is prescribed to warm the middle *jiao* and disperse cold. In a prolonged case of diarrhea complicated by the sinking of spleen *qi* and the prolapse of the anus, Decoction for Strengthening Middle *Jiao* and Benefiting *Qi* (154) is used to improve the tone of *qi*, send the clear *qi* upwards, invigorate the spleen and stop diarrhea.

(3) Deficiency of kidney *yang*

Clinical manifestations: Diarrhea at dawn following abdominal pain and borborygmus, both of which are relieved after bowel movements, cold limbs, soreness and weakness in the lumbus and knees, a pale tongue with a white coating, and a deep and thready pulse.

Analysis: Deficient kidney *yang* fails to warm the spleen and stomach. *Yang-qi* is deficient and *yin* cold is in excess at dawn, this explains diarrhea at dawn following abdominal pain and borborygmus. Since intestinal and gastric *qi* circulates more smoothly after bowel movements, abdominal pain and borborygmus subside. Cold limbs, soreness and weakness in the lumbus and knees, a pale tongue with white coating, and a deep and thready pulse are signs of splenic and gastric *yang-qi* deficiency.

Treatment: To warm the kidneys, invigorate the spleen, promote astringency and stop diarrhea.

Prescription: Pill of Four Miraculous Drugs (94) with additional drugs. In the formula, Fructus Psoraleae warms and tonifies kidney *yang*; Fructus Evodiae and Semen Myristicae warm the middle *jiao* and disperse cold; and Fructus Schisandrae constricts the intestines and stops diarrhea. The addition of Radix Aconiti Lateralis Preparata and Rhizoma Zingiberis further warms the spleen and kidneys. In cases of incessant diarrhea due to a weak constitution in old age, manifesting sinking of *qi* in the middle *jiao*, add Radix Astragali, Radix Codonopsis, Radix Bupleuri and Rhizoma Cimicifugae to improve the tone of *qi* and send *qi* upward. These herbs can be used together with *Taohua* Decoction (232) to further induce astringency and check diarrhea.

(4) Fluid retention in the intestines

Clinical manifestations: Emaciation, borborygmus, diarrhea with clear watery or frothy stools, vomiting of clear fluid, abdominal distention, small amounts of urine, a pale tongue with a white and slippery coating, and a soft, smooth pulse.

Analysis: Water and fluid retention in the intestines due to overdrinking and the inability to absorb the water lead to borborygmus and diarrhea with watery or frothy stools. It also explains abdominal distention and the lack of urine. The upward movement of the fluid gives rise to vomiting of clear fluid. Splenic dysfunctions prevent water and food from being transformed into essence, thus the muscles are deprived of nourishment and emaciation occurs. A slippery white tongue coating and a soft, smooth pulse are signs of internal water and fluid retention.

Treatment: To invigorate the spleen, eliminate dampness and stop diarrhea by promoting diuresis.

Prescription: Decoction of Poria, Cinnamomi, Atractylodis Macrocephalae, and Glycyrrhizae (170) and Pill of Stephaniae Tetrandrae, Zanthoxyli, Lepidii seu Descurainiae and Rhei (31). In the formula, Ramulus Cinnamomi invigorates *yang*; Poria and Rhizoma Atractylodis Macrocephalae invigorate the spleen and eliminate dampness; Radix Glycyrrhizae harmonizes the middle *jiao*; Radix Stephaniae Tetrandrae and Pericarpium Zanthoxyli promote diuresis; Semen Lepidii seu Descurainiae disperses heat from the lungs and promotes diuresis; and Radix et Rhizoma Rhei removes retained water through the anus. If there is abdominal pain, the above prescription combined with Decoction of Cinnamomi (224) will harmonize the nutrient *qi* and check pain. The patient should be advised not to eat raw or cold food, and drink as little tea or water as possible.

(5) Stagnant blood in the intestinal vessels

Clinical manifestations: Prolonged diarrhea, a feeling of incomplete defecation after each bowel movement, a stabbing pain in the abdomen with a fixed location and which is aggravated by pressure, dark complexion, dry mouth with desire to drink a small quantity of water, a dark red tongue or dark spots on the edge of the tongue, and a taut and slightly unsmooth pulse.

Analysis: Prolonged diarrhea leads to the stagnation of blood in the intestinal vessels, thus causing a stabbing pain in the abdomen. Stagnant *qi* and blood stasis produce a feeling of incomplete defecation. A dry mouth with desire to drink, dark complexion, a dark red tongue or dark spots on the edge of the tongue, and a taut, and slightly unsmooth pulse are signs of blood stagnation.

Treatment: To remove blood stasis, smooth the vessels, harmonize the nutrient *qi* and relieve pain.

Prescription: Decoction for Removing Blood Stasis in the Lower Abdomen (68). In the recipe, Pollen Typhae, Faeces Trogopterori, Radix Angelicae Sinensis and Rhizoma Chuanxiong are the main herbs. Rhizoma Corydalis and Myrrha activate blood circulation and relieve pain; Cortex Cinnamomi, Fructus Foeniculi and Rhizoma Zingiberis warm the meridians and remove stasis. When blood stagnation is relieved, diarrhea and abdominal pain will cease spontaneously. If there are mucus and blood in the stool due to stagnant *qi* and blood, the above formula is combined with Decoction of Pulsatillae (100) to disperse heat and cool the blood.

Remarks

The above syndromes may occur separately or in combination, and one syndrome often turns into another. Complicated syndromes caused by deficiency and excess can be treated by improving the tone of the spleen and eliminating pathogenic factors. Complicated syndromes caused by cold and heat can be treated by warming the spleen and stomach, and despelling cold at the same time. Tonics and astringents should not be prescribed in acute diarrhea. Herbs that promote diuresis should not be used in large doses when treating chronic diarrhea. Herbs that are bitter and cold should not be used too often to disperse heat because they may damage the spleen. Finally, sweet and warm herbs should not be used exclusively to treat syndromes caused by deficiencies because they produce dampness and thus cause fullness. In addition, the patient is advised to keep a proper diet and avoid raw, cold, or greasy food.

Case Studies

Name: Zhang XX; Sex: Male; Age: 52.

First visit (June 18, 1963): The patient had loose stools for 15 days, with bowel movements four to five times a day. Other clinical manifestations were poor appetite, pale tongue with a sticky white coating, retarded but strong pulse, and absence of abdominal pain or any arthralgia on rainy days. The disease was due to improper diet complicated by strain and stress, which then impaired the splenic function and produced dampness. Treatment aimed at regulating the spleen and stomach, invigorating *yang* and eliminating dampness. The following drugs were prescribed:

Rhizoma Atractylodis (stir-baked)	4.5 g;
Cortex Magnolicae Officinalis	3 g;
Pericarpium Citri Reticulatae	4.5 g;

Radix Glycyrrhizae Preparata	1.5 g;
Caulis Agastaches	6 g;
Pericarpium Arecae	4.5 g;
Fructus Amomi Rotundus	4.5 g;
Herba Artemisiae Scopariae	6 g;
Testa Lablab Album	6 g;
Fructus Hordei Germinatus (stir-baked)	6 g;
Massa Medicata Fermentata	6 g.

Three doses were prescribed.

Second visit (July 8, 1963): The bowel movements became normal, but the patient felt distention in the lower abdomen after sitting for a long time, which was alleviated after flatus. The pulse was deep, thready and slightly taut. There was no coating on the tongue. All this was due to deficiency of the middle *jiao* complicated by retained dampness. Treatment aimed to improve *qi*, harmonize the middle *jiao*, resolve dampness and disperse heat. The following drugs were prescribed:

Rhizoma Atractylodis Macrocephalae	4.5 g;
Poria	9 g;
Rhizoma Alismatis	9 g;
Cortex Magnoliae Officinalis	4.5 g;
Pericarpium Arecae	4.5 g;
Radix Aucklandiae	2.1 g;
Pericarpium Citri Reticulatae	4.5 g;
Caulis Akebiae	3 g;
Caulis Agastaches	4.5 g;
Herba Artemisiae Scopariae	6 g.

Four doses were prescribed, one dose every other day.
All symptoms disappeared.

Name: Qiao XX; Sex: Male; Age: 44.

First visit (July 24, 1964): Diarrhea with watery stool began on July 13, with seven to eight bowel movements that night, and the same the next day. Stool culture was negative. The diarrhea improved following intravenous injection of glucose saline, oral administration of chloromycetin, Decoction of Puerariae, Scutellariae and Coptidis (293) and acupuncture. But it worsened at night and increased in frequency. There was no abdominal pain or tenesmus. The other symptoms and signs included borborygmus, thirst with preference for hot drinks, lassitude, a red tongue with thin and sticky coating exfoliated at the root, and a soft and smooth pulse.

The disease was due to splenic and gastric disharmony complicated by retention of heat and dampness in the intestines. The treatment aimed to harmonize the middle *jiao*, dry dampness, regulate *qi* and disperse intestinal heat. The following drugs were prescribed:

Herba Agastaches	9 g;
Herba Eupatorii	9 g;
Semen Lablab Album	9 g;
Rhizoma Atractylodis Macrocephalae (stir-baked)	9 g;
Radix Aucklandiae	4.5 g;

Pericarpium Citri Reticulatae	6 g;
Radix Glycyrrhizae Preparata	2.4 g;
Fructus Crataegi (charred)	9 g;
Massa Medicata Fermentata (charred)	9 g;
Folium Nelumbinis	a small piece;
Pill of Aucklandiae and Coptidis (to be taken separately, 2.25 g each time)	4.5 g.

Seven doses were prescribed.

Second visit (August 1, 1964): The diarrhea began to improve after two doses and ceased for the past two days, but borborygmus developed after midnight and continued till dawn. The patient's appetite was good. He had red tongue with exfoliated coating at the root, and a soft and small pulse. The spleen was then invigorated and the middle *jiao* harmonized by prescribing the following drugs:

Rhizoma Atractylodis Macrocephalae (stir-baked)	9 g;
Radix Codonopsis (stir-baked)	9 g;
Radix Glycyrrhizae Preparata	3 g;
Radix Aucklandiae	4.5 g;
Pericarpium Citri Reticulatae	4.5 g;
Massa Crataegi Fructus (charred)	9 g,
Herba Agastaches	9 g;
Folium Nelumbinis	a small piece.

Seven doses were prescribed.

Discussion: Diarrhea was due to exposure to summer-heat and dampness. It had not been completely cured by the first course of treatment, because the splenic and gastric functions were not yet fully restored, and dampness still remained. Herba Agastaches, Herba Eupatorii, Folium Nelumbinis and Pill of Aucklandiae and Coptidis resolve turbid dampness and disperse heat from the intestines. Semen Lablab Album, Rhizoma Atractylodis Macrocephalae, Radix Aucklandiae, Pericarpium Citri Reticulatae, Radix Glycyrrhizae, Fructus Crataegi and Massa Fermentata Medicinalis invigorate the spleen, harmonize the middle *jiao* and resolve dampness. It was not advisable to prescribe herbs that produce *yin* fluid, even though the patient showed signs of *yin* consumption such as a red tongue with exfoliated coating. *Yin* fluid would recover naturally when diarrhea stopped and the patient began eating. If the diarrhea did not respond to the treatment, manifesting a syndrome of deficiency-cold, *yin* consumption, or a deficiency syndrome complicated by excess, other methods of treatment should be adopted.

XXII. Dysentery

Dysentery is marked by frequent bowel movements, abdominal pain, tenesmus, and mucus and blood in the stools. Its main cause is invasion by external pathogenic dampness-heat or infectious factors. It often occurs in the summer and autumn, and only occasionally in the spring and winter.

The Inner Canon of the Yellow Emperor describes dysentery as a disease marked by the passage of dirty, greasy and pus-like liquid in the stool accompanied by *pipi* noises during bowel movements. *Synopsis of Prescriptions of the Golden Chamber* says, "In the treatment of dysentery with mucus and blood in the stools, *Taohua* Decoction (232) is prescribed. If dysentery is due to heat and shows the symptom of tenesmus, Decoction of Pulsatillae (100) should then be chosen." For the first time in the history of Chinese medicine, this book recommends warming the middle *jiao* and inducing astringency in the treatment of dysentery of the cold type marked by incontinence of feces; and dispersing heat and eliminating toxins in dysentery of the hot type marked by tenesmus. *The Pathogenesis and Manifestations of Diseases* names red (blood) and white (mucus) dysentery, bloody dysentery, purulent bloody dysentery, cold dysentery, hot dysentery, and recurrent dysentery. Medical classics during the Jin and Yuan dynasties, such as *Danxi's Experience on Medicine*, recognize dysentery as an infectious disease.

Dysentery corresponds to acute and chronic bacillary dysentery, acute and chronic amebiasis, and chronic non-specific ulcerative colitis in Western medicine.

Etiology and Pathogenesis

This disease is the result of damage to the spleen, stomach and intestines by external pathogenic dampness-heat, or infectious factors or as the result of an improper diet. Pathogenic factors are closely related to the condition of the body's *yang-qi*. In cases of constitutional *yang* deficiency, cold-dampness is likely to invade. In some cases dampness invades, which is then transformed to cold within the body. In cases of constitutional excess, dampness-heat is likely to invade, or else dampness invades and is then transformed into heat. Thus either dampness-heat or cold-dampness predominates in dysentery.

1. External Pathogenic Factors

The invasion of the stomach and intestines by summer-heat and dampness or infectious factors leads to the stagnation of *qi* and blood. The combination of summer-heat, dampness, pestilential factors, and stagnant *qi* and blood produces purulent blood, thus giving rise to dampness-heat dysentery or epidemic toxic dysentery.

2. Improper Diet

Greasy, sweet and spicy food taken in excess produce dampness-heat, impairing the function of the large intestine and causing the *qi* and the blood to stagnate. The combination of dampness-heat and the stagnation of *qi* and blood forms pus and blood, giving rise to dampness-heat dysentery. Raw and cold food taken in excess impair the splenic and gastric functions and produce cold-dampness. Unclean food damages the stomach and intestines, and causes the *qi* and the blood to stagnate. The stagnation of *qi* and blood, combined with dirty and turbid substances in the intestines turns into pus and blood, thus giving rise to cold-dampness dysentery.

External pathogenic factors and improper diet often combine to cause dysentery.

This disease is located in the intestines. Pestilential factors, dampness-heat, or cold-dampness damage the vessels and then combine with stagnant *qi* and blood to produce pus and blood. This causes abdominal pain, tenesmus, and dysentery with mucus and blood in the stools. Gastric disturbance by infectious factors and dampness-heat causes gastric deficiencies and the upward movement of stomach *qi*. A lowered resistance following prolonged dysentery leads to the same problem. Thus the stomach fails to receive food, and anorectic dysentery develops. A prolonged case of dysentery weakens the resistance, and pathogenic factors may be retained in the body for a long time. In this case, either chronic or intermittent dysentery results. In a prolonged case of damage to the spleen and stomach, both splenic and renal deficiencies will develop, the pathological conditions will then be even more stubborn and lingering.

Differentiation and Treatment

Dysentery in its initial stage is often caused by excesses. Delayed or incorrect treatment or an excess of pathogenic factors may produce critical conditions such as cold limbs and mental confusion. In chronic cases, complicated conditions combining both deficiencies and excesses, or else pure deficiency conditions may occur. In the latter, the disease is marked by a deficiency of both *yin* and *yang*, involving the spleen and kidneys. In the treatment of a heat syndrome of the excess type, treatment primarily aims heat, relieve dampness and eliminate toxins; its secondary aims are to regulate *qi* and the circulation of blood. Herbs that induce astringency should not be used. A proper quantity of herbs that relieve the exterior syndrome should be added if this syndrome is present. Herbs that assist digestion and relieve stagnation should be added in cases where food retention occurs. Purgative herbs should be added in an interior hot syndrome marked by excesses.

Chronic dysentery is often caused by deficiencies. For a cold syndrome of this type, treatment warms the spleen and kidneys, improving their tone. *Yin* is nourished and heat dispersed in a hot syndrome.

For the treatment of complicated syndromes involving both deficiencies and excesses, techniques of eliminating pathogenic factors should be combined with promoting bodily resistance, and both the cause and the symptoms should be treated.

1. Dampness-Heat Dysentery

Clinical manifestations: Abdominal pain, tenesmus, dysentery with mucus and blood in the stool, a burning sensation in the anus, small amounts of deep yellow urine, a red tongue with a sticky yellow coating, and a smooth and rapid pulse.

Analysis: The combination of dampness-heat and food in the intestines blocks the *qi* and impairs intestinal functioning. This explains abdominal pain and tenesmus. Pathogenic dampness-heat damages the intestinal vessels and thus produces the stagnation of *qi* and blood, which causes mucus and blood in the stool. The downward movement of dampness-heat produces a burning sensation in the anus, and small amounts of deep yellow urine. A sticky tongue coating suggests dampness, and a red tongue with a yellow coating suggests heat. A smooth pulse indicates a syndrome of the excess type, and a rapid pulse indicates heat.

Treatment: To disperse heat, relieve dampness, regulate *qi* and circulate blood.

Prescription: Decoction of Paeoniae (121). Radix et Rhizoma Rhei, Radix Scutellariae and Rhizoma Coptidis reduce fire, eliminate toxins, dissipate heat, relieve dampness and dispel stagnation; Radix Paeoniae, Radix Angelicae Sinensis and Radix Glycyrrhizae harmonize the nutrient *qi* and relieve pain; and Cortex Cinnamomi, Radix Aucklandiae and Semen Arecae regulate *qi* to relieve tenesmus.

If excess internal heat is accompanied by exterior symptoms (e.g., fever, aversion to cold or headache), then Decoction of Puerariae, Scutellariae and Coptidis (293) should be prescribed to relieve exterior symptoms and dissipate heat. In cases of excess heat with more blood than mucus in the stool or else the passage of pure blood, along with fever and thirst, Decoction of Pulsatillae (100) can be used to disperse heat and get rid of retained toxins.

If herbs that remove retained food and promote digestion are needed, choose Fructus Crataegi, Massa Medicata Fermentata and Fructus Aurantii immaturus; if herbs that disperse heat are needed, choose Flos Lonicerae and Fructus Forsythiae; if herbs that relieve exterior symptoms are needed, then Herba Schizonepetae and Radix Ledebouriellae should be used.

If *yin* blood has been damaged in a prolonged case, and there is mucus and blood in the patient's stool or the patient is suffering from restlessness, irritability, hectic fever, a red tongue or a thready and rapid pulse, prescribe *Zhuju* Pill (187) to nourish *yin* blood and clear dampness-heat.

2. Fulminant Dysentery

Clinical manifestations: An abrupt onset, high fever, thirst, headache, restlessness, irritability, or even coma or convulsions in severe cases, severe abdominal pain, tenesmus, passage of purple, purulent and bloody stool, a crimson tongue with a dry yellow coating, and a smooth and rapid pulse.

Analysis: Infectious factors invade the body in a drastic manner, producing an abrupt onset of severe symptoms. Consumption of fluid by excess internal heat causes a high fever, thirst and headache. Pathogenic heat disturbs the nutrient and blood systems and then blocks the clear cavity, thus causing restlessness, irritability and even coma. Extreme heat produces wind, which causes convulsions. Infectious factors are more offensive than dampness-heat in causing diseases, and that is why abdominal pain, tenesmus and bloody stool occur. A crimson tongue with a dry yellow coating and a smooth, rapid pulse are signs of excess toxin-heat.

Treatment: To disperse heat, cool blood and eliminate toxins.

Prescription: Decoction of Pulsatillae (100) with additional drugs. Radix Pulsatillae primarily cools blood and eliminates toxins; Rhizoma Coptidis, Cortex Phellodendri and Cortex Fraxini, bitter and cold in nature, resolve dampness and disperse heat. To further eliminate toxins and check dysentery, add Flos Lonicerae, Radix Scutellariae, Radix Paeoniae Rubra, Cortex Moutan and Radix Sanguisorbae.

A high fever and mental confusion are critical signs, suggesting invasion of the nutrient and blood systems by toxin-heat. 1-2 g of Purple-Snow Pellet (299) or Pill of Precious Drugs (124) should then be administered. Convulsions are also a critical sign resulting from toxin-heat stirring the liver wind. For this treatment, add Ramulus Uncariae cum Uncis and Concha Haliotidis to calm the liver wind. If signs of collapse are present (e.g., pallor, cold limbs, sweating, shortness of breath, and a thready and weak pulse), Decoction of Ginseng and Aconiti Lateralis Preparata (188) should be administered urgently to restore *yang* and prevent collapse. This should be fed through the nose if oral administration is impossible. Acupuncture can also be used in combination with this. When the collapse has been treated, curative measures can focus on the primary disease.

Fulminant dysentery often occurs in children. Abdominal pain and abnormal bowel movements may precede convulsions and even coma. Since this condition is so severe, emergency treatment must be given combining Chinese and Western medicine.

3. Cold-Dampness Dysentery

Clinical manifestations: More mucus than blood in the stool or pure mucus, abdominal pain, tenesmus, poor appetite, fullness in the epigastrium, lassitude, a pale tongue with a sticky white coating, and a soft and retarded pulse.

Analysis: Retained food and cold-dampness in the intestines block *qi*, giving rise to dysentery with abdominal pain and tenesmus. Cold-dampness is likely to damage the *qi* system; this explains the preponderance of mucus. Retained cold-dampness in the middle *jiao* impairs transportation and transformation, thus leading to poor appetite, fullness and lassitude. A pale tongue with a white coating and a soft and retarded pulse are signs of excess internal cold-dampness.

Treatment: To eliminate cold, dry out dampness, circulate *qi* and relieve stagnation.

Prescription: Modified *Weiling* Decoction (204). Rhizoma Atractylodis, Rhizoma Atractylodis Macrocephalae, Cortex Magnolicae Officinalis and Pericarpium Citri Reticulatae dry dampness and invigorate the spleen; Cortex Cinnamomi, Rhizoma Zingiberis Recens and Poria eliminate cold and relieve dampness; and Radix Aucklandiae, Fructus Aurantii Immaturus and Fructus Crataegi relieve food retention.

In a prolonged case marked by splenic *yang*-deficiency and symptoms including mucus in loose stool, dull pain in the abdomen, slight tenesmus, aversion to cold and cold limbs, Pill for Regulating Middle *Jiao* (258) is prescribed with additional drugs to warm the middle *jiao*, disperse the cold, invigorate the spleen and relieve dampness.

If there are heat signs, add a proper amount of Cortex Fraxini and Radix Scutellariae to the previous prescription to disperse cold and relieve dampness on the one hand, and to dissipate heat on the other.

In cases of splenic and renal deficiency with stagnant cold exhibiting prolonged dysentery, incontinence and a weak constitution, *Taohua* Decoction (232) or *Zhenren* Decoction for Nourishing Viscera (222) can be prescribed to warm and improve the tone of the patients' organs, and induce astringency.

Prolapse of the anus following prolonged dysentery is due to the sinking of spleen *qi*. Modified Decoction for Strengthening Middle *Jiao* and Benefiting *Qi* (154) can be used to improve the tone of the *qi* and to elevate it.

4. Recurrent Dysentery

Clinical manifestations: Dysentery occurs intermittently and lingers. Other symptoms include lassitude, an aversion to cold, a poor appetite, abdominal pain, tenesmus, mucus or possibly blood in the stool, a pale tongue with a sticky coating, and a soft and thready pulse.

Analysis: Splenic *yang*-deficiency in prolonged dysentery gives rise to lassitude, an aversion to cold and a poor appetite. Retained dampness-heat allows external pathogenic factors or an improper diet to induce a new attack, with symptoms of abdominal pain, tenesmus and mucus in the stool. A deficiency of anti-pathogenic factors and retained pathogenic dampness are the cause of a pale tongue with a sticky coating and a soft and thready pulse.

Treatment: To warm the middle *jiao*, invigorate the spleen, dissipate heat and relieve dampness.

Prescription: Decoction of Coptidis for Regulating Middle *Jiao* (147) with additional drugs. In this formula, Radix Ginseng, Rhizoma Atractylodis Macrocephalae, Rhizoma Zingiberis and Radix Glycyrrhizae warm the middle *jiao* and invigorate the spleen; and Rhizoma Coptidis dissipates heat in the intestines and dries dampness. The addition of Radix Angelicae Sinensis, Radix Paeoniae Rubra and Radix Sanguisorbae harmonizes the nutrient system and cools blood; and the addition of Radix Aucklandiae regulates *qi* and checks pain. In cases of deficient spleen-*yang* and cold retained in the intestines, with symptoms of feeling cold, abdominal pain and mucus in the stool, replace Rhizoma Coptidis with Radix Aconiti Lateralis Preparata and Cortex Cinnamomi to warm the spleen and disperse the cold. During the remission stage, Decoction of Six Mild Drugs with Aucklandiae and Amomi (211) should be administered to prevent recurrence.

If the stool of a patient with lingering dysentery is dark red and jam-like, accompanied by abdominal pain and mild tenesmus, Fructus Bruceae is recommended. The shell of this fruit should be removed, and its kernel wrapped in a capsule, dried longan pulp or a piece, bread. This should be taken orally three times a day, 15 pieces a time after meals, for seven to ten days in succession. This checks dysentery by stimulating the gastrointestinal tract. Be sure not to break the kernel when removing the shell.

5. Anorectic Dysentery

Clinical manifestations: Mucus and blood in the stool, refusal to eat, nausea, vomiting, emaciation, listlessness, restlessness, insomnia, a sticky yellow tongue coating, and a soft and rapid pulse.

Analysis: This type of dysentery originates from dampness-heat or fulminant dysentery. Toxin-heat damages the *qi*, the blood and the intestinal vessels, giving rise to dysentery with mucus and blood in the stool. The toxin-heat damages the stomach *qi*, which causes the refusal to eat. The upward movement of stomach *qi* leads to nausea and vomiting. Refusal to eat implies a deficient source of *qi* and blood; this explains the emaciation and listlessness experienced by the patient. Pathogenic heat disturbing the heart and mind results in restlessness and insomnia. A sticky yellow tongue coating and a soft and rapid pulse are the results of excess dampness-heat.

Treatment: To harmonize the stomach, conduct the unhealthy *qi* downward, dissipate heat and resolve the turbid *qi*.

Prescription: Modified Powder for Treating Food-Refusal Dysentery (42). In the recipe, Radix Ginseng, Poria and Pericarpium Citri Reticulatae improve *qi* tone and harmonize the stomach; Semen Caesalpiniae Minacis, Rhizoma Acori Tatarinowii, Semen Benincasae and Petiolus Nelumbinis conduct the unhealthy *qi* downward and resolve the turbid *qi*; and Rhizoma Coptidis and Radix Salviae Miltiorrhizae relieve heat and calm the mind. If oral administration is impossible, 0.5-1.0 gram of *Yushu* Pill (72) should be taken first to resolve the turbid *qi* and stop any vomiting. Then the previous decoction should be taken bit by bit.

If the stomach *yin* is severely damaged, the patient will show signs such as a dry crimson tongue and a thready, rapid pulse. Then herbs that nourish body fluids, such as Herba Dendrobii, Radix Ophiopogonis, and Radix Adenophorae, should be added to Powder for Treating Food-Refusal Dysentery (42). Frequent vomiting, hiccups and the refusal to take food are critical signs that the stomach *qi* has been exhausted. In this case, herbs that nourish *qi* and *yin* can be used. These primarily include Radix Ginseng, Radix Ophiopogonis and Herba Dendrobii; aromatics that resolve the turbid *qi*, such as Folium Cymbidii Ensifolii, Folium Eupatorii and Flos Rosae Multiflorae, can be used secondarily.

Remarks

The main symptoms of dysentery (e.g., mucus and blood in stool, abdominal pain and tenesmus) will disappear after several days of herbal treatment, but treatment should continue for another five to seven days in order to prevent any relapses from occurring.

Prophylactic measures include avoiding unclean or rotten food, not eating excessive quantities of raw or cold food, refrain from voracious eating and paying attention to weather changes to avoid external pathogenic factors. It is advisable to eat a proper amount of garlic in summer and autumn.

Case Studies

Name: Zhong XX; Sex: Male; Age: 41.

First visit (June 6, 1962): In May 1959, the patient suffered from bacillary dysentery, for which he took sulfonamides. The medication was discontinued as soon as his bowel movements became normal. From then on, symptoms such as abdominal pain and diarrhea with pus and blood in the stool were often induced by exposure to cold or an improper diet. Treatment with streptomycin and sintomycin used to be effective, but less so over the past year. The most recent attack occurred two weeks ago, when the patient exhibited abdominal distention and pain, loose stool with mucus and blood, four to seven bowel movements a day with a weighted sensation in the anus, an absence of fever, an aversion to cold and yellow urine. His appetite was still normal. The disease was treated with streptomycin one week ago, but in vain. The patient still had a thready pulse and a sticky white tongue coating. The stool examination revealed undigested food and both red and white blood cells. The disease was diagnosed as splenic deficiency and stagnant *qi*, complicated by residual dampness-heat. Treatment aimed to invigorate the spleen, regulate the *qi*, dissipate the heat and eliminate any dampness. The prescription was based on Decoction of Coptidis for Regulating Middle *Jiao* (147), consisting of Radix Codonopsis, Rhizoma Atractylodis Macrocephalae, Poria, Rhizoma Zingiberis, Rhizoma Coptidis, Radix Glycyrrhizae Preparata, Fructus Aurantii, Radix Aucklandiae and Rhizoma Alismatis.

Six doses were prescribed.

Second visit (June 12, 1962): Tenesmus and abdominal pain had disappeared. The frequency of the patient's bowel movements had decreased to once daily, and the stool had gained form. However, there was still a little yellowish mucus in the stool and abdominal distention was still present after eating. The tongue coating and pulse remained unchanged. The same method of treatment was adopted. The prescription was based on Powder of Ginseng, Poria and Atractylodis Macrocephalae (190), consisting of Radix Codonopsis, Rhizoma Atractylodis Macrocephalae, Poria, Rhizoma Dioscoreae, Semen Lablab Album, Pericarpium Citri Reticulatae, Semen Nelumbinis, Semen Coicis, Radix Platycodi, Fructus Amomi, Radix Glycyrrhizae Preparata, Massa Medicata Fermentata, Fructus Hordei Germinatus, and Fructus Crataegi.

Four doses were prescribed.

Third visit (June 19, 1962): Abdominal pain and diarrhea returned three days ago. The patient had three to five bowel movements a day with mucus in loose stool. Tenesmus was not present. The pulse was thready, and the tongue coating was thin and yellow. Decoction of Coptidis for Regulating Middle *Jiao* (147) was resumed, and the following herbs were prescribed:

Radix Codonopsis, Rhizoma Atractylodis Macrocephalae, Poria, Rhizoma Coptidis, Rhizoma Zingiberis, Radix Paeoniae Alba, Radix Glycyrrhizae Preparata, Fructus Aurantii, Radix Aucklandiae, and Massa Medicata Fermentata.

Fourth visit (June 23, 1962): From yesterday on, the patient's bowel movements had became normal at a frequency of once daily, with formed stool. But he still complained of lower abdominal distention, occasional abdominal pain, and a poor appetite. The tongue coating was thin and yellow, and his pulse thready. Fructus Hordei Germinatus and Fructus Crataegi were added to the last prescription. Another four doses were prescribed.

Fifth visit (June 27, 1962): Bowel movements remained normal over the past week. The stool examination was negative. But the patient still felt that his digestion was poor if he ate a little bit more than usual. The tongue coating was thin, and his pulse was taut and thready. So Pill of Ginseng, Poria and Atractylodis Macrocephalae (190) were prescribed to be taken twice a day, nine grams a time, to consolidate the therapeutic results.

Discussion: An incomplete recovery from acute dysentery meant that residual dampness-heat was retained in the intestines, causing abdominal pain, tenesmus, mucus and blood in the stool and yellow urine; this occurred when the patient was exposed to cold or had an improper diet. Repeated attacks caused *yang* deficiency in the middle *jiao* marked by an aversion to cold, abdominal distention and a thready pulse.

Name: Liu XX; Sex: Male; Age: 50.

First visit (October 28, 1960): The patient suffered from relapses of dysentery following an acute attack. The most recent relapse occurred nine days ago, with symptoms of difficult bowel movements with mucus in the stool at a frequency of four to seven times a day and tenesmus. Other symptoms included pain if pressure was exerted on the lower left-hand side of the abdomen, lassitude, reduced weight, slightly yellow urine, a pale tongue with a red tip and a dirty sticky coating. There was a deep and soft pulse at *cun* position on both sides, a deep and slow pulse at the right *guan* position, a deep and taut pulse at the left *guan* position, and a deep, smooth and strong pulse at *chi* position on both sides. Red and white blood cells were present in the stool, but no bacteria were found in culture.

The disease was due to deficiency of the middle *jiao* complicated by dampness. Treatment aimed to warm the middle *jiao* and eliminate dampness. The following herbs were prescribed:

Radix Codonopsis	30 g;
Rhizoma Atractylodis (stir-baked with rice water)	6 g;
Rhizoma Zingiberis (baked)	3 g;
Radix Glycyrrhizae Preparata	3 g;
Pericarpium Citri Reticulatae	6 g;
Herba Artemisiae Scopariae	9 g;
Semen Coicis	12 g;
Poria	9 g;
Rhizoma Alismatis	3 g;
Cortex Cinnamomi	1.5 g.

Three doses were prescribed; each was decocted twice, and 100 ml of medicine was made each time. A small amount of brown sugar was added before oral administration.

Second visit (October 31, 1960): The stool was formed, and the frequency of bowel movements and the amount of mucus in the stool were both reduced; but the patient still complained of abdominal distention and a weighted sensation. His tongue was slightly red but the coating was normal. His pulse was a bit slow but strong. Another three doses were prescribed, and the following herbs, based on Decoction for Regulating Middle *Jiao* (258), were administered in the form of a bolus to warm the middle *jiao*, invigorate the spleen, regulate *qi*, and treat dampness.

Radix Codonopsis	30 g;
Rhizoma Atractylodis Macrocephalae	30 g;
Rhizoma Zingiberis (baked)	15 g;
Radix Glycyrrhizae Preparata	15 g;
Cortex Cinnamomi	6 g;
Semen Arecae	15 g;
Fructus Aurantii Immaturus (stir-baked)	15 g;
Radix Aucklandiae	9 g;
Poria	60 g;
Fructus Toosendan (baked)	15 g;
Radix Linderae	15 g;
Fructus Foeniculi (stir-baked in salty water)	6 g;
Fructus Amomi	15 g.

These herbs were ground to make a powder and made into honey boluses, each weighing six grams. One bolus was taken with warm water twice a day.

Discussion: This case exhibited a cold syndrome caused by deficiencies complicated by dampness, making the disease protracted and relapses likely to occur. The oral administration of boluses consolidated the therapeutic results.

Name: Bai XX; Sex: Male; Age: 28.

The patient suffered from dysentery in 1952 for the first time when the frequency of his bowel movements was five to eight times a day. Since the disease was not completely cured at that time, he experienced frequent relapses afterwards. The most recent one was induced by heavy physical labor during the harvest season. A diagnosis of chronic dysentery was established. He had received various kinds of treatment in the past, such as oral sintomycin and sulfonamides, acupuncture, Pill of Four Miraculous Drugs (94) taken orally and digestive herbs, but in vain. He currently had frequent bowel movements (three to four times a day) with undigested food and mucus in the stool, abdominal pain alleviated by warmth and pressure, borborygmus, severe tenesmus, lumbar soreness, lassitude, a poor appetite, emaciation, a pale and swollen tongue with a slippery white coating, and a pulse which was deep, but thready and weak.

The disease was due to the deficiency of spleen *yang* and kidney fire, and the failure of clear *yang* to ascend. Treatment sought primarily to warm and improve the splenic and renal tone, and secondarily to raise the clear *qi*. The following herbs were prescribed:

Radix Codonopsis	9 g;
Radix Paeoniae Alba	9 g;
Rhizoma Dioscoreae	9 g;
Fructus Psoraleae	6 g;
Rhizoma Atractylodis Macrocephalae	6 g;
Radix Glycyrrhizae Preparata	6 g;
Rhizoma Zingiberis Preparata	3 g;
Fructus Schisandrae	3 g;
Rhizoma Cimicifugae	0.6 g.

Abdominal pain and frequent bowel movements both lessened after five doses. The patient was discharged from hospital with all symptoms resolved after another six doses in increased amounts.

Discussion: It is generally recognized that recurrent dysentery is marked by the deficiency of the body's anti-pathogenic factors and residual pathogenic factors retained in the intestines. The most common treatment is to warm the spleen and kidneys and improve their tone, and secondarily to relieve stagnation. The tenesmus this patient had may mislead people into thinking that this treatment should be adopted. But further inquiry showed that the patient had more severe tenesmus after bowel movements. This was due to the deficiency and sinking of *qi*. Excessive tenesmus is often alleviated temporarily by bowel movements; therefore herbs that promote digestion and relieve stagnation were not used in this case. Rhizoma Cimicifugae was instead added to herbs that warm and improve tone, and good results were gained.

XXIII. Abdominal Pain

Abdominal pain occurs between the epigastrium and the hairy pubic region. The abdominal cavity contains the liver, the gallbladder, the spleen, the large and small intestines, the urinary bladder, and the uterus. The abdomen is traversed by all *yin* meridians, the Meridian of Foot-*Shaoyang*, the Meridian of Foot-*Yangming*, and the *Ren* (Conception Vessel), *Chong* (Thoroughfare Vessel), and *Dai* (Belt Vessel). Abdominal pain is caused by retarded *qi* or retarded blood circulation in these meridians due to external factors or internal damage, or to lack of nourishment and warmth in these *zang-fu* organs and meridians caused by deficient *qi* or deficient blood.

Abdominal pain is a symptom of many diseases, such as acute pancreatitis, gastrointestinal spasms, incarcerated hernia in its early stages, neurosis, and dyspepsia. In these cases, it can be distinguished and treated according to the descriptions that follow. For abdominal pain occurring in acute gastritis, duodenal ulcer, acute gastroenteritis, cholecystitis, appendicitis, biliary ascariasis, and chronic cystitis, please refer to the the chapters on "Epigastric Pain," "Hypochondriac Pain," "Parasitosis" and "Stranguria" in this volume.

Etiology and Pathogenesis
1. Pain due to Cold

If the abdomen is invaded by external cold, or if damage is done to *yang* of the middle *jiao* by excess consumption of raw or cold food, then the splenic functions may be impaired, causing *qi* stagnation of the middle *jiao*, along with abdominal pain. The invasion of the *Jueyin* meridians also causes abdominal pain.

2. Pain due to Heat

This results from external pathogenic summer-heat or heat, the transformation of long-retained abdominal cold to heat, or the retention of dampness-heat and food blocking the circulation of *qi* in the large intestine. The latter may occur after eating pungent or highly-flavored food.

3. Pain Caused by Deficiencies

Abdominal pain caused by deficiencies may originate from a deficiency of *yang-qi*, which means a deficiency of spleen *yang* and the impaired function of the spleen to transport and transform. It may also result from prolonged retention of cold-dampness, which causes a deficiency of *yang* of the middle *jiao* and a deficiency of *qi* and blood, thus depriving *zang-fu* organs in the abdominal cavity of warmth and nourishment.

4. Pain Caused by Excesses

This type of abdominal pain is the result of voracious eating, or excessive eating of sweet, greasy or highly-flavored food, or eating unclean food. In all these circumstances, the stomach and intestines become damaged, food is retained, and thus *qi* circulation is hindered. This kind of pain can also be the consequence of mental depression or anger, because emotional stress damages the liver and causes liver *qi* to invade the spleen and stomach. Another cause of this pain can be from an operation or contusions to the abdomen. In this case, stagnation of *qi* and blood results. Round worms can also cause abdominal pain by disturbing the intestines and gallbladder, as well as the *qi* and blood.

These four types of abdominal pain are not clearly distinguishable clinically. They often combine together, thus creating conditions such as complications combining both heat and cold, both deficiencies and excesses, cold syndromes caused by deficiencies, and heat syndromes caused by excesses. A correct diagnosis and treatment should be based on actual clinical symptoms.

Diagnosis

Abdominal pain in different regions of the abdomen can be diagnosed as the following:

1. Pain in Both Sides of the Lower Abdomen.

Pain in the left or (and) right lower abdomen is a symptom of the Liver Meridian diseases. Pain in the right-hand side of the lower abdomen, which is aggravated by pressure, and accompanied by lying with the legs curled up, fever, nausea, and difficulty in passing bowel motions, suggests acute appendicitis.

2. Pain Around the Umbilicus.

This suggests three conditions: dry cholera, ascariasis, and periumbilical colic due to the invasion of cold. Dry cholera produces a colicky pain in the intestines, nausea, an absence of vomiting, a frequent desire to move the bowels, an absence of diarrhea, restlessness, irritability, and in severe cases, a cyanotic complexion, cold limbs, head sweats, and a deep and hidden pulse.

Ascariasis is marked by intermittent severe pain, vomiting of yellow-greenish fluid or round worms, and the restoration of normal appetite when the pain is over. This condition is often present in children.

Periumbilical colic due to the invasion of cold leads to pain around the umbilicus, the contracture of the abdomen, a cold feeling and sweating, cold limbs, and a deep, tense pulse.

3. Pain in the Lower Abdomen.

If pain below the umbilicus is accompanied by distention, hardness and contracture, and mania in severe cases, but urination is normal, this may be caused by stagnation of blood in the lower *jiao*. Acute intermittent pain in the lower abdomen accompanied by dysuria suggests stranguria due to retention of heat in the urinary bladder.

Differentiation and Treatment

Different kinds of abdominal pain can be distinguished according to etiological factors, as well as the location and the nature of the pain. Etiological factors include external wind, cold, summer-heat, dampness, an improper diet, the stagnation of *qi*, the stagnation of blood, parasitosis, urine retention, and lumps. So far as painful areas are concerned, pain above the umbilicus suggests diseases of the spleen, stomach and intestinal tract, while pain below the umbilicus indicates disorders of the Liver Meridian of Foot-*Jueyin*. Pain due to ascariasis is often felt around the umbilicus, and pain because of appendicitis is often located around the lower right-hand side of the abdomen. In terms of the nature of the pain, pain caused by excesses is aggravated by pressure; pain on a full stomach is caused by excesses; pain on an empty stomach by deficiencies; pain with visible pathological products is caused by excesses; pain without them by deficiencies; continuous violent pain, which is alleviated by warmth, is due to cold; intermittent pain, which is alleviated by cold and is accompanied by dry stool, is due to heat; intermittent pain around the umbilicus implies ascariasis; abdominal pain aggravated by pressure, accompanied by fullness at the epigastrium and abdomen, foul belching and acid regurgitation, is caused by retention of food; intermittent spreading pains without any fixed location are the result of stagnation of *qi*; and abdominal pain, stabbing in nature, with a fixed location, and accompanied by a palpable lump, is due to the stagnation of blood. In addition, the characteristics of the functions carried out by various *zang-fu* organs, and the symptoms accompanying abdominal pain should be considered when diagnosing the nature of the pain.

One principle in the treatment of abdominal pain is to remove any obstructions. *True Medical*

Record says, "When the obstruction is removed, the pain is relieved. There are various methods to remove obstructions, such as regulating *qi* for harmonizing the blood, regulating the blood for harmonizing *qi*, conducting the unhealthy *qi* downwards, dispersing any stagnation in the middle *jiao*, improving the tone of any deficiency, and providing warmth for a cold condition. It is wrong to think that purgation is the only method to remove an obstruction." Ye Tianshi of the Qing Dynasty holds that a protracted illness penetrates the meridians. In the treatment of a protracted illness, therefore, the commonly-used method is to activate blood circulation and remove any obstruction of the meridians by prescribing herbs which are acrid and moist in nature.

1. Pain due to Cold

Clinical manifestations: Acute and violent abdominal pain which is alleviated by warmth and aggravated by cold, an absence of thirst, clear urine, loose stool, a sticky white tongue coating, and a deep, tense pulse.

Analysis: Invasion of external pathogenic cold hinders *yang-qi* and blocks the circulation of both *qi* and blood, thus causing acute and violent abdominal pain. Since warmth disperses cold, and further exposure to cold makes the obstruction worse, abdominal pain is alleviated by warmth and aggravated by cold. Loose stool is the result of a deficiency of *yang* in the middle *jiao*, which means impaired splenic function with regard to transportation and transformation. An absence of thirst, clear urine, a white tongue coating, and a deep, tense pulse are signs of the retention of cold in the interior.

Treatment: To warm the middle *jiao*, disperse cold, regulate *qi* and relieve pain.

Prescription: Pill of Alpiniae Officinarum and Cyperi (151) combined with Fragrant Power for Strengthening Anti-Pathogenic *Qi* (74) is the main prescription. In the recipe, Rhizoma Alpiniae Officinarum, Rhizoma Zingiberis and Folium Perillae warm the middle *jiao* and disperse cold; and Radix Linderae, Rhizoma Cyperi, and Pericarpium Citri Reticulatae regulate *qi* and relieve pain. Intolerable pain around the umbilicus, which is alleviated by pressure and warmth, suggests deficiency of kidney *yang* complicated with invasion of the interior by pathogenic cold. In this case, Decoction for Dredging Meridian and Cold Extremities (252) is prescribed to warm and invigorate kidney *yang*.

2. Pain due to Heat

Clinical manifestations: Abdominal pain aggravated by pressure, fullness and distention of the abdomen, constipation, restlessness, thirst, spontaneous sweating, small amounts of deep yellow urine, a sticky yellow tongue coating, and a bounding, rapid pulse.

Analysis: Retention of heat in the interior causes the stagnation of *qi* and blood, so the circulation of *qi* in the large intestine is blocked. This explains the abdominal pain aggravated by pressure and the fullness and distention of the abdomen. Pathogenic heat consumes body fluids and impairs the function of the intestines in transmission, thus ensuing symptoms of constipation, thirst and restlessness. The heat forces the fluid out of the body, which is the cause of spontaneous sweating. Deep yellow urine, a yellow tongue coating and a rapid pulse are signs of an excessive heat.

Treatment: To dissipate heat and promote purgation.

Prescription: Modified Decoction for Potent Purgation (26). In this formula, Radix et Rhizoma Rhei, bitter and cold in nature, disperses heat and solves the problem of dry stool; Natrii Sulfas, salty and cold in nature, moistens dryness and relieves stagnation; and Cortex Magnoliae Officinalis and Fructus Aurantii Immaturus end the stagnation of the *qi* and discharge any accumulated substance. If the heat is more pronounced than the retention of dry stool, remove Natrii Sulfas from the prescription, and add Radix Scutellariae and Flos Lonicerae. If abdominal pain refers to the hypochondrium on both sides, add Radix Bupleuri and Radix Curcumae to the prescription.

Abdominal pain in febrile diseases is often acute, and is characterized by an abrupt onset and the rapid development of pathological conditions. Refer to the relevant chapters on distinction and treatment.

3. Pain Caused by Deficiencies

Clinical manifestations: Abdominal pain is protracted and occurs intermittently. It is alleviated by warmth, pressure, eating and rest, and is aggravated by cold, hunger and fatigue. Other manifestations include loose stool, lassitude, shortness of breath, an aversion to cold, a pale tongue with a white coating, and a deep and thready pulse.

Analysis: Abdominal pain as described here suggests a cold syndrome caused by deficiencies. A deficiency of spleen *yang* leads to impaired splenic functions in transportation and transformation, thus giving rise to loose stool. A deficiency of *qi* in the middle *jiao* and a weakness of the defensive *yang* lead to lassitude, shortness of breath, and an aversion to cold. A pale tongue with a white coating and a deep and thready pulse are signs of a cold syndrome caused by deficiencies.

Treatment: To replenish the relevant organs with sweet warming herbs, benefit *qi*, and disperse cold.

Prescription: Decoction for Mildly Warming Middle *Jiao* (34) is the main formula. In the recipe, Rhizoma Cinnamomi combined with Saccharum Granorum, and Rhizoma Zingiberis combined with Fructus Jujubae, warm the middle *jiao* and provide replenishment; Radix Paeoniae Alba and Radix Glycyrrhizae harmonize the interior and relieve acute symptoms. In case of a deficiency of *qi* with symptoms of lassitude, difficult bowel movements with loose stool, Radix Astragali should be added to nourish *qi*. In severe cases of abdominal pain caused by deficiencies with the stagnation of cold, Decoction for Potently Warming Middle *Jiao* (25) is used to warm the middle *jiao* and disperse cold. In cases where there is a deficiency of *yang* in both the spleen and the kidneys, Bolus of Aconiti Lateralis Preparata for Regulating Middle *Jiao* (163) is then prescribed to warm and replenish both the spleen and kidneys.

4. Pain Caused by Excesses

(1) Stagnation of *qi* and blood

Clinical manifestations: If the stagnation of *qi* predominates, clinical manifestations include epigastric and abdominal distention or pain, which has no fixed location, but occurs on the sides of the lower abdomen, and is alleviated by belching or flatus, and aggravated by anger. The pulse is taut, and the tongue coating is thin. If the stagnation of blood is more pronounced than the stagnation of *qi*, the pain is violent with a fixed location. The tongue is purplish, and the pulse is taut or unsmooth.

Analysis: The stagnation of *qi* leads to spreading pain at the epigastrium and abdomen. This pain has no fixed location as it is caused by the dysfunction of *qi* in ascending and descending. Belching and flatus help *qi* to circulate, thus alleviating pain, and anger makes the stagnation of *qi* worse, thus aggravating pain. The stagnation of liver *qi* causes the taut pulse. This *qi* stagnation becomes a stagnation of the blood in a prolonged case. Pain with a fixed location, a purplish tongue and an unsmooth pulse are signs of the stagnation of the blood.

Treatment: To soothe the liver, relieve stagnation, regulate *qi* and stop pain in cases where *qi* has stagnated; to activate blood circulation, remove blood stasis, nourish nutrient *qi* and relieve pain in cases where the stagnation of the blood is more pronounced than the stagnation of *qi*.

Prescription: Powder of Bupleuri for Releasing Stagnant Liver-*Qi* (239) is the main formula if stagnation of *qi* predominates. In this formula, Radix Bupleuri, Rhizoma Cyperi and Fructus Aurantii soothe the liver, relieve stagnation, regulate *qi* and stop any pain; Radix Paeoniae Alba and Radix Glycyrrhizae harmonize the interior of the body and relieve acute pain; and Rhizoma Chuanxiong helps *qi* to circulate, activates blood circulation and relieves pain.

Decoction for Removing Blood Stasis in the Lower Abdomen (68) can be used, if the stagnation of the blood is more pronounced than the stagnation of *qi*. In this formula, Radix Angelicae Sinensis, Rhizoma Chuanxiong, and Radix Paeoniae Rubra nourish the nutrient *qi* and activate blood circulation;

Pollen Typhae, Faeces Trogopterori, Myrrha, and Rhizoma Corydalis remove blood stasis and relieve pain; and Cortex Cinnamomi, Rhizoma Zingiberis and Fructus Foeniculi warm the meridians and relieve pain. If abdominal pain is due to intestinal adhesion following an abdominal operation, Herba Lycopi and Flos Carthami can be added to activate blood circulation and remove blood stasis. If the pain results from a contusion or a traumatic damage, add Herba Centellae and Semen Vaccariae; also Radix Notoginseng (powder) can be administered by mouth separately to help the blood to circulate and remove blood stasis.

(2) Retention of food

Clinical manifestations: Abdominal distention, fullness and pain, which are aggravated by pressure, lack of appetite, foul-smelling belching, acid regurgitation, possibly diarrhea which alleviates pain or constipation, a dirty, sticky tongue coating, and a smooth and forceful pulse.

Analysis: Retention of food in the stomach and intestines gives rise to distention, fullness and pain at the epigastrium and abdomen, aggravated by pressure. The upward disturbance of the turbid *qi* due to the retention of food is the cause of nausea, foul-smelling belching and acid regurgitation. Retention of food in the middle *jiao* impairs the functions of the stomach and spleen in transportation and transformation, thus resulting in abdominal pain and diarrhea. However, bowel movements pass the turbid *qi*, thus alleviating pain. The retention of food blocks *qi* circulation in the intestines, giving rise to constipation. A dirty, sticky tongue coating and a smooth and forceful pulse are signs of retention of food and dampness in the middle *jiao*.

Treatment: To promote digestion and relieve stagnation.

Prescription: Modified Pill for Promoting Digestion (216) or Pill of Aurantii Immaturus for Relieving Stagnation (196). In the recipe, Radix et Rhizoma Rhei, Fructus Aurantii Immaturus and Massa Medicata Fermentata promote digestion and relieve stagnation; Radix Scutellariae, Rhizoma Coptidis and Rhizoma Alismatis clear heat and resolve dampness; and Rhizoma Atractylodis Macrocephalae and Poria invigorate the spleen and stomach. If the retention of food is complicated with ascariasis which shows symptoms of intermittent abdominal pain, then refer to the chapter "Parasitosis".

Remarks

Cold, heat, deficiency and excess are four principles for differentiating abdominal pain. Clinically, transformation from one syndrome to another often takes place, further complicating conditions. For example, a lingering pain caused by cold may turn into heat; pain due to heat in a prolonged case may become pain caused by cold, which in turn is caused by deficiencies, thus creating a complicated condition involving both cold and heat. An improper diet may change a condition caused by splenic deficiency with symptoms of lassitude and poor appetite to a syndrome complicated by simultaneous deficiencies and excesses with symptoms such as spreading pain at the epigastrium and abdomen, foul-smelling belching and a sticky tongue coating due to retention of food. The stagnation of *qi* can become the stagnation of blood, and vice versa. Ascariasis is likely to be complicated with retention of food, and vice versa. However, the main points and chief manifestations should be clarified in diagnosis.

Case Studies

Name: Tang XX; Sex: Female; Age: 34.

First visit (May 17, 1975): The patient complained of a dull pain and distention at the epigastrium and abdomen. The pain wandered and radiated to the shoulder and back. Both appetite and defecation were normal. The patient's tongue was purple with a sticky coating, and her pulse was thready and taut. The patient was mentally depressed. She had suffered from bacillary dysentery last autumn.

The disease was due to the stagnation of liver *qi*, and prolonged pain affecting the meridians. The method of treatment was to soothe the liver, regulate the *qi*, remove blood stasis and relieve pain. The following herbs were prescribed:

Radix Bupleuri	6 g;
Rhizoma Corydalis	9 g;
Rhizoma Cyperi Preparata	9 g;
Radix Aucklandiae	6 g;
Radix Curcumae	9 g;
Lignum Dalbergiae Odoriferae	6 g;
Pericarpium Citri Reticulatae	9 g;
Rhizoma Pinelliae Preparata	9 g;
Radix Angelicae Sinensis	9 g;
Flos Carthami	4.5 g.

Six doses were prescribed.

Second visit (May 24, 1975): Abdominal distention had disappeared, and the pain was markedly improved, rarely reaching the shoulder or the back. The patient's tongue was still purple, and her pulse was thready and taut. Treatment following the same principles was employed. Pericarpium Citri Reticulatae and Rhizoma Pinelliae were removed from the prescription, and nine grams of Radix Salviae Miltiorrhizae was added. Another six doses were prescribed.

Discussion: In the past, this patient had taken more than thirty doses of herbs that tonify the *qi* and blood, but in vain. Mental depression impaired the function of the liver in promoting the free flow of *qi*, and the resulting obstruction caused the pain. The hyperactivity of liver *qi* caused a dysfunction in the ascending and descending of *qi*, thus a wandering pain followed. A purple tongue was the result of prolonged abdominal pain which turned the stagnation of *qi* to the stagnation of the blood, thus it was not a syndrome where *qi* or blood was deficient.

The main ingredients in the above prescription promote the liver's function in regulating the free flow of *qi*; Pericarpium Citri Reticulatae, Rhizoma Pinelliae and Lignum Dalbergiae Odoriferae harmonize the stomach and conduct the unhealthy *qi* downwards; and Radix Angelicae Sinensis and Flos Carthami activate blood circulation and remove blood stasis.

Name: Zhu XX; Sex: Female; Age: 40.

First visit (March 22, 1955): The patient complained of an intermittent pain in the left-hand side of the abdomen, a poor appetite, lumbar soreness, and leukorrhea. The coating of her tongue was sticky, and her pulse was taut. Powder for Regulating the Liver and Spleen was prescribed primarily to harmonize the liver and spleen, tonify the kidneys and check leukorrhea. The following herbs were prescribed:

Radix Bupleuri (vinegar prepared)	3 g;
Radix Paeoniae Alba (baked)	4.5 g;
Fructus Aurantii Immaturus (charred)	3 g;
Radix Glycyrrhizae Preparata	2.4 g;
Rhizoma Pinelliae Preparata	6 g;
Pericarpium Citri Reticulatae	4.5 g;
Pericarpium Amomi	4 g;
Rhizoma Atractylodis Macrocephalae (stir-baked)	4.5 g;
Radix Dipsaci (stir-baked)	6 g;

Cortex Eucommiae (stir-baked)	6 g;
Zuojin Pill (81) (to be taken separately)	1.5 g;
Fructus Setariae Germinatus (stir-baked)	12 g;
Folium Citri Reticulatae (stir-baked)	4.5 g;
Semen Cardamomi Rotundi (stir-baked)	12 g.

Three doses were prescribed.

Second visit: The previous method of treatment proved effective. So a new prescription based on the original one was made up.

Radix Bupleuri (vinegar prepared)	3 g;
Radix Paeoniae Alba (baked)	4.5 g;
Fructus Aurantii Immaturus (charred)	3 g;
Radix Glycyrrhizae Preparata	2.4 g;
Rhizoma Pinelliae Preparata	4.5 g;
Poria	9 g;
Pericarpium Amomi	3 g;
Massa Medicata Fermentata	4.5 g;
Cortex Eucommiae (stir-baked)	6 g;
Radix Dipsaci (stir-baked)	9 g;
Fructus Citri Sarcodactylis	4.5 g;
Zuojin Pill (to be taken separately)	1.5 g;
Folium Citri Reticulatae	4.5 g;
Pericarpium Citri Reticulatae	4.5 g;
Fructus Aurantii (stir-baked)	12 g.

Three doses were prescribed.

Discussion: The pathogenesis of this case is liver dysfunction in promoting the free flow of *qi*, and the subsequent invasion of the spleen and stomach by liver *qi*. The impaired function of the spleen and stomach in transportation and transformation gives rise to a poor appetite and abdominal pain. Since the spleen and stomach are not deficient, it is not advisable to tonify the middle *jiao*. Radix Bupleuri, which soothes the liver, and Radix Paeoniae Alba, which nourishes it, are combined to treat the liver. Fructus Aurantii Immaturus, which promotes digestion, and Radix Glycyrrhizae, which harmonizes the middle *jiao*, are combined to treat the spleen. Proper quantities of herbs that invigorate the spleen and conduct the unhealthy *qi* downwards should be used to ensure the potency of the medication. Cortex Eucommiae and Radix Dipsaci strengthen the kidneys, allowing them to control the *Dai* Meridian (Belt Vessel). All the symptoms ceased after two visits.

XXIV. Constipation

Constipation refers to difficulty in passing stools. The main cause of constipation is the dysfunction of the large intestine in transmission. In this condition, the stools are retained in the intestinal tract for too long, and their fluid is absorbed, producing dry and hard stools. Weakness of the body in passing stools is another cause of constipation. In this case, the stools are not necessarily dry.

Treatise on Cold Diseases classifies this disease into constipation of the *yang* type caused by excesses and heat, that of the *yin* type caused by deficiencies and cold, and that caused by deficiencies of the spleen and lack of fluid. *A Complete Collection of Jingyue's Treatise* holds that constipation of the *yang* type is due to fire; and constipation without fire is of the *yin* type.

Habitual constipation and constipation due to the body's inability to pass stools, neurosis, weak intestinal peristalsis at the restoration stage of inflammation of the intestinal tract, anal fissure, hemorrhoids, inflammation of the rectum, or as a side effect of drugs, should be diagnosed and treated according to the following descriptions. Constipation due to high fever is dealt with in the same way on the basis of its primary disease.

Etiology and Pathogenesis

The stomach receives food, and both the stomach and spleen transform food into essence to be absorbed and then transported throughout the body. The residue from the food is turned into feces in the large intestine which is to be excreted from the body. The normal functioning of the stomach and intestines ensures normal bowel movements. However, diseases of the stomach and intestines and the dysfunctioning of the stomach and intestines due to other causes can both lead to constipation.

1. Accumulation of Heat in the Stomach and Intestines

An excess of *yang*, excessive alcoholic drinking, overindulgence in pungent and spicy foods or the accumulation of heat in a febrile illness may all cause dryness and heat in the stomach and intestines. The large intestine is then deprived of moisture, thus producing dry and hard stools.

2. Stagnation of *Qi*

Excessive anxiety or a lack of physical exercise is liable to cause the stagnation of *qi*. Dysfunctions of the stomach and intestines in digestion and transmission do not allow the food residue to pass downwards.

3. *Qi* and Blood Deficiencies

These are the results of strain and stress, severe illness, or old age. *Qi* deficiency refers to the weakened function of the large intestine in transmission. Blood deficiency implies that the body fluid has been exhausted and that there is a lack of moisture in the large intestine.

4. Retention of *Yin* Cold

This occurs in people with *yang* deficiency or in elderly men. A deficiency of *yang-qi* may produce cold in the interior of the body. The retention of turbid *yin* in the stomach and intestines weakens their functions in transmission.

The first two conditions are caused by excesses, while the last two by deficiencies.

Diagnosis

Constipation may produce cord-like masses which can be felt on the left abdomen. These masses of varying sizes may also palpable on other regions of the abdomen if constipation is prolonged. These masses shrink or disappear completely as soon as constipation is relieved.

Abdominal masses from other causes than constipation will still remain after passing stools.

Differentiation and Treatment

Constipation generally refers to dry stools and difficulty in passing them at a frequency of every three to eight days. Some patients suffer from dry stools and difficulty passing them at the normal frequency of bowel movements. Very few patients note difficulty in passing stools, which are not dry. Prolonged constipation may produce other symptoms such as abdominal distention, abdominal pain, dizziness, a distending sensation in the head, a poor appetite and insomnia due to the blockage of the *qi* passage of the large intestine. Hemorrhoids and anal fissures are possible consequences of constipation.

1. Constipation due to Excesses

(1) Constipation due to heat

Clinical manifestations: Constipation with dry stools, one bowel movement every several days, small amounts of deep yellow urine, possible abdominal pain and distention, foul breath, restlessness, insomnia, a red tongue with a sticky yellow or dry yellow coating, and a smooth and rapid pulse.

Analysis: The large intestine is in charge of transmission, and is moistened by body fluid. An accumulation of heat in the stomach and intestines consumes the body fluid and thus causes constipation with dry stools. The movement of heat to the urinary bladder causes only small amounts of deep yellow urine to be produced. The retention of food in the stomach and intestines does not allow the turbid *qi* to move downwards. The results are abdominal pain and distention, thirst and foul breath. The disturbance of the mind by excess heat is the cause of restlessness and insomnia. A red tongue with a yellow coating and a smooth and rapid pulse are signs of the accumulation of heat in the stomach and intestines.

Treatment: To disperse heat and moisten the intestines.

Prescription: Bolus of Cannabis (271). In this formula, Fructus Cannabis and Semen Armeniacae Amarum moisten the intestines; Radix et Rhizoma Rhei, Fructus Aurantii immaturus and Cortex Magnolicae Officinalis which together make up of Decoction for Mild Purgation (35) disperse heat and relieve constipation; and Radix Paeoniae Alba and Mel, in nature sour and sweet respectively, relieve acute pain and moisten the intestines. This is a mild formula for relieving constipation.

If symptoms of irritability, redness of the eyes and a taut pulse are present, three grams of *Gengyi* Pill (146) can be taken once or twice a day in order to disperse heat from the liver and remove any obstructions in the intestines.

(2) Constipation due to the stagnation of *qi*

Clinical manifestations: Constipation with difficulty in passing stools although there is an urge to defecate, frequent belching, fullness in the costal and hypochondriac regions, a distending pain in the abdomen in severe cases, a poor appetite, a sticky tongue coating, and a taut pulse.

Analysis: The stagnation of liver and spleen *qi* following emotional stress impairs their functions to transport, and this causes the retention of the food residue in the interior and the difficulty in passing stools, though there is an urge to defecate. The invasion of liver *qi* to the stomach prevents the stomach *qi* from descending, which is the cause of frequent belching and the fullness in the costal and hypochondriac regions. The stagnation of *qi* also causes the retention of food in the stomach and intestines, thus leading to abdominal pain and a poor appetite. A sticky tongue coating and a taut pulse are both signs of disharmony between the liver and spleen, complicated by the retention of food.

Treatment: To circulate *qi* and relieve stagnation.

Prescription: Decoction of Six Ground Ingredients (57). In this formula, Radix Aucklandiae and Radix Linderae circulate *qi*; Fructus Aurantii Immaturus disperses stagnant *qi*; Lignum Aquilariae Resinatum sends *qi* downward; and Semen Arecae and Radix et Rhizoma Rhei send *qi* downward and relieve stagnation. When *qi* circulates smoothly, the constipation will be relieved.

2. Constipation due to Deficiencies

(1) Constipation due to a deficiency of *qi*

Clinical manifestations: Stools are not necessarily dry and hard. There is an urge to defecate, but actual defecation requires some effort. Sweating and shortness of breath occur after a bowel movement. Other symptoms include a pale complexion, listlessness, a pale tongue with a white coating, and a feeble pulse.

Analysis: A deficiency of *qi* in the lungs and spleen accounts for this syndrome. The lungs control the *qi* throughout the entire body, and are externally and internally related to the large intestine. A deficiency of lung *qi* is related to the weakness of the large intestine in transmission, and so constipation occurs. The weakness of the defensive *qi* causes sweating and shortness of breath when efforts are made to defecate. Splenic deficiency means that the sources of *qi* and blood are insufficient, which explains the paleness of the complexion and the lassitude. A pale tongue with a white coating and a feeble pulse are signs of *qi* and blood deficiency.

Treatment: To replenish *qi* and moisten the intestines.

Prescription: Decoction of Astragali (266). In this formula, Radix Astragali tonifies the lung and spleen *qi*; Pericarpium Citri Reticulatae conducts the unhealthy *qi* downwards; and Fructus Cannabis and Mel moisten the intestines and relieve constipation. Radix Codonopsis and Radix Glycyrrhizae are added to further replenish *qi* and relieve constipation. In cases caused by deficiencies and the sinking of *qi* with a weighted sensation in the anus, add Rhizoma Cimicifugae and Radix Bupleuri to elevate *qi* and cure drooping.

(2) Constipation due to a deficiency of blood

Clinical manifestations: Constipation, a pale complexion, dizziness, a blurring of vision, palpitations, pale lips, a pale tongue, and a thready and soft pulse.

Analysis: A deficiency of blood means that body fluid has been exhausted. In this condition, the large intestine fails to be moist and constipation then occurs. A deficiency of blood deprives the head and face of nourishment, thus resulting in a pale complexion, dizziness, a blurring of vision, a pale tongue and a thready pulse. A deficiency of blood also deprives the heart of nourishment, which may cause palpitations.

Treatment: To nourish the blood and moisten dryness.

Prescription: Bolus for Lubricating Intestine (242) should be prescribed. In this formula, Radix Angelicae Sinensis tonifies the blood and *yin*; Semen Persicae and Fructus Cannabis activate blood circulation and moisten the intestines; and Fructus Aurantii relieves the stagnation of *qi* and sends the unhealthy *qi* downwards. In cases of heat due to a deficiency of blood with symptoms of thirst, restlessness, an exfoliated tongue coating and a thready and rapid pulse, add Radix Polygoni Multiflori, Radix Polygalae Odorati and Rhizoma Anemarrhenae to produce body fluid and disperse heat. If body fluid has been restored but the stools are still too dry, use Pill of Five Kinds of Seed (48) to moisten the intestinal tract.

Since deficiencies of *qi* and blood often occur in combination with each other, the above two methods of treatment should be used together, depending on which condition is predominant.

(3) Constipation due to a deficiency of *yang*

Clinical manifestations: Constipation, a cold feeling and pain in the abdomen, an increased amount of clear urine, cold limbs, soreness and a feeling of cold in the lumbar region and knees, a pale tongue with a moist white coating, and a deep and slow pulse.

Analysis: A deficiency of *yang* is the result of severe illness or old age. In either case, the retention of *yin* cold in the stomach and intestines impairs their transmitting functions, and constipation then occurs. The retention of *yin* cold also may cause a feeling of cold in the kidneys and a pain in the abdomen. A deficiency of splenic and renal *yang* is the cause of the clear urine, cold limbs and the soreness and feelings of cold in the lumbar region and knees. A pale tongue with a white coating is a sign of *yang* deficiency leading to the retention of cold in the interior.

Treatment: To warm *yang* and relieve constipation.

Prescription: *Jichuan* Decoction (205) to be combined with Pill of Pinelliae and Sulfur (109). In the former, Herba Cistanches warms *yang*, nourishes the kidneys, moistens the intestines and relieves constipation; Radix Angelicae Sinensis, which is acrid and moist in nature, nourishes blood and moistens the intestines; Radix Achyranthis Bidentatae nourishes the liver and kidneys to assist with the downward movement of the turbid *qi*; Rhizoma Alismatis sends the turbid *qi* downwards; Fructus Aurantii conducts the *qi* downwards; and Rhizoma Cimicifugae raises the *yang-qi*. In the latter, Sulfur removes any obstructions in the intestinal tract, strengthens fire, and relieves stagnation; and Rhizoma Pinelliae harmonizes the stomach and sends *qi* downwards. Three grams of this pill should be taken twice a day.

The following two simple methods are often adopted in the treatment of constipation due to heat:

Six grams of Radix et Rhizoma Rhei is soaked in boiling water and taken orally.

Three to six grams of Folium Sennae is soaked in boiling water and taken orally.

The following two simple methods are often adopted in the treatment of constipation due to lack of moisture in the intestinal tract during old age or habitual constipation which fails to respond to purgatives:

Thirty grams of Radix Polygoni Multiflori should be decocted to be taken twice a day or it can be made into pills to be taken twice a day, ten grams a time.

Semen Sesami Nigrum or Semen Juglandis can be stir-baked over a mild fire after being cleaned, and then pounded. Then they should be mixed with a proper amount of Mel and taken orally with boiled water.

Remarks

The above syndromes may occur separately or in combination. For instance, deficiencies of blood and *qi* often appear at the same time; and a deficiency of *qi* may exist alongside a deficiency of *yang*. Thus constipation will not be relieved if only purgatives are taken. In the treatment of habitual constipation, the patient should be free from emotional stress, do proper exercises, pay attention to their diet, and go to the toilet regularly. It is not advisable to administer purgatives to those patients who have not had any bowel movements for a period of time due to insufficient food intake in the case of febrile diseases or prolonged illness. When stomach *qi* is promoted and the patient's appetite improves, they will have regular bowel movements. If constipation does not respond to any treatment over a period of time and the patient's body weight drops sharply, a further examination must be made to rule out the possibility of malignant tumors.

Case Studies

Name: Liu XX; Sex: Male; Age: 34.

First visit (February 26, 1966): The patient had suffered from pulmonary tuberculosis ten months ago, but the disease was now under control and the patient was no longer coughing. However, constipation made him quite uncomfortable, and he had to take purgatives. Other symptoms included abdominal spreading pain which was aggravated by pressure, a distending pain in the lower abdomen after bowel movements, insomnia, a red tongue with a thick, sticky, yellow coating, and a taut and smooth pulse, which was slightly larger on the right-hand side.

The cause of this illness was the dryness of the intestines and the stagnation of *qi*. The method of treatment was to regulate the *qi* of the middle *jiao*, harmonize the stomach and moisten the intestines. The following prescription was formulated:

Radix Polygoni Multiflori	15 g;
Rhizoma Polygonati Odorati	9 g;
Pericarpium Arecae	12 g;
Pericarpium Citri Reticulatae Viride	6 g;
Fructus Aurantii	9 g;
Radix Linderae	9 g;
Folium Citri Reticulatae	9 g.

The stool began to turn moist, and the distending sensation at the abdomen was partially relieved after five doses of the above prescription. The distending sensation at the abdomen disappeared after another five doses.

Discussion: In this case, constipation was due to a deficiency of lung *yin*, which causes the dryness of the intestines and the stagnation of *qi*. Radix Polygoni Multiflori and Rhizoma Polygonati Odorati nourish *yin* and moisten the dryness; and Pericarpium Arecae and Fructus Aurantii relieve the stagnation of *qi*.

Name: Ke XX; Sex: Male; Age: 65.

First visit (September 20, 1973): The patient was found to have a dark yellow complexion, lassitude, a blurring of vision, an aversion to cold, weakness in all four limbs, dizziness when standing up from a squatting position, chest discomfort, abdominal pain, one bowel movement only every two to three days with difficulty passing hard stools, a pale and swollen tongue with purple spots on the edges and a thin coating, and a taut pulse.

The pathogenesis was splenic deficiency due to a lack of fluid and renal deficiency with a stagnation of cold. The method of treatment was to promote purgation with herbs which are warm in nature by prescribing a decoction for warming the spleen.

Radix Aconiti Lateralis Preparata	6 g;
Rhizoma Zingiberis	3 g;
Radix Codonopsis	9 g;
Radix Glycyrrhizae Preparata	4.5 g;
Radix Polygoni Multiflori	9 g;
Herba Cistanchis	6 g;
Radix et Rhizoma Rhei	6 g.

Three doses were prescribed.

Second visit (September 24, 1973): Constipation was relieved and the daily frequency of bowel movements increased to two, with soft stools. Discomfort in the chest, abdominal pain and the aversion to cold all improved. Nevertheless, the patient still felt tired. The condition of both his tongue and his pulse had improved. All this showed that the previous method of treatment had been correct. Herbs that replenish the liver and kidneys were added to regulate *yin* and *yang*. Rhizoma Zingiberis, Radix et Rhizoma Rhei and Radix Polygoni Multiflori were removed from the prescription, and one and a half grams of Cortex Cinnamomi, 12 grams of Radix Rehmanniae Preparata, and nine grams of Radix Polygoni Multiflori Preparata were added.

Five doses were prescribed.

Discussion: Constipation in old age is often caused by splenic deficiency due to a lack of fluid, and renal deficiency due to the stagnation of cold. Thus herbs which were warm in nature were prescribed to promote purgation. Kidney *yin* and *yang* are the root of the *yin* fluid and *yang-qi* of the entire body. Herbs that replenish kidney *yin* and *yang* should therefore be prescribed to regulate *yin* and *yang* and restore body resistance.

Name: Chen XX; Sex: Female; Age: 45.

First visit (January 29, 1975): The patient told the doctor that she had developed constipation after bacillary dysentery. She had a bowel movement every seven or eight days with mucus in the dry stools. She also felt abdominal pain and distention, a poor appetite, stuffiness in her chest, nausea and a headache. Her sputum was sticky and her tongue was dark red and swollen with a thin and slightly sticky coating. Her pulse was deep and taut.

The pathogenesis was retention of food and dampness complicated by the stagnation of blood. In this case, the turbid *qi* was not able to descend, nor the clean *qi* to ascend. The method of treatment was to deal with the retained food, resolve the problem of dampness, remove the blood stasis, regulate *qi* and send the turbid *qi* downwards. A decoction for removing blood stasis from below the diaphragm was prescribed.

Radix Angelicae Sinensis	9 g;
Radix Paeoniae Rubra	9 g;
Rhizoma Chuanxiong	4.5 g;
Semen Persicae	9 g;
Flos Carthami	9 g;
Faeces Trogopterori	3 g;
Radix Aucklandiae	4.5 g;
Massa Medicata Fermentata	9 g.

Second visit (February 5, 1975): The patient did defecate until she had taken the decoction for one week. The stools were hard and tinged with blood and mucus. Her appetite had returned. Her tongue was red and swollen with a thin coating, and her pulse was deep but thready, and became stronger on pressure. A decoction for mild purgation was added to the previous prescription.

Radix Angelicae Sinensis	9 g;
Radix Paeoniae Rubra	9 g;
Rhizoma Chuanxiong	4.5 g,
Semen Persicae	9 g;
Flos Carthami	3 g;
Faeces Trogopterori	9 g;
Radix Aucklandiae	4.5 g;
Semen Arecae	12 g;
Radix et Rhizoma Rhei	9 g;
Cortex Magnolicae Officinalis	9 g;

Fructus Aurantii Immaturus (stir-baked)	9 g;
Semen Coicis	12 g;
Massa Medicata Fermentata	9 g;
Fructus Cannabis	9 g.

Third visit (March 17, 1975): The frequency of bowel movement had increased to one every two or three days, with no mucus in the stools, and at the same time abdominal pain was alleviated. But abdominal distention still existed. The patient had not menstruated for three months, and showed insomnia and restlessness with the condition of her tongue and pulse remaining unchanged. This was due to the continuing blood stasis which prevented new blood from being produced and nourished, although the turbid dampness was gradually being eliminated. Large dosages of herbs which nourish the blood and moisten dryness were prescribed.

Radix Angelicae Sinensis	9 g;
Rhizoma Chuanxiong	6 g;
Radix et Rhizoma Rhei	12 g;
Radix Paeoniae Rubra	12 g;
Semen Persicae	9 g;
Radix Glycyrrhizae Preparata	4.5 g;
Fructus Tritici Levis	30 g;
Fructus Jujubae	8 pieces;
Radix et Rhizoma Rhei Preparata	9 g;
Pericarpium Arecae	9 g;
Semen Arecae	9 g.

Fourth visit (March 26, 1975): Abdominal pain had been further alleviated but the patient still had difficulty passing stools, having bowel movements at intervals of four or five to ten days, and the patient had still not menstruated. Her tongue was red with tooth marks on the edge and a thin coating, and the pulse was thready and slightly taut. All this showed a deficiency syndrome complicated by excesses. The method of treatment was to nourish blood, regulate menstruation, moisten dryness and remove any obstructions in the large intestine.

Radix Angelicae Sinensis	9 g;
Radix Rehmanniae	9 g;
Radix Achyranthis Bidentatae	9 g;
Fructus Tritici Levis	30 g;
Fructus Jujubae	6 pieces;
Pericarpium Citri Reticulatae Viride	6 g;
Radix Platycodi	4.5 g;
Herba Cistanchis	9 g;
Fructus Aurantii	9 g;
Radix et Rhizoma Rhei Preparata	9 g;
Rhizoma Alismatis	9 g;
Natrii Sulfas Exsiccatus (to be mixed with the prepared decoction)	9 g.

Fifth visit (April 2, 1975): Menstrual flow had begun, bowel movements were normal at a frequency of one per day with no mucus in the stools, and all other symptoms had disappeared. The condition of the tongue and pulse remained the same as before. The patient still felt dull pains on both sides of the lower abdomen. Since the Liver Meridian runs through the lower abdomen, herbs that soothe the liver and regulate *qi* were added to the previous prescription.

Radix Angelicae Sinensis	9 g;
Radix Rehmanniae	9 g;
Herba Cistanchis	9 g;
Fructus Tritici Levis	30 g;
Fructus Jujubae	6 pieces;
Fructus Aurantii (stir-baked)	9 g;
Radix Bupleuri	4.5 g;
Pericarpium Citri Reticulatae Viride	6 g;
Radix Platycodi	4.5 g;
Rhizoma Alismatis	9 g;
Natrii Sulfas Exsiccatus (to be mixed with the prepared decoction)	9 g;
Radix Achyranthis Bidentatae	9 g.

Discussion: This is a case of the *yang*-type constipation due to heat-consuming *yin*. Since it is a deficiency syndrome complicated by excesses, elimination and nourishment are combined to achieve good results.

XXV. Parasitosis

Parasitosis has two meanings in traditional Chinese medicine. Broadly speaking, it refers to diseases resulting from various kinds of parasites, such as schistosomiasis, filariasis, pulmonary trematodiasis, clonorchiasis, fasciolopsiasis, ascariasis, enterobiasis, taeniasis and ancylostomiasis. In a more narrow sense, it refers to intestinal parasitic diseases. The following discussion focuses on ascariasis, enterobiasis and taeniasis.

There are explicit descriptions of parasitosis in medical classics. *The Inner Canon of the Yellow Emperor* says, "The symptoms of the 'stomach cough' include vomiting on coughing, and roundworms may be vomited." It also states, "Wandering abdominal pain, intermittent pain, a hot sensation in the abdominal region, the desire to drink and an excessive flow of saliva, may all be caused by the presence of roundworms." Zhang Zhongjing of the Eastern Han Dynasty was one of the first to try and diagnose and treat ascariasis on the basis of relevant descriptions in *The Inner Canon of the Yellow Emperor*. In the *Treatise on Cold Diseases*, he writes, "Vomiting of roundworms occurs if they disturb the stomach. Severe pain in the precordial region and abdomen is present, as well as cold limbs, if the roundworms have entered the biliary tract. In these cases, Bolus of Mume should be prescribed." He also recognized the fact that eating half-cooked pork and beef can cause taeniasis. *Clandestine Essentials from the Imperial Library* holds, "Enterobiasis most often affects children, and occasionally adults." It recommends Decoction of Meliae for the treatment of ascariasis. *Zhang's Medical Treatise* discusses the cravings of patients with ascariasis. "They have a liking for raw rice, paper, tea-leaves and soil." All these descriptions in the medical classics have laid a solid foundation for later medical scholars to understand parasitosis. Some of the formulas recommended by the medical classics are still used today.

Etiology and Pathogenesis

The main cause of parasitosis is unclean food and disharmony of the spleen and stomach. Ascariasis and enterobiasis are contracted after eating food contaminated by parasitic eggs. Once they enter the body, they will grow and remain in the intestinal tract. Taeniasis is caused by half-cooked meat in which hidden cysticerci are still living.

1. Eating Unclean Food

This refers to food contaminated by parasitic eggs and pork or beef contaminated by cysticerci.

2. Disharmony Between the Spleen and Stomach

An improper diet, such as too much raw, cold, greasy or unclean food, damages the spleen and stomach and impairs transportation and transformation. This produces dampness-heat and causes a deficiency of the *zang-fu* organs, creating a good environment for parasites. *Prescriptions of Wonderful Effectiveness* says, "Nine kinds of parasitosis are caused by the deficiency of the *zang-fu* organs, the spleen and stomach in particular, and complicated by improper diet, such as eating too much raw, cold, sweet or greasy food, or else eating vegetables, fruits or offal contaminated by parasitic eggs."

Parasites living in the intestinal tract disturb the *qi* circulation there and then produce dampness-heat and food retention. Moreover, the consumption of *qi* and blood by the parasites further damages the *zang-fu* organs, including the spleen and stomach.

Disturbance of the *qi* circulation in the intestinal tract causes intermittent abdominal pain, and *qi* and blood consumption by the parasites produces a sallow complexion, emaciation and listlessness in prolonged cases.

Clinical manifestations of parasitosis may vary. Roundworms tend to twist together; when they block the intestinal tract, violent abdominal pain, severe vomiting and constipation occur. If the environment of the intestinal tract is unfavorable, they will move in various directions. When they enter the biliary tract, abrupt pain will be felt in the hypochondriac region, as well as cold limbs. Pinworms live in the large intestine and often come out of the anus to lay eggs at night. This produces pruritus of the anus, thus disturbing sleep. Tapeworms are discharged from the anus when gravid segments become detached. They also may cause pruritus of the anus and additionally consume essence and blood, thus giving rise to deficiencies of the *qi* and blood.

Differentiation and Treatment

Symptoms are usually out of sight during the initial stage of a disease caused by parasitosis and therefore parasitosis is often neglected even though in actual fact it is occurring. In chronic cases, however, the consumption of body essence causes emaciation, which is often accompanied by a poor appetite, intermittent abdominal pains and insomnia. Diagnosis can be made with stool examinations. In the treatment of parasitosis, conditions caused by deficiencies and excesses should be differentiated. Condition caused by excesses can be treated in their initial stage by expelling or killing the parasites. If resistance is weak in prolonged cases, the spleen and stomach should be regulated first, and then the parasites can be expelled. Alternately, both treatments can be combined.

1. Ascariasis

Clinical manifestations: An empty and uncomfortable sensation in the stomach, intermittent pain around the umbilicus, polyphagia coupled with emaciation and a sallow complexion, possibly itching in the nose, grinding of the teeth during sleep, millet-like granules on the lips, white spots on the face, vomiting of roundworms, or discharge of roundworms through the anus.

Analysis: Roundworms in the intestinal tract disturb gastric and intestinal *qi* circulation, and thus cause the empty sensation and pain around the umbilicus. When roundworms remain dormant, this pain disappears. The consumption of *qi* and blood by the roundworms leads to a sallow complexion, emaciation and lassitude in spite of the fact that the patient eats a lot. Disharmony between the spleen and stomach and the functional disturbance of these organs cause polyphagia and paroxia. The Large Intestine Meridian of Hand-*Yangming* originates from through the lower gum, and passes through the lips and the nose; while the Stomach Meridian of Foot-*Yangming* originates from the nose and enters the upper gum. Roundworms living in the gastrointestinal tract produce dampness-heat that is displaced upwards along the meridians, thus causing grinding of teeth during sleep, itching in the nose, and granules on the lips. Both of the meridians run through the cheek; this explains the white spots on the face. Roundworms tend to move, which results in vomiting or anal discharge of roundworms. The pulse is unsteady, alternately large and small, because of the disturbance of *qi* circulation.

Treatment: Primarily to expel roundworms, secondarily to regulate *qi* and resolve dampness.

Prescription: Pill for Pursuing Parasites (220), Pill for Killing Parasitosis (58), and Powder of Quisqualis (176). The first formula should be used in ascariasis marked by excess heat and constipation. In the recipe, Semen Arecae, Omphalia, Cortex Meliae, Fructus Gleditsiae expel the roundworms and relieve stagnation; Radix Aucklandiae regulates the *qi* and harmonizes the middle *jiao*; and Semen Pharbitidis and Herba Artemisiae Scopariae disperse heat, relieve dampness and put a halt to constipation. The second formula can be used in cases of ascariasis without pronounced abdominal pain. In the recipe, Fructus Carpesii, Semen Arecae, Cortex Meliae and Pulvis Minium expel the roundworms and relieve stagnation, and Alumen Exsiccatum eliminates dampness. In the last formula, Fructus Quisqualis,

Fructus Ulmi Preparata and Fructus Toosendan expel roundworms; and Radix Glycyrrhizae harmonizes the middle *jiao* and eliminates toxins. After the roundworms have been expelled, Pill of Six Mild Drugs with Aucklandiae and Amomi (211) is administered to invigorate the spleen and stomach if the spleen is suffering from deficiencies.

Bolus of Mume (66) is administered to calm roundworms if there is severe abdominal pain or violent upper abdominal pain accompanied by sweating, cold limbs and vomiting of clear fluid or worms. In this formula, Fructus Mume, naturally sour, pacifies them; Pericarpium Zanthoxyli and Herba Asari warm the *zang* organs and expel the roundworms; Cortex Phellodendri and Rhizoma Coptidis, both bitter, send the roundworms downwards; Ramulus Cinnamomi, Radix Aconiti Lateralis Preparata and Rhizoma Zingiberis warm the *zang* organs and pacify them; and Radix Ginseng and Radix Angelicae Sinensis replenish the *qi* and the blood. As a saying goes, "Roundworms calm down when exposed to sour tastes, hide themselves in safe places when exposed to pungent tastes, and move downwards when exposed to bitter tastes." When they have calmed down, administer drugs that expel them.

2. Taeniasis

Clinical manifestations: A dull pain or distending sensation in the abdomen, itching of the anus, diarrhea, presence of white noodle-like or tape-like movable segments of worms or tapeworm eggs in the stool, or else tapeworm segments in the patient's underwear and bedclothes. In chronic cases, symptoms include a sallow complexion, emaciation, dizziness, lassitude, insomnia, a pale tongue, and a thready pulse.

Analysis: The disturbance of the intestines by tapeworms produces distention or a dull abdominal pain. Impaired transport and transformation systems produce diarrhea. The consumption of nutrient substances by worms in chronic cases causes a sallow complexion, emaciation, lassitude, dizziness, insomnia, a pale tongue and a thready pulse. Itching of the anus is caused by the discharge of tapeworm segments giving rise to irritation.

Treatment: To first kill the tapeworms and regulate *qi*, afterward to invigorate the spleen and stomach.

Prescription: Proven formulas contain Semen Arecae and Semen Cucurbitae or Gemma Agrimoniae, or else Decoction of Arecae (317). Semen Arecae is effective for 90% of diseases caused by Taenia solium and 30-50% of those caused by Taenia fenestrata. This herb may help paralyze the head and anterior segment of the tapeworms, but not the middle or posterior section. Semen Cucurbitae has the opposite function. The head segment can be found in 30-50% of patients who have taken only Semen Arecae. Oral administration of both herbs at the same time will soften the whole body and discharge all segments through the anus within three hours. Symptoms such as nausea, vomiting and abdominal pain occur in only a few patients after taking these herbs; but these herbs are not suitable for pregnant women or patients with heart diseases.

Agrimophol is most effective in Gemma Agrimoniae, a herb which is most effective in spring and autumn, and least effective in summer; it is not water soluble and its efficacy is destroyed by exposure to heat. This herb expels tapeworms by causing them to have convulsions and then die rapidly. It acts on the head, neck and body of adult worms, especially the head. Since it has purgative effects, other purgatives are not needed. Generally, worms are discharged from the body five or six hours after oral administration. Such side effects as nausea may occur. Pill of Six Mild Drugs with Aucklandiae and Amomi (211) can be taken to invigorate the spleen and stomach after the worms have been expelled.

3. Enterobiasis

Clinical manifestations: Itching of the anus which is more pronounced at night, insomnia, and thready worms creeping out from the anus at night. Chronic cases exhibit dull abdominal pain, a poor appetite, emaciation and lassitude. This disease most often occurs in children, occasionally in adults.

Analysis: Pinworms do not lay their eggs in the intestinal tract, instead they creep out of the anus at night. Their wriggling movement produces itching, which makes the patient unable to sleep. The pinworms also impair the functions of the gastrointestinal tract, giving rise to dull pain and a poor appetite. The consumption of essential body substances by the pinworms leads to lassitude and emaciation.

Treatment: To expel the pinworms and relieve the itching by combining oral and external administration of herbal preparations.

Prescription: Pill for Pursuing Parasites (220) by mouth combined with Decoction of Stemonae (117) in enema form. The patient should pay attention to personal hygiene, changing their clothes and bedclothes frequently, keeping their fingernails clean, and boiling their underwear to kill eggs.

Case Studies

One day, a girl surnamed Bao came to complain of intermittent abdominal pain which was accompanied by emaciation. She said that she had suffered from whooping cough two months before, and lately she had started to feel abdominal cramps in the morning, which were aggravated by pressure and the frequent vomiting of roundworms. Other symptoms were a poor appetite, constipation, a swollen and hard abdomen, a blue complexion, cold limbs, restlessness, irritability, a tongue with red spots and a thick sticky coating, and a taut and unsmooth pulse.

The disease was due to roundworms. Treatment aimed to expel them and calm the stomach by prescribing sour, bitter, acrid, laxative and warm drugs. Fifty grams of uncooked rape-seed oil were taken first, then the following prescription:

Pericarpium Zanthoxyli (stir-baked, wrapped)	4.5 g;
Radix Glycyrrhizae Preparata	4.5 g;
Fructus Ulmi Preparata (wrapped)	9 g;
Omphalia	12 g;
Radix Stemonae (steamed)	6 g;
Fructus Evodiae	18 g;
Folium Eriobotryae (stir-baked)	12 g;
Fructus Crataegi	12 g;
Radix Peucedani Preparata	6 g;
Radix Angelicae Sinensis Preparata	9 g;
Semen Arecae	9 g.

Second visit: The patient had had three bowel movements, discharging over 50 roundworms. After that the limbs had warmed up, and the patient's blue complexion had subsided. At the same time, her abdominal pains had improved slightly and her abdomen was not as swollen as before. The patient could drink thin porridge and sleep at night. Her pulse was taut and smooth, and the tongue coating was less thick and sticky.

All this showed that the roundworms had not been completely expelled. To achieve this and harmonize the middle *jiao*, the following were prescribed:

Radix Codonopsis (stir-baked with rice)	9 g;
Radix Glycyrrhizae Preparata	4.5 g;
Angelicae Sinensis Preparata	9 g;
Semen Arcae	9 g;

Fructus Mume	9 g;
Omphalia	9 g;
Pericarpium Zanthoxyli (stir-baked, wrapped)	4.5 g;
Radix Paeoniae Alba (stir-baked)	6 g;
Pericarpium Citri Reticulatae Preparata	9 g;
Radix Aucklandiae (roasted)	4.5 g;
Cortex Meliae	15 g.

Third visit: The patient had discharged over 40 roundworms during the past two days. Both abdominal distention and pain had disappeared. The tongue had fewer red spots and a thin sticky coating, and the pulse was slightly taut. The *qi* of the middle *jiao* had not yet been restored. Treatment aimed at invigorating the spleen and regulating the middle *jiao*.

Explanation: At the time, the patient was hospitalized with the diagnosis of intestinal obstruction. Since her pathological condition was severe, she was about to receive surgery. But the disease was relieved by the Chinese herbal medicines described above. Uncooked rape-seed oil circulates the *qi*, making the intestinal tract slippery, dispersing any masses and killing parasites. It renders immediate therapeutic results in the treatment of intestinal blockage by roundworms.

XXVI. Hypochondriac Pain

Hypochondriac pain may occur in one or both sides of the chest. *The Inner Canon of the Yellow Emperor* attributes it to disorders of the liver and the gallbladder: "Pathogenic factors attacking the liver cause hypochondriac pain on both sides." It also states, "Pathogenic factors attacking the meridians of foot-*Shaoyang* lead to incessant pain in the hypochondrium." This is because the Meridians of the Liver and the Gallbladder run through the costal and hypochondriac region.

Hypochondriac pain in disorders of the liver and gallbladder, and in intercostal neuralgia, can be diagnosed and treated according to the following descriptions.

Etiology and Pathogenesis

Emotional stress, an improper diet, exposure to dampness-heat, contusions, and a weak constitution are among the causes of hypochondriac pain. The liver and the gallbladder become diseased causing hypochondriac pain. The liver is located in the hypochondrium, and its meridians extends on both sides of the hypochondrium; the gallbladder is attached to the liver. The Liver and Gallbladder Meridians are externally and internally related.

1. Liver *Qi*-Stagnation

Either mental depression or anger damages the liver and impairs its ability to promote the free flow of *qi*. Stagnant *qi* in the Liver Meridian leads to hypochondriac pain.

2. Blood Stagnation

Stagnant liver *qi* causes blood stagnation in the meridians at the hypochondrium, thus leading to pain. Damage to the meridians at the hypochondrium due to contusions or sprains may also have the same effect.

3. Dampness-Heat of the Liver and Gallbladder

This originates from either external pathogenic dampness-heat or an improper diet. When dampness-heat is retained in these organs, their ability to promote the flow of *qi* is impaired, and pain in the hypochondrium region ensues.

4. Liver *Yin* (Blood)-Deficiency

A weak constitution due to chronic illness, stress or excessive sexual intercourse consumes body essence and blood. Hepatic *yin* deficiency deprives the liver collaterals of nourishment, thus causing hypochondriac pain.

Differentiation and Treatment

The state of *qi* and blood, and whether there are excesses or deficiencies should be clarified in order to diagnose the condition correctly. Stagnant liver *qi* causes distending hypochondriac pain, while stagnant blood produces a stabbing pain with a fixed location in the hypochondrium. Liver *yin* (blood)-deficiency results in a dull hypochondriac pain alleviated by pressure. Pain in the hypochondrium region caused by excesses is due to dampness-heat in the liver and gallbladder; this pain is violent, and accompanied by a bitter taste in the mouth and jaundice.

These four conditions are closely related; one may become or complicate another. For example, *qi* stagnation over a long time is often accompanied by blood stagnation; the latter prevents the production of new blood and thus develops into blood deficiency; and dampness-heat in the liver and gallbladder can be complicated by *qi* stagnation.

1. Liver *Qi*-Stagnation

Clinical manifestations: Distending, wandering pain in the hypochondrium region closely related to emotional factors. Other symptoms are stuffiness in the chest, frequent belching, a poor appetite, a thin tongue coating, and a taut pulse.

Analysis: Liver *qi*-stagnation implies the blockage of *qi* circulation in the hypochondriac region; this explains the occurrence of distending pains there. This type of pain wanders because the *qi* is non-substantial, alternately accumulating and dispersing. Since emotional changes directly affect *qi*, hypochondriac pain in this syndrome is closely related to emotional factors. Stuffiness in the chest is another result of *qi* stagnation. If liver *qi* attacks the spleen and stomach, then a poor appetite and belching will result. A taut pulse indicates the stagnation of *qi*.

Treatment: To soothe the liver and regulate *qi*.

Prescription: Modified Powder of Bupleuri for Releasing Stagnant Liver-*Qi* (239). In this formula, Radix Bupleuri promotes the liver's ability to regulate the flow of *qi*; Rhizoma Cyperi and Fructus Aurantii regulate *qi*; Rhizoma Chuanxiong activates blood circulation; and Radix Paeoniae Alba and Radix Glycyrrhizae relieve acute pain. If the pain is violent, drugs like Rhizoma Corydalis, Radix Curcumae, Pericarpium Citri Reticulatae Viride, Olibanum and Myrrha can be added to help regulate *qi* and relieve pain. In cases of stagnant *qi* turning into fire with symptoms of costal and hypochondriac pain, restlessness, a hot sensation, thirst, difficulty in passing urine and stools, a red tongue with a yellow coating and a taut and rapid pulse, Powder of Toosendan (183), Cortex Moutan and Fructus Gardeniae should be added to disperse any heat in the liver and regulate *qi*. If liver *qi* invades the spleen, causing hypochondriac pain, borborygmus, abdominal pain and diarrhea, then Rhizoma Atractylodis Macrocephalae, Radix Ledebouriellae and Pericarpium Citri Reticulatae can be added to invigorate the spleen and soothe the liver. If the stomach's ability to descend is impaired and hypochondriac pain, nausea and vomiting appear, then Flos Inulae, Haematitum and Rhizoma Pinelliae should be added to harmonize the stomach, conduct the unhealthy *qi* downward and stop vomiting. If the patient's appetite becomes poor and a distending sensation occurs after eating, then Endothelium Corneum Gigeriae Galli, Massa Medicata Fermentata, Fructus Crataegi and Fructus Amomi should be added to invigorate the spleen, harmonize the stomach and improve digestion. If there is acid regurgitation, Concha Arcae and Concha Bellamya Quadratae can be added to regulate *qi* and check acid secretion.

2. Blood Stagnation

Clinical manifestations: Stabbing pain in the hypochondrium which is worse at night and fixed in location. There may be palpable masses in the hypochondrium. The patient's tongue is dark purple or has purple spots, the pulse is taut or unsmooth.

Analysis: Stagnant blood originating from stagnant *qi*, or due to contusions or sprains causes a stabbing pain with a fixed location. Because blood belongs to *yin*, the pain becomes worse at night. Accumulations of blood form palpable masses. A dark purple tongue and an unsmooth pulse are both indications of internal blood stasis.

Treatment: To activate blood circulation, remove stasis, circulate *qi*, and remove any obstruction of the meridians.

Prescription: Modified Decoction of Inulae (276). In the recipe, *Xinjiang* (dark reddish silk dyed with madder) can be replaced by Radix Rubiae to activate blood circulation and remove any obstruction of the meridians; Flos Inulae regulates *qi* and relieves pain. To further activate blood circulation and remove stasis, Terminalis Angelicae Sinensis Radix, Semen Persicae and Radix Curcumae can be added. If blood stagnation is pronounced, Decoction for Activating Blood Circulation and Dredging Meridian

(213) should be prescribed. In this formula, Radix Bupleuri regulates liver and gallbladder *qi*; Radix Angelicae Sinensis, Semen Persicae and Flos Carthami nourish the blood, activate circulation and produce new blood; Squama Manitis moves stagnant blood and removes any vascular obstructions; Fructus Trichosanthis moistens dryness and disperses blood; Radix Glycyrrhizae relieves acute symptoms; and Radix et Rhizoma Rhei removes stasis and produces new blood. When blood is stagnant, there is always stagnant *qi*. "*Qi* controls the blood," and "the circulation of *qi* leads to circulation of blood." So drugs that regulate *qi* should be added to improve the problem of blood stagnation. In cases of palpable masses in the costal and hypochondriac region, drugs that circulate blood and disperse masses should be added if the patient's body resistance is strong; these include Rhizoma Sparganii, Rhizoma Curcumae and Eupolyphaga seu Steleophaga. It is also advisable to take Bolus of Carapax Trionycis (325).

3. Dampness-Heat of the Liver and Gallbladder

Clinical manifestations: Violent pain in the hypochondrium region, a bitter taste in the mouth, red eyes, stuffiness in the chest, a poor appetite, nausea, vomiting, possibly yellow sclera and yellow skin, deep yellow urine, a sticky yellow tongue coating, and a taut and rapid pulse.

Analysis: The retention of dampness-heat in the liver and gallbladder impairs the free flow of *qi*, thus giving rise to pain in the hypochondrium and a bitter taste in the mouth. The liver opens into the eyes, and so if the liver fire has flared up, the eyes will be red. The retention of dampness-heat in the middle *jiao* impairs transportation and transformation by the spleen, as well as gastric descent; this explains the stuffiness in the chest, poor appetite, nausea and vomiting. Dampness-heat compels the bile to flow outside the normal route, resulting in yellow sclera and yellow skin. The downward movement of dampness-heat to the urinary bladder causes deep yellow urine. A sticky yellow tongue coating and a taut and rapid pulse are indications of dampness-heat in the liver and gallbladder.

Treatment: To dissipate heat and eliminate dampness.

Prescription: Modified Decoction of Gentianae for Purging Liver-Fire (78). In the recipe, Radix Gentianae disperses excess fire in the liver and gallbladder and eliminates dampness-heat; Radix Scutellariae and Fructus Gardeniae dissipate heat and reduce fire; Caulis Aristolochiae Manshuriensis, Semen Plantaginis and Rhizoma Alismatis eliminate dampness-heat; Radix Rehmanniae and Radix Angelicae Sinensis nourish liver blood, since hyperactive fire definitely damages *yin*; Radix Bupleuri regulates the liver and gallbladder *qi*; and Radix Glycyrrhizae harmonizes the middle *jiao*, eliminates toxins and coordinates all the ingredients of the prescription. In cases of fever and jaundice, Herba Artemisiae Scopariae and Cortex Phellodendri should be added to dissipate heat, eliminate dampness and relieve jaundice. When dampness-heat condenses the bile to stones which block the biliary tract, causing hypochondriac pain extending to the shoulders and back, Herba Lysimachiae, Spora Lygodii, Radix Curcumae and Powder of Nitrum and Alumen (298) should be added to ease the gallbladder and expel the stones. In cases of dry-heat in the gastrointestinal tract with constipation and abdominal distention and fullness, Radix et Rhizoma Rhei and Natrii Sulfas should be added to disperse the heat and relieve constipation. In cases of violent pain with the vomiting of roundworms, Bolus of Mume (66) should first be administered to pacify the roundworms, then other formulas can be used to expel them.

4. Liver *Yin*-Deficiency

Clinical manifestations: Dull pain in the costal and hypochondriac region aggravated by stress and alleviated by pressure, thirst, dry throat, restlessness, a hot sensation in the chest, dizziness, blurred vision, a red tongue with a small amount of coating, and a thready, taut and rapid pulse.

Analysis: Two conditions may cause a dull pain, either the stagnant liver *qi* may turn into heat, which consumes heat or after a chronic illness the body resistance is weak and there is a deficiency of *yin* blood depriving the liver meridians of nourishment. A deficiency of *yin* produces internal heat, which results in thirst, a dry throat, restlessness and a hot sensation. Deficiencies of essence and blood prevent the upward supply of nourishment, thus giving rise to dizziness and blurred vision. A red tongue with a small amount of coating and a thready, taut and rapid pulse are indications of *yin* deficiency leading to internal heat.

Treatment: To nourish liver *yin*.

Prescription: *Yiguan* Decoction (1) is the main formula. In the recipe, Radix Rehmanniae and Fructus Lycii nourish the liver and kidneys; Radix Adenophorae, Radix Ophiopogonis and Radix Angelicae Sinensis nourish liver *yin*; and Fructus Toosendan soothes the liver, regulates *qi* and relieves pain. To strengthen the analgesic effect, Rhizoma Corydalis is added. In cases of a bitter taste and dry throat, or epistaxis, Radix Scutellariae, Rhizoma Imperatae and Pollen Typhae can be added to disperse heat and check bleeding. In cases of palpitation and insomnia, Semen Ziziphi Spinosae and Fructus Tritici Levis should be added to nourish the heart and calm the mind. In cases of distensive costal and hypochondriac pain, Fructus Akebiae, Rhizoma Cyperi and Radix Curcumae soothe the liver and regulate *qi*. In cases of dizziness and blurred vision, Fructus Ligustri Lucidi and Herba Ecliptae fortify the liver and kidneys. In cases of yellow urine, Cortex Phellodendri dissipates heat.

5. Wood (the Liver) Overpowering Earth (the Spleen)

Clinical manifestations: Dull pain in the costal and hypochondriac region, listlessness, shortness of breath, a poor appetite, epigastric distention after eating, dizziness, general aching, loose stools, a sallow complexion, a thin tongue coating, and a taut pulse.

Analysis: Liver *qi* is likely to attack the spleen. When this occurs, spleen *qi* becomes insufficient. As a result, the liver loses nourishment and the dull pains, listlessness, and shortness of breath ensue. The impaired functions in transporting and transforming explain the lack of appetite, the epigastric distention and the loose stools. Dizziness, general aching and a sallow complexion are signs of simultaneous disorders of the liver and spleen.

Treatment: To nourish *qi*, invigorate the spleen, replenish blood and reinforce liver *yin*.

Prescription: Decoction of Four Mild Drugs (91) added with Radix Angelicae Sinensis and Radix Paeoniae Alba. In the recipe, Radix Ginseng, Radix Atractylodis Macrocephalae, Poria and Radix Glycyrrhizae invigorate the spleen and replenish *qi*; Radix Angelicae Sinensis and Radix Paeoniae Alba nourish the blood and reinforce liver *yin*. When the spleen is strengthened, liver *qi* will become smooth. The addition of Fructus Toosendan and Rhizoma Corydalis regulate the *qi* and relieve pain. In cases of loose stool, Radix Ledebouriellae and Rhizoma Zingiberis (charred) raise the clear *qi* and check diarrhea. If epigastric distention takes place after eating, Fructus Aurantii and Endothelium Corneum Gigeriae Galli can be added to circulate *qi* and relieve distention. In cases of nausea and vomiting, Rhizoma Pinelliae and Pericarpium Citri Reticulatae should be added to harmonize the stomach and conduct the unhealthy *qi* downward.

Case Studies

Name: Chen XX; Sex: Male; Age: 44.

First visit: The patient complained of long-term hypochondriac pain. This was due to stagnant liver *qi*. Treatment sought to soothe the liver and remove any obstructions. The following drugs were prescribed:

Radix Bupleuri	3 g;
Radix Angelicae Sinensis	6 g;
Radix Paeoniae Alba	6 g;
Cortex Moutan	4.5 g;

Fructus Aurantii	4.5 g;
Fructus Gardeniae	9 g;
Radix Curcumae	9 g;
Folium Citri Reticulatae	4.5 g;
Retinervus Citri Reticulatae	4.5 g;
Fructus Rhizoma Cyperi Preparata	9 g;
Radix Glycyrrhizae Preparata	1.8 g;
Fructus Tribuli	9 g;
Pericarpium Citri Reticulatae Viride (vinegar prepared)	3 g.

Second visit: Hypochondriac pain had improved and the patient could twist his body. Treatment now sought to relieve acute symptoms with sweet drugs, promote astringency with sour drugs, and remove obstructions with acrid ones:

Radix Glycyrrhizae Preparata	3 g;
Radix Paeoniae Alba	6 g;
Radix Curcumae	9 g;
Rhizoma Cyperi	9 g;
Fructus Aurantii	4.5 g;
Folium Citri Reticulatae	4.5 g;
Retinervus Luffae Fructus	4.5 g;
Pericarpium Citri Reticulatae Viride	3 g;
Fructus Tribuli	4.5 g;
Radix Angelicae Sinensis	6 g;
Cortex Moutan	6 g;
Radix Bupleuri	2.4 g.

Explanation: This disease was caused by liver *qi*-stagnation. Ye Tianshi said, "Long-standing pain affects the vessels." Thus drugs that nourish blood and remove vascular obstruction were added.

Name: Zhang XX; Sex: Male; Age: 44; Occupation: Office worker.

The patient had experienced pains in the hypochondrium region over the past year. Examinations showed that the liver had become enlarged 2.5-3.0 cm below the ribs, and that the spleen was not palpable. Tests revealed that the liver function was normal. The patient felt pain in both sides, but it was worse on the right-hand side. Other clinical manifestations included lassitude and the distention of the epigastrium and the abdomen. The patient had taken more than 80 doses of drugs that soothe the liver, regulate *qi*, resolve dampness and remove blood stasis, without favorable results. He now exhibited emaciation, a bitter taste in the mouth, a dry throat, dizziness, insomnia, severe hypochondriac pain and constipation. His pulse was taut at the *guan* position and weak at the *chi* position. His tongue was crimson and cracked in the middle with a thin coating.

The pathogenesis was *yin* deficiency and dry blood complicated by liver *qi* attack. Treatment aimed to dissipate heat, nourish liver *yin* and moisten dryness. The following drugs were prescribed:

Radix Glehniae	12 g;
Radix Rehmanniae	15 g;
Radix Ophiopogonis	9 g;

Fructus Lycii	12 g;
Terminalis Angelicae Sinensis Radix	4.5 g;
Fructus Toosendan (roasted)	4.5 g;
Rhizoma Coptidis	0.9 g;
Semen Ziziphi Spinosae	12 g;
Semen Platycladi	12 g;
Fructus Hordei Germinatus	3 g;
Fructus Trichosanthis (pounded)	15 g.

After five successive doses, the constipation was relieved, the hypochondriac pain had improved greatly, and other symptoms had disappeared. The treatment continued for a month, during which the patient took more than 20 doses. After that, all the clinical symptoms had disappeared, and the enlargement of the liver was reduced to 1.5 cm.

Explanation: Hypochondriac pain due to liver *qi*-stagnation gave rise to symptoms of *yin* deficiency and dry blood. *Yiguan* Decoction (1) was most effective in nourishing *yin* and soothing the liver.

XXVII. Jaundice

Jaundice refers to the condition when the eyeballs, face, skin and urine become abnormally yellow. The yellow discoloration of the eyeballs is the most important symptom of the disease; without that discoloration a patient cannot be considered to be suffering from jaundice.

In the Chinese medical classics, three methods are used to classify jaundice. The first is based on etiology as shown in *Synopsis of Prescriptions of the Golden Chamber*. According to this book, jaundice falls into five categories: jaundice, jaundice due to improper diet, jaundice due to excessive alcohol, jaundice due to excessive sex, and chronic jaundice. The second method of classifying jaundice focuses on its clinical manifestations. Bright yellow jaundice is *yang* type, and dark yellow is *yin* type. Since this way of classification is simple, it is still used in traditional Chinese medicine. The third method of classification is a combination of etiology and clinical manifestations. For instance, 28 kinds of jaundice are classified in *The Pathogenesis and Manifestations of Diseases*; and nine kinds with 36 different colors are described in *Imperial Medical Encyclopedia*. Since this is complicated and confusing, it is rarely used by doctors nowadays.

The direct cause of jaundice is the dysfunction of the gallbladder in storing and excreting bile. The pathogenesis is the dysfunction of the spleen and stomach in transportation and transformation, and of the liver in promoting the free flow of *qi*, thus spreading bile to the surface of the body. This was discovered by Zhang Jingyue as long ago as the the Ming Dynasty.

The condition is severe if jaundice breaks out abruptly and the patient exhibits bright yellow skin coloration, irritability, fever, restlessness, and even mental confusion, delirium and mania. This is described in *The Pathogenesis and Manifestations of Diseases* and *Essentially Treasured Prescriptions* as acute yellow discoloration with a poor prognosis. Shen Jin'ao of the Qing Dynasty considered it to be an epidemic disease.

In Western medicine, jaundice is classified as hepatocellular jaundice, obstructive jaundice and hemolytic jaundice. Diseases such as viral hepatitis, hepatocirrhosis, diseases of the biliary tract, leptospirosis, hemolytic anemia and septicemia are differentiated and treated according to the following descriptions.

Etiology and Pathogenesis

Jaundice can be caused by both external and internal factors. External factors include attacks by dampness-heat, toxins or an improper diet, while internal factors refer to a weak spleen and stomach and prolonged *qi* and blood stagnation. These two types of cause are different yet interrelated.

1. Dampness-Heat Retention

The main cause of jaundice is attacks by dampness-heat. This blocks the middle *jiao* and hinders the excretion of the bile. Dampness-heat also impairs the free flow of *qi*, causing the bile to flow a different route from normal. When the bile reaches the skin, muscles, eyes and bladder, then the skin, eyeballs and urine will become abnormally yellow.

The appearance of dampness-heat can be attributed to irregular food intake or excessive alcohol intake. In these cases, the spleen and stomach are damaged and their functions impaired, producing dampness. Prolonged stagnation of dampness generates heat. The combination of dampness and heat further impairs the functions of the liver and gallbladder, causing the bile to stray from its normal route.

2. Weak Spleen and Stomach

Dampness may either be caused by splenic or gastric deficiency with stagnant cold or by a deficiency of spleen *yang* following protracted illness. This dampness may then be transformed into cold. Cold-dampness blocks the middle *jiao* and hinders the excretion of bile.

The weakness of the spleen and stomach leads to impaired digestion and impaired *qi* and blood production; *qi* and blood deficiency deprives the skin and muscles of nourishment. The exposure of the color of the spleen (earth) on the body surface gives rise to jaundice.

3. *Qi* Stagnation

Blood stasis resulting from long-term *qi* stagnation blocks the biliary tract, thus causing jaundice.

Mental depression affects the liver and gallbladder, and impairs the free flow of *qi*. Moreover, pathogenic dampness turns into heat, which condenses body fluid into stones. As long as these stones remain in the biliary tract, the excretion of bile is hindered.

4. Hyperactive Toxin-Heat

External pathogenic dampness is associated with toxin-heat or invasive infectious factors. The latter are violently offensive; they attack the *ying* and *xue* systems, affect the liver and kidneys, penetrate the pericardium and disturb the mind, thus causing acute jaundice.

In short, pathogenic dampness is the principal factor. It causes jaundice of the *yang* type through heat, that of the *yin* type through cold and that of the acute type through toxin-heat and infectious factors. The kind of jaundice caused by splenic deficiency with insufficient blood production also belongs to the *yin* type, and jaundice caused by stagnation may be of either type.

Diagnosis

1. General Edema with Yellow Skin

This condition can often be seen in ancylostomiasis. If hookworms remain in the intestines for a long time, they consume *qi* and blood, causing a puffy, yellow face, yellow-whitish skin, lassitude, possible nausea, vomiting of yellow fluid, bristling hair all over the body, and a preference for eating raw rice, tea leaves and clay. The fact that the eyeballs are not yellow should alert the practitioner to this diagnosis.

2. Sallow Complexion

This is often caused by *qi* and blood deficiency after a severe or chronic illness, or excessive blood loss. Deficient *qi* and blood means an inability to nourish the muscles and skin, producing dry, withered, yellow skin, dizziness and palpitations. However, eyeballs are still not yellow.

Differentiation and Treatment

Each type of jaundice has its own characteristic features, and should be distinguishable from other types. Jaundice of the *yang* type occurs abruptly and does not last long, and its color is bright yellow, exhibiting a heat-syndrome caused by excesses. Jaundice of the *yin* type has a slow onset and a long duration, its color is dark yellow, and it exhibits a cold-syndrome caused by deficiencies. Severe acute jaundice is marked by an abrupt onset and rapid changes, its the color is golden yellow and it exhibits a complicated syndrome caused by the combination of deficiencies, excesses, cold and heat.

Attention should next be paid to the pathological changes. If the patient's bright yellow color grows lighter, and he is in fairly good spirits, then his condition is improving. On the contrary, if the color turns darker or deeper, and restlessness and irritability are present, that shows his condition is getting worse.

The early stages of the disease shows symptoms such as fever, an aversion to cold, a lack of appetite, nausea, vomiting, lassitude and dysuria with yellow urine; then the eyeballs become yellow, followed by the entire body in severe cases.

Since pathogenic dampness is the main cause, the therapeutic principle is to eliminate dampness and promote diuresis. When urination increases, pathogenic dampness will be discharged downwards, and pathogenic heat or cold will be eliminated more easily. In addition, treatment that dissipates the heat and eliminates toxins can be adopted for *yang*-type jaundice. Methods of invigorating the spleen, dispersing the cold, replenishing *qi* and blood, soothing the liver and activating blood circulation can be used for *yin*-type jaundice; and those which dissipate heat, eliminate toxins, cool the blood and nourish *yin* for severe acute jaundice.

1. *Yang*-Type Jaundice

(1) In cases where heat is more severe than dampness

Clinical manifestations: Bright yellow eyeballs and skin, fever, thirst, small amounts of deep yellow urine the same color as strong tea, nausea, a poor appetite, epigastric and abdominal distention, constipation, a sticky yellow tongue coating, and a taut and rapid pulse.

Analysis: Dampness-heat impairs the free flow of *qi*, and thus spreads the bile to the muscles and skin, and to the eyes through the Liver Meridian, resulting in yellow skin, face and eyeballs. Heat is a *yang* factor, so the yellow color it causes is bright. Excess pathogenic heat consumes fluid and thereby causes fever and thirst. Dampness-heat retained in the middle *jiao* impairs transportation and transformation, and causes the turbid *qi* of the stomach to ascend; this is the reason for nausea and poor appetite. Excess heat in the stomach and intestines blocks the *qi*, producing distention and constipation. The downward movement of dampness-heat to the bladder causes the small amounts of deep yellow urine. A sticky yellow tongue coating and a taut and rapid pulse are indications of dampness-heat in the liver and gallbladder.

Treatment: To dissipate heat, eliminate dampness and relieve constipation.

Prescription: Decoction of Artemisiae Scopariae (200) with additional drugs. In this formula, Herba Artemisiae Scopariae is used in large doses because it is the main ingredient for dispersing heat, eliminating dampness and relieving jaundice; Fructus Gardeniae dissipates dampness-heat in the triple *jiao*; Radix et Rhizoma Rhei relieves constipation; the combination of Herba Artemisiae Scopariae and Fructus Gardeniae eliminates dampness-heat through urination; and the combination of Herba Artemisiae Scopariae and Radix et Rhizoma Rhei relieves retained heat through bowel movements. Drugs that eliminate dampness through urination, such as Semen Plantaginis, Polyporus and Rhizoma Alismatis, are added with drugs that disperse heat and eliminate toxins, such as Herba Sedi Sarmentosi, Herba Hyperici Japonici, Herba Abri Fruticulosi and Radix Isatidis.

In cases of restlessness and nausea, Rhizoma Coptidis and Caulis Bambusae in Taeniam are added to disperse heat which has accumulated in the heart, relieve restlessness, conduct the unhealthy *qi* downwards and check vomiting. In cases of epigastric and abdominal distention, Fructus Aurantii Immaturus and Cortex Magnoliae Officinalis should be added to help the *qi* to circulate and relieve stagnation. If there is pain in the right hypochondrium, Radix Bupleuri, and Radix Curcumae can be added to soothe the liver, relieve stagnation and kill pain. When bowel movements are unobstructed, and the sticky tongue coating is gradually subsiding, drugs that invigorate the spleen and eliminate dampness, such as Rhizoma Atractylodis Macrocephalae and Poria, should be added; at the same time bitter and cold drugs, used for dispersing heat, should be reduced to protect spleen *yang*.

(2) In cases where dampness is more severe than heat

Clinical manifestations: The skin, face and eyeballs are all yellow, but less of a bright color than in the previous condition. Other clinical manifestations include a recessive fever, a heaviness of the head, sluggishness, epigastric fullness, a poor appetite, thirst coupled with the desire to drink only small quantities, loose stools with difficult bowel movements, small amounts of yellow urine, a thick and sticky or yellowish-white tongue coating, and a soft, retarded, taut and smooth pulse.

Analysis: Dampness is a *yin* factor. When dampness is more severe than heat, the color of the patient is less bright than in the opposite case. Dampness-heat with heat retention gives rise to recessive fever, which means that when the patient's skin is touched, it does not feel hot initially but only after a relatively long time. When the middle *jiao* is attacked by pathogenic dampness, this impairs the splenic and gastric abilities to transport and transform, which results in the feeling of heaviness in the head, as well as the sluggishness, epigastric fullness, poor appetite, and loose stools with difficult bowel movements. Internal excess dampness and consumption of fluid by heat cause the thirst. A thick and sticky or yellow-white tongue coating and a soft, retarded, taut and smooth pulse are due to the attack of the spleen by dampness.

Treatment: To eliminate dampness, soothe the turbid *qi* and disperse heat.

Prescription: Powder of Artemisiae Scopariae and Four Ingredients with Poria (198) combined with additional drugs. In the recipe, Herba Artemisiae Scopariae dissipates heat, eliminates dampness and relieves jaundice; Polyporus Poria and Rhizoma Alismatis eliminate dampness through diuresis; and Rhizoma Atractylodis Macrocephalae invigorates the spleen and eliminates dampness. Aromatics for soothing the turbid *qi* such as Herba Agastaches and Fructus Amomi Rotundus, can be added to promote the smooth circulation of *qi* so as to dry dampness and relieve jaundice.

In cases of nausea and vomiting due to the upward movement of the turbid *qi* in the stomach, Rhizoma Pinelliae and Pericarpium Citri Reticulatae should be added. If abdominal distention is severe, Pericarpium Arecae and Fructus Aurantii Immaturus can be added to circulate *qi* and relieve distention.

If dampness and heat are both severe in *yang*-type jaundice, Detoxification Pill should be prescribed in combination in order to eliminate dampness, soothe the turbid *qi*, disperse heat and eliminate toxins.

(3) Obstruction of the biliary tract

Clinical manifestations: Jaundice occurs rapidly. Violent pains occur on the right-hand side of the hypochondrium, which often spread to the right shoulder and back. Other clinical manifestations include alternate fever and chilliness, a bitter taste, dry throat, nausea, abdominal distention, a poor appetite, light gray stools, small amounts of yellow urine, a burning sensation when urinating, a red tongue with a sticky yellow coating, and a taut and rapid pulse. There is usually a history of relapses.

Analysis: Due to an obstruction of the biliary tract, the outflow of bile causes the rapid onset of jaundice. The hypochondrium is where the liver and gallbladder are housed; heat retained in the liver and gallbladder accordingly causes hypochondriac pain that may spread along the Gallbladder Meridian to the shoulder and the back. Alternate fever and chilliness, a bitter taste in the mouth and a dry throat are the main symptoms that the Gallbladder Meridian of Foot-*Shaoyang* has been affected. Nausea, abdominal distention and a poor appetite result from the impaired splenic and gastric functions due to the disorders of the liver and the gallbladder. The obstruction of the biliary tract prevents the bile from entering the intestinal tract, this causes the grayish-white stools. Small amounts of yellow urine, a burning sensation when urinating, a red tongue with sticky yellow coating, and a taut and rapid pulse are all indications of excess heat in the liver and the gallbladder.

Treatment: To soothe the liver and the gallbladder, disperse heat and relieve stagnation.

Prescription: Modified Decoction of Bupleuri for Regulating *Shaoyang* and *Yangming* Meridians (28). In this formula, Radix Bupleuri and Radix Paeoniae Alba soothe the liver and relieve pain; Radix Scutellariae and Rhizoma Pinelliae disperse heat and harmonize the middle *jiao*; and Radix et Rhizoma Rhei and Fructus Aurantii Immaturus relieve constipation and promote the flow of bile. If the obstruction of the biliary tract is caused by stones, Herba Artemisiae Scopariae, Herba Lysimachiae, Radix

Curcumae, Rhizoma Polygoni Cuspidati and Powder of Nitrum and Alumen (298) can be added to help disperse the heat, promote the flow of bile, dispel the stones and relieve jaundice.

If jaundice occurs suddenly and is accompanied by alternate fever and chills, along with intermittent pains in the right hypochondrium that produce an upward boring sensation and the vomiting of roundworms, this suggests a blockage caused by worms in the biliary tract. Bolus of Mume (66) and Herba Artemisiae Scopariae should then be prescribed to promote the flow of bile, relieve jaundice, pacify roundworms and check any pain. Drugs that expel worms, help the *qi* to circulate and relieve pain should be added, such as Fructus Toosendan, Semen Arecae and Fructus Quisqualis.

2. *Yin*-Type Jaundice

(1) Cold-dampness stagnation

Clinical manifestations: Dark yellow eyeballs and skin, a poor appetite, epigastric discomfort or abdominal distention, loose stools, listlessness, an aversion to cold, a pale tongue with a sticky white coating, and a deep, thready and slow pulse.

Analysis: Retained cold-dampness hinders *yang-qi* and causes the stagnation of liver and gallbladder *qi*. In this case, the normal flow of bile is blocked and the bile spreads to the muscles and skin, causing jaundice. Since both cold and dampness are *yin* factors, the yellow color is dark. Because the spleen has been attacked by cold-dampness, this impairs its ability to transport and transform, and thus gives rise to a poor appetite, epigastric discomfort, abdominal distention and loose stools. The prolonged retention of cold-dampness causes *yang-qi* deficiency as well as deficiencies of both *qi* and blood. The body is consequently deprived of warmth and nourishment, and symptoms of listlessness and aversion to cold occur. A pale tongue with a sticky white coating results from the retention of turbid dampness. A deep, thready and slow pulse is an indication of retained cold-dampness in the *ying* system.

Treatment: To invigorate the spleen, harmonize the stomach, disperse cold and resolve dampness.

Prescription: Decoction of Artemisiae Scopariae, Atractylodis Macrocephalae and Aconiti Lateralis Preparata (199) with additional drugs. In the recipe, Herba Artemisiae Scopariae is combined with Radix Aconiti Lateralis Preparata and Rhizoma Zingiberis to warm the middle *jiao*, disperse cold and dry dampness; Radix Atractylodis Macrocephalae and Radix Glycyrrhizae, sweet and warm in nature, invigorate the spleen. Poria and Rhizoma Alismatis are added to aid the elimination of dampness. In cases where abdominal distention occurs and the tongue has a thick and sticky coating, Rhizoma Atractylodis and Cortex Magnoliae Officinalis can be added, and Radix Glycyrrhizae and Radix Atractylodis Macrocephalae removed from the prescription.

If the liver and spleen are diseased at the same time due to liver *qi*-stagnation and splenic deficiency, with symptoms of epigastric and abdominal distention, dull pain in the costal and hypochondriac regions, a poor appetite, lassitude, alternate loose stools and constipation and a taut and thready pulse, then treatment aims to assist the spleen and soothe the liver by prescribing modified *Xiaoyao Powder* (250).

(2) Splenic hypofunction and blood deficiency

Clinical manifestations: The color of the face, the eyeballs and the skin is light and lusterless. Other clinical manifestations are weak limbs, lassitude, palpitations, shortness of breath, a poor appetite, loose stool, a pale tongue with a thin coating, and a soft and thready pulse.

Analysis: Splenic and gastric hypofunction and blood deficiency mean the inability of the blood to nourish the muscles and skin on the exterior and the *zang-fu* organs in the interior. The color of the spleen is therefore exposed on the surface. *Qi* deficiency gives rise to short breath. Weak limbs, lassitude, a poor appetite, loose stools and a soft and thready pulse are indications of splenic hypofunction and blood deficiency.

Treatment: To invigorate the spleen, warm the middle *jiao*, replenish *qi* and blood.

Prescription: Decoction for Mildly Warming Middle *Jiao* (34) combined with additional drugs. In this formula, Ramulus Cinnamomi are combined with Rhizoma Zingiberis Recens and Fructus Jujubae, both acrid and sweet, to assist *yang* and warm the middle *jiao*; Radix Paeoniae Alba and Radix Glycyrrhizae, both sour and sweet in nature, nourish *yin*; and Saccharum Granorum invigorates the spleen and relieves pain. The whole prescription nourishes both *yin* and *yang*, and produces both *qi* and blood. Once the function of the spleen and stomach are restored, jaundice gradually subsides. If *qi* deficiency is more pronounced, Radix Astragali and Radix Codonopsis are added; if blood deficiency is more pronounced, Radix Angelicae Sinensis and Radix Rehmanniae are added. In case of *yang* deficiency with cold, Ramulus Cinnamomi is replaced by Cortex Cinnamomi.

(3) Blood stagnation

Clinical manifestations: Dark yellow skin and eyeballs, dark complexion, palpable masses and distending pain in the hypochondriac region, red threads on the skin, a purple tongue or purple spots on the tongue, and a taut and unsmooth or thready and unsmooth pulse.

Analysis: Prolonged jaundice or recurrent attacks of jaundice produces blood stasis in the hypochondriac region, which forms palpable masses and blocks the vessels, subsequently giving rise to red threads on the skin. Stagnant blood prevents the production of new blood and thereby deprives the face of nourishment; this explains the dark complexion. A purple tongue or purple spots on the tongue, and a taut and unsmooth or a thready and unsmooth pulse are indications of blood stagnation.

Treatment: To activate blood circulation, remove stasis, soothe the liver, and relieve jaundice.

Prescription: Bolus of Carapax Trionycis (325). In the recipe, Carapax Trionycis, as the main ingredient, softens the hardness, disperses the masses and removes vascular obstruction; Radix et Rhizoma Rhei, Eupolyphaga seu Steleophaga and Semen Persicae break blood stasis and remove any obstructions in the vessels of the Liver Meridian; Cortex Magnoliae Officinalis, Radix Bupleuri and Catharsius Molossus circulate *qi*, relieve stagnation and promote smooth blood circulation; Herba Dianthi and Folium Pyrrosiae eliminate dampness and promote diuresis; Rhizoma Zingiberis and Radix Scutellariae regulate *yin* and *yang*; and Radix Ginseng and Colla Corii Asini replenish *qi* and blood. Other ingredients in this formula may either enter the *xue* system to remove stasis or enter the *qi* system to relieve *qi* stagnation, or else assist the body's anti-pathogenic *qi* or eliminate pathogenic factors. The whole prescription combines replenishment and elimination, cooling and warming in order to regulate *qi* and blood.

Prolonged jaundice may cause the accumulation of turbid dampness and the disharmony of *qi* and blood, with symptoms including the enlargement of the liver and spleen, scaly skin and a distended abdomen with engorged veins. In this case, refer to the chapter on Tympanites.

3. Acute Jaundice

(1) Hyperactive toxin-heat

Clinical manifestations: The patient's facial color becomes deep yellow within a short space of time. Other clinical manifestations are high fever, restlessness, thirst, frequent vomiting, distention and fullness in the epigastrium and abdomen along with pain which is aggravated by pressure, constipation, small amounts of urine, irritability, a tongue which is red at the tip and edges with a coarse yellow coating, and a taut and rapid or bounding and large pulse.

Analysis: Toxin-heat attacks the liver and gallbladder, causing the bile to overflow; that is why the yellow color deepens. Hyperactive toxin-heat consumes the body fluid, and thereby gives rise to a high fever, restlessness, thirst and small amounts of urine. Retained toxin-heat in the gastrointestinal tract blocks intestinal *qi*, causing constipation, epigastric and abdominal distention, fullness and pain. The failure of stomach *qi* to descend causes frequent vomiting. Disturbance of the mind by hyperactive toxin-heat causes irritability and restlessness. A coarse yellow tongue coating and a taut and rapid or bounding and large pulse are indications of fluid consumption due to hyperactive toxin-heat.

Treatment: To disperse heat, eliminate toxins, reduce fire, and relieve jaundice.

Prescription: Modified Decoction of Artemisiae Scopariae (200), Decoction of Coptidis for Detoxification (263) and Decoction of Five Ingredients for Detoxification (52). Decoction of Artemisiae Scopariae dissipates heat, eliminates dampness, and relieves jaundice through urination and bowel movements. Radix Scutellariae dissipates fire in the upper *jiao*, as does Rhizoma Coptidis in the middle *jiao*, and Cortex Phellodendri in the lower *jiao*. Decoction of Five Ingredients for Detoxification disperses heat and eliminates toxins. The combination of the three formulas dissipates hyperactive fire and heat in all three *jiao* and relieves toxin-heat in the *xue* system.

(2) Deep penetration of toxin-heat

Clinical manifestations: The onset is acute, and pathological conditions change rapidly. The skin becomes as yellow as gold. Other clinical manifestations include a high fever, the retention of urine, epistaxis, bloody stool, ecchymosis and petechiae, restlessness and delirium, a crimson tongue with a dirty coating, and a taut, thready and rapid pulse.

Analysis: Attacked by violent and changeable toxin-heat, this type of jaundice usually comes on abruptly and undergoes rapid pathological changes. The bile is made to spread to the surface and produces a bright yellow color. At the same time fluid is consumed and the bladder's ability to control urine is impaired. All these cause a high fever and the retention of urine. When toxin-heat attacks the *ying* and *xue* systems, this causes the extravasation of blood to the muscles and skin, resulting in ecchymosis and petechiae. Its upward movement gives rise to epistaxis, while its downward one causes bloody stools. When toxin-heat agitates liver wind, tremors occur in mild cases, mania and convulsion in more severe ones. The deep penetration of toxin-heat into the pericardium disturbs the mind, thus giving rise to absent-mindedness and restlessness in mild cases, mental confusion and delirium in severe ones. A crimson tongue with a dirty coating and a taut, thready and rapid pulse are signs of the consumption of *yin* essence due to the deep penetration of toxin-heat into the *ying* and *xue* systems.

Treatment: To dissipate heat, eliminate toxins, cool blood and rescue *yin*.

Prescription: Powder of Cornu Rhinocerotis (307) with additional drugs. In this formula, Cornu Rhinocerotis, as the main ingredient, disperses heat, eliminates toxins and cools the blood. When Rhizoma Coptidis, Fructus Gardeniae and Rhizoma Cimicifugae are combined, this effect is strengthened. Herba Artemisiae Scopariae dissipates heat, eliminates dampness and relieves jaundice. Since Cornu Rhinocerotis is a rare animal drug, it is often replaced by Cornu Bubali, which should be prescribed in a larger dosage, generally 30-60 grams per dose, to be decocted first. Alternately, drugs that disperse heat and eliminate toxins are used, such as Folium Isatidis, Rhizoma Smilacis Glabrae, Herba Taraxaci, Herba Ardisiae Japonicae and Herba Sedi Sarmentosi, and drugs that nourish *yin* and cool blood are added, such as Radix Rehmanniae, Radix Scrophulariae, Herba Dendrobii and Cortex Moutan. In cases of hematemesis, hemafecia and ecchymosis or petechiae, Decoction of Cornu Rhinocerotis and Rehmanniae (306) should be prescribed and added to Cacumen Platycladi, Rhizoma Imperatae, Herba Agrimoniae and Radix Sanguisorbae (charred) to cool the blood and check bleeding. If toxin-heat agitates the liver wind, causing tremors or convulsions, Cornu Saigae Tataricae, Ramulus Uncariae cum Uncis and Concha Margaritifera Usta can be added to disperse heat, cool the liver and subdue wind. In cases of mental confusion and delirium, Pill of Precious Drugs (124), Purple-Snow Pellet (299), or Bolus of Calculus Bovis for Resurrection (127) should be administered immediately to disperse any heat in the heart and restore consciousness.

Remarks

The patient should eat light, easily digestible food instead of greasy or sweet food in order to avoid dampness. On the other hand, measures should be taken against food-borne infections.

Case Studies

Name: Wang XX; Sex: Female; Age: 54.
First visit: January 14, 1976.

The patient was admitted into hospital when her illness was diagnosed as acute icterohepatitis. She had felt tired and her appetite had been poor for two weeks, and she had had jaundice for two days. GPT was 400 units on admission. Her total bilirubin increased to 14 mg% four days after admission, and one minute bilirubin 13 mg%. Prothrombin time was 28 seconds. Alkaline phosphatase AKP was 25.5 units %. A-G ratio was 29/29. HAA (-). Glutamyl-transpeptidase was 9.5 units. The patient had deep yellow skin and eyeballs, abdominal fullness and distention, a poor appetite, a bitter taste in the mouth, a preference for cold drinks, edema of the lower limbs, slight edema of the hands, poor sleep with dreams, a pale and swollen tongue with a white coating, and a slightly smooth pulse.

Treatment aimed primarily to activate the blood circulation, remove stasis, circulate *qi*, eliminate dampness, and secondarily to cool the blood. The following drugs were prescribed:

Radix et Rhizoma Rhei	24 g;
Semen Persicae	9 g;
Eupolyphaga seu Steleophaga	6 g;
Lacca Sinica Exsiccatae	15 g;
Radix Notoginseng	15 g;
Cornu Rhinocerotis	9 g;
Radix Paeoniae Rubra	9 g;
Herba Lysimachiae	30 g;
Pericarpium Arecae	15 g;
Pericarpium Citri Reticulatae Viride	9 g;
Radix Aucklandiae	9 g;
Poria	30 g.

Two doses were prescribed.
Second visit: January 17, 1976.

Urination had increased, and bowel movements took place once or twice a day. The color of the skin and eyeballs seemed less yellow. In addition, abdominal distention was relieved, the patient's appetite had improved, and sleep had become normal. However, her tongue was dark red with a thin, white, dry coating, and her pulse was quite smooth. Three grams of Radix Ginseng were added, and another three doses were prescribed.

On January 21, the patient had another blood test. The total bilirubin had become normal. GPT was 43 units, and TFT was normal. Another 17 doses were prescribed.

Explanation: The patient had deep yellow skin and eyeballs, abdominal fullness and distention, and a dark red tongue; this indicated blood stagnation in the liver and gallbladder. Retained dampness-heat, stagnant *qi* and stagnant blood impaired the *qi* activity in the triple *jiao*. *Didang* Pill, Decoction for Purging Stagnated Blood, and Lacca Sinica Exsiccatae and Radix Paeoniae Rubra all relieve blood stagnation and remove stasis.

Name: Yang XX; Sex: Female; Age: 19.

On October 26, 1960, the patient's face and eyeballs were slightly yellow, and she felt discomfort in the chest and epigastrium, accompanied by a poor appetite, vomiting and lassitude. Two days later, she took a turn for the worse, repeatedly losing consciousness and talking in a confused manner. She was then rushed into hospital.

Examination: The patient's body temperature was 38.8°C, respiration 24/m, and pulse rate 96/m. The patient looked distressed, exhibiting mental confusion and restlessness. She was not cooperative during the examination. Her skin and the eyeballs were yellow, and the both her pupils were dilated. There was no reaction to light and no corneal reflex. There was fetid hepatic odor. The abdomen was slightly distended, and on percussion the sound produced was tympanic and fixed in location. The spleen was not palpable.

Laboratory tests showed bilirubin 4 mg, icteric index 45 units, GOT more than 200 units, GPT more than 400 units, and urine bilirubin and urobilin were positive.

Diagnosis: Infectious hepatitis, acute hepatic necrosis, hepatic coma.

The patient was treated with Western medicine soon after admission, but to no avail. On October 30th, doctors trained in traditional Chinese medicine were invited to make a diagnosis.

First visit: The patient exhibited mental confusion, coma, yellow skin and eyeballs, mania, convulsions, abdominal fullness, constipation for five days, deep yellow urine, sweating, a crimson tongue, and a rapid forceful pulse. This was diagnosed as severe acute jaundice. Decoction for Potent Purgation (26) was prescribed to relieve constipation straight away and protect the body's *yin*; and Purple-Snow Pellet (299) was also administered to eliminate toxin-heat:

Cortex Magnoliae Officinalis	6 g;
Fructus Aurantii Immaturus	9 g;
Radix et Rhizoma Rhei	12 g;
Natrii Sulfas Exsiccatus (to be taken separately in the form of infusion)	9 g;
Purple-Snow Pellet (to be mixed with prepared decoction for nasal feeding)	3 g.

Second visit: October 31.

The patient's constipation remained unchanged, and her fever continued. The tongue coating had begun to fade, although the tongue itself was still crimson. The patient sweated a lot, but urinated less than before. She was still comatose. All this showed that toxin-heat was retained in the *Yangming* Meridians and *fu* organs, and had already dried out. White Tiger Decoction and Purple-Snow Pellet were prescribed:

Gypsum Fibrosum	60 g;
Rhizoma Anemarrhenae	9 g;
Radix Glycyrrhizae	4.5 g;
Fructus Oryzae Sativae	30 g;
Herba Lophatheri (fresh)	50 pieces;
Radix Trichosanthis	9 g;
Radix Rehmanniae (fresh)	30 g;
Purple-Snow Pellet	3 g.

Third visit: November 1.

The patient had moved her bowels, passing half a spittoon of dark stools. Heat signs immediately began to subside, her mind became clear and her eyes shiny. She felt hungry and wanted to eat. Her tongue coating was moist. However, her pulse was still rapid, her skin and eyeballs yellow, and her urine yellow. All this showed that toxic fire was still hyperactive, and residual pathogenic factors still had not been eliminated. White Tiger Decoction with additional drugs was prescribed:

Gypsum Fibrosum	30 g;
Rhizoma Anemarrhenae	6 g;
Radix Glycyrrhizae	3 g;
Fructus Oryzae Sativae	18 g;
Radix Rehmanniae (fresh)	15 g;
Radix Scutellariae	9 g;
Talcum (wrapped)	15 g.

Fourth visit: November 2.

The patient's mind was fully clear, and her appetite had improved. Her skin color had become less yellow, and her pulse slower. Her urine flowed smoothly and was light yellow in color. The patient was out of danger now. Treatment sought to eliminate the residual pathogenic factors and regulate stomach *qi*:

Herba Artemisiae Scopariae	9 g;
Fructus Forsythiae	9 g;
Folium Eupatorii	9 g;
Radix Glycyrrhizae	2.4 g;
Radix Scutellariae	6 g;
Talcum	12 g;
Pericarpium Citri Reticulatae	3 g;
Fructus Setariae Germinatus	9 g.

Two doses were prescribed.

The patient then took both Chinese herbal medicine and Western drugs for some time. Her liver function was tested, and the results showed icteric index 10 units, bilirubin 0.5 mg, GOT 38.5 units, GPT 41 units, urine bilirubin and urobilin negative, and the jaundice of the eyeballs had subsided. She left hospital on December 4.

Explanation: This was a case of severe acute jaundice, exhibiting inward transmission of toxin-heat caused by the blockage of the *Yangming fu* organs and the coma. Since her urination was unobstructed, *yin* had not yet been depleted. The failure of Decoction for Potent Purgation was due to the fact that "the boat had stopped moving due to lack of water." White Tiger Decoction and Purple-Snow Pellet, acrid and cool, eliminate pathogenic factors; and Radix Rehmanniae and Radix Trichosanthis produce body fluid. When the retained feces were discharged and excess fire was reduced, she immediately became conscious. Treatment concluded by dispersing heat and relieving dampness.

Name: Liu XX; Sex: Male; Age: 20.

The patient's disease began with alternating fevers and chilliness, followed by his face and eyeballs turning yellow. It was diagnosed as hemolytic jaundice and treated with Western medicine, including a blood transfusion of 2,000 ml. Since his pathological condition remained serious, Chinese doctors were invited to the consultation.

The patient exhibited a slightly yellow face and eyeballs, listlessness, pale lips and tongue, lassitude, a dislike of speaking, feeble breathing, dizziness, palpitations, inability to rise from the bed, night sweating, loose stools, yellow urine, a feverish sensation caused by deficiencies, an inability to taste anything, poor appetite, and a large, retarded and soft pulse.

Decoction of Astragali for Strengthening Middle *Jiao* (267), sweet and warm, was prescribed to replenish *qi* and blood, and invigorate the spleen:

Radix Astragali	12 g;
Ramulus Cinnamomi	6 g;
Radix Paeoniae Alba	12 g;
Radix Glycyrrhizae Preparata	4.5 g;
Rhizoma Zingiberis Recens	6 g;
Fructus Jujubae	5 pieces;
Sacchrum Granorum	30 g.

The symptoms became less obvious after more than 20 doses. Treatment then continued for another two months, adding to the previous prescription Radix Codonopsis, Radix Angelicae Sinensis, Herba Artemisiae Scopariae, Radix Aconiti Lateralis Preparata, Poria and Rhizoma Atractylodis Macrocephalae. Thus the symptoms further improved. Subsequently, Decoction for Invigorating Spleen and Nourishing Heart (110) was administered to conclude the treatment. Laboratory tests six months later showed that the patient was functioning almost normally, with red blood cells increased to 4,060,000/mm from 1,080,000/mm at the beginning of traditional treatment, hemochrome increased to 72% from 30%, and icteric index decreased to 11 units from 50 units. The disease was cured.

Explanation: This disease was principally caused by splenic deficiency, thus being different to *yang*-type jaundice due to dampness-heat. It was advisable to treat it by replenishing *qi* and blood, and invigorating the spleen with sweet and warm drugs. Decoction of Astragali for Strengthening Middle *Jiao* was the right treatment in this case. When the symptoms were gone and the spleen and stomach were functioning better, drugs that replenish *qi* and blood and drugs that warm *yang* and relieve jaundice could be be added. Thus satisfactory therapeutic results were achieved. Last of all, the disease was treated by administering Decoction for Invigorating Spleen and Nourishing Heart.

XXVIII. Abdominal Masses

The most marked symptoms of abdominal masses, which are called *jiju* in Chinese, are abdominal distention and pain. *Ji* refers to visible abdominal masses, which produce pain with a fixed location. They involve the *xue* system and are generally caused by disorders of the *zang* organs. Since *ji* forms over a period of time, the pathological condition is severe and so *ji* is difficult to cure. *Ju* refers to invisible masses, which produce pain without a fixed location. It involves the *qi* system, and is mostly caused by disorders of the *fu* organs. *Ju* feels like a mass when *qi* accumulates; but this mass disappears when *qi* disperses. Since this type of mass forms over a short period, its pathological condition is mild and it is generally easier to deal with than *ji*.

Abdominal tumors, enlargement of the liver and spleen, hyperplastic intestinal tuberculosis, functional gastrointestinal disturbances, and incomplete intestinal obstructions can be diagnosed and treated according to the following descriptions.

Etiology and Pathogenesis

Among the causes of abdominal masses are mental depression, an improper diet, and attacks by pathogenic cold-dampness or toxin-heat. The internal cause of abdominal masses is a deficiency in the body's anti-pathogenic *qi*. Classics on traditional Chinese medicine hold that "People with strong resistance do not have abdominal masses, only weak people are likely to suffer from them." Abdominal masses gradually develop when the body's anti-pathogenic *qi* fails in its struggle against the attacking pathogenic factors. This disease is principally related to the liver and spleen. The stagnation of the *qi* and the blood and phlegm retention play a major role in the pathogenesis of abdominal masses.

1. Mental Depression and *Qi* and Blood Stagnation

Mental depression causes the stagnation of liver *qi*, which produces *ju* lumps. This leads to blood stagnation, which over a long period forms masses, thus producing *ji* masses.

2. Improper Diet and Production of Turbid Phlegm

An improper diet refers to overindulgence in alcohol or voracious eating. This damages the spleen and stomach, producing turbid dampness whose accumulation forms phlegm; this further results in *qi* and blood stagnation. These combine with phlegm to cause abdominal masses.

3. Attack and Retention of Pathogenic Factors

When pathogenic cold, dampness, heat, or toxins attack, they may remain there for a long time. This impairs the functions of the affected *zang-fu* organs, causing *qi* and blood stagnation and turbid phlegm. Over a long time, abdominal masses are produced.

Any one or combination of these causes may produce abdominal masses. For example, abdominal masses can be caused by pathogenic wind-cold and phlegm due to improper diet, or by mental depression coupled with wind-cold and phlegm.

Diagnosis

1. Distress and Fullness in the Epigastrium and Abdomen

In this case, there is neither a visible accumulation of *qi* nor any palpable masses.

2. Tympanites

Tympanites is characterized by a distention of abdomen with tympanic resonance on percussion. Palpable masses can be felt in both tympanites and *jiju*. However, there is also fluid accumulation in tympanites, which serves to distinguish between the two.

Differentiation and Treatment

The pathological changes which occur with *ji* and *ju* are different. In the *ju* syndrome, the disease is located in the *qi* system and the basic principle of treatment is to soothe the liver, regulate and circulate *qi* and disperse accumulation, with the major focuses on regulating *qi*. In the *ji* syndrome, the *xue* system is affected and treatment seeks to activate blood circulation and remove stasis, soften hardness and disperse the masses, with the major focuses on treating the blood. If *ju* syndrome is treated properly in its initial stages, then the symptoms will improve and the disease may even be cured. A prolonged *ju* syndrome produces blood stagnation, thus transforming itself into a *ji* syndrome. According to the duration of the disease and its pathological manifestations, *ji* syndrome is divided into initial, middle and late stages. Since the abdominal masses are small and soft during the initial stage, and the resistance is still strong, treatment aims at eliminating pathogenic factors. The masses increase in size and become harder during the middle stage, because the body's resistance is weaker than the pathogenic factors, elimination of the masses must therefore combined with reinforcing the resistance. At the late stage, the abdominal mass becomes very hard, and the resistance is greatly damaged. Treatment then focuses on strengthening the resistance, and strong drugs for eliminating pathogenic factors should not be used.

1. *Ju* Syndromes

(1) Liver *qi*-stagnation

Clinical manifestations: *Qi* accumulates and flows to the chest, hypochondrium, epigastrium and abdomen, causing pain in these areas. This condition changes according to the patient's emotional state. Other manifestations include mental depression, a thin and sticky tongue coating, and a taut pulse.

Analysis: Mental depression leads to liver *qi*-stagnation, which causes the accumulation of *qi* and its movement in all directions, resulting in distensive pain. This syndrome involves the *qi* system. *Qi* accumulates following mental depression and disperses when the patient is free of emotional stress. A taut pulse suggests liver disorders.

Treatment: To soothe the liver, relieve stagnation, circulate *qi* and disperse the accumulation.

Prescription: Modified Powder of Aucklandiae for Promoting Smooth Circulation of *Qi* (44). In the recipe, Radix Aucklandiae, Pericarpium Citri Reticulatae, Pericarpium Citri Reticulatae Viride, Fructus Aurantii, Fructus Toosendan, Radix Linderae, Fructus Amomi, Rhizoma Atractylodis, Rhizoma Chuanxiong and Rhizoma Cyperi help the *qi* to circulate and soothe the liver; Cortex Cinnamomi, acrid and warm in nature, disperses cold and helps the *qi* to circulate; and Radix Glycyrrhizae, sweet and mild, relieves pain in the middle *jiao*. If there are any indications of heat, such as a bitter taste in the mouth and a red tongue, then Cortex Cinnamomi should not be used and *Zuojin* Pill (81) should be added to dissipate any hepatic heat. The presence of grief, weeping and absent-mindedness is due to liver *qi*-stagnation and heart *qi*-deficiency. In this case, Decoction of Glycyrrhizae, Tritici Levis and Jujubae (84) can be prescribed to nourish the heart, calm the mind and relieve *qi* stagnation.

(2) Retention of food and phlegm

Clinical manifestations: Abdominal distention or pain, constipation, a poor appetite, a sticky tongue coating, and a taut and smooth pulse. Occasionally, there are visible cord-like masses on the abdomen which are tender to the touch.

Analysis: Retained food in the intestinal tract impairs transportation and transformation, and thus produces phlegm-dampness, which combined with retained food blocks the *qi* circulation, thereby causing abdominal pain, constipation and a poor appetite. When this condition is combined with stagnant *qi*, the cord-like masses occur on the abdomen; these disappear when the *qi* of the *fu* organs circulates freely and retained food is sent downwards.

Treatment: To relieve stagnation and constipation, regulate *qi* and cure phlegm.

Prescription: Decoction of Six Ground Ingredients (57) is the main formula. In the recipe, Radix et Rhizoma Rhei, Fructus Aurantii Immaturus and Semen Arecae separate retained food from stagnant *qi* by relieving constipation; and Lignum Aquilariae Resinatum, Radix Aucklandiae and Radix Linderae circulate *qi*. If liver *qi* combines with phlegm to block the throat, Decoction of Pinelliae and Magnoliae Officinalis (107) can be added to circulate *qi* and cure phlegm.

Although in most cases *ju* syndrome is caused by an excess of pathogenic factors, repeated attacks may damage the spleen *qi*. In this case, Decoction of Six Mild Drugs with Aucklandiae and Amomi (211) can be prescribed at the same time as the other drugs to replenish *qi* and invigorate the spleen.

2. *Ji* Syndromes

(1) Initial stage (*qi* and blood stagnation)

Clinical manifestations: Abdominal masses are soft and produce distensive pain. The tongue is blue and the pulse is taut.

Analysis: Stagnant *qi* and blood form abdominal masses. At this stage, pathogenic factors move to the *xue* system from the *qi* system. The masses have only recently formed and so they are still soft to touch. Distensive pain, a blue tongue and a taut pulse are indications of stagnant blood caused by liver *qi*-stagnation.

Treatment: To circulate *qi*, relieve stagnation, harmonize the blood and remove any obstruction of the meridians.

Prescription: Decoction for Relieving Stagnation Syndrome (20) combined with Powder for Dissipating Blood Stasis (98). In the former, Pericarpium Citri Reticulatae Viride, Pericarpium Citri Reticulatae, Radix Platycodi and Herba Agastaches circulate *qi* and disperse masses; and Ramulus Cinnamomi, Rhizoma Sparganii, Rhizoma Curcumae and Rhizoma Cyperi remove vascular obstruction by providing warmth. In the latter, Pollen Typhae and Faeces Trogopterori activate blood circulation, remove stasis and relieve pain.

(2) Middle stage (retention of stagnant blood)

Clinical manifestations: Abdominal masses increase in size and feel hard; the pain caused by them has a fixed location. Other clinical manifestations include a dark grey complexion, emaciation, lassitude, a poor appetite, fever and aversion to cold in some cases, a bluish-purple tongue or a tongue with purple spots, a taut and smooth, or a thready and unsmooth pulse. Amenorrhea occurs with women.

Analysis: The protracted presence of abdominal masses and gradual aggravation of blood stagnation explain the hard enlarged masses and fixed pain. The stagnation of *qi* and blood impairs the ability of the spleen and stomach to transport and transform, giving rise to a dark gray complexion, emaciation, lassitude and a poor appetite. The accumulation of stagnant *qi* and blood causes disharmony between the nutrient *qi* and the defensive *qi*, which brings fever and an aversion to cold. Amenorrhea, a purple tongue and an unsmooth pulse are all caused by the internal accumulation of stagnant blood. A taut and smooth pulse suggests hepatic hyperactivity.

Treatment: To remove blood stasis, soften the masses, invigorate the spleen and replenish *qi*.

Prescription: Decoction for Resolving Blood Stasis Under Diaphragm (318) is the main formula. In the recipe, Semen Persicae, Flos Carthami, Radix Angelicae Sinensis, Rhizoma Chuanxiong, Faeces Trogopterori and Radix Paeoniae Rubra activate blood circulation and remove stasis; Rhizoma Cyperi, Radix Linderae and Rhizoma Corydalis circulate *qi*, relieve pain and assist in the removal of stasis; and Radix Glycyrrhizae replenishes *qi* and relieves pain in the middle *jiao*. Fructus Toosendan, Rhizoma Sparganii and Rhizoma Curcumae can be added. If abdominal masses are hard and produce pain that is aggravated on pressure, Bolus of Carapax Trionycis (325) is administered orally with water to remove blood stasis, soften the masses and relieve pain. In order to eliminate pathogenic factors and reinforce resistance, the above two formulas can be taken alternately with Decoction of Six Mild Drugs (55). If the abdominal masses increase in size and feel hard and painful, such drugs as Eupolyphaga seu Steleophaga, Squama Manitis and Sargassum should be added to resolve stasis, relieve accumulation and soften the masses.

(3) Late stage (anti-pathogenic *qi* deficiency and accumulation of blood stasis)

Clinical manifestations: The abdominal masses are hard and the pain is increasingly violent. Other clinical manifestations include a sallow or dark yellow complexion, emaciation, a greatly reduced appetite, a light purple tongue with a coarse gray coating, or a glossy red tongue with no coating, and a thready and rapid or taut and thready pulse.

Analysis: Prolonged accumulation of blood stasis in the vessels gives rise to hard masses and violent pain. This also damages splenic and gastric *qi* and impairs transport and transformation; thus the appetite is greatly reduced and emaciation results. Accumulation of blood stasis also prevents the production of new blood, leading to extreme deficiency of nutrient *qi*; its symptom is a sallow or a dark-yellow complexion. A purple tongue is the result of blood stasis. A gray and coarse tongue coating or a red and glossy tongue without coating, a thready and rapid or taut and thready pulse are indications of fluid depletion and consumption of *qi* and blood.

Treatment: To markedly replenish *qi* and blood, activate blood circulation and remove stasis.

Prescription: Eight Precious Ingredients Decoction (13) combined with Pill for Relieving Masses (60). In the former, Decoction of Four Mild Drugs (91) and Four Drugs Decoction (93) greatly replenish *qi* and blood. In cases of extreme *yin*-fluid deficiency with signs of a glossy red tongue without a coating, Radix Rehmanniae, Radix Adenophorae and Herba Dendrobii are prescribed to nourish *yin* and produce fluid. The latter softens the masses, resolves stasis and activates blood circulation. This prescription gradually achieves therapeutic results.

In the treatment of *ji* syndromes at any stage, external application of drugs can also be adopted. For instance, Plaster of Resina Ferulae (165) or Plaster of Polygoni Orientalis (69) both help to disperse the masses and remove stasis.

Case Studies

A patient surnamed Ma suffered from a protracted illness. An improper diet caused intestinal dysfunction in transmission, resulting in the production of dampness that turned into heat over a period of time. The combination of dampness-heat and retained food in the intestines produced a *ju* syndrome. The following drugs were prescribed:

        Rhizoma Coptidis;
        Aloe;
        Endothelium Corneum Gigeriae Galli;
        Radix Aucklandiae (roasted);
        Pericarpium Citri Reticulatae Viride;
        Semen Raphani;
        Fructus Crataegi;
        Cortex Magnoliae Officinalis.

Pills for oral administration were made up of these drugs.

Explanation: Rhizoma Coptidis and Aloe dissipate heat. Radix Aucklandiae and Cortex Magnoliae Officinalis regulate the *qi*. Endothelium Corneum Gigeriae Galli, Pericarpium Citri Reticulatae Viride,

Semen Raphani and Fructus Crataegi relieve retained food. Since it was a chronic case, they were taken in the form of pills to achieve gradual elimination.

A patient surnamed Du had a mass on the right side of his abdomen; it felt slightly painful on pressure, and a similar pain might also occur on the left side. Other manifestations were interior heat, listlessness, a thin and sticky tongue coating, and a deep and taut pulse.

Yang deficiency in the middle *jiao* prevented the blood from nourishing the liver, leading to hepatic *qi* and blood stagnation. The clinical manifestations suggested that this was neither mild nor shallow. Since exclusive elimination might cause tympanites, a variation of Decoction of Six Mild Drugs with Aucklandiae and Amomi (211) was prescribed, primarily to invigorate the spleen and stomach and secondarily to disperse the mass:

Radix Codonopsis (stir-baked)	9 g;
Rhizoma Cyperi Preparata	4.5 g;
Fructus Jujubae	5 pieces;
Poria	9 g;
Exocarpium Amomi	1.5 g;
Radix Glycyrrhizae Preparata	2.4 g;
Rhizoma Atractylodis Macrocephalae (stir-baked)	6 g;
Pericarpium Citri Reticulatae	3 g.

Second visit: After 20 doses, both internal heat and listlessness improved, the mass was no longer painful. Its size had decreased slightly, and the patient's appetite had improved. All this suggested that *yang* was starting to be restored to the middle *jiao*. The new prescription was based on the old one:

Radix Codonopsis (stir-baked)	9 g;
Radix Glycyrrhizae Preparata	2.4 g;
Pericarpium Citri Reticulatae	3 g;
Poria	9 g;
Rhizoma Cyperi Preparata	4.5 g;
Pericarpium Arecae	9 g;
Rhizoma Atractylodis Macrocephalae (stir-baked)	6 g;
Exocarpium Amomi	1.5 g;
Fructus Hordei Germinatus (stir-baked)	9 g;
Fructus Jujubae	5 pieces;
Arillus Longan	5 pieces.

Explanation: A palpable mass had already formed in this case. Since the spleen and stomach were weak and the *yang* of the middle *jiao* was insufficient, drugs that eliminate pathogenic factors could damage the the body's anti-pathogenic *qi* if used by themselves. Decoction of Six Mild Drugs with Aucklandiae and Amomi (211) was prescribed as the main formula to invigorate the spleen and stomach, and secondarily to regulate *qi*. When *yang* was invigorated and its transporting and transforming functions restored, the abdominal mass gradually shrank.

XXIX. Tympanites

Tympanites is characterized by the distention of the abdomen like a drum. *The Inner Canon of the Yellow Emperor* describes it thus, "Tympanites is marked by a distended abdomen, greenish-yellow in color, with exposed veins."

Many different names are given to this disease in the medical classics, such as tympanites due to fluid retention, tympanites due to *qi* stagnation, tympanites due to blood stagnation, simple abdominal tympanites marked by the thinness of the head, face and limbs and the distention of the abdomen, spider tympanites, and parasitic tympanites.

With regard to the causes of tympanites, *The Inner Canon of the Yellow Emperor* holds, "The accumulation of turbid *qi* in the upper part of the body produces distention and stuffiness in the chest and diaphragm." *The Pathogenesis and Manifestations of Diseases* believes that it is related to an internal accumulation of toxic water and *qi*. Both *Danxi's Experience on Medicine* and *A Complete Collection of Jingyue's Treatise* attribute tympanites to mental depression, irregular food intake, or indulgence in alcohol.

Disorders of *qi*, blood and water often combine with each other to cause tympanites with one of them taking the dominant position; that is because it is possible that they can change from one to another. For instance, water turns into *qi*, *qi* into water, and the retained water does not allow the body fluid to be transformed into blood, thus the blood deficiency depletes essence and causes water retention. There are sayings in the medical classics: "*Qi* circulates like flowing water" and "retarded blood circulation leads to water retention." Therefore, *qi* stagnation may give rise to blood stagnation and water retention; blood stagnation produces *qi* stagnation and water retention; and water retention causes *qi* and blood stagnation. As one medical classic points out, "*Qi*, water and blood often combine to cause disease. There are cases in which *qi* stagnation occurs first and blood stagnation afterwards, cases in which blood stagnation occurs first and *qi* stagnation afterwards, cases in which water retention occurs first and blood stagnation afterwards, and cases in which blood stagnation occurs first and water retention afterwards."

The following description classifies this disease into two types, caused by deficiencies or by excesses. As a matter of fact, these two syndromes often occur in conjunction with one another, and so their methods of treatment are often combined.

Conditions known as ascites present in hepatocirrhosis, tumors of the abdominal cavity and tuberculous peritonitis in Western medicine all fall into the category of tympanites in traditional Chinese medicine.

Etiology and Pathogenesis

Pathologically, tympanites is caused by the retention of *qi*, blood and water in the abdomen when the liver, spleen and kidneys are diseased. There are four causes.

1. Mental Depression

Mental depression causes kidney *qi*-stagnation and retarded blood circulation. Stagnant blood retained in the vessels of the liver damages this organ. At the same time, stagnant liver *qi* impairs the splenic and gastric abilities to transport and transform, producing water and dampness. Finally, retained water and stagnant blood combine to block the middle *jiao*. If this occurs, the liver and the spleen are diseased at the same time, and the kidneys are gradually affected as well.

2. Improper Diet

Either excessive alcohol or irregular food intake damages the spleen and stomach and then produces dampness-heat. In a chronic case, or in a case due to excessive sex, both the spleen and kidneys suffer. The turbid dampness is retained, preventing the upward movement of clear *yang* and the downward movement of turbid *yin*. The combination of the clear *yang* and the turbid *yin* impairs the liver's ability to promote the free flow of *qi*, thus causing water and fluid accumulation. In addition, renal deficiency leads to an inability to discharge water or fluid from the body and their accumulation makes the abdomen swollen.

3. Contact with Contaminated Water

Fishing, washing, or swimming in a river contaminated with schistosome causes infection. During the later stages of schistosomiasis, the liver and spleen are damaged, the vessels blocked, and the ascending and descending functions impaired. The combination of the clear and the turbid *qi* gradually causes tympanites. *The Pathogenesis and Manifestations of Diseases* says, "Accumulated toxin-water causes a swollen abdomen, a splashing sound in the abdomen when the patient moves their body, a frequent desire to drink, and a dark yellow skin." Toxin-water possibly includes cercariae or schistosome.

4. Jaundice and Abdominal Masses

In a chronic case of jaundice or abdominal masses, *qi* and blood stagnate in the meridians, often leading to water retention and dampness. Palpable masses in the abdomen, regardless of their location, inevitably hinder the circulation of splenic and renal *qi*, and impair the ability of the kidneys and bladder to control urine. As a result, tympanites gradually occurs. *Rules for Physicians* says, "Abdominal masses are the root cause of tympanites. Over a long time, the abdomen becomes as big as a dustpan or even as a jar, and this is known as simple tympanites."

Diagnosis

Differentiation between tympanites and edema.

Tympanites is marked by simple abdominal swelling with greenish-yellow skin and exposed blue veins. It is sometimes accompanied by the swelling of the lower limbs. Edema often involves the head, face and four limbs, and the whole body. Abdominal distention and a pale complexion are symptoms which may accompany edema.

Differentiation and Treatment

The clinical manifestations of this disease include abdominal enlargement; a soft abdomen during the initial stage, which gradually becomes hard on palpation. Severe cases are marked by exposed blue veins, a protruding umbilicus, a greenish-yellow or dark yellow complexion, yellow eyeballs, red spots or threads on the face, neck and chest, dry skin, a poor appetite, epigastric distention after eating, constipation or loose stools, small amounts of urine, epistaxis, bleeding of the gums or bloody stools, and coma. These symptoms are different in different patients.

The initial stage often presents a syndrome caused by excesses. It is treated by soothing the liver, eliminating dampness, relieving fullness, dispelling retained water and relieving blood stasis. When signs caused by excesses gradually subside and the body's anti-pathogenic *qi* becomes insufficient, it is treated by nourishing the liver and kidneys and invigorating the spleen. In a prolonged case exhibiting *qi* deficiency in the *zang-fu* organs and excessive pathogenic factors, both causative and symptomatic treatments are adopted at the same time by promoting the body's anti-pathogenic *qi* and eliminating pathogenic factors.

1. Tympanites Caused by Excesses

(1) Stagnation of *qi* and retention of dampness

Clinical manifestations: A distended abdomen with the skin tightly stretched, distention and fullness or pain at the hypochondrium, small amounts of urine, a poor appetite, epigastric distention after eating, belching, a sticky white tongue coating, and a taut pulse.

Analysis: Disharmony between the liver and the spleen causes *qi* stagnation and dampness retention, and hinders the normal ascent and descent of *qi*. When the abdomen fills with the turbid *qi*, it becomes distended with the skin tightly stretched. Renal *qi* stagnation leads to hypochondriac distention and fullness or pain. The blocked water passage of water due to stagnant *qi* and retained dampness causes the patient to only urinate small amounts. Spleen and stomach dysfunctions are the causes of the poor appetite, epigastric distention after eating, and belching. A sticky white tongue coating suggests the retention of dampness, and a taut pulse indicates hyperactivity of the liver.

Treatment: To soothe the liver, regulate *qi*, eliminate dampness and relieve fullness.

Prescription: Modified Powder of Bupleuri for Releasing Stagnant Liver-*Qi* (239) and *Weiling* Decoction (204). In the former, Radix Bupleuri, Fructus Aurantii, and Rhizoma Cyperi release the liver and regulate *qi*; Rhizoma Chuanxiong activates blood circulation and circulates *qi*; and Radix Paeoniae Alba and Radix Glycyrrhizae harmonize the liver and spleen and relieve pain. The latter formula consists of Powder for Regulating the Function of Stomach and Powder of Five Drugs Containing Poria (51), which serves to eliminate dampness, relieve fullness, invigorate *yang* and promote diuresis. In a severe case of abdominal distention, Radix Aucklandiae and Semen Arecae can be added to relieve *qi* stagnation. If the patient spits clear fluid, then Rhizoma Pinelliae and Rhizoma Zingiberis can be added to harmonize the stomach and conduct the unhealthy *qi* downwards.

(2) Attack of the spleen by cold-dampness

Clinical manifestations: The abdomen is large and distended, on palpitation it feels like a bag full of water. Other symptoms include stuffiness in the chest and epigastric fullness alleviated by warmth, listlessness, an aversion to cold, small amounts of urine, loose stools, a sticky white tongue coating, and a retarded pulse.

Analysis: The retention of water and dampness due to spleen *yang*-deficiency following an attack by cold-dampness causes the large and distended abdomen, and also explains the stuffiness in the chest and epigastric fullness. The hindrance of *yang-qi* by cold-dampness results in listlessness and an aversion to cold. The impaired ability to transport and transform leads to loose stools. Splenic deficiency means the inability to control water, resulting in the production of small amounts of urine. A sticky white tongue coating and a retarded pulse are signs of excessive dampness and deficient *yang*.

Treatment: To warm the middle *jiao* and relieve dampness.

Prescription: Decoction for Invigorating Spleen (180) is the main formula. In the recipe, Radix Aconiti Lateralis Preparata, Rhizoma Zingiberis, Rhizoma Atractylodis Macrocephalae, Radix Glycyrrhizae and Fructus Jujubae warm *yang* and invigorate the spleen; Rhizoma Zingiberis Recens, Radix Aucklandiae, Cortex Magnoliae Officinalis, Fructus Tsaoko, Semen Arecae, Fructus Chaenomelis and Poria disperse the cold, circulate *qi* and relieve dampness. When only small amounts of urine are produced, Ramulus Cinnamomi or Cortex Cinnamomi can be added to strengthen the effect of promoting *qi* and circulating water. If there is a distensive costal or hypochondriac pain, then Pericarpium Citri Reticulatae Viride, Rhizoma Cyperi and Rhizoma Corydalis should be added to release the liver, regulate *qi* and relieve pain.

(3) Accumulation of dampness-heat

Clinical manifestations: A large, hard, and full abdomen, a bursting pain in the epigastrium and abdomen, restlessness, a hot sensation, a bitter taste in the mouth, a dry mouth with no desire to drink, difficulties in urination, constipation or loose and fetid stools, a tongue with a red tip and red edges, and a sticky yellow or dark gray coating, a taut pulse, and in some cases yellow eyeballs and skin.

Analysis: Accumulated dampness-heat causes water retention, which in its turn is the cause of a large, hard and full abdomen, and bursting pain. The upward displacement of dampness-heat complicated by retained water and dampness explains restlessness, the hot sensation, the bitter taste, and the dryness. Its movement down to the bladder gives rise to difficult urination. Retention of dampness-heat in the gastrointestinal tract leads to constipation or loose and fetid stools. Dampness-heat acting on the surface produces yellow sclera and skin. A red tongue with a sticky yellow or dark gray coating and a taut pulse are signs of hepatic and splenic disorders due to excessive dampness-heat.

Treatment: To disperse heat, eliminate dampness, promote purgation, and dispel water.

Prescription: For dispersing heat and eliminating dampness, Pill for Relieving Epigastric Fullness (46) and Decoction of Artemisiae Scopariae (200); for promoting purgation and dispelling water, *Zhouju* Pill (136). In the former, Radix Scutellariae, Rhizoma Coptidis and Rhizoma Anemarrhenae disperse heat and relieve dampness; Cortex Magnoliae Officinalis, Fructus Aurantii, Rhizoma Pinelliae and Pericarpium Citri Reticulatae regulate *qi* and dry dampness; and Poria, Polyporus and Rhizoma Alismatis eliminate dampness through diuresis. If heat is severe and accompanied by yellow skin, then Radix Ginseng and Rhizoma Zingiberis should not be used, and Decoction of Artemisiae Scopariae (200) can be prescribed with additional drugs to dissipate heat and eliminate dampness. In cases where urination is difficult, Fructus Lagenariae Sicerariae, Talcum and powder of Gryllodes should be added and taken separately. If a distended abdomen is unbearable and there is very little urine, *Zhouju* Pill (136) should be prescribed. Since this formula is drastically purgative, it should be stopped immediately when the urine and stool increase and the abdomen becomes slightly loose. Long-term administration damages the body's anti-pathogenic *qi*.

(4) Stagnant blood in the liver and spleen

Clinical manifestations: The abdomen is large, hard and distended, with markedly exposed blue veins. Other clinical manifestations include hypochondriac and abdominal pain, dark yellow complexion and skin, red threads on the head, neck, chest and arms, red marks on the palms, purple lips, dry mouth with no desire to drink, black stools, a purple-red tongue or a tongue with purple spots, and a thready and unsmooth or a thready, taut and smooth pulse.

Analysis: Stagnant blood in the vessels of the liver and spleen blocks the passage of water and makes it accumulate; this is the cause of the distended abdomen with exposed blue veins, as well as the pain. Stagnant *qi* and blood give rise to the dark yellow complexion and skin, the red threads and marks and the purple lips. Retained water and dampness prevent body fluid from nourishing upwards, resulting in a dry mouth with no desire to drink. Black stools are due to hemorrhaging following vascular damage. A purple tongue and an unsmooth pulse are both signs of stagnant *qi* and blood. In the case of massive loss of blood, a hollow pulse is present.

Treatment: To activate blood circulation and remove stasis.

Prescription: Modified Decoction for Regulating Nutrient System (248). In this formula, Rhizoma Chuanxiong, Radix Angelicae Sinensis and Radix Paeoniae Rubra activate blood circulation and remove stasis; Rhizoma Cucurmae, Rhizoma Corydalis and Radix et Rhizoma Rhei disperse *qi* and resolve stasis; and Herba Dianthi, Semen Arecae, Semen Lepidii seu Descurainiae, Poria and Cortex Mori circulate water and promote diuresis. This formula is for symptomatic treatment in an acute case. In cases with black stools, drugs that remove blood stasis and stop bleeding, such as Radix Notoginseng and Cacumen Platycladi, are added. If abdominal distention and fullness are severe, the pulse is taut, rapid and strong, and the constitution is still good, *Zhouju* Pill (136) can be used temporarily. In the course of elimination, constant attention should be paid to the condition of splenic and gastric *qi*. It will not do to apply this treatment excessively. Signs of blood stasis can still be present following elimination; these should be dealt with in a smooth and gradual way, or by combining elimination with nourishment. Exacerbation of pathological conditions will exhibit such critical signs as spitting of blood, bloody stools, and coma.

2. Tympanites Caused by Deficiencies

(1) Splenic and renal *yang* deficiency

Clinical manifestations: The abdomen is large, distended and full; this is more pronounced in the evening than in the morning. Other manifestations include a greenish-yellow complexion, epigastric distress, a poor appetite, lassitude, an aversion to cold, cold limbs or edema of the lower limbs, dysuria with small amounts of urine, a swollen and light purple tongue, and a deep, thready and taut pulse.

Analysis: Splenic and renal *yang* deficiency means water stagnation, cold in nature, which causes the large and distended abdomen which is more serious in the evening. Deficient spleen *yang* implies the inability to transport and transform food, resulting in epigastric distress and poor appetite. The failure of *yang-qi* in being distributed around the body explains the lassitude, aversion to cold and cold limbs. Deficient kidney *yang* means that the urinary bladder is unable to control urine; thus dysuria with small amounts of urine and edema of the lower limbs ensue. A greenish-yellow complexion is due to splenic and renal *yang* deficiency. A swollen and light purple tongue and a deep, thready and taut pulse are signs of splenic and renal *yang* deficiency complicated by blood stagnation.

Treatment: To warm and nourish the spleen and kidneys, promote *qi* and circulate water.

Prescription: Bolus of Aconiti Lateralis Preparata for Regulating Middle *Jiao* (163) combined with Powder of Five Drugs Containing Poria (51), if splenic *yang* deficiency is more obvious; *Jisheng* Pill for Invigorating Kidney-*Qi* (206) if renal *yang* deficiency is more pronounced.

(2) Hepatic and renal *yin* deficiency

Clinical manifestations: The abdomen is large, distended and full, with exposed blue veins in severe cases. Other manifestations include a sallow complexion, purple lips, dry mouth, restlessness; possibly epistaxis and bleeding of the gums, small amounts of hot urine, a crimson tongue with little fluid, and a taut, thready and rapid pulse.

Analysis: This syndrome is present at the late stage of tympanites. Damage to both the liver and kidneys causes an accumulation of water and stagnation of the blood, with the ensuing signs of a large, distended abdomen, and exposed blue veins in severe cases. *Qi* and blood stagnation causes a sallow complexion and purple lips. Depleted *yin* fluid and blood extravasation due to hyperactive internal fire caused by deficiencies lead to small amounts of hot urine, restlessness, dry mouth, epistaxis, a red tongue with little fluid and a taut, thready and rapid pulse.

Treatment: To nourish the liver and kidneys, cool blood and remove stasis.

Prescription: Pill of Six Drugs Containing Rehmanniae Preparata (56), or *Yiguan* Decoction (1) combined with Decoction for Removing Blood Stasis Under Diaphragm (318). The first formula nourishes the liver and kidneys; the second one nourishes *yin* blood and promotes the smooth circulation of liver *qi*; and the third activates blood circulation and removes stasis. In cases of thirst and a crimson tongue with little fluid due to internal heat, add Radix Scrophulariae and Herba Dendrobii to disperse heat and produce fluid. If afternoon fever and restlessness are present, Radix Stellariae, Cortex Lycii, Carapax Trionycis and Herba Lophatheri are added to disperse heat and relieve restlessness. If urine is only in small amounts, then Polyporus, Talcum and a small amount of Cortex Cinnamomi should be added to invigorate *yang* and circulate water. In case of epistaxis and bleeding of the gums, drugs that cool the blood and check bleeding, such as fresh Rhizoma Imperatae and Herba Agrimoniae, can be added.

In addition, if pathogenic water is difficult to eliminate and the body's anti-pathogenic *qi* is reasonably strong, the following drugs can be selectively prescribed, as they eliminate retained water and promote diuresis.

Powder of Pharbitidis: to be taken once or twice a day, 1.5-3.0 grams a time.

Powder of Pharbitidis and Foeniculi (203): 120 grams of Semen Pharbitidis and 30 grams of Fructus Foeniculi, to be ground into powder and taken once or twice a day, 1.5-3.0 grams a time.

Powder of Kansui: 1.0-1.5 grams in capsules to be taken with boiled water.

The first two formulas are mild, and the third is stronger. The dosage can increase or decrease according to actual conditions.

Chronic tympanites is often complicated by the following symptoms:

(a) Hematemesis and hemafecia

In chronic cases of tympanites, liver *yin* is insufficient, and liver fire hyperactive. Damage to the vessels causes extravasation of blood, and the liver's ability to store blood is also impaired. The patient will have a taut, thready and rapid pulse and a red tongue.

Treatment aims to cool the blood, remove blood stasis and check bleeding. Decoction of Cornu Rhinocerotis and Rehmanniae (306) should be taken together with powder of Notoginseng. If signs of splenic failure to control blood are present — such as a pale complexion, sweating, cold limbs, a pale tongue and a deep and thready pulse — primordial *qi* is promoted and collapse is prevented by prescribing Decoction of Ginseng (218). If the patient shows critical signs such as spitting large quantities of blood or tarry stools, accompanied by restlessness, upper abdominal distress, dizziness, palpitations, a pale complexion, dry mouth and lips, and cold limbs, the patient should rest in bed and try to avoid worrying, and emergency treatment should be given immediately.

(b) Coma

In the late stage of tympanites, both liver *yin* and kidney *yin* are extremely deficient, and liver wind becomes agitated with symptoms including tremors, the twitching of the lips, foul-smelling breath, restlessness and coma. Treatment aims to subdue the liver wind, produce fluid, moisten dryness, disperse cardiac heat, and restore consciousness. Modified Decoction of Cornu Saigae Tataricae (277) should be prescribed. In the recipe, Cornu Saigae Tataricae and Concha Haliotidis disperse heat in the liver and subdue liver wind; and Radix Rehmanniae, Radix Paeoniae Alba and Carapax et Plastrum Testudinis nourish *yin* and produce fluid. Rhizoma Acori Tatarinowii, Radix Curcumae and Fructus Forsythiae can be added to disperse cardiac heat and restore consciousness. In order to relieve convulsions, subdue liver wind and restore consciousness, Purple-Snow Pellet (299) or Bolus of Calculus Bovis for Resurrection (127) can also be used. In cases when the turbid phlegm mists the clear cavity, with symptoms including coma, a gurgling sound in the throat, a sticky white tongue coating and a soft, thready and smooth pulse, resolve turbid phlegm-dampness and restore consciousness by prescribing modified Decoction for Cleansing Phlegm (243). In this prescription, Rhizoma Pinelliae, Arisaema cum Bile and Exocarpium Citri Rubrum dry dampness and cure phlegm; Fructus Aurantii Immaturus and Caulis Bombusae in Taeniam relieve *qi* stagnation and remove phlegm; Rhizoma Acori Tatarinowii removes phlegm and restore consciousness; and Radix Ginseng, Poria and Radix Glycyrrhizae invigorate the spleen, replenish *qi*, eliminate dampness and remove phlegm. Bolus of Styrax (143) can also be administered in order to restore consciousness by means of aromatics.

Premonitory symptoms of coma include abruptly blurred vision, good spirits or indifference, disorientation, and abnormal behavior, such as lying in bed all the time with no desire to get up, or walking around with no desire to go to bed, or shouting, weeping, or laughing without reason. If tympanites is accompanied by coma, the pathological conditions are critical, and the prognosis is poor.

Remarks

In the treatment of tympanites, the administration of drugs should be combined with proper nursing. *Shen's Treatise on the Importance of Life Preservation* says, "The patient should first avoid salty food, pay special attention to staying warm, refrain from worry, and try to avoid becoming angry." Salt is astringent, and thus exacerbates water retention. Food with low salt content is usually recommended, and salt-free food should be taken if the amount of urine has decreased considerably. Salt intake should increase gradually after abdominal distention has been relieved. At the same time, the patient should set aside all misgivings and be confident that the disease can be cured. The patient should also pay special attention to staying warm because weak resistance is likely to induce attack by external pathogenic factors, leading to a high fever and other pathological changes.

Case Studies

Name: Zhang XX; Sex: Male; Age: 30.
First visit: January 30, 1961.
Case history: Over the past two years, the patient often noticed a bitter taste in his mouth, a poor appetite, abdominal distention after eating, a distensive pain in the right hypochondrium, loose stools at a frequency of one to five bowel movements a day, a low fever in the afternoon, dizziness, blurred vision, impaired hearing, insomnia and lassitude. Recently, the abdominal distention had become aggravated and the patient's urine had decreased. There was edema of the lower limbs, and the patient's appetite was rather poor. Examinations showed that the spleen was enlarged 3 cm below the ribs and it felt hard on palpation. There were positive signs of ascites, pitting edema of the lower limbs, and the icteric index was 12 units. The disease was then diagnosed as hepatocirrhosis complicated by ascites.

Thirteen years ago, the patient suffered from acute infectious hepatitis, which improved upon treatment during hospitalization. However, since then he often had an uncomfortable feeling in the hepatic region, poor digestion, abdominal distention after eating, and occasional low-grade fever. Three years ago, he had duodenal drainage, contrast examination of the biliary tract and liver puncture. The diagnosis of hepatocirrhosis and chronic cholecystitis was then established.

Examination: Emaciation, a dark yellow complexion, a red tongue with a thin yellow coating and a taut and unsmooth pulse.

Diagnosis: Splenic and renal *yang* deficiency, stagnation of liver *qi*, and internal dampness-heat retention.

Treatment: To nourish the kidneys, invigorate the spleen, soothe the liver, regulate *qi*, disperse heat and eliminate dampness.

Prescription:

Semen Ziziphi Spinosae (stir-baked)	30 g;
Semen Cuscutae	24 g;
Rhizoma Dioscoreae	18 g;
Pericarpium Citri Reticulatae Viride	9 g;
Fructus Corni	9 g;
Carapax Trionycis	15 g;
Rhizoma Cyperi	9 g;
Herba Agrimoniae	9 g;
Herba Abri Fruticulosi	9 g;
Herba Hyperici Japonici	9 g;

Fructus Amomi	6 g;
Cortex Eucommiae	9 g;
Rhizoma Atractylodis Macrocephalae	12 g;
Radix Gentianae	3 g;
Semen Citri Reticulatae	9 g;
Fructus Psoraleae	9 g;
Poria	12 g;
Rhizoma Corydalis	9 g;
Radix Stellariae	9 g.

(These drugs were decocted twice and taken warm.)

Second visit: February 5, 1961.

The patient took four doses. His urine had increased considerably, both abdominal distention and edema had improved, as had his appetite. Sleep was normal, and the patient moved his bowels once a day with formed stools. His tongue coating was thin and white, his pulse thready and weak. Three grams of Endothelium Corneum Gigeriae Galli were added to the previous prescription.

Third visit: March 1, 1961.

The patient took another ten doses, which relieved the ascites and brought his body temperature back to normal. He still had slight abdominal distention and a dull pain in the right hypochondrium. The patient's tongue and pulse remained unchanged. Twelve grams of Radix Curcumae and 12 grams of Radix Astragali were added.

On December 2, 1961, the patient wrote to the doctor, saying that after taking several dozen doses his condition had begun to improve and that the ascites had not developed again, so he had gone back to work more than six months before.

Discussion: The doctor thought that the etiology of this disease was very complicated. It could have been due to damage done to the spleen and kidneys following excessive intake of alcohol, or it is possible that mental depression caused the liver *qi* to attack the spleen. A chronic hepatic and splenic disorder then further affected the kidneys. Deficient kidney *yang* means the inability to warm and nourish the spleen, and deficient kidney *yin* implies a lack of nourishment for the liver and spleen. Disorders of the liver, spleen and kidneys impair the circulation of *qi*, blood and water. These accumulate in the abdomen, leading to its gradual enlargement and swelling. Hence, tympanites occurs.

The following are the principles observed by the doctor in the treatment of this disease.

First, the method of treatment was primarily to reinforce the body's resistance and secondarily to eliminate pathogenic factors. The doctor believed that this disease is often caused by deficiencies or deficiencies complicated by excesses, and so nourishment should be adopted as the primary treatment. *Medical Mirror* by Gu Xuyuan says, "Tympanites is caused by a deficiency of spleen *qi*, so potent tonics should principally be prescribed to reinforce resistance, and proper quantities of drugs promoting smooth circulation of *qi* should be used secondarily to relieve stagnation. In cases of food retention, drugs that assist digestion should also be used. In cases of heat retention, drugs that are cold and cool can also be applied to dissipate heat. If only potent tonics are prescribed, stagnation will become worse and so will tympanites." The principal methods of nourishment include nourishment of the middle *jiao* and invigoration of the spleen, nourishment of the liver and kidneys, warming the kidneys and assisting *yang*. The secondary methods include soothing the liver and regulating *qi*, activating blood circulation, removing stasis and softening hardness, dissipating heat, relaxing the middle *jiao*, eliminating dampness, promoting diuresis, nourishing the heart and calming the mind. Drugs that are commonly used to nourish the liver and kidneys include Semen Cuscutae, Fructus Corni, Radix Aconiti Lateralis Preparata,

Radix Morindae Officinalis, Radix Polygoni Multiflori, Herba Cistanches, Fructus Psoraleae, Fructus Lycii, Radix Rehmanniae Preparata, Rhizoma Polygonati and Cortex Eucommiae. Drugs that replenish *qi* and invigorate the spleen include Rhizoma Atractylodis Macrocephalae, Radix Codonopsis, Radix Astragali and Endothelium Corneum Gigeriae Galli. Drugs that eliminate dampness and retained water include Radix Stephaniae Tetrandrae, Aloe, Radix Kansui and Flos Genkwa. Drugs that soothe the liver and regulate *qi* include Radix Bupleuri, Rhizoma Cyperi, Pericarpium Citri Reticulatae Viride, Radix Aucklandiae, Pericarpium Arecae, Semen Citri Reticulatae and Semen Raphani. Drugs that activate blood circulation and remove stasis include Rhizoma Corydalis, Radix Curcumae, Radix Salviae Miltiorrhizae, Semen Persicae, Flos Carthami and Rhizoma Sparganii. Drugs that eliminate dampness and disperse heat include Herba Hyperici Japonici, Herba Dianthi, Radix Gentianae, Herba Artemisiae Scopariae, Herba Abri Fruticulosi and Radix et Rhizoma Rhei. Drugs that regulate *qi* and relax the middle *jiao* include Cortex Magnoliae Officinalis, Fructus Amomi, Fructus Aurantii Immaturus, Fructus Tsaoko and Lignum Aquilariae Resinatum. Drugs that nourish the heart and calm the mind include Semen Ziziphi Spinosae and Succinum.

Second, if this disease is complicated by general edema, or if ascites continues after resistance has been reinforced, induced sweating should be combined with the promotion of diuresis. *Synopsis of Prescriptions of the Golden Chamber* says, "Edema below the lower back is treated by promoting diuresis, and edema above it by sweating." To induce sweating, modified Decoction for Relieving Edema (297) is prescribed. To promote diuresis, Decoction of Stephaniae Tetrandrae and Astragali (332), Decoction of Stephaniae Tetrandrae and Poria (333), Powder of Five Drugs Containing Poria (51), or Decoction Containing Five Kinds of Peel (50) can be used. According to the doctor's experience, no marked effects can be expected if these treatments are used separately. Thus, the doctor often combines them and adds a small amount of drugs that promote the lungs' dispersive function in order to obtain good results. In severe cases, the doctor recommends using this simple formula to assist with the treatment. Either crucian carp or carp cooked with Pericarpium Citri Reticulatae, Bulbus Allii, Filamentum Usneae, and Fructus Amomi should be taken as food in order to relieve the swelling, promote diuresis, and dispel water retained in the abdomen.

Third, drastic purgatives for eliminating retained water should be used as little as possible. This is because the disease is often caused by deficiencies or deficiencies complicated by excesses, and rarely by excesses. When talking about the aftereffects of drastic purgatives, Zhang Jingyue says, "Ill-trained people often use drastic purgatives in the treatment of edema. Diarrhea occurs in the morning if they are taken the previous evening, and in the evening if they are taken in the morning. With a decalitre of water discharged from the body, swelling is immediately relieved. Therapeutic results seem quick; but these people disregard the strength of the patient's resistance and pay no attention to the patient's life. What they aim to do is to discharge the retained water as quickly as possible. They do not know that swelling may recur as soon as it is relieved, and within a few days it will become even worse than it was before." This doctor seldom prescribes drastic purgatives. Only when there is dry stool and clinical manifestations exhibit that the syndrome is caused by excesses does he use a small amount of drugs, such as Radix Euphobriae Pekinensis, Flos Genkwa, Radix Kansui and Semen Pharbitidis. He never forgets that "The spleen should be invigorated first to treat disorders of the liver." Drugs that invigorate the spleen and replenish *qi* are thus prescribed.

Fourth, coma in tympanites is often the result of dampness-heat in the liver and gallbladder, which spreads to the triple *jiao*, disturbing the brain and misting the clear cavity. Treatment aims primarily to dissipate heat and eliminate dampness, and secondarily to resolve phlegm-heat and restore consciousness by using aromatics. The commonly used drugs include Fel Ursi, Indigo Naturalis, Gypsum Fibrosum, Rhizoma Anemarrhenae, Carapax Eretmochelydis, Cornu Saigae Tataricae, Calculus Bovis, Arisaema cum Bile, Concretio Silicea Bambusae and Rhizoma Acori Tatarinowii. If *yin* is damaged by heat caused by excesses, then Radix Panacis Quinquefolii, Herba Dendrobii, Radix Adenophorae, Bulbus Lilii, Radix Ophiopogonis, Radix Asparagi, Radix Rehmanniae, Radix Scrophulariae, and Radix Trichosanthis should be used to nourish *yin*, reduce fire, moisten dryness and relieve thirst.

XXX. Headache

Headaches may involve the entire head or the anterior, posterior, or lateral portions of the head. As a common subjective symptom, headaches occur in a variety of acute and chronic diseases. The following discussion focuses on cases when a headache is the predominant symptom and not an accompanying one, since in the latter case, the headache will go away when the disease itself is cured.

Throughout the ages, medical practitioners have classified headaches in the following ways:

First, in terms of etiology: headache due to external pathogenic factors and headache due to internal disorders.

Second, in terms of the six meridians: *Taiyang*, *Yangming*, *Shaoyang*, *Taiyin*, *Shaoyin* and *Jueyin* headaches.

Third, in terms of disease: chronic headache, one-sided headache, severe headache, and headache due to cold.

It is for this reason that diagnosis seems more important in the treatment of this disease than in the treatment of most other diseases.

Headaches may occur in many diseases in internal medicine, surgery, neurology, psychiatry and five sensory organs (ears, eyes, lips, nose and tongue). As a predominant symptom in infectious febrile diseases, hypertension, intracranial diseases and neurosis in internal medicine, it can be diagnosed and treated according to the following descriptions.

Etiology and Pathogenesis

The head is the confluence of various *yang* meridians of the body. It is also where the blood and the clear *yang-qi* of the five *zang* and six *fu* organs converge.

1. Headache due to External Pathogenic Factors

External factors contributing to headaches include wind, cold, dampness, and heat. These attack the head along the surface meridians, hindering the clear *yang-qi*. When pathogenic wind attacks, the head is affected first; this is the most frequent cause of headaches. If wind associates with cold, blood coagulates in the vessels, a headache then follows. If it associates with heat, *qi* and blood are disturbed; this affects the clear cavity and causes a headache. If it associates with dampness, the clear cavity is blocked and this also can cause headaches.

2. Headache due to Internal Disorders

The brain is the sea of marrow, and it is nourished with essence and blood from the liver and kidneys, and food essence from the spleen and stomach. Headaches due to internal disorders are therefore related to the liver, spleen and kidneys, Emotional stress impairs the liver's ability to promote the free flow of *qi*, and turns stagnant liver *qi* into fire, which disturbs the clear cavity and leads to a headache. Liver fire consumes *yin* and deprives the liver of nourishment; or renal deficiency prevents water from nourishing wood. In either case, hepatic and renal *yin* are both insufficient, causing the liver *yang* to rise, and a headache to occur. In addition, any congenital deficiency of renal essence implies a lack of brain marrow, which subsequently leads to a headache. *Yin* deficiency can affect *yang*, and renal *yang* deficiency means that clear *yang-qi* is not able to nourish the head, thus producing a headache. Finally, the deficiency of the spleen and stomach due to stress or to chronic infection results in insufficient *qi* and blood production, and the lack of nourishment of the brain marrow subsequently results in a headache. This kind of headache can also be the result of massive blood loss. An excessive intake of greasy or sweet food impairs the spleen's ability to transport and transform, and produces internal phlegm-dampness that disturbs the clear cavity and hinders clear *yang*, bringing on a headache.

If the vessels are affected by stagnant *qi* and blood due to traumatic injuries or chronic illness, this is another etiological factor which may cause headaches.

Diagnosis
1. Thunder-Headache

Thunder-headache is marked by a thundering sound in the head, the presence of nodules on the head and face, or a red and swollen face. It often results from climatic factors or from the upward displacement of dampness-heat complicated by phlegm. Treatment aims primarily to disperse heat and eliminate toxins. A general headache does not show symptoms such as nodules or swelling.

2. A Heavy Sensation in the Head

With this type of headache, the patient experiences a heavy sensation or a feeling that the head is tightly wrapped, which is aggravated on rainy days; it is not accompanied by pain. Attention should be paid to distinguishing this from a headache caused by pathogenic dampness.

Differentiation and Treatment

The duration, location and nature (deficiency or excess) of the headache should be ascertained.

Headaches caused by external pathogenic factors usually occur abruptly. In this type of headache, the patient will feel continuous sensations of cramping, throbbing, burning, distending or heaviness, and these are signs of a syndrome caused by excesses. Treatment aims to eliminate wind and other pathogenic factors. In contrast, headaches caused by internal damage usually have a slow onset. They are often intermittent and are characterized by dull, lingering sensations, accompanied by feelings of emptiness or dizziness, and aggravated by stress. These are signs of a syndrome caused by deficiencies. Treatment seeks to reinforce the body's resistance. Headaches due to the retention of turbid phlegm or blood stagnation are often due to syndromes caused by deficiencies and complicated by excesses. Different methods of treatment can be adopted.

With three *yang* and *Jueyin* meridians going through the head, tracing the headache according to which meridian has been affected helps to pin down its etiological factors. A headache of the *Taiyang* Meridians will be located in the posterior portion of the head and neck; a headache of the *Yangming* Meridians will be concentrated around the forehead and the superciliary region; a headache of the *Shaoyang* Meridians will be located on either side of the head and around the ear region; and a headache of the *Jueyin* Meridians on the top of the head or around the eyes.

A headache due to stagnant blood is stabbing and has a fixed location. A history of trauma around the head can help in making a correct diagnosis. A headache due to retained turbid phlegm is often accompanied by nausea and vomiting.

1. Headaches due to External Pathogenic Factors

(1) Wind-cold headache

Clinical manifestations: Frequent attacks, spreading to the neck and back, which are aggravated by exposure to the wind and alleviated by warmth; an aversion to wind and cold, a preference for wearing hats, an absence of thirst, a thin white tongue coating and a superficial pulse.

Analysis: When pathogenic factors attack the head, this hinders the clear *yang-qi* and causes headaches. Since the *Taiyang* Meridians go from the top of the head to the neck and back, the pain spreads to those areas. Wind-cold prevents the defensive *yang-qi* from reaching the exterior; this causes an aversion to wind and cold. Warmth reduces cold, and so alleviates the headaches. Since there is no heat, thirst is not present. A thin white tongue coating and a superficial pulse are signs that the body surface has been attacked by wind-cold.

Treatment: To eliminate wind and disperse cold.

Prescription: Modified Powder of Chuanxiong with Folium Camelliae Sinensis (29). In the recipe, Rhizoma Chuanxiong, Herba Schizonepetae, Radix Ledebouriellae, Rhizoma seu Radix Notopterygii, Radix Angelicae Dahuricae and Herba Asari, all acrid and warm in nature, eliminate wind, disperse cold and relieve pain. Rhizoma Chuanxiong circulates the *qi* in the blood, eliminates wind in the blood, and acts on the head and eyes; thus it is important for the treatment of headaches due to external factors.

If pathogenic cold affects the *Jueyin* Meridians and brings about symptoms such as a headache in the vertex, retching, spitting of saliva, cold limbs in severe cases, a white tongue coating, and a taut pulse, then a prescription based on Decoction of Evodiae (148) can be used with Radix Ginseng and Fructus Jujubae removed and Rhizoma Pinelliae Preparata, Rhizoma Ligustici, and Rhizoma Chuanxiong added. This produces warmth, dispersing the cold, as well as conducting the unhealthy *qi* downwards.

(2) Wind-heat headache

Clinical manifestations: Distending headache that produces bursting sensations in severe cases. Other clinical manifestations include fever, aversion to wind, a flushed face and red eyes, thirst, constipation, deep yellow urine, a red tongue with a yellow coating, and a superficial and rapid pulse.

Analysis: Heat is a *yang* factor, and it is marked by upward flaring. When wind-heat blocks the meridians, the headache will be distensive and produce sensations of bursting in severe cases. A flushed face and red eyes are also caused by the upward movement of heat. Fever and aversion to wind are the consequences of wind-heat attacking the body surface. Thirst is due to fluid consumption by pathogenic heat. Constipation, deep yellow urine, a red tongue with a yellow coating and a superficial and rapid pulse are signs of excessive wind-heat.

Treatment: To eliminate wind and disperse heat.

Prescription: Modified Decoction of Chuanxiong, Angelicae Dahuricae, and Gypsum Fibrosum (120). In the recipe, Rhizoma Chuanxiong, Radix Angelicae Dahuricae, Flos Chrysanthemi and Gypsum Fibrosum, which make up the main ingredients, are used to eliminate wind and disperse heat. Since Rhizoma seu Radix Notopterygii and Rhizoma Ligustici are acrid and warm, they should be removed if the patient is suffering from excessive heat. In order to disperse heat and eliminate toxins, acrid and cool drugs, such as Radix Scutellariae, Herba Menthae and Fructus Gardeniae, can be added. In cases of excess heat that consumes body fluid, accompanied by a red tongue and little fluid, Herba Dendrobii, Radix Trichosanthis and Rhizoma Phragmitis should be added to promote the production of fluid and relieve thirst.

If the large intestines are blocked with dry stools and ulcers are present in the mouth and nose, Pill of Coptidis for Clearing Away Heat (260), which is bitter and cold in nature, can be prescribed to reduce fire; or Radix et Rhizoma Rhei and Natrii Sulfas can be added to disperse heat and relieve constipation.

(3) Wind-dampness headache

Clinical manifestations: Headache accompanied by a tight feeling in the head, as if it were wrapped in a towel. Other clinical manifestations are a heavy sensation in the body and limbs, a poor appetite, stuffiness in the chest, dysuria, loose stools, a sticky white tongue coating, and a soft pulse.

Analysis: Attack of the head by external wind-dampness clouds the clear cavity and thus causes a headache accompanied by a tight feeling of the head as if it were wrapped in a towel. Dampness is characterized by heaviness and viscosity. If the spleen is attacked by dampness, this impairs its ability to transport and transform and to control the limbs; therefore stuffiness, a poor appetite, and a heavy sensation ensue. The internal retention of dampness does not allow the division of the clear and the turbid *qi*; the result is dysuria and loose stools. A sticky white tongue coating and a soft pulse are signs of excess dampness.

Treatment: To eliminate wind and dampness.

Prescription: Modified Decoction of Notopterygii for Eliminating Dampness (175). In the recipe, Rhizoma seu Radix Notopterygii, Radix Angelicae Pubescentis, Rhizoma Chuanxiong, Radix Ledebouriellae, Fructus Viticis and Rhizoma Ligustici are the main ingredients. They serve to relieve headaches caused by wind-dampness. If this dampness is serious, and stuffiness in the chest and a lack of appetite are present, then Rhizoma Atractylodis, Cortex Magnoliae Officinalis, Fructus Aurantii and Pericarpium Citri Reticulatae should be added to dry dampness and relax the chest. If the patient is nauseous or vomiting, Rhizoma Pinelliae (ginger prepared) can be added to conduct the unhealthy *qi* downward and check vomiting.

If summer-heat and dampness combine to cause a headache accompanied by fever, sweating and thirst, then treatment aims to disperse summer-heat and resolve dampness by prescribing Decoction of Coptidis and Elsholtziae (262) plus Herba Agastachis, Herba Eupatorii and Folium Nelumbinis.

2. Headaches due to Internal Disorders

(1) Hyperactive liver *yang*

Clinical manifestations: Headache, blurred vision, restlessness, irritability, insomnia, a flushed face and red eyes, a bitter taste in the mouth, a red tongue with a thin yellow coating, and a taut and strong pulse.

Analysis: The rising liver *yang* disturbs the head and eyes and causes a headache and blurred vision. Liver *yang* turns into fire, which disturbs the heart and mind, resulting in restlessness, irritability, and insomnia. The condition of the liver is reflected in the eyes; thus when the liver *yang* is hyperactive, the face becomes flushed and the eyes red. If the fire of the liver and gallbladder is hyperactive, there is a bitter taste in the mouth; if the pulse is taut, the liver is in a state of disorder. In addition, a red tongue with a thin yellow coating is also a sign of hyperactive liver fire.

Treatment: To calm the liver and suppress *yang*.

Prescription: Decoction of Gastrodiae and Uncariae cum Uncis (40) with Concha Haliotidis and Concha Margaritifera Usta. In the recipe, Rhizoma Gastrodiae and Ramulus Uncariae cum Uncis calm the liver; and Concha Haliotidis and Concha Margaritifera suppress *yang*. If the headache is serious, Cornu Saigae Tataricae should be added. If the headache is accompanied by a flushed face, a bitter taste in the mouth, constipation, deep yellow urine, a yellow tongue coating, and a taut and rapid pulse, it suggests liver fire. Treatment aims to dissipate heat and suppress hepatic fire by prescribing a variation of Decoction of Gentianae for Purging Liver-Fire (78).

If the headache is dull and lingering, and does not respond readily to treatment, and if it is accompanied by blurred vision, lower back pain, a red tongue and a thready pulse, we can say that hepatic and renal *yin* deficiency and hyperactive fire are playing their parts. In this case, Bolus of Lycii, Chrysanthemi and Rehmanniae Preparata (144) is prescribed to nourish the liver and kidneys.

(2) Renal deficiency

Clinical manifestations: Headache and an empty sensation in the head, dizziness, tinnitus, soreness and weakness in the lumbar region and knees, nocturnal emissions, leukorrhea, a red tongue, and a deep, thready and weak pulse.

Analysis: The brain is the sea of marrow, which is dominated by the kidneys. Renal deficiency leads to an inability to nourish the brain, which causes a headache with an empty sensation, dizziness and tinnitus. The lower back is where the kidneys reside, and so renal deficiency causes some weakness in the lower back and knees. It also implies the weakness of the gate of essence and of the *Dai* Meridian (Belt Vessel); thus nocturnal emissions and leukorrhea occur. A red tongue is a sign of *yin* deficiency, and a deep, thready and weak pulse suggests renal deficiency.

Treatment: To replenish *yin* and nourish the kidneys.

Prescription: Decoction for Potently Invigorating *Qi* and Blood (21) is the main formula. In the recipe, Radix Rehmanniae Preparata, Rhizoma Dioscoreae, Fructus Corni and Fructus Lycii nourish kidney *yin*; Radix Ginseng and Radix Angelicae Sinensis replenish *qi* and blood; and Cortex Eucommiae strengthens the lower back and nourishes the kidneys. All these drugs are used together to replenish renal *yin*.

In cases of renal *yang* deficiency accompanied by a headache, an aversion to cold, a pale complexion, cold limbs, a pale tongue and a deep, thready and weak pulse, *Yougui* Pill (82) is prescribed to warm and replenish kidney *yang*.

(3) *Qi* deficiency

Clinical manifestations: A lingering headache aggravated by stress, lassitude, a poor appetite, a pale tongue, and a thready and weak pulse.

Analysis: *Qi* deficiency means the failure of clear *yang* to ascend; the clear cavity is thus not well nourished, and this leads to a lingering headache. The hindrance of *yang-qi* leads to a *qi* deficiency in the middle *jiao*, which means impaired transportation and transformation, resulting in lassitude and a poor appetite. A pale tongue and a thready and weak pulse are signs of *qi* deficiency.

Treatment: Primarily to replenish *qi*.

Prescription: Decoction for Promoting the Smooth Circulation of *Qi* and Regulating the Middle *Jiao* (215) is the main formula; it consists of Decoction for Strengthening the Middle *Jiao* and Benefiting *Qi* (154) along with Herba Asari, Fructus Viticis and Rhizoma Chuanxiong. Since it nourishes the middle *jiao* and also has a dispersive effect, it is effective for headaches caused by *qi* deficiency.

(4) Blood deficiency

Clinical manifestations: Headache, dizziness, palpitations, pale complexion, a pale tongue, and a thready and feeble pulse.

Analysis: The headache and dizziness are due to blood deficiency complicated by fire which flares up. Deficient heart blood leads to palpitations. It also explains the pale complexion, pale tongue and thready and feeble pulse.

Treatment: Primarily to nourish blood.

Prescription: Four Drugs Decoction with Additional Drugs (112) is the main formula. This consists of Four Drugs Decoction (93) with Flos Chrysanthemi, Fructus Viticis and Radix Glycyrrhizae. Their function is to nourish the blood and suppress wind.

(5) Retention of turbid phlegm

Clinical manifestations: Headache, dizziness, epigastric fullness, stuffiness in the chest, nausea, vomiting of a sputum-like substance, a sticky white tongue coating, and a smooth pulse.

Analysis: Turbid phlegm clouds the clear cavity, blocks the meridians and inhibits clear *yang*, thus giving rise to headache and dizziness. Phlegm retained in the chest and diaphragm inhibits hepatic and splenic *yang-qi*, and thereby causes epigastric fullness and stuffiness. The upward movement of turbid phlegm leads to nausea and vomiting of a sputum-like substance. A white and sticky tongue coating, and a smooth pulse are signs of internal turbid phlegm retention.

Treatment: To resolve phlegm and regulate the spleen.

Prescription: Modified Decoction of Pinelliae, Atractylodis Macrocephalae and Gastrodiae (106). In this prescription, Rhizoma Pinelliae, Rhizoma Atractylodis Macrocephalae, Poria, Pericarpium Citri Reticulatae and Rhizoma Zingiberis Recens invigorate the spleen, resolve phlegm, conduct the unhealthy *qi* downwards and check vomiting; and Rhizoma Gastrodiae, important for the treatment of headaches and dizziness, calms the liver and suppresses wind. If phlegm-dampness turns into heat over a period of time, producing a bitter taste in the mouth, a sticky yellow tongue coating and constipation, then Rhizoma Atractylodis Macrocephalae should be removed and drugs that disperse heat and resolve stagnation, such as Radix Scutellariae, Caulis Bambusae in Taeniam and Fructus Aurantii Immaturus, should be added.

(6) Stagnation of blood

Clinical manifestations: A prolonged and lingering headache which is fixed in location and causes a stabbing pain. There may be a history of head trauma, as well as a dark purple tongue and a thready and unsmooth pulse.

Analysis: Blood stagnation in the vessels following a chronic illness leads to lingering, fixed and stabbing headache. A dark purple tongue and a thready and unsmooth pulse are signs of blood stagnation.

Treatment: To activate blood circulation and blood stasis.

Prescription: Modified Decoction for Opening Orifice and Activating Blood Circulation (253). In the recipe, Semen Persicae, Flos Carthami, Rhizoma Chuanxiong and Radix Paeoniae Rubra activate blood circulation and solve stasis; Moschus clears the cavity, activates blood circulation, and removes any obstructions from the meridians; Rhizoma Zingiberis Recens and Fructus Jujubae harmonize the nutrient and defensive *qi*, and Bulbus Allii Fistulosi invigorates *yang* and conducts the effects of the drugs to the diseased spot. If the headache is violent, dried insects such as Scorpio, Scolopendra, and Lumbricus are added.

In addition, medicine that conducts the effects of the drugs to the diseased meridians is selected according to the location of headache. For example, in the treatment of a headache of the *Taiyang* Meridians, Rhizoma seu Radix Notopterygii, Fructus Viticis and Rhizoma Chuanxiong are used; for a headache of the *Yangming* Meridians, Radix Puerariae and Radix Angelicae Dahuricae are prescribed; for a headache of the *Shaoyang* Meridians, Radix Bupleuri and Radix Scutellariae are administered; and for a headache of the *Jueyin* Meridians, Fructus Evodiae is used.

Remarks

A headache due to external pathogenic factors is caused by excesses, while a headache due to internal disorders may have a variety of causes, either being due to deficiencies, or to excesses, or to deficiencies complicated by excesses. For example, headaches due to renal, *qi* or blood deficiencies are, of course, caused by deficiencies; while headaches due to turbid phlegm retention or blood stagnation are caused by excesses; and headaches due to hyperactive liver *yang* are caused by complicated syndromes combining deficiency and excess. Some cases exhibit very complicated pathogenesis. For example, hepatic and renal *yin* deficiency is likely to be complicated by rising liver *yang*, which may be further complicated by the movement of turbid phlegm and, in a severe case, external wind-heat as well.

Case Studies

Name: Xu XX; Sex: Male; Age: 30.
First visit: April 25, 1971.

The patient had a severe headache on the left-hand side of his head for a year. Examination of the brain revealed nothing abnormal. Other clinical manifestations were a feeling of heavy pressure in the head, hypertension, a red tongue with a thin yellow coating, and a taut pulse. The patient could hardly sleep because he had used his brain too much. The most recent headache had already lasted one month, though it was alleviated by means of medication now and then. The pathogenesis was rising liver *yang* and blood stagnation in the vessels. Treatment aimed to calm the liver, suppress *yang*, promote blood circulation and remove vascular obstruction:

Rhizoma Gastrodiae	4.5 g;
Concha Haliotidis (decocted first)	30 g;
Ramulus Uncariae cum Uncis	15 g;
Radix Paeoniae Rubra	9 g;
Radix Paeoniae Alba	9 g;
Fructus Viticis	12 g;
Folium Mori	9 g;
Flos Chrysanthemi	9 g;
Semen Persicae	9 g;
Powder of Scorpio (to be taken separately in capsule)	1.5 g.

When the headache was violent, 0.9 gram of Powder of Cornu Saigae Tataricae was also administered.

Seven doses were prescribed.

Second visit: May 16, 1971.

The patient's headache had reduced in severity and frequency, and his appetite had become normal. However he was still short of energy, and slept poorly. His tongue was red and his pulse was taut.

Although liver *yang* was being suppressed, *qi* and *yin* had not yet been restored. Treatment focused on nourishing *qi* and *yin*, and suppressing liver *yang* to prevent any relapses:

Radix Glehniae	12 g;
Radix Paeoniae Rubra	9 g;
Radix Paeoniae Alba	9 g;
Concha Haliotidis (decocted first)	12 g;
Radix Ophiopogonis	9 g;
Flos Chrysanthemi	9 g;
Semen Persicae	9 g;
Caulis Spatholobi	12 g;
Caulis Polygoni Multiflori	30 g.

Fourteen doses were ordered.

Explanation: The patient's headache was due to rising liver *yang*. *The Inner Canon of the Yellow Emperor* says, "Stress expands the body's *yang-qi*." Since the recent headache had continued over a long period of time in a fixed location and was accompanied by a feeling of heavy pressure in the head, vascular blood stagnation was suggested. Therefore, drugs that activate blood circulation and remove stasis were added. The headache disappeared after one month.

Name: Gong XX; Sex: Female; Age: 41.

First visit: The patient was weak and mentally depressed. She had suffered from a headache for two months when she went to see the doctor. She said that she could feel pain all over her head including the vertex, the teeth and the cheeks. This disease had been wrongly diagnosed as an attack of the *Taiyang* Meridians by external wind, and she had not responded to drugs like Rhizoma seu Radix Notopterygii and Radix Ledebouriellae. Moreover, the disease recently took a turn for the worse and was accompanied by vomiting, muscular twitching and spasms. The patient's pulse was taut, thready and rapid.

Medical classics say, "In cases when wind is agitated, with symptoms of involuntary body movement and dizziness, then liver disorders are suggested." Thus, this headache was due to rising liver *yang*.

Deficient water produced floating *yang* and the failure of water to nourish wood. Treatment was to nourish *yin* and suppress *yang*:

Cornu Saigae Tataricae	1.5 g;
Radix Rehmanniae	15 g;
Radix Paeoniae Alba	9 g;
Zuojin Pill (81)	2.4 g;
Colla Corii Asini	12 g;
Concha Ostreae	24 g;
Carapax et Plastrum Testudinis	12 g;
Flos Chrysanthemi	4.5 g;
Ramulus Uncariae cum Uncis	12 g;
Fructus Gardeniae	9 g;
Radix Glycyrrhizae	2.4 g;
Cortex Moutan	6 g;
Magnetitum	24 g.

Three doses were prescribed.

Second visit: The patient's headache was greatly reduced, and she no longer suffered from vomiting, muscular twitching or spasms. Cornu Saigae Tataricae and *Zuojin* Pill (81) were removed and 24 grams of Concha Haliotidis, and nine grams of Radix Scrophulariae were added. The problems disappeared after another five doses were administered.

XXXI. Vertigo

Vertigo refers to a feeling of great unsteadiness, as though one's head were spinning around. In mild cases, it disappears as soon as the eyes are closed. But sometimes the spinning feeling is continuous and accompanied by nausea, vomiting, sweating, and even fainting.

This disease is closely related to the brain. The pathogenesis is either invasion of the brain by various pathogenic factors or malnutrition of the brain due to deficiencies of the *qi* and blood and emptiness of the marrow.

There are many descriptions in the medical classics concerning the etiology and treatment of dizziness. *The Inner Canon of the Yellow Emperor* links this disease to the following factors: (1) Disorders of the liver, as "endogenous winds marked by vertigo, spasms and convulsions are related to the liver." (2) Invasion of external pathogenic factors to the head and brain. (3) Deficiency, referring to the emptiness of the sea of the marrow and malnutrition of the brain.

Zhu Danxi of the Yuan Dynasty attributed this disease to the retention of phlegm-dampness in the interior which prevents the clear *yang-qi* from ascending. He put forward the view that vertigo cannot occur if there is no phlegm in the body. In his opinion, when dealing with vertigo, phlegm should be treated. Zhang Jingyue of the Ming Dynasty said, "Most of the time, vertigo is caused by the body's weakened resistance." In other words, "only in rare cases does vertigo occur when the body's resistance is not weak." He therefore suggested that efforts be made to improve resistance in treating vertigo.

Clinically, vertigo usually belongs to the deficiency-type, and this syndrome is caused by the increase of liver *yang* due to *yin*, the malnutrition of the brain due to blood deficiency, and the lack of essence and marrow due to a deficiency of turbid phlegm or phlegm-fire misting the clear cavity. Different methods are adopted in the treatment of this disease, such as calming the liver and suppressing *yang*, invigorating the spleen and replenishing *qi* and blood, and nourishing the kidneys. If vertigo is caused by phlegm and fire, a better method is to get rid of the phlegm and suppress the fire.

As a common symptom in clinical practice, vertigo can be seen in many diseases.

Aural vertigo (Meniere's disease and labyrinthitis), cerebral vertigo (cerebral atherosclerosis and hypertensive encephalopathy), and other diseases with vertigo as the main symptom (hypertension, hypotension, anemia and neurasthenia) can be diagnosed and treated according to the following descriptions.

Etiology and Pathogenesis

1. Hyperactivity of Liver *Yang*

The hyperactivity of *yang* is likely to cause the liver *yang* to increase. The liver *qi* stagnates due to mental depression and then turns to fire over a period of time, which then consumes liver *yin* and stirs up liver *yang*. In other cases, a deficiency of kidney *yin* means that the kidneys fail to nourish the liver, thereby causing liver *yang* to increase.

2. Deficiencies of *Qi* and Blood

Deficiencies of *qi* and blood may result from prolonged illnesses which consume *qi* and blood, massive blood loss which exhausts *qi*, or deficiencies of the spleen and stomach which lead to the inability to produce *qi* and blood. The *qi* deficiency means the failure of clear *yang-qi* to ascend, while blood deficiency implies that the brain may suffer from malnutrition.

3. Insufficient Kidney Essence

The kidney is the basis of the human constitution, storing essence and producing marrow. A deficiency of kidney essence due to congenital weakness, old age, or excessive sexual activity has an unfavorable effect on the production of marrow; the lack of marrow may cause vertigo.

4. Retention of Turbid Phlegm in the Middle *Jiao*

Eating too much greasy or sweet food, or working too much may damage the spleen and stomach and impair their ability to transport and transform. As a result, food cannot be transformed into essence, and phlegm-dampness is produced. Retention of phlegm-dampness in the middle *jiao* hinders *yang-qi* from ascending.

To conclude, dizziness is mostly caused by internal disorders, which can be manifested as both deficiencies and excesses. The former refers to deficiencies of *qi*, blood, *yin* and *yang*, while the latter is shown by excesses of phlegm and fire. The diseased organs include the liver, spleen and kidneys. In all these conditions, the function of the brain is impaired.

Diagnosis

1. *Jue*-Syndrome

Fainting may occur both in cases of vertigo and *jue*-syndrome. However, *jue*-syndrome is characterized by coma, loss of consciousness, cold limbs, or even death when it becomes severe, while vertigo does not have these symptoms and signs.

2. Apoplexy

Fainting may occur when vertigo and apoplexy are severe. However, apoplexy is marked by the loss of consciousness, which is accompanied by hemiplegia and contortions of the patient's facial muscles.

3. Epilepsy

Dizziness can be seen in both vertigo and epilepsy (in particular in protracted cases). However, fainting in an epileptic seizure is followed by foaming at the mouth, staring upward, convulsions, grunting and making noises similar to pigs and sheep, something that would never happen to anyone suffering from vertigo.

Differentiation and Treatment

In the diagnosis of dizziness, attention is paid to ascertaining whether the root cause of the illness is due to deficiencies or excesses. If the pathogenic factors are caused by excesses, this refers to excesses of phlegm and fire, while deficiencies imply deficiencies of *qi*, blood and *yin* of the liver and kidneys. The chief principle of treatment is to nourish the kidneys and calm the liver, tonify *qi* and blood, invigorate the spleen and get rid of the phlegm.

1. Hyperactivity of Liver *Yang*

Clinical manifestations: Dizziness, tinnitus and a distending headache, all of which are aggravated by stress or anger. Other clinical manifestations include a facial flush, restlessness, irritability, poor sleep with many dreams, a red tongue, and a taut pulse.

Analysis: The disturbance of the brain due to an increase in liver *yang* leads to vertigo. An increase in liver *yang* also explains the facial flush, irritability and restlessness. Fire disturbing the mind gives rise to poor sleep with many dreams. A red tongue and a taut pulse are both signs of an increase in liver *yang*.

Treatment: To calm the liver and suppress *yang*, and disperse fire and eliminate wind.

Prescription: Modified Decoction of Gastrodiae and Uncariae cum Uncis (40). In this formula, Rhizoma Gastrodiae, Ramulus Uncariae cum Uncis and Concha Haliotidis calm the liver and suppress *yang*; Radix Scutellariae and Fructus Gardeniae dissipate liver fire; Radix Achyranthis Bidentatae, Cortex Eucommiae and Herba Taxilli nourish the liver and kidneys; Caulis Polygoni Multiflori and Lignum Pini Poriaferum replenish the heart and calm the mind. In order to further calm the liver and suppress *yang*, Flos Chrysanthemi, Fructus Tribuli and Spica Prunellae can be added to the prescription. In cases of hyperactivity of fire as shown by red eyes, a coarse yellow tongue coating and a taut and rapid pulse, add Radix Gentianae and Cortex Moutan to clear liver fire. In cases of constipation, add Pill of Angelicae Sinensis, Gentianae and Aloe (130) to disperse heat in the liver and remove obstructions in the large intestines. If there are signs of liver wind such as aggravation of dizziness, nausea or vomiting, numbness of the four limbs, tremors in the hands and feet and muscular twitching, add Os Draconis, Concha Ostreae and Concha Margaritifera Usta to suppress liver wind. Use Cornu Saigae Tataricae if necessary. Patients showing these symptoms should receive immediate treatment, especially those who are middle aged or elderly, in order to prevent apoplexy.

If the accompanying symptoms and signs include soreness and weakness in the lower back and knees, nocturnal emissions, lassitude, a taut, thready and rapid pulse and a glossy red tongue, prescribe Bolus for Serious Endogenous Wind-Syndrome (24) to nourish *yin* and suppress *yang*. This formula is applicable to severe cases of dizziness due to extreme deficiency of *yin* of the liver and kidneys, and hyperactivity of liver wind and liver *yang*.

When symptoms and signs are alleviated after the above treatment, administer Bolus of Lycii, Chrysanthemi and Rehmanniae Preparata (144) twice daily to consolidate the therapeutic results.

2. Deficiencies of *Qi* and Blood

Clinical manifestations: Vertigo and blurred vision which are aggravated by strain or by standing up suddenly. Other clinical manifestations include pale a complexion, pale lips and nails, palpitations, insomnia, lassitude, a dislike of speaking, a poor appetite, a pale tongue, and a thready and weak pulse.

Analysis: Malnutrition of the brain due to deficiencies of *qi* and blood leads to dizziness and blurring of vision, which are aggravated by stress or by standing up suddenly. Malnutrition due to blood deficiencies gives rise to a pale complexion, pale lips and pale nails. Malnutrition of the heart produces palpitations and insomnia. A deficiency of *qi* explains the lassitude and dislike of speaking. The impaired functions of the spleen and stomach cause a lack of appetite. A pale tongue and a thready and weak pulse are signs of *qi* and blood deficiency.

Treatment: To replenish *qi* and blood, and invigorate the spleen and stomach.

Prescription: Decoction for Invigorating Spleen and Nourishing Heart (110). This prescription invigorates the spleen, replenishes *qi* and blood, and nourishes the heart. If the patient's stools are loose due to the impaired splenic function, then Radix Angelicae Sinensis should be stir-baked to reduce its lubricant property. Radix Aucklandiae can be roasted to help check diarrhea. Herbs that invigorate the spleen and assist digestion can be added, such as Poria, Rhizoma Dioscoreae and Massa Medicata Fermentata. If the body is cold due to the hypofunction of the spleen and stomach with cold manifestations, add Cortex Cinnamomi and Rhizoma Zingiberis to warm the middle *jiao* and assist *yang*. If the blood deficiency is more pronounced, add Radix Rehmanniae Preparata, Colla Corii Asini and Powder of Placenta Hominis (to be taken separately with water), and prescribe large doses of Radix Codonopsis and Radix Astragali.

If the *qi* of the middle *jiao* is deficient and the clear *yang-qi* fails to ascend, symptoms will be frequent attacks of dizziness, the dislike of doing any form of exercise, a pale complexion, a lack of vigor, a poor appetite, loose stools, the prolapse of the rectum and a thready and weak pulse. The method of treatment is to replenish the *qi* of the middle *jiao* and raise clear *yang* by prescribing Decoction for Strengthening Middle *Jiao* and Benefiting *Qi* (154) with some modifications.

3. Insufficient Kidney Essence

Clinical manifestations: Dizziness, a poor memory, soreness and weakness in the lower back and knees, nocturnal emissions and tinnitus. If *yin* deficiency is more pronounced, the accompanying symptoms include restlessness, a hot sensation in the palms, soles and chest, a red tongue, and a taut and thready pulse. If *yang* deficiency is more pronounced, then the signs include cold limbs, impotence, a pale tongue and a deep and thready pulse.

Analysis: A deficiency of kidney essence means the inability of the kidneys to produce enough marrow to fill the brain, thus causing dizziness and a poor memory. Since the kidneys dominate the bones and the lumbus is the residence of the kidneys, deficiency of the kidneys produces soreness in the lumbus and the knees. Weakness of the gate of essence causes nocturnal emissions. The kidneys lead to a specific body opening in the ear, so kidney deficiencies lead to tinnitus. A deficiency of *yin* produces internal heat, which explains restlessness, a hot sensation in the palms, soles and chest, a red tongue, and a taut and thready pulse. *Yang* deficiency produces internal cold, which causes cold limbs, a pale tongue, and a deep and thready pulse. Because fire is declining from the life gate, impotence occurs.

Treatment: To replenish kidney *yin* in the case of *yin* deficiency; and to nourish kidney *yang* in the case of *yang* deficiency.

Prescription: *Zuogui* Pill (79) is the main formula to replenish kidney *yin*. In the recipe, Radix Rehmanniae Preparata, Fructus Corni, Semen Cuscutae, Radix Achyranthis Bidentatae and Carapax et Plastrum Testudinis replenish kidney *yin*; Colla Cornus Cervi nourishes essence and produces marrow. If a deficiency of *yin* produces internal heat with the symptoms of restlessness, a hot sensation in the palms, soles and chest, a red tongue and a taut and thready pulse, add Carapax Trionycis Preparata, Rhizoma Anemarrhenae, Radix Rehmanniae and Cortex Phellodendri to nourish *yin* and dissipate heat.

To replenish kidney *yang*, *Yougui* Pill (82) can be prescribed. In this prescription, Radix Rehmanniae Preparata, Fructus Corni and Cortex Eucommiae are the main ingredients for replenishing the kidneys; and Radix Aconiti Lateralis Preparata, Cortex Cinnamomi and Colla Cornus Cervi strengthen fire and assist *yang*. Since Radix Aconiti Lateralis Preparata and Cortex Cinnamomi are drastic herbs, dry in nature, they can only be administered for a short period of time. For long-term treatment, Radix Morindae Officinalis and Herba Epimedii are recommended, because they are warm and moist in nature, and they replenish *yang* without damaging *yin*. If vertigo is severe, add Os Draconis, Concha Ostreae and Magnetitum to the above two formulae to suppress floating *yang*.

4. Retention of Phlegm-Dampness in the Middle *Jiao*

Clinical manifestations: Dizziness accompanied by a heavy sensation in the head. Other clinical manifestations include stuffiness in the chest, nausea, a poor appetite, lethargy, a sticky white tongue coating, and a soft and smooth pulse.

Analysis: Phlegm-dampness retained in the middle *jiao* prevents clear *yang* from ascending; and the upward disturbance of wind-phlegm gives rise to dizziness accompanied by a heavy sensation in the head. Retention of phlegm-dampness in the middle *jiao* blocks the circulation of *qi*, causing stuffiness in the chest and nausea. The dampness in the spleen weakens the *yang* of the middle *jiao*, causing a poor appetite and lethargy. A sticky white tongue coating and a soft and smooth pulse are signs that phlegm-dampness are being retained.

Treatment: To dry up dampness, eliminate phlegm, invigorate the spleen, and harmonize the stomach.

Prescription: Modified Decoction of Pinelliae, Atractylodis Macrocephalae and Gastrodiae (106). In this prescription, *Erchen* Decoction (3) resolves dampness and eliminates phlegm; Rhizoma Atractylodis Macrocephalae invigorates the spleen; and Rhizoma Gastrodiae subdues wind. If vertigo is severe and vomiting occurs frequently, add Haematitum to conduct the unhealthy *qi* downwards; prescribe Poria in large doses, and add Rhizoma Alismatis and Semen Plantaginis for the purpose of eliminating phlegm-dampness from the middle *jiao* through urination. In cases of epigastric distress and lack of appetite, add Fructus Amomi Rotundus and Fructus Amomi to resolve dampness, circulate *qi* and harmonize the stomach. In cases of tinnitus and deafness, add Rhizoma Acori Tatarinowii to eliminate phlegm and soothe the ears.

If the phlegm turns to fire, producing symptoms of distending pains in the head and eyes, restlessness, palpitations, a bitter taste in the mouth, a sticky yellow tongue coating and a taut and smooth pulse, Decoction of Coptidis for Clearing Away Gallbladder-Heat (264) is prescribed to dissipate fire and relieve phlegm. In cases when the liver *yang* is rising, the formula for calming the liver and suppressing *yang* is also used.

Case Studies

Name: Su XX; Sex: Female; Age: 36.
First visit: December 6, 1971.
The patient had epigastric and abdominal distention, dizziness, numbness and heaviness of the hands during sleep, a taut pulse, and a glossy tongue. Her blood pressure was high. The method of treatment was to promote the liver's function in regulating the free flow of *qi*, suppress liver *yang* and harmonize the stomach. The following prescription was formulated.

Herba Taxilli	9 g;
Ramulus Uncariae cum Uncis	12 g;
Spica Prunellae	12 g;
Concha Margaritifera Usta	15 g;
Flos Inulae (wrapped)	9 g;
Haematitum	12 g;
Fructus Akebiae	9 g;
Radix Bupleuri	4.5 g;
Radix Paeoniae Alba	9 g;
Radix Linderae	6 g;
Rhizoma Cyperi Preparata	9 g.

Four doses were prescribed.
Second visit: December 13, 1971.
The clinical manifestations shown by the patient included dizziness, epigastric and abdominal distention, numbness of the hands, a slightly taut pulse, and a thin tongue coating. The blood pressure was 200/135 mm Hg. The method of treatment was to promote the liver's function in regulating the free flow of *qi*, harmonize the stomach and decrease blood pressure. The following herbs were prescribed.

Flos Inulae (wrapped)	9 g;
Haematitum	12 g;
Radix Paeoniae Alba	3 g;
Fructus Amomi Rotundus	3 g;
Cortex Magnolicae Officinalis	4.5 g;
Pericarpium Arecae	9 g;
Radix Bupleuri	4.5 g;
Rhizoma Cyperi Preparata	9 g;
Massa Aquilariae Resinatum Lignum	12 g.

Four doses were prescribed.

Third visit: December 20, 1971.

Blood pressure was slightly lowered (160/100 mm Hg). The face was red. There was stagnation of *qi* in the abdomen and epigastrium with the symptom of belching. The pulse was slightly taut and rapid. The tongue was dark red with glossy coating. The method of treatment was to suppress liver *yang* and conduct the unhealthy *qi* downward. The following herbs were prescribed.

Spica Prunellae	24 g;
Herba Leonuri	15 g;
Ramulus Uncariae cum Uncis	9 g;
Fructus Gardeniae (charred)	9 g;
Concha Margaritifera Usta	30 g;
Herba Taxilli	12 g;
Haematitum	12 g;
Radix Paeoniae Alba	9 g;
Carapax et Plastrum Testudinis Preparata	15 g;
Semen Cassiae	12 g.

Seven doses were prescribed.

Discussion: The head is the meeting place of all *yang* meridians of the body. The ears and eyes are clear orifices. The increase of liver *yang* is likely to cause vertigo. The transverse movement of liver *yang* leads to numbness in the four limbs. Stagnant liver *qi* may damage the spleen, causing flatulence. The raised blood pressure and taut pulse are both signs of hyperactivity of liver *yang*. To dissipate heat from the liver and suppress liver *yang*, Herba Taxilli, Ramulus Uncariae cum Uncis, Spica Prunellae and Concha Margaritifera Usta were prescribed. To harmonize the liver and spleen, Rhizoma Cyperi, Radix Linderae, Lignum Aquilariae Resinatum and Fructus Akebiae were used. Flos Inulae and Haematitum conduct the unhealthy *qi* downward; and Radix Bupleuri and Radix Paeoniae Alba calm the liver. Since signs of liver *qi*-stagnation improved during the third visit, herbs that promote the smooth circulation of *qi* were removed from the prescription. Radix Bupleuri was replaced by Fructus Gardeniae for the purpose of conducting heat in the liver downward. Carapax et Plastrum Testudinis and Semen Cassiae were added in order to decrease blood pressure.

Name: Li XX; Age: 20; Occupation: Farm worker.

First visit: December 13, 1974.

Over the past few months, the patient had suffered vertigo, tinnitus, nausea and stuffiness in the chest, all of which occurred intermittently. His sputum was plentiful. These symptoms were not alleviated after taking medicine, because the emphasis of the treatment was laid upon calming the liver and preventing an increase of *yang*. At the time of his first visit, his pulse was thready and rapid, his tongue coating was white and sticky. This was due to the clear cavity being disturbed by liver *yang* containing phlegm. The method of treatment used was to calm the liver, harmonize the stomach, resolve phlegm and conduct the unhealthy *qi* downward. The following herbs were used.

Concha Margaritifera Usta	30 g;
Testa Glycine	9 g;
Flos Chrysanthemi	9 g;
Radix Paeoniae Alba	9 g;
Caulis Bambusae in Taeniam (ginger prepared)	9 g;

Poria	9 g;
Pericarpium Citri Reticulatae Viride	9 g;
Pericarpium Citri Reticulatae	9 g;
Fructus Tribuli	9 g;
Flos Inulae (wrapped)	9 g;
Haematitum	30 g;
Rhizoma Zingiberis Recens	3 slices;
Fructus Citri Sarcodactylis	9 g.

Six doses were prescribed.

Second visit: December 20, 1974.

Sputum had increased, vomiting disappeared, and the vertigo had been relieved, but the patient complained of throbbing pain in his temples. His pulse and tongue coating remained unchanged. All this showed the gradual resolution of turbid phlegm and unchecked liver *yang*. The same method of treatment was adopted and Caulis Bambusae in Taeniam was removed from the prescription. Another six doses were prescribed.

Third visit: December 27, 1974.

Vertigo and stuffiness in the chest had gradually disappeared. But the patient noted lassitude and lethargy. His pulse was thready and soft and his tongue coating was thin and white. This was chiefly because his gastric and splenic functions had been impaired by the disturbance of liver *yang* and phlegm. Herbs that invigorate the spleen and harmonize the stomach were added. The following prescription was formulated:

Flos Inulae (wrapped)	9 g;
Pericarpium Citri Reticulatae Viride	9 g;
Pericarpium Citri Reticulatae	9 g;
Rhizoma Atractylodis Macrocephalae	9 g;
Poria	9 g;
Fructus Citri Sarcodactylis	9 g;
Fructus Tribuli	9 g;
Concha Margaritifera Usta	30 g;
Radix Paeoniae Alba	9 g;
Flos Chrysanthemi	9 g.

Seven doses were prescribed.

Discussion: This patient suffered from aural vertigo with the symptoms of tinnitus, excessive sputum, a sticky white tongue coating and a thready and rapid pulse. The pathogenesis was the increase in liver *yang* complicated with the retention of turbid phlegm. Since herbs that suppress liver *yang* did not work in the previous treatment, herbs that resolve phlegm and conduct the unhealthy *qi* downwards were added to the prescription, such as Caulis Bambusae in Taeniam, Pericarpium Citri Reticulatae and Flos Inulae, and good results were achieved.

XXXII. Apoplexy

Apoplexy, known as *zhongfeng* in Chinese, is a condition which may cause the sufferer to fall to the ground all of a sudden, losing consciousness. The symptoms that follow are contortion of the facial muscles, dysphasia and hemiplegia. In some cases, the facial muscles become contorted and the patient experiences hemiplegia, but without any obvious signs of disturbed consciousness. Apoplexy is characterized by its abrupt onset with pathological changes taking place over a very short space of time, like the time it takes for the nature of the wind to change. It is for this reason that its Chinese name is "*zhongfeng*", literally meaning "wind stroke." Etiologically, wind (either external or internal) is the principal factor.

The earliest description of apoplexy in China's medical classics can be found in *The Inner Canon of the Yellow Emperor*, which calls it by a different name. The *Synopsis of Prescriptions of the Golden Chamber* was the first of the Chinese medical classics to use the term *zhongfeng* to describe apoplexy.

Theories concerning apoplexy were developed over two stages in traditional Chinese medicine. Before the Tang and Song dynasties, external wind was thought to be the principal factor contributing to apoplexy. Scholars maintained that when the body resistance is weak, *qi* and blood are insufficient and the meridians are empty, thus the invasion of the meridians by external wind could lead to fits, facial contortions, hemiplegia and numbness in the affected half of the body. Moreover, according to the severity and scope of the disease, an attack on the meridians could be distinguished from an attack on the *zang-fu* organs. During the period following the Tang and Song dynasties, especially in the Jin and Yuan dynasties many medical scholars put forward a different theory concerning apoplexy, that internal wind was the cause of the disease. Another theory took hold in the Ming Dynasty when Zhang Jingyue thought that apoplexy was caused by the imbalance of *yin* and *yang* owing to weakened *zang-fu* organs. Ye Tianshi of the Qing Dynasty further expounded the pathology of the disease, holding that when the essence and the blood of the body had been exhausted, the kidneys would fail to nourish the liver, thus leading to an increase in liver *yang* and the agitation of liver wind. Zhang Bolong and Zhang Shanlei of the Qing Dynasty believed that apoplexy developed as a result of the wind being stirred by liver *yang*. This was further complicated by the upward movement of *qi* and blood to the brain. All these theories show the way in which people gained understanding of this disease.

Different methods of treating this disease were adopted in the light of the different findings concerning the etiological factors. Before the Tang and Song dynasties, the main treatment for apoplexy consisted of eliminating wind and other pathogenic factors and assisting the body's resistance. Attention was given to nourishing *yin* in order to check the increase of *yang*, subduing the hyperactivity of the liver to calm endogenous wind, removing any obstructions of the *fu* organs to resolve phlegm, promoting blood flow to remove any obstructions from the meridians, dispersing heat and resolving phlegm, invigorating the spleen to relieve dampness, benefiting *qi* and nourishing blood. Yi Tianshi used Pill of Precious Drugs (124) to induce resuscitation when dealing with syndromes caused by excesses and Decoction of Ginseng and Aconiti Lateralis Preparata (188) to restore *yang* after it has been exhausted. In treating the aftereffects of apoplexy, he adopted the method of nourishing the *qi* and the blood, dissipating phlegm-fire and removing any obstructions from the meridians. Wang Qingren developed the Decoction for Invigorating *Yang* (156) to replenish *qi* and promote blood flow in treating hemiplegia, a decoction which is still widely used nowadays.

This disease is similar to hemorrhagic and ischemic cerebrovascular diseases. Thus cerebral hemorrhage, thrombosis, embolism, and transient cerebral ischemia can be diagnosed and treated according to the following descriptions.

Etiology and Pathogenesis

Apoplexy is closely related to the kidneys, heart, spleen, and particularly the liver. Its pathological factors include deficiencies, wind, phlegm and fire. Here deficiencies refer to *yin* deficiencies of the liver and kidneys, which result from stress, excessive sexual activity, or old age. It also refers to *qi* and blood deficiencies, which may be complicated by stagnant *qi* and blood in the meridians, and shown by the contortion of the facial muscles and hemiplegia. Wind denotes both external and internal wind. The former comes from the natural environment, while the latter refers to liver wind resulting from *yin* deficiencies in the liver and kidneys and the hyperactivity of liver *yang*. Phlegm implies phlegm-dampness, which is produced by excess alcohol intake, stress, or too much greasy or sweet food, causing impaired transportation and transformation; obese people usually have excessive amounts of phlegm. Fire indicates fire of the heart and liver, which originates in emotional upsets or deficiencies of liver and kidney *yin*. In addition, unhealthy *qi* and stagnant blood also play an important role in apoplexy.

1. Invasion by External Pathogenic Wind

When the resistance is weak and the meridians are empty, pathogenic wind can invade them, hindering the circulation of *qi* and blood and depriving the muscles, skin and tendons of nourishment. In other cases, the patient has turbid phlegm, which, induced by external wind, enters the meridians. This numbs the muscles and skin, and causes the contortion of facial muscles and hemiplegia.

2. Deficiency of *Yin* and Agitated Wind

In cases of excessive sexual activity, weakness following a prolonged illness, or old age, essence and blood become depleted and liver and kidney *yin* insufficient. Since the liver is deprived of nourishment, liver *yang* increases. Induced by emotional upset, excess alcohol, stress, or abnormal weather, liver *yang* agitates wind; this causes both *qi* and blood to disturb the clear cavity.

3. Upward Displacement of Turbid Phlegm

An improper diet or strain damages the spleen and stomach, and impairs transportation and transformation, thus producing phlegm-dampness. Long-standing phlegm-dampness turns into heat, blocks the meridians, and mists the clear cavity. Phlegm can also result from the invasion of the spleen by liver fire. Liver fire itself may condense fluid into phlegm. Subsequently, liver wind, coupled with phlegm-fire, invades the meridians transversely and mists the clear cavity in an upward direction.

4. Hyperactive Fire of the Heart and Liver

Emotional upsets are the direct cause of hyperactive heart fire. Excess anger impairs the liver, causes the liver *yang* to increase, and further induces heart fire. Wind and fire work together with *qi* and blood as they move upward.

The pathogenesis of apoplexy is very complicated. However, deficient *yin* of the liver and kidneys is the root cause, and phlegm, fire, wind, *yang* and stagnant blood are secondary factors. All these pathogenic factors often combine to induce a stroke. Although both external and internal wind can lead to disease, the type of apoplexy caused by internal wind is more common.

Diagnosis

1. Epilepsy

Both apoplexy and epilepsy manifest themselves in the form of fits, when the patient is prostrated. Epilepsy is paroxysmal, and when a patient suffering epilepsy falls down, he grunts like pigs or sheep, foaming at the mouth and shaking convulsively. After regaining consciousness, the patient will look like a normal healthy person, displaying no visible aftereffects. However, the patient may experience repeated epileptic seizures.

Things are a little bit different for patients suffering from apoplexy. When they suffer fits, they do not scream, shake convulsively or foam at the mouth. Furthermore, after regaining consciousness, there will be aftereffects. Sometimes convulsions accompany attacks of apoplexy. In these cases, only one side of the body is affected, because the other side of the body suffers from paralysis. Epileptic patients often have systemic convulsions.

2. Flaccid Paralysis of Limbs

If hemiplegia remains for a long time after an attack, the patient will become thin, their muscles will atrophy and their tendons become flaccid. Therefore attention should be given to distinguishing apoplexy from the flaccid paralysis of the limbs. The latter is usually marked by its slow onset and exhibits motor impairment of the lower limbs on both sides of the body, or muscular atrophy of the limbs.

3. *Jue*-Syndrome

Jue-syndrome is marked by fits where the patient is prostrated, loss of consciousness, sometimes accompanied by cold limbs. The patient usually regains consciousness very quickly, without any aftereffects. However, attacks can be fatal in particularly serious cases and patients suffering from apoplexy will experience aftereffects after regaining consciousness, including the contortion of facial muscles and hemiplegia.

Differentiation and Treatment

Apoplexy can be caused by a deficient bodily constitution or excess pathogenic factors. Clinically, the following points should be clarified: whether the meridians or the *zang-fu* organs have been attacked, scope and severity of the disease, and whether the disease is caused by a deficient constitution or by pathogenic factors. If the meridians have been attacked, then the disease is often superficial, the pathological conditions are mild and there are no abnormal changes in consciousness. In this case, the contortions of the facial muscles, dysphasia and hemiplegia are the only symptoms. If the *zang-fu* organs have been attacked, then the patient's state is more severe, and symptoms such as loss of consciousness, contortion of the facial muscles and hemiplegia can be seen. There are other premonitory symptoms and sequelae as well as these.

1. Attack on the Meridians

(1) Emptiness of the meridians and collaterals, and invasion by pathogenic wind

Clinical manifestations: Numbness of the hand and foot, or the abrupt onset of deviation of the mouth and eye, dysphasia, and hemiplegia. The accompanying symptoms may include aversion to cold, fever, stiffness of the limbs and arthralgia. The tongue coating is thin and white, and the pulse is superficial and taut or taut and thready.

Analysis: In cases where resistance is weak and the meridians are empty, pathogenic wind may invade the meridians and block the circulation of *qi* and blood, depriving the tendons of nourishment. As a result, contortions of the facial muscles, hemiplegia and dysphasia occur. Invasion by pathogenic wind causes disharmony between nutrient and defensive *qi*, resulting in an aversion to cold, fever and stiffness of the limbs. A thin white tongue coating and a superficial and taut pulse are signs that the surface of the body has been invaded by pathogenic factors. A taut and thready pulse suggests *qi* and blood deficiencies.

Treatment: To eliminate wind, remove obstructions from the meridians, nourish blood and harmonize nutrient and defensive *qi*.

Prescription: Modified Decoction of Gentianae Macrophyllae (27). Radix Gentianae Macrophyllae,

Rhizoma seu Radix Notopterygii, Radix Angelicae Pubescentis, Radix Ledebouriellae and Radix Angelicae Dahuricae relieve exterior symptoms and eliminate wind; and Radix Rehmanniae, Radix Angelicae Sinensis, Rhizoma Chuanxiong, and Radix Paeoniae Rubra nourish the blood and harmonize nutrient and defensive *qi*. Herbs that eliminate wind and remove obstructions from the meridians can be added, such as Caulis Piperis Kadsurae, Caulis Spatholobi, Scorpio and Scolopendra. If there is no internal heat, herbs that disperse heat, such as Radix Scutellariae and Gypsum Fibrosum, should not be used. If the exterior syndrome of wind-heat is present, choose herbs that eliminate wind and disperse heat, such as Folium Mori, Flos Chrysanthemi and Herba Menthae. In cases where the neck is stiff, add Radix Puerariae and Ramulus Cinnamomi to eliminate wind and relax the muscles. If there is excessive sputum and a sticky white tongue coating, remove Radix Rehmanniae and add herbs that eliminate phlegm and dry dampness, such as Caulis Bambusae in Taeniam, Rhizoma Pinelliae, Rhizoma Arisaematis, Exocarpium Citri Rubrum, etc.

(2) Deficient *yin* of the liver and kidneys, and upward movement of liver wind and *yang*

Clinical manifestations: Vertigo, headache, tinnitus, blurring of vision, a numbness of the four limbs, irritability, a hot sensation on the face, and soreness in the lower back and knees. Contortions of the facial muscles, numbness in one side of the body, sluggishness, dysphasia, and hemiplegia may occur abruptly. The tongue will be red with a sticky yellow coating, and the pulse is taut, thready and rapid, or taut and smooth.

Analysis: The upward displacement of liver wind and *yang* due to deficient *yin* of the liver and kidneys leads to dizziness, tinnitus, blurred vision, a hot sensation and soreness. If the meridians are invaded by liver wind, then the *qi* and blood flow will be blocked, and the muscles will be deprived of nourishment, thus producing numbness, contortion of the facial muscles and hemiplegia. A red tongue with a sticky yellow coating, and a taut and rapid, or taut and smooth pulse are signs of *yin* deficiency and *yang* excess complicated by retained phlegm-heat.

Treatment: To nourish *yin*, suppress *yang* and tranquilize liver wind.

Prescription: Modified Decoction of Gastrodiae and Uncariae cum Uncis (40) and Decoction for Calming Liver-Wind (328). Rhizoma Gastrodiae, Ramulus Uncariae cum Uncis, Concha Haliotidis, Os Draconis, Concha Ostreae and Haematitum tranquilize liver wind; Carapax et Plastrum Testudinis, Radix Paeoniae Alba, Herba Taxilli and Radix Scrophulariae nourish the liver and kidney; and large dosages of Radix Achyranthis Bidentatae should be used to conduct blood downwards. In cases where restlessness and a hot sensation in the chest occur, Fructus Gardeniae and Radix Scutellariae should be added into the prescription. If phlegm-heat is pronounced, Arisaema cum Bile and Succus Bambusae can also be added. In case of insomnia or when the patient's sleep is disturbed by dreams, add Dens Draconis, Caulis Polygoni Multiflori and Lignum Pini Poriaferum to calm the mind and soothe the heart.

2. Attack on the *Zang-Fu* Organs

This exhibits critical signs such as fits when the patient loses consciousness and is prostrated; this syndrome can be classified into two categories, syndromes caused by excesses and syndromes caused by exhaustion. The former is marked by an excess of pathogenic factors, so treatment aims to eliminate them and restore consciousness. The latter is chiefly manifested by the exhaustion of *yang-qi*, and thus is a condition caused by deficiencies. This condition should be urgently treated by restoring *yang* and thus preventing it from being exhausted. These two syndromes are entirely different, and they should be carefully diagnosed in order to determine the correct method of treatment.

(1) Syndrome caused by excesses

This syndrome is characterized by fits when the patient is prostrated, loss of consciousness, a locked jaw, clenched fists, constipation, retention of urine, and stiffness and spasms of the limbs.

Since internal wind may complicate phlegm-fire or phlegm-dampness, the syndrome caused by excesses may be further divided into *yang* and *yin* type.

(i) *Yang*-type syndrome caused by excesses

Clinical manifestations: In addition to the principal manifestations of the excess-syndrome, symptoms of this also include a flushed face, coarse breathing, restlessness, foul-smelling breath, fever, a red tongue and lips, a sticky yellow tongue coating, and a taut, smooth and rapid pulse.

Analysis: An increase in liver *yang* agitates wind, which is accompanied by *qi*, blood and phlegm-fire as it moves upward. The misting of the clear cavity leads to fits and the loss of consciousness. Internal wind complicated by phlegm-fire produces a flushed face, fever, coarse breathing, foul-smelling breath and constipation. A red tongue with a sticky yellow coating and a taut, smooth and rapid pulse are signs of internal wind complicated by phlegm-fire.

Treatment: To restore consciousness with acrid and cool herbs, dissipate heat in the liver and suppress wind.

Prescription: First of all, Pill of Precious Drugs (124) is administered via the mouth or nose to restore consciousness. If heat is pronounced, prescribe Bolus of Calculus Bovis for Resurrection (127) and modified Decoction of Cornu Saigae Tataricae (277) to disperse heat in the liver, calm the wind, nourish *yin* and suppress *yang*. In this prescription, Cornu Saigae Tataricae, Flos Chrysanthemi and Spica Prunellae relieve heat in the liver and calm the wind; Radix Paeoniae Alba, Carapax et Plastrum Testudinis and Concha Haliotidis nourish *yin* and suppress *yang*; and Radix Rehmanniae and Cortex Moutan cool the blood and disperse heat. Radix Achyranthis Bidentatae can be added to conduct the blood downwards. In cases where spasms occur, add Scorpio, Scolopendra and Bombyx Batryticatus to calm wind. If there is excessive sputum, add Arisaema cum Bile, Concretio Silicae Bambusae and Succus Bambusae to eliminate phlegm. In cases of constipation, foul-smelling breath and abdominal distention, add Radix et Rhizoma Rhei, Natrii Sulfas, and Fructus Aurantii Immaturus to remove any obstructions from the *fu* organs and disperse heat.

(ii) *Yin*-type syndrome caused by excesses

Clinical manifestations: In addition to the principal manifestations of conditions caused by excesses, symptoms also include a pale complexion, dark lips, excessive sputum and saliva, an absence of restlessness, cold limbs, a sticky white tongue coating, and a deep, smooth and retarded pulse.

Analysis: Internal wind complicated by phlegm-dampness disturbs the clear cavity, thus giving rise to excessive sputum and saliva and an absence of restlessness. Retained turbid phlegm prevents *yang-qi* from warming the body; this causes a pale complexion, dark lips and cold limbs. A sticky white tongue coating, and a deep, smooth and retarded pulse are signs of retained phlegm-dampness.

Treatment: To restore consciousness with acrid and warm herbs, eliminate phlegm, and calm wind.

Prescription: First of all, Bolus of Styrax (143) is administered via the mouth or nose to restore consciousness. In the meantime, modified Decoction for Cleansing Phlegm (243) is taken. In the latter Rhizoma Pinelliae, Poria, Exocarpium Citri Rubrum and Caulis Bambusae in Taeniam eliminate dampness and phlegm; Rhizoma Acori Tatarinowii and Arisaema cum Bile eliminate phlegm and restore consciousness; and Fructus Aurantii Immaturus conducts the unhealthy *qi* downward, and harmonizes the middle *jiao*. To calm liver wind, Rhizoma Gastrodiae, Ramulus Uncariae cum Uncis, and Bombyx Batryticatus should be added.

(2) Syndrome caused by exhaustion

Clinical manifestations: Fall in a fit, loss of consciousness, closed eyes, open mouth, feeble breathing, relaxed hands, cold limbs, profuse and incessant sweating, incontinence, flaccid limbs, hypokinesia of the tongue, and a feeble, thready and fainting pulse.

Analysis: The collapse of anti-pathogenic *qi* and *qi* of the five *zang* organs affects eyes, mouth, breathing and hands, and produces incontinence. The exhaustion of *yang-qi* produces a tendency for *yin* and *yang* to separate; the resultant symptoms include cold limbs, profuse and incessant sweating, a hypokinetic tongue, and a feeble and fainting pulse.

Treatment: To replenish *qi*, restore *yang*, promote resistance and prevent exhaustion.

Prescription: Decoction of Ginseng and Aconiti Lateralis Preparata (188) with additional herbs. In this prescription, Radix Ginseng replenishes *qi*; and Radix Aconiti Lateralis Preparata restores *yang* and prevents exhaustion. In the case of profuse and incessant sweating, add Os Draconis, Concha Ostreae, and Fructus Schisandrae to check sweating and prevent exhaustion.

If signs of wind, phlegm, stagnant *qi* and fire are present after *yang* has been restored, treatment should aim at calming wind, resolving phlegm, circulating *qi* and dissipating fire. If signs of prostration are still present but not pronounced, herbs that replenish *qi* and prevent exhaustion should also be used to prevent *yang-qi* from being exhausted once again. Red face, cold feet, restlessness and an extremely weak or superficial and large pulse with no root suggest deficiencies of kidney *yang* and floating *yang*. In these cases, Decoction of Rehmanniae (118) should be prescribed. Radix Rehmanniae Preparata, Radix Ophiopogonis, Herba Dendrobii, Radix Morindae Officinalis, Herba Cistanches, Fructus Corni, and Fructus Schisandrae replenish kidney *yin* and essence; Rhizoma Acori Tatarinowii and Radix Polygalae eliminate phlegm and restore consciousness; and a small dose of Radix Aconiti Lateralis Preparata and Cortex Cinnamomi warms the kidneys and restores floating *yang*.

To conclude, both the aforementioned syndromes of apoplexy exhibit critical signs. Generally, the syndrome caused by excesses is more common. However, they may change from one to the other or even be present simultaneously. A syndrome caused by excesses can be complicated by one caused by exhaustion and vice versa. If a syndrome caused by excesses is not treated correctly, the body's anti-pathogenic *qi* will be weakened, and a syndrome caused by exhaustion will gradually occur. With the rehabilitation of the anti-pathogenic *qi* of the body following emergency treatment, the syndrome caused by exhaustion will gradually disappear but it may be replaced by the syndrome caused by excesses.

In the treatment of the syndrome caused by excesses, emphasis falls on eliminating pathogenic factors and, additionally, restoring consciousness. To deal with the exhaustion syndrome, attention should be paid to promoting the resistance and preventing exhaustion. If both excess and prostration syndromes are present, the resistance and the pathogenic factors should be dealt with at the same time. If the excess syndrome predominates, elimination of pathogenic factors is primary and strengthening of the resistance is secondary; the opposite applies if the exhaustion syndrome is predominant.

3. Sequelae

The sequelae of apoplexy include hemiplegia, dysphasia and contortions of the facial muscles. Efforts should be made to treat these as early as possible. In addition to herbs prescribed on diagnosis, herbs that activate blood circulation, relieve stasis, and remove any obstructions of the meridians should be used. Acupuncture, massage and physical exercises can also be used for better results.

(1) Hemiplegia

(i) Deficient *qi* and stagnant blood in the meridians

Clinical manifestations: Motor impairment, numbness or total loss of sensation on one side of the body, a sallow complexion, weak limbs, a purple tongue or a tongue with purple spots, and a thready and unsmooth or weak pulse.

Analysis: Insufficient *qi* leads to difficulties in circulating blood, resulting in stagnant *qi* and blood in the meridians. This causes hemiplegia.

Treatment: To replenish *qi*, activate blood circulation and remove any obstructions of the meridians.

Prescription: Modified Decoction for Invigorating *Yang* (156). Large dosages of Radix Astragali can be used to replenish *qi*; Radix Angelicae Sinensis, Radix Paeoniae Rubra, Rhizoma Chuanxiong,

Semen Persicae and Flos Carthami all activate blood circulation; and Lumbricus removes obstructions.

In cases of incontinence, add Fructus Alpiniae Oxyphyllae and Oötheca Mantidis to warm the kidneys and control urine. If the upper limbs are paralyzed, add Ramulus Mori, and Ramulus Cinnamomi to remove any obstructions of the meridians. In cases of weakness and motor impairment of the lower limbs, add Radix Achyranthis Bidentatae, Radix Dipsaci, Herba Taxilli and Cortex Eucommiae to strengthen the tendons and bones of the lower back and knees. If hemiplegia persists, add Hirudo, Tabanus and Squama Manitis to resolve stagnant blood and remove obstructions of the meridians.

(ii) An increase in liver *yang* and stagnant blood in the meridians

Clinical manifestations: Stiffness, rigidity and impaired movement of the limbs on the affected side, headaches, vertigo, a flushed face, tinnitus, a red tongue with a yellow coating, and a taut and strong pulse.

Analysis: Liver fire and wind induced by an increase in liver *yang* are accompanied by *qi* and blood as they move upwards; these block the meridians and subsequently produce hemiplegia. Headaches and a flushed face are both signs of an increase in liver *yang*.

Treatment: To suppress liver *yang*, calm wind, and remove any obstructions of the meridians.

Prescription: Modified Decoction for Calming Liver-Wind (328) or Decoction of Gastrodiae and Uncariae cum Uncis (40). In the former, Carapax et Plastrum Testudinis, Radix Paeoniae Alba, Radix Scrophulariae and Radix Asparagi nourish *yin* and suppress *yang* so as to calm wind; and Haematitum, Os Draconis and Concha Ostreae calm liver wind. In the latter, Rhizoma Gastrodiae, Ramulus Uncariae cum Uncis and Concha Haliotidis calm liver wind; Cortex Eucommiae and Herba Taxilli nourish kidney *yin* and liver *yin*; and Fructus Gardeniae and Radix Scutellariae clear fire. Radix Achyranthis Bidentatae in both prescriptions conducts blood downward. To remove obstructions, add Lumbricus and Caulis Spatholobi.

(2) Dysphasia

(i) Wind-phlegm blocking the meridians

Clinical manifestations: Hypokinesia of the tongue, dysphasia, numbness of the limbs, a sticky white tongue coating, and a taut and smooth pulse.

Analysis: The blockage of the tongue meridians by liver wind mixed with phlegm leads to dysphasia. Retained phlegm-dampness in the meridians hinders *qi* and blood circulation and deprives the limbs of nourishment; this causes numbness.

Treatment: To eliminate wind and phlegm, and remove obstructions.

Prescription: Pill for Relieving Slurred Speech (312). Rhizoma Gastrodiae, Scorpio, Rhizoma Arisaematis and Concretio Silicae Bambusae calm liver wind and eliminate phlegm; Radix Polygalae, Rhizoma Acori Tatarinowii, Radix Curcumae and Radix Aucklandiae ease the tongue, regulate *qi*, and remove obstructions. If headaches or vertigo is present due to an increase in liver *yang*, modified Decoction of Gastrodiae and Uncariae cum Uncis (40) or Decoction for Calming Liver-Wind (328) can be prescribed.

(ii) Deficiencies of the kidneys and essence

Clinical manifestations: Dysphasia or aphonia, soreness in the lower back and knees, palpitations, shortness of breath, a thin tongue coating, and a thready and weak pulse.

Analysis: In cases of renal deficiency, the essence and *qi* fail to nourish the Lung Meridians, thus leading to aphonia. Soreness and weakness of the lower back and knees, palpitations, and shortness of breath are signs of these deficiencies.

Treatment: To nourish kidney *yin* and relieve aphonia.

Prescription: Decoction of Rehmanniae (118) omitting Cortex Cinnamomi, and Radix Aconiti Lateralis Preparata in order to replenish the kidneys and essence. To promote vocalization and relieve aphonia, Semen Oroxyli, Membrana Follicularis Ovi and Radix Platycodi should be added.

(3) Contortions of the facial muscles

Clinical manifestations: Numbness and weakness of the facial muscles on the affected side, the affected half of the face will be contorted towards the healthy side, drooling and dysphasia. When the patient eats, food will collect in the affected side of the mouth.

Analysis: Blockage of the meridians by wind-phlegm causes disharmony of *qi* and blood, thus leading to the contortion of facial muscles.

Treatment: To eliminate wind, resolve phlegm, activate blood circulation and remove any obstructions of the meridians.

Prescription: Powder for Treating Face Distortion (202) with additional drugs. Rhizoma Typhonii eliminates wind, resolves phlegm, suppresses convulsion and removes obstructions; Bombyx Batryticatus and Scorpio both calm wind and suppress convulsions. To activate blood circulation, Radix Angelicae Sinensis and Rhizoma Chuanxiong can be added. To calm liver wind, add Rhizoma Gastrodiae, Ramulus Uncariae cum Uncis, and Concha Haliotidis.

To conclude, treatment for the sequelae of apoplexy aims to promote resistance, activate blood circulation and remove any obstructions from the meridians. In cases when the liver *yang* is increased, liver wind should be calmed. In cases when the wind-phlegm is blocking the meridians, wind should be eliminated and phlegm resolved. Various sequelae are often present at the same time, so during treatment consideration should be given to all sequelae.

Remarks

1. If apoplexy is induced by external wind, no premonitory symptoms are present, but there are exterior signs. The opposite often applies in cases of internal wind.

2. Apoplexy may be recurrent.

Case Studies

Name: Zu XX; Sex: Female; Age: 39; Admission: July 9, 1963.

This patient has a history of hypertension. When she was working two days before, she was prostrated by a fit, suffering hemiplegia on the left side and dysphasia.

Examination: The patient's blood pressure was 260/190 mm Hg. She had almost lost consciousness and the pupil on the affected side of the body was dilated and not responding to light. The left half of the body paralyzed and the cerebrospinal fluid pressure had increased.

Diagnosis: Cerebral hemorrhage.

After being admitted to the hospital, the patient received a slow intravenous injection of 10 ml of 20% magnesium sulfate and 40 ml of 25% glucose solution. She had an intravenous drip of 500 ml of 10% glucose solution with 50 mg of chlorpromazine; and 4 mg of verticil was orally administered three times a day. Her condition did not improve and at 11 a.m. on July 10, it deteriorated. Thus, it was decided that Chinese herbal remedies should be used on the patient.

First visit: July 10, 1963.

The patient exhibited lockjaw, loss of consciousness, excessive sputum and saliva, hemiplegia of the left side, a flushed face, coarse breathing, a sticky yellow tongue coating, and a taut, smooth and strong pulse. All this showed that a syndrome of apoplexy caused by excesses due to an increase in liver *yang* and complicated by phlegm-heat misting the clear cavity. The method of treatment used was to calm liver wind, dissipate heat, eliminate phlegm and restore consciousness. Decoction of Cornu Saigae Tataricae and Ramulus Uncariae cum Uncis (278) and modified Decoction of Acori Tatarinowii and

Curcumae was prescribed.

Prescription:

Powder of Cornu Saigae Tataricae (to be taken separately)	3 g;
Spica Prunellae	15 g;
Concha Haliotidis (decocted first)	30 g;
Ramulus Uncariae cum Uncis (decocted later)	12 g;
Scorpio	6 g;
Radix Achyranthis Bidentatae	30 g;
Rhizoma Acori Tatarinowii	15 g;
Radix Curcumae	9 g;
Bulbus Fritillariae Cirrhosae	6 g;
Exocarpium Citri Rubrum	9 g;
Concretio Silicae Bambusae	6 g;
Succus Bambusae (to be taken separately)	15 g
Radix Glycyrrhizae	6 g.

All these herbs were decocted in water and taken nasally. Purple-Snow Pellet (299) was also administered twice daily, three grams a time.

Second visit: July 12.

The patient's blood pressure was 210/160 mm Hg, and the amount of sputum and saliva had reduced after two doses. But she remained unconscious, and her limbs were still spastic. Her pulse was taut and rapid.

Prescription:

Rhizoma Coptidis	6 g;
Fructus Gardeniae	6 g;
Cortex Moutan	9 g.

These were added to the previous prescription. Purple-Snow Pellet (299) was replaced by Bolus of Calculus Bovis for Resurrection (127) which was taken twice daily, one bolus a time.

Third visit: July 15.

After three doses, she had regained consciousness, and the sputum and saliva were returned to normality. The patient's lockjaw was relieved, her blood pressure lowered to 180/110 mm Hg, and movement was restored in the left side of her body. But the limbs remained spastic. Treatment now aimed at nourishing blood and *yin*, and calming liver wind.

Prescription:

Radix Paeoniae Alba	15 g;
Concha Haliotidis	15 g;
Radix Rehmanniae	24 g;
Lignum Pini Poriaferum	12 g;
Caulis Trachelospermi	15 g;
Concha Ostreae	15 g;
Radix Achyranthis Bidentatae	24 g;
Rhizoma Gastrodiae	12 g;
Radix Glycyrrhizae Preparata	6 g.

Results: Spasms stopped after four doses. The same treatment continued for a few more days to consolidate the results. The patient left hospital on July 23, and was advised to receive acupuncture and moxibustion in her native town.

Discussion: Cerebral hemorrhage is a kind of apoplexy in traditional Chinese medicine, and should be treated as an excess syndrome. For this reason, liver wind was calmed, heat dissipated, phlegm eliminated and consciousness restored. As soon as the patient regains consciousness and has a normal blood pressure, then treatment focuses on nourishing *yin* and blood and calming the liver wind.

Name: Zhao Junchuan; Sex: Male; Age: 59.

First visit: September 18, 1939.

The patient was prostrated with a fit and lost consciousness one month before his first visit. At the time of his first visit, he exhibited numbness in the left side of the body, difficulty in walking, contortion of the facial muscles, incessant drooling, dysphasia, a gurgling sound in the throat, and a deep and thready pulse. Treatment aimed to promote the resistance, remove obstructions from the meridians and eliminate phlegm.

Prescription:

Radix Astragali	60 g;
Radix Paeoniae Rubra	9 g;
Radix Angelicae Sinensis	9 g;
Lumbricus	6 g;
Rhizoma Chuanxiong	3 g;
Ramulus Cinnamomi	4.5 g;
Semen Persicae	3 g;
Flos Carthami	6 g;
Succus Bambusae	12 g;
Succus Zingiberis Recens	3 drops;
Pill for Relaxing Muscles and Tendons and Activating Blood Circulation (to be taken separately)	1 piece.

Second visit: September 19.

The left side of the body was still paralyzed, and the patient could not sit up. After taking the above herbs, he still felt numb on the diseased side, though a little warmer than before. The dosage was increased.

Prescription:

Radix Astragali	60 g;
Radix Paeoniae Rubra	9 g;
Radix Angelicae Sinensis	9 g;
Succus Zingiberis Recens	3 drops;
Ramulus Cinnamomi	4.5 g;
Rhizoma Chuanxiong	4.5 g;
Lumbricus	9 g;
Pill for Relaxing Muscles and Tendons and Activating Blood Circulation (to be taken separately)	2 pieces.

Third visit: September 20.

The patient could move and turn the diseased side of his body. Drooling had stopped, though contortion of the muscles around his mouth was still present. He could drink unaided. His speech was still slurred. The same treatment was adopted.

Prescription:

Radix Astragali	60 g;
Radix Paeoniae Rubra	9 g;
Rhizoma Chuanxiong	6 g;
Lumbricus	9 g;
Semen Persicae	6 g;
Retinervus Citri Reticulatae Fructus	4.5 g;
Ramulus Mori	9 g;
Ramulus Cinnamomi	4.5 g;
Succus Bambusae	9 g;
Succus Zingiberis Recens	3 drops;
Pill for Relaxing Muscles and Tendons and Activating Blood Circulation (to be taken separately, one piece each time)	2 pieces.

Fourth visit: September 21.

The symptoms had improved markedly. The patient could get up and walk by himself. His speech was clearer, and his pulse stronger. The same treatment was adopted.

Prescription:

Radix Astragali	60 g;
Radix Paeoniae Rubra	9 g;
Radix Angelicae Sinensis	9 g;
Flos Carthami	9 g;
Lumbricus	6 g;
Ramulus Cinnamomi	4.5 g;
Rhizoma Chuanxiong	4.5 g;
Semen Persicae	9 g;
Rhizoma Pinelliae	6 g;
Arisaema cum Bile	6 g;
Retinervus Citri Reticulatae Fructus	4.5 g;
Rhizoma seu Radix Notopterygii	3 g;
Succus Bambusae	12 g;
Succus Zingiberis Recens	3 drops;
Pill for Relaxing Muscles and Tendons and Activating Blood Circulation (to be taken separately)	2 pieces.

After taking the above prescription, the patient could walk and speak normally, and the problems around his mouth had also disappeared. Six grams of Exocarpium Citri Rubrum and nine grams of Ramulus Mori were added.

XXXIII. Goiter

Goiters result from stagnant *qi*, retained phlegm, and stagnant blood in the neck due to emotional trauma, an improper diet or unsuitable living conditions. The main symptom of goiters is a swollen mass on both sides of the Adam's apple.

There are many names for goiter in the Chinese medical classics. The first book to call this disease "goiter" was *The Pathogenesis and Manifestations of Diseases* compiled by Chao Yuanfang living in the Sui Dynasty.

A Handbook of Prescriptions for Emergencies recommends Thallus Laminariae seu Eckloniae and Sargassum as a treatment. *The Pathogenesis and Manifestations of Diseases* attributes this disease to emotional trauma and unsuitable living conditions, saying: "Goiters are caused by stagnant *qi* due to worry. It is also said that drinking sandy water causes sand to enter the meridians along with the *qi*, and sand and stagnant *qi* to stay in the neck, thus leading to goiters." Several dozen formulae are prescribed as treatment in the medical classics such as *Essentially Treasured Prescriptions* and *Clandestine Essentials from the Imperial Library*. The recommended herbs include Sargassum, Thallus Laminariae seu Eckloniae, and the thyroid glands of sheep or deer. *Imperial Medical Encyclopedia* states that goiters are more common in mountainous areas. *A Medical Text for Confucianists to Serve Family Members and Relatives* says: "Sargassum and Thallus Laminariae seu Eckloniae all grow in the sea. Keep them in a jar and eat them frequently. In this way, goiters can be relieved." *The Great Herbalism* clearly points out that Rhizoma Dioscoreae Bulbiferae cools blood, subdues fire, relieves goiters and eliminates toxins. *Orthodox Treatise on External and Surgical Disorders* describes the main pathogenic factors causing goiters as stagnant *qi*, phlegm and blood, and treats them by circulating *qi* and blood, removing phlegm, conducting the unhealthy *qi* downward, activating blood circulation and curing masses. Decoction of Sargassum for Goiter (241), recommended in this book, is still used today.

Etiology and Pathogenesis
Emotional trauma, an improper diet and inappropriate living conditions are the three main causes of goiters. Goiters are also closely related to the body's constitution.

1. Emotional Trauma

Long-standing mental depression, anger or anxiety blocks the circulation of *qi* and results in abnormal liver *qi* movement. Stagnant *qi* condenses with fluid to become phlegm, which subsequently combines with the *qi* in the neck to form goiters. The size of the goiters changes along with the emotional state. Stagnant *qi* and phlegm hinder blood circulation, and the stagnant blood thus produced results in hard goiters or nodules.

2. Improper Diet and Unsuitable Living Conditions

A bad diet, or living in a mountainous area where the patient is not able to adapt to the local conditions may impair the ability of the spleen and stomach to transport and transform, thus producing phlegm. Additionally, the normal circulation of *qi* and blood is hindered. Stagnant *qi*, phlegm and blood in the neck all combine to form goiters.

3. Constitution

Women's physiological characteristics, such as menstruation, pregnancy, giving birth, and breastfeeding, are closely related to the *qi* and blood of the Liver Meridians. Induced by emotional trauma and a bad diet, pathological changes such as stagnant *qi* and phlegm, stagnant *qi* and blood and stagnant liver *qi* turning into fire are likely to occur. Thus, women are more likely to suffer from goiters than men. A constitutional *yin* deficiency may cause stagnant *qi* and phlegm to turn into fire, which further consumes *yin*, prolonging the disease.

To conclude, the stagnation of *qi* and phlegm in the neck is the basic pathogenesis of goiters. Some cases exhibit *yin* deficiency complicated by hyperactive fire due to phlegm-heat. The liver and heart are particularly affected by deficient *yin* and hyperactive fire.

During their initial stages, goiters are usually caused by excesses. In prolonged cases, excesses may become deficiencies (chiefly deficiencies of *yin* and *qi*) forming a complicated syndrome combining both deficiencies and excesses.

Diagnosis

Goiters, which are basically manifested by swelling in the anterior part of the neck, often occur in women. This complaint can be diagnosed by close inspection and palpation. The swollen mass moves when the patient swallows. Its size changes greatly, so it may be as small as a cherry or a fingertip at the beginning, but as large as an orange during its later stages. It grows slowly, and feels soft and smooth. In prolonged cases, the mass becomes hard, or turns into a palpable nodule.

Masses in the neck are also symptoms of tuberculosis of the lymph nodes, but these differ from goiters in location, nature and shape. Goiters are located at the front of the neck, and are usually big. The masses seen in tuberculosis of the lymph nodes are on both sides of the neck, are as small as walnuts, and vary in number.

Differentiation and Treatment

The basic principles of treatment are to regulate *qi*, resolve phlegm, and get rid of the growth. If the goiter is hard and nodular, herbs that activate blood circulation and remove stasis should be added. In cases of deficient *yin* and hyperactive fire, the main aim of treatment is to nourish *yin* and suppress fire.

1. Stagnant *Qi* and Phlegm

Clinical manifestations: Swelling at the front of neck, which feels soft and produces a distending sensation, but without pain. Other clinical manifestations include stuffiness in the chest, sighing, and sometimes wandering pains in the costal and hypochondriac regions. This disease is closely related to the emotions. The tongue coating is thin and white and the pulse is taut.

Analysis: Stagnant *qi* and phlegm in the front of the neck causes a swelling there, which feels soft and produces a distensive sensation, but without pain. Stagnant *qi* due to mental depression leads to stuffiness, sighing and wandering pain. A taut pulse is a sign of stagnant liver *qi*.

Treatment: To regulate *qi*, relieve stagnation, resolve phlegm and get rid of the goiter.

Prescription: Modified Pill of Marine Drugs for Relieving Goiter (95). Radix Aristolochiae and Pericarpium Citri Reticulatae promote the free flow of *qi*; Thallus Laminariae seu Eckloniae, Sargassum, Os Sepiae and Concha Meretricis seu Cyclinae resolve phlegm, soften masses and remove the goiter. In cases of stuffiness in the chest and hypochondriac pain, add Radix Bupleuri, Radix Curcumae and Rhizoma Cyperi to regulate *qi* and relieve stagnation. In cases of discomfort in the throat, add Radix Platycodi, Fructus Arctii, Semen Oroxyli, and Rhizoma Belamcandae to ease the throat and relieve swelling.

2. Stagnant Phlegm and Blood

Clinical manifestations: A hard mass or nodule in the front of the neck, which stays there over a long period of time. Other clinical manifestations include stuffiness in the chest, a poor appetite, a dark purple tongue with a thin or sticky white coating, and a taut or unsmooth pulse.

Analysis: Over a long period of time, stagnant *qi* and phlegm give rise to stagnant blood. Accumulated *qi*, phlegm and blood in the front of the neck produce a hard mass or nodule, which stays there over a long period of time. This also impairs transportation and transformation, causing stuffiness in the chest and a poor appetite. A sticky white tongue coating, and a taut or unsmooth pulse are signs of retained phlegm-dampness complicated by stagnant *qi* and blood.

Treatment: To regulate *qi*, activate blood circulation, resolve phlegm and remove the goiter.

Prescription: Modified Decoction of Sargassum for Goiter (241). Sargassum and Thallus Laminariae seu Eckloniae resolve phlegm, soften the mass and remove the goiter; Pericarpium Citri Reticulatae Viride, Rhizoma Pinelliae, Bulbus Fritillariae Cirrhosae, Fructus Forsythiae and Radix Glycyrrhizae regulate *qi*, resolve phlegm and disperse masses; and Radix Angelicae Sinensis and Rhizoma Chuanxiong nourish the blood and activate circulation. If there is a hard mass or a nodule, add proper amounts of Rhizoma Dioscoreae Bulbiferae, Rhizoma Sparganii, Rhizoma Cucurmae, Nidus Vespae, Squama Manitis and Radix Salviae Miltiorrhizae to help activate circulation, soften masses and remove the goiter. In cases where the patient feels stuffiness in the chest, add Radix Curcumae and Rhizoma Cyperi to regulate *qi* and relieve stagnation. If stagnant *qi* turns into fire over a long period of time, producing restlessness, a hot sensation in the chest, a red tongue with a yellow coating and a rapid pulse, add herbs that clear heat and fire, such as Spica Prunellae, Cortex Moutan and Radix Scrophulariae. In cases of poor appetite and loose stools, add Rhizoma Atractylodis Macrocephalae, Poria and Rhizoma Dioscoreae to invigorate the spleen and replenish *qi*.

3. Hyperactive Liver Fire

Clinical manifestations: Mild or moderate swelling in the front of the neck, which feels soft and smooth. Other clinical manifestations include restlessness, a hot sensation in the chest, a liability to sweat, irritability, bulging pupils, trembling hands, a hot sensation on the face, a bitter taste in the mouth, a red tongue with a thin yellow coating, and a taut and rapid pulse.

Analysis: This syndrome is mainly caused by stagnant *qi*, stagnant phlegm and the transformation of stagnant *qi* into fire. Hyperactive liver fire resulting from *qi* which has long been stagnant is the cause of restlessness, the hot sensation, irritability, and the bitter taste. Fire forces the fluid out, thus causing sweating. Agitated liver wind and hyperactive liver *yang* due to the flaring up of liver fire produce the bulging eyes and trembling hands. A red tongue with a yellow coating and a taut pulse are signs of hyperactive liver fire.

Treatment: To disperse fire from the liver.

Prescription: Modified Decoction of Gardeniae for Clearing Liver-Fire (269) and Powder of Sargassum and Dioscoreae Bulbiferae (324). In the former, Radix Bupleuri and Radix Paeoniae Alba promote the liver's ability to regulate the flow of *qi*, and also act to dissipate heat; Poria, Radix Glycyrrhizae, Radix Angelicae Sinensis and Rhizoma Chuanxiong invigorate the spleen, nourish the blood and activate circulation; Fructus Gardeniae and Cortex Moutan clear liver fire; and Fructus Arctii clears heat, eases the throat and relieves swelling. In the latter, Sargassum and Rhizoma Dioscoreae Bulbiferae both relieve goiters and disperse masses, and Rhizoma Dioscoreae Bulbiferae also cools the blood and subdues fire. In cases of hyperactive liver fire with restlessness, irritability and a taut and rapid pulse, add Spica Prunellae and Radix Gentianae to disperse liver fire. If liver *yang* is hyperactive and liver wind is agitated, accompanied by trembling hands, add herbs that calm liver wind such as Concha Haliotidis, Ramulus Uncariae cum Uncis, Fructus Tribuli and Concha Ostreae. If the patient eats large quantities but feels hungry soon afterwards due to excessive gastric heat, add Gypsum Fibrosum and Rhizoma Anemarrhenae to clear this.

4. Deficiency of Heart and Liver *Yin*

Clinical manifestations: The goiter is soft and grows slowly, varying in size. Other clinical manifestations include palpitations, restlessness, poor sleep, a tendency to sweat, trembling hands, dry eyes, blurred vision, lassitude, a trembling red tongue, and a taut, thready and rapid pulse.

Analysis: Stagnant phlegm and *qi* at the front of the neck produce goiters. Deficient heart *yin* caused by the consumption of *yin* by fire deprives the heart of nourishment, resulting in palpitations, restlessness, and poor sleep. Deficient liver *yin* leads to malnutrition in the muscles and tendons, which causes lassitude. Since the liver opens into the eyes, deficient liver *yin* leads to dry eyes and blurred vision. The agitation of liver wind due to deficient liver *yin* produces trembling hands and a trembling tongue. The color of the tongue and the taut, thready and rapid pulse are signs of heat due to *yin* deficiency.

Treatment: To nourish *yin* and essence, soothe the heart, and nourish the liver.

Prescription: Modified King of Heaven Tonic Pill for Mental Discomfort (39). Radix Rehmanniae, Radix Scrophulariae, Radix Ophiopogonis, and Radix Asparagi nourish *yin* and disperse heat; Radix Ginseng, Poria, Fructus Schisandrae and Radix Angelicae Sinensis replenish *qi* and produce blood; and Radix Salviae Miltiorrhizae, Semen Ziziphi Spinosae, Semen Platycladi, and Radix Polygalae nourish the heart and calm the mind. In cases of disharmony of the Liver Meridian accompanied by a dull pain due to deficient liver *yin*, prescribe *Yiguan* Decoction (1) adding Fructus Lycii and Fructus Toosendan to nourish the liver and promote the free flow of *qi*. For agitated wind as caused by deficiencies, with symptoms including trembling hands and tongue, add Ramulus Uncariae cum Uncis, Fructus Tribuli and Radix Paeoniae Alba to calm liver wind. In cases when loose stools occur and the frequency of bowel movements is increased due to impaired functions of transportation and transformation, add herbs that invigorate the spleen and stomach, such as Rhizoma Atractylodis Macrocephalae, Semen Coicis, Rhizoma Dioscoreae and Fructus Hordei Germinatus. If kidney *yin* is deficient, exhibiting tinnitus along with soreness and weakness of the lower back and knees, add herbs that nourish it, such as Carapax et Plastrum Testudinis, Herba Taxilli and Radix Achyranthis Bidentatae. If the body's anti-pathogenic *qi* has been depleted and essence and blood have become insufficient, as in prolonged cases, with symptoms including emaciation, lassitude, oligomenorrhea or amenorrhea and impotence, add proper amounts of herbs that replenish anti-pathogenic *qi*, and nourish essence and blood, such as Radix Astragali, Fructus Corni, Radix Rehmanniae Preparata, Fructus Lycii and Radix Polygoni Multiflori Preparata.

All the syndromes when goiters occur are interrelated. Phlegm and blood stagnation often appear when stagnant *qi* and phlegm reach a new stage of development; hyperactive liver fire and deficiencies of heart and liver *yin* usually occur at the same time. In the treatment of the first two syndromes, regulate *qi*, resolve phlegm, activate blood circulation, soften masses and remove the goiter. In the treatment of the other two, attention should be given to nourishing *yin* and subduing fire. When herbs that remove the goiter and disperse masses are needed, Rhizoma Dioscoreae Bulbiferae is usually chosen. Since the treatment generally takes place over a long period of time, it is advisable to prescribe no more than 12 grams for each dose in order to prevent damage to the liver.

The prognosis is good for the most part. Small and soft goiters are curable, but large ones do not go away so easily. If the mass is hard, grows fast and moves little, the prognosis is poor. If hyperactive liver fire and deficiency of heart and liver *yin* are moderate, good results can be achieved. Symptoms of deficient *yin* and hyperactive fire will aggravate the disease. Restlessness, a high fever and a swift pulse suggest critical pathological conditions.

Emotional stability and a proper diet should be maintained to prevent goiters. In areas where goiters are liable to occur, people should often eat Thallus Laminariae and iodized salt (salt to which 0.01% of sodium iodine and potassium iodine is added).

Case Studies

Name: Huang XX; Sex: Female; Age: 36.
First visit: September 12, 1968.

Two years ago, the patient had her first child. Afterwards, she noted palpitations, stuffiness in the chest, shortness of breath, sweating, a shortened menstrual cycle, trembling hands, irritability, slightly bulging eyes, and an enlargement of the thyroid which was more pronounced on the right-hand side. Examinations showed a basal metabolism of +26, an isotope I^{131} uptake test of 62, and blood pressure of 160/90 mm Hg. The pulse was thready and rapid, with the pulse rate being 106 beats per minute. The tongue coating was thin. Treatment aimed at resolving phlegm, softening the mass, and relieving goiter.

Prescription:

Spica Prunellae	12 g;
Thallus Laminariae seu Eckloniae	12 g;
Sargassum	12 g;
Pumex	15 g;
Concha Ostreae	30 g;
Radix Paeoniae Alba	9 g;
Rhizoma Chuanxiong	6 g;
Rhizoma Pinelliae	6 g;
Radix Ophiopogonis	9 g;
Bulbus Fritillariae Thunbergii	9 g;
Pericarpium Citri Reticulatae	6 g;
Semen Aesculi	9 g.

Second visit: After 21 doses, the sweating and palpitations had improved, and the pulse rate had decreased to 92 beats per minute. The tongue coating was thin. A variation of the previous prescription was formulated.

Third visit: Herbal treatment had continued for over two months. The patient's basal metabolism had dropped to +16, and all the symptoms had improved. Since the patient hated herbal decoctions, Prunellae Extract and Pill of Rhizoma Colocasiae Esculentae were recommended instead. She was advised to eat food with as high an iodine content as possible, such as jellyfish and kelp.

XXXIV. Malaria

The symptoms of malaria are chills and high fever at regular intervals. Malaria, which is caused by plasmodium, usually occurs in the summer and autumn. The incidence of malaria in rural areas is much higher than in cities.

Malaria is called *"nueji"* in the Chinese language. The character *"nue"* can be found on inscriptions on bones and tortoise shells dating back to the Shang Dynasty over 1,200 years ago. *The Inner Canon of the Yellow Emperor* gives a description of malaria's etiology, symptoms and the methods of treatment. It says: "Malaria starts from the tiny hair, and it will cause yawning by stretching the body, shivering, shaking of the lower jaw, pain in both loins and spine; when cold is gone, heat will step in both internally and externally, with the patient experiencing a headache as severe as if the head were going to explode, and violent thirst with the desire for cold drinks." It also says: "In malaria, when the patient feels cold, neither a hot bath nor sitting in front of a fire will succeed in warming the patient; and when the patient feels hot, neither ice nor cold water will succeed in cooling him down." According to *Shennong's Classic of Herbalism*, Radix Dichroae can be used to treat warm malaria and Ramulus et Folium Dichroae to deal with malaria in general. *Synopsis of Prescriptions of the Golden Chamber* lists a taut pulse as a characteristic of malaria, and tells how to differentiate cold and heat according to the frequency of the pulse. It also advises on how to classify malaria into high-fever malaria, warm malaria and cold malaria on the basis of the severity of the chills and fever. The same book recommends White Tiger Decoction with Cinnamomi (104) for warm malaria, and Powder of Dichroae for cold malaria. It also states that if malaria is not cured over a long period of time, masses will form in the hypochondrium; and that Bolus of Carapax Trionycis (325) can be prescribed for their treatment. *A Handbook of Prescriptions for Emergencies* discusses dampness-heat malaria in the mountainous areas, and recommends arsenicum for this. Anti-malarial therapies were very popular in the Tang Dynasty. For example, in both *Essentially Treasured Prescriptions* and *Clandestine Essentials from Imperial Library*, Radix Dichroae and Ramulus et Folium Dichroae are used as primary herbs and are combined with Radix Bupleuri, Herba Artemisiae Annuae, Fructus Mume, Rhizoma Anemarrhenae, Radix Scutellariae, and Concha Ostreae to stop malarial attacks. The author of *A Medical Text for Confucianists to Serve Family Members and Relatives* holds that this disease is infectious, and that it is incorrect to believe that ghosts and gods are responsible.

In malaria, sometimes attacks may occur at intervals of one, two, or three days. When the fever is more pronounced than the chills, it is called warm malaria. When only fever is present, it is known as high-fever malaria. When the chills are more pronounced than the fever, or only chills are present, it is referred to as cold malaria. The form caused by dampness-heat is called miasmic malaria. The chronic form with emaciation due to exhaustion is known as malaria with general debility; and there is another type of chronic malaria characterized by splenomegaly. Typical malaria is marked by alternate chills and fever at regular intervals.

Treatment primarily aims at harmonizing the *Shaoyang* meridians and putting an end to malarial attacks. If malaria is prolonged, and the anti-pathogenic *qi* is weak, the resistance should be promoted and pathogenic factors eliminated. In cases of splenomegaly, phlegm should be resolved, stasis removed and masses softened.

Etiology and Pathogenesis

1. Invasion by External Pathogenic Factors

Principal factors leading to malaria include a specific malarial pathogen and toxic miasma. Malaria was initially thought to be caused by external wind, cold, summer-heat and dampness. *The Inner Canon of the Yellow Emperor* says, "Malaria is caused by wind," and "exposure to summer-heat in the summer leads to malaria in the autumn." As medical practice developed, medical scholars began to recognize a special malarial pathogen. Yu Jiayan of the Qing Dynasty says, "The malarial pathogen hides somewhere between the exterior and the interior of the body. When it goes deep into the interior and fights against *yin*, chills are produced. When it comes out to the exterior and contends with *yang*, fever results. The *Shaoyang* meridians travel between the exterior and interior, thus are responsible for the alternate occurrence of chills and fever. Malaria is the result of disorders of the *Shaoyang* meridians and can be accompanied by symptoms in other meridians. If the *Shaoyang* meridians are not involved, then the illness is not malaria."

The Pathogenesis and Manifestations of Diseases points out that miasmic malaria most commonly occurs in the mountainous areas in south China; and that, caused by toxic miasma and pathogenic dampness, exhibits acute and serious symptoms. Since the malaria pathogen and toxic miasma are associated with wind, cold, summer-heat, or dampness, symptoms will vary accordingly.

2. Weakness of the Body's Anti-Pathogenic *Qi*

A bad diet, irregular food intake and too much raw, cold, or greasy food damage the spleen and stomach, produce phlegm-dampness, and impair transportation and transformation. As a result, *qi* and blood both suffer from deficiencies and the body's anti-pathogenic *qi* becomes weakened.

Stress or an unsuitable lifestyle consumes the body's *qi*, and exhausts the nutrient and defensive *qi*. In either condition, the malarial pathogen finds that the body's resistance is depleted, so it is easier to invade the body.

The pathogenesis of malaria is that such pathogenic factors as the malaria pathogen, toxic miasma, wind, cold, summer-heat, and dampness hide between the exterior and interior, and travel in and out between the nutrient and defensive *qi*. The struggle between the invading pathogenic factors and the body's anti-pathogenic *qi* produces a malarial attack. When the pathogenic factors hide, chills and fever cease. Once an attack occurs, the factors go deep inside to struggle with the nutrient *yin* and prevent the defensive *yang* from reaching the surface, thus causing contractions of the pores and muscles, resulting in chills and tremors. The pathogenic factors then struggle with the defensive *yang*, causing high temperatures and fever. If the body's anti-pathogenic *qi* wins, the factors withdraw and hide between the exterior and interior, and the fever subsides after sweating. The length of the intervals at which attacks occur is related to the depth at which the factors hide. If they are shallow, attacks occur every day or every other day; if they are deep inside the body, attacks occur every three days. Decreased intervals between attacks suggest the outward movement of factors and quick recovery; prolonged intervals imply inward movement and slow recovery.

Differentiation and Treatment

Typical symptoms include chills and fever at regular intervals. Gooseflesh, yawning and lassitude are the initial indications, followed by chills, shivering of the jaw and sore limbs. The patient will feel cold, even when covered with thick bedclothes. After the chills, fever affects the patient. The patient will feel like burning charcoal. Fever will be accompanied by severe headaches, a flushed face and lips, restlessness, and thirst. The patient sweats heavily all over the body as the fever subsides and the body cools down. Clinically, typical malaria, warm malaria, cold malaria and chronic malaria with general debilities can all be distinguished according to the severity of the chills and the fever. The basic principle of treatment is to cause the malarial attacks to cease. If pathogenic factors affect the *Shaoyang* meridians, then the harmonization of the meridians will eliminate pathogenic factors. If fever is more pronounced than chills, disperse heat in order to relieve the external symptoms; if chills are more pronounced than fever, acrid and warm herbs should be prescribed to disperse pathogenic factors. If the cause of malaria is exposure to toxic miasma, this should be eliminated; if there is phlegm, this too should be eliminated; and if food is retained, this should be relieved. If in prolonged cases, signs of deficiencies can be seen, then the body's resistance can be strengthened by either invigorating the spleen and stomach or replenishing *qi* and blood. If splenomegaly is produced, then the masses should be softened, and the stasis and the phlegm should be relieved.

1. Typical Malaria

Clinical manifestations: Chills and fever at regular intervals. The disease starts with yawning, lassitude and sore limbs, followed by chills and shivering of the jaw. When these symptoms go away, a burning heat spreads over the whole body, accompanied by a headache, a flushed face and thirst. When the fever subsides, profuse sweating occurs. The tongue coating is thin and white or yellow and sticky. The pulse is mostly taut, and may become more tense when the patient is suffering from chills. When fever is present, the pulse is rapid.

Analysis: When a malarial episode starts, the pathogenic factors affect *yang* first. The hindrance of the *yang-qi* and deficiencies of the nutrient and defensive *qi* cause yawning and lassitude. Then the pathogenic factors penetrate the body and affect *yin*. Excess *yin* and deficient *yang* cause chills and a shivering jaw. When the pathogenic factors have left *yin* and reached *yang* again, *yin* becomes deficient and an excess of *yang* is produced. Excess *yang* leads to fever; this explains the burning heat, headache and flushed face. Consumption of fluid by excess heat causes thirst. After this, the pathogenic factors withdraw and hide as the pores open due to the heat, and sweating occurs. In this way, fever subsides and the body cools down. A thin white tongue coating is present at the beginning of the disease when pathogenic factors are on the surface. A sticky yellow tongue coating suggests that the pathogenic factors are moving inward and the production of heat. A taut pulse is usually present in malaria. A taut and tense pulse suggests cold, and a taut and rapid one suggests heat.

Treatment: To harmonize the *Shaoyang* Meridians and put a halt to malarial attacks.

Prescription: Decoction of Bupleuri for Regulating *Shaoyang* Meridians (36) with Radix Dichroae and Fructus Tsaoko. In this prescription, Radix Bupleuri eliminates pathogenic factors between the exterior and interior of the body; Radix Scutellariae disperses heat; Rhizoma Pinelliae dries dampness and resolves phlegm; Radix Ginseng and Radix Glycyrrhizae replenish *qi* and harmonize the middle *jiao*; and Radix Dichroae and Fructus Tsaoko eliminate pathogenic factors and put a halt to malarial attacks. If chills are pronounced and there is little sweating, add Ramulus Cinnamomi, Rhizoma seu Radix Notopterygii and Radix Ledebouriellae to relieve the external symptoms and produce sweating. In cases when the patient experiences distress, fullness in the chest and epigastrium and a sticky tongue coating, remove Radix Ginseng and add Rhizoma Atractylodis, Cortex Magnoliae Officinalis and Pericarpium Citri Reticulatae Viride to regulate *qi* and resolve dampness. In cases of thirst, add Radix Puerariae and Herba Dendrobii to produce fluid.

2. Warm Malaria

Clinical manifestations: High fever and mild chills, or fever without chills, irregular sweating, headache, painful joints, restlessness, thirst, constipation, deep yellow urine, a red tongue with a yellow coating, and a taut and rapid pulse.

Analysis: Hyperactive *yang* complicated by exposure to malarial pathogens, or excess internal heat after exposure to summer-heat, gives rise to high fever and mild chills or fever without chills.

Consumption of fluid by internal heat causes thirst, constipation and deep yellow urine. Summer-heat usually causes profuse sweating, but since people like to relax in cool places on hot summer days, this allows the wind-cold to invade the body. As a result, the dispersion of heat is impaired, and irregular perspiration, a headache and painful joints occur. A red tongue with a yellow coating and a taut and rapid pulse are signs of excess pathogenic heat.

Treatment: To dissipate heat and relieve exterior symptoms.

Prescription: The primary prescription is White Tiger Decoction with Cinnamomi (104). Heat can be dispersed by using Gypsum Fibrosum and Rhizoma Anemarrhenae, which are cold in nature; Ramulus Cinnamomi eliminates wind-cold. To harmonize the *Shaoyang* meridians and stop malarial attacks, add Radix Bupleuri and Herba Artemisiae Annuae. If excess heat consumes *yin*, add Radix Rehmanniae, Carapax Trionycis and Radix Scrophulariae to nourish *yin* and produce body fluid. In cases of excess dampness-heat with symptoms of stuffiness in the chest and nausea, add Radix Scutellariae, Rhizoma Coptidis, Talcum and Poria to disperse dampness-heat. In cases of fever without chills, prescribe White Tiger Decoction. If *qi* is damaged, add Radix Ginseng.

If pathogenic heat persists, and *yin* fluid is consumed, with symptoms of emaciation and a glossy crimson tongue, *yin* can be nourished and heat dispersed by prescribing Decoction of Artemisiae Annuae and Carapax Trionycis (168). In the formula Carapax Trionycis nourishes *yin*, lowers fever and eliminates pathogenic factors from the meridians; Herba Artemisiae Annuae disperses heat, eliminates pathogenic factors and checks malarial attacks; Rhizome Anemarrhenae and Radix Rehmanniae nourish *yin* and dissipate heat; and Cortex Moutan cools blood and dissipates heat.

3. Cold Malaria

Clinical manifestations: Chills without fever, or severe chills and mild fever, absence of thirst, distress and fullness in the costal and hypochondiac region, lassitude, a sticky white tongue coating, and a taut and slow pulse.

Analysis: Deficient *yang* complicated by exposure to malarial pathogen and pathogenic wind-cold produces excess internal cold and disordered circulation of *yang-qi*. The failure of the *yang-qi* to reach the body surface gives rise to chills without fever, or severe chills and mild fever. Invasion of the spleen by cold-dampness impairs transport and transformation, thus thirst disappears and lassitude occurs. The disharmony of *qi* of the *Shaoyang* meridians leads to distress and fullness in the costal and hypochondriac region. A sticky white tongue coating and a taut and slow pulse are signs of retained cold-dampness and of malarial pathogens deep in the *yin* system.

Treatment: To eliminate pathogenic factors with acrid and warm herbs.

Prescription: Modified Decoction of Bupleuri, Cinnamomi and Zingiberis (238). Radix Bupleuri harmonizes the *Shaoyang* meridians; Ramulus Cinnamomi eliminates deeply retained pathogenic cold; and Rhizoma Zingiberis, acrid and warm, helps disperse cold. In cases of irregular sweating, remove Concha Ostreae. When there is excess cold-dampness in the interior, with symptoms of distress in the chest and abdomen and a sticky white tongue coating (as if there were an accumulation of powder on the tongue), add Fructus Tsaoko, Semen Arecae and Cortex Magnoliae Officinalis to regulate *qi* and resolve dampness; or prescribe modified Decoction of Seven Treasured Drugs for Relieving Malaria (313). Radix Dichroae, Semen Arecae and Fructus Tsaoko all check malarial attacks; Cortex Magnoliae Officinalis, Pericarpium Citri Reticulatae Viride, and Pericarpium Citri Reticulatae relieve dampness, invigorate the spleen, regulate *qi* and resolve phlegm; and Radix Glycyrrhizae harmonizes the middle *jiao*. If a sputum-like substance is expectorated, add Radix Aconiti Lateralis Preparata and Ramulus et Folium Dichroae to disperse cold-phlegm.

4. Miasmic Malaria

In mountainous areas, excess dampness-heat and exposure to miasmic toxins lead to miasmic malaria. This has an acute onset, and delirium and coma are its main symptoms. The accompanying symptoms include a violent headache, restlessness and convulsions. Some patients exhibit mental disturbances and mania. Most patients suffer from a high fever, while in a few cases body temperature can be lower than normal. Since miasmic malaria is infectious and it produces a critical pathological condition, a combination of traditional Chinese and Western medicine should be applied without delay.

Miasmic malaria can be classified into two types, hot and cold. When miasmic toxins invade the body, if the patient suffers from excess *yang* then hot miasmic malaria breaks out because heat is more severe than dampness, or dampness turns into heat. Cold miasmic malaria appears if dampness is more severe than heat, or if dampness turns into cold, producing retained cold-dampness.

(1) Hot miasmic malaria

Clinical manifestations: High fever and mild chills, or high fever without chills, a headache, flushed face, red eyes, stuffiness in the chest, nausea, restlessness, thirst with a preference for cold drinks, mental confusion and delirium in severe cases, constipation, hot deep yellow urine, a crimson tongue or a tongue with a dark and dirty coating, and a bounding and rapid or taut and rapid pulse.

Analysis: Invasion by miasmic toxins produces excess internal heat, which, if unrelieved by sweating, causes a high fever with or without chills. The upward movement of toxin-heat leads to a headache, flushed face and red eyes. Retained toxin-heat in the middle *jiao* impairs the stomach's ability to descend, resulting in stuffiness in the chest and nausea. Consumption of fluid by excess heat causes restlessness and thirst. Accumulated heat in the *Yangming* meridians results in constipation. The downward movement of heat to the bladder produces hot, deep yellow urine. The misting of the clear cavity and damage to the nutrient blood due to toxin-heat bring about restlessness, mental confusion and delirium. A crimson tongue or a tongue with a dark and dirty coating and a bounding and rapid or taut and rapid pulse are signs of excess toxin-heat.

Treatment: To eliminate miasmic toxins, disperse heat and protect body fluid.

Prescription: Modified Decoction for Clearing Away Miasmic Toxins (284). Radix Bupleuri and Herba Artemisiae Annuae harmonize the *Shaoyang* meridians and eliminate pathogenic factors; Rhizoma Pinelliae, Pericarpium Citri Reticulatae, Poria and Caulis Bambusae in Taeniam dry dampness, harmonize the stomach and control the flow of unhealthy *qi*; Radix Scutellariae, Rhizoma Coptidis and Rhizoma Anemarrhenae disperse heat and eliminate toxins. Radix Dichroae checks malarial attacks; Fructus Aurantii Immaturus relieves distress and fullness; and Powder for Clearing Away Summer-Heat and Dampness relieves restlessness and dampness. If signs of dryness appear due to fluid consumption, add Radix Rehmanniae, Radix Scrophulariae and Radix Ophiopogonis to nourish *yin* and produce body fluid. In cases of mental confusion or delirium, administer Purple-Snow Pellet (299) straight away to disperse heat in the heart and restore consciousness. If vomiting is severe, administer *Yushu* Pill (72) to eliminate toxins.

(2) Cold miasmic malaria

Clinical manifestations: Severe chills and mild fever, or chills without fever. A severe case may exhibit mental confusion and aphasia. The tongue coating is white, thick, and sticky; the pulse is taut.

Analysis: A deficiency of *yang* complicated by invasion of miasmic toxins and turbid dampness prevents *yang-qi* from spreading to the surface, thus causing severe chills with or without fever. In a severe case, miasmic toxins and turbid dampness mist the heart, and mental confusion and aphasia result. A white, thick and sticky tongue coating and a taut pulse are signs of failure to disperse retained cold-dampness.

Treatment: To resolve turbid dampness with aromatics, eliminate pathogenic factors and regulate *qi*.

Prescription: Powder for Restoring Anti-Pathogenic *Qi* (75). Herba Agastachis, Herba Eupatorii and Folium Nelumbinis are used as aromatics to resolve turbid dampness and eliminate miasmic toxin; Cortex Magnoliae Officinalis, Rhizoma Atractylodis, Rhizoma Pinelliae and Pericarpium Citri Reticulatae dry dampness, relieve fullness, regulate *qi* and deal with phlegm. Rhizoma Acori Tatarinowii restores consciousness; Fructus Tsaoko checks malarial attacks; and Radix Glycyrrhizae Preparata harmonizes the middle *jiao*. In cases of mental confusion and aphasia due to misting of the heart by phlegm-dampness, add Bolus of Styrax (143) to restore consciousness.

5. Malaria with General Debility

Clinical manifestations: Frequent attacks of alternate chills and fever, lassitude, poor appetite, spontaneous sweating, a sallow complexion, emaciation, possibly splenomegaly, a pale tongue, and a thready and weak pulse.

Analysis: The consumption of *qi* and blood and the disharmony between the nutrient and defensive *qi* in prolonged cases explain the frequent chills and fevers. In protracted cases, the consumption of *qi* leads to a deficiency of *qi* in the spleen, which means impaired transportation and transformation; this causes a poor appetite, lassitude, a sallow complexion, and emaciation. Stagnant blood and retained phlegm in a prolonged case give rise to splenomegaly. The disharmony between the nutrient and defensive *qi* causes the weakness of the pores and the result is spontaneous sweating. A pale tongue and a thready and weak pulse, are signs of *qi* and blood deficiency.

Treatment: To promote the anti-pathogenic *qi* and harmonize the nutrient and defensive *qi*.

Prescription: Decoction of Polygoni Multiflori and Ginseng for Malaria (160). Radix Polygoni Multiflori replenishes the liver and kidneys and nourishes essence and blood; Radix Ginseng and Radix Angelicae Sinensis replenish *qi* and blood; Rhizoma Zingiberis Recens disperses cold; and Pericarpium Citri Reticulatae regulates *qi*. If dampness results from splenic deficiencies, with symptoms of sweating and lassitude, Decoction for Various Kinds of Malaria (87) is prescribed. In this prescription, Decoction of Six Mild Drugs (55) invigorates the spleen and relieves dampness; Fructus Tsaoko, warm in nature, disperses cold and relieves dampness; Fructus Mume relieves restlessness, heat in the chest and thirst; and Rhizoma Zingiberis Recens and Fructus Jujubae harmonize the nutrient and defensive *qi*. In cases of splenomegaly, resolve phlegm, eliminate stasis and soften masses by combining Bolus of Carapax Trionycis (325) with herbs that regulate and replenish *qi* and blood.

In the treatment of all these malarial syndromes, special formulas are applicable. Commonly-used formals include Decoction of Seven Treasured Drugs for Relieving Malaria (313) and Decoction of Dichroae (289), both with Radix Dichroae and Fructus Tsaoko as main ingredients. The former is selected if phlegm-dampness is pronounced, the latter if dampness-heat is severe. Commonly-used herbs for checking malarial attacks include Radix Dichroae, Ramulus et Folium Dichroae, Herba Artemisiae Annuae and Herba Verbenae. Artemisinine extracted from Herba Artemisiae Annuae is made into pills and injection; it renders immediate and satisfactory results, without causing any obvious toxic reactions or side effects. One gram of artemisinine pill or injection should be administered every day for two days. It is advisable to take anti-malarial drugs two to three hours before an attack occurs.

Case Studies

A patient by the name of Ma Zuo was exposed to summer-heat in the summer and to wind-cold in the autumn. Cold is a pathogenic factor of the *yin* type, which affects the defensive *qi*. Invasion by wind-cold gives rise to deficient *yang* and excess *yin*. Summer-heat is a pathogenic factor of the *yang* type, which affects the nutrient *qi*. Invasion by summer-heat leads to deficient *yin* and excess *yang*. Excess *yin* causes chills, while excess *yang* causes fever. This patient had chills when his jaw shivered, followed by high fever and a headache. All symptoms went away after sweating. The patient noted that he had suffered similar episodes for the past 20 days. Other symptoms included stuffiness in the chest, a poor appetite, a sticky tongue coating, and a taut and smooth pulse. A taut pulse is one of the *Shaoyang* meridians, and a smooth pulse suggests phlegm-dampness. The pathogenesis was invasion of the *Shaoyang* meridians by pathogenic factors and retained phlegm-dampness in the middle *jiao*. Decoction for Clearing Away Spleen-Heat was prescribed to harmonize the *Shaoyang* meridians and resolve phlegm-dampness. The following prescription was formulated.

Radix Bupleuri	3 g;
Rhizoma Pinelliae	6 g;
Cortex Magnoliae Officinalis	2.4 g;
Fructus Tsaoko (roasted)	2.4 g;
Pericarpium Citri Reticulatae Viride	3 g;
Radix Glycyrrhizae	1.2 g;
Massa Medicata Fermentata	9 g;
Herba Eupatorii	6 g;
Rhizoma Zingiberis Recens	1 piece.

Discussion: This is a case of typical malaria characterized by alternate chills and fever in a repeated pattern of 24 hours. The disease is caused by exposure to malarial pathogen, summer-heat in summer, and wind-cold in autumn.

XXXV. Edema

Edema refers to abnormal fluid retention in the tissue. This may affect the head, face, eyelids, limbs, abdomen and back, and even the entire body. Severe edema can be accompanied by hydrothorax and ascites.

Descriptions of edema can be found in *The Inner Canon of the Yellow Emperor*: "When edematous abdominal swelling begins, there is light swelling around the eyelids. When waking in the morning, there is a visible rising and falling of the pulse in the neck, a constant cough, a cold sensation on the medial side of the thigh, swelling in the tibia, and abdominal enlargement." This book also says that an accumulation of pathogenic factors in the lung, spleen and kidney meridians cause edema. Edema can be classified into wind, stone and pouring edema. *Synopsis of Prescriptions of the Golden Chamber* discusses this disease in a special essay, classifying edema into wind, skin, systemic and stone edema according to the patient's etiology and pulse, and into heart, liver, lung, spleen and kidney edema according to the five *zang* organs. Since these classifications are too complicated, Zhu Danxi of the Yuan Dynasty proposed two categories: *yang* and *yin* edema.

Danxi's Experience on Medicine says, "Systemic edema accompanied by restlessness, thirst, dysuria with deep yellow urine and constipation is referred to as edema of the *yang* type, but systemic edema with no restlessness or thirst, or oliguria but without dysuria or deep yellow urine is called edema of the *yin* type." This theory later helped medical scholars to gain a further understanding of this condition.

Edema was treated by sweating or diuresis prior to the Han and Tang dynasties. These methods gradually developed to include invigorating the spleen, nourishing the kidneys, warming *yang* and combining elimination and nourishment.

Edema usually breaks out in acute and chronic nephritis, congestive heart failure, endocrine disturbance and dystrophy.

Etiology and Pathogenesis

The lung regulates the water passages, the spleen governs the transportation and transformation of body fluid, and the kidneys dominate water metabolism. The normal functioning of these organs enables the triple *jiao* to drain the water passages and the bladder to control urination. However, if these organs do not work well, the functioning of the triple *jiao* will be impaired. The upper *jiao* will fail to disperse sweat or to send water to the urinary bladder. The obstruction in the middle *jiao* will lead to water retention and dampness. Finally, the obstruction in the lower *jiao* will weaken its control over urination. These are the reasons why edema appears.

1. Invasion by External Pathogenic Wind and Dysfunction of Pulmonary Dispersion

The lungs, the upper source of water, dominate the exterior of the body, relating externally to the skin and hair. The lungs possess the functions of dispersing and descending lung *qi*, as well as regulating the water passages. If lung *qi* is invaded by external pathogenic wind, then it will not be dispersed, the pores will be closed and the body will not be able to excrete its fluid as sweat. At the same time, lung *qi* will fail to descend, and fluid will not be discharged from the urinary bladder as urine. Because of this, the fluid will spread to the muscles and skin and give rise to edema.

Edema can also be caused by skin infections. *Clandestine Essentials from Imperial Library* by Wang Tao of the Tang Dynasty says, "If skin ulcers fester, edema will enter the whole body." *Shen's Treatise on the Importance of Life Preservation* by Shen Jin'ao of the Qing Dynasty says, "Edema is caused by skin ulcers due to heat in the blood." In his medical records, Ye Tianshi says, "Wind-warm pathogens lead to edema." All this shows the relationship between edema and external factors.

2. Invasion of Water and Dampness and Dysfunction of the Spleen in Transportation

The spleen transports and transforms water and dampness, and promotes the circulation and excretion of body fluid; in this it relies on the strength of spleen *qi* and spleen *yang*. The spleen likes dryness and dislikes dampness. Invasion by water and dampness may follow if the patient lives in a damp place, wades in water, or is caught in the rain. When this occurs, transportation and transformation will be impaired, and excess water will spread to the muscles and skin, causing edema. An accumulation of pathogenic dampness in the middle *jiao* may be the result of excess alcohol, irregular food intake or too much raw or cold food. In this condition, the splenic functions are impaired, the clear *qi* cannot ascend and the turbid *qi* (including water and dampness) cannot descend. Retained water and dampness in the muscles and skin give rise to edema. If dampness is retained for a long time, it will turn into heat; this combination impairs the function of the bladder, resulting in edema.

3. Stress and Improper Diet

The spleen sends fluid and essence produced from food to the lungs, through which it spreads to various parts of the body. Stress or an improper diet causes deficient spleen *qi* and spleen *yang*, as well as an accumulation of fluid. The overflow gives rise to edema.

4. Excessive Sexual Activity and Childbirth

These cause kidney *qi*-deficiency. Prolonged deficiency of spleen *qi* due to stress may affect the kidneys over a long time, resulting in a deficiency of spleen and kidney *qi*. Renal deficiency means an impaired ability to disperse *qi* and circulate water, while splenic deficiency implies impaired transportation and transformation of water and dampness. In either case, edema results.

In summary, edema caused by the invasion of pathogenic wind, water and dampness, excess alcohol or too much raw or cold food belongs to the *yang* type, while edema caused by splenic and renal deficiencies after stress or excessive sexual activity is of the *yin* type. These two types are interchangeable. For example, in a prolonged case of *yang*-type edema, retained water and dampness may weaken the body's anti-pathogenic *qi*, giving rise to deficiencies of spleen and kidney *yang* with lingering pathological conditions. Here *yang*-type edema turns into *yin* type. On the contrary, exposure to external pathogenic factors impairs the lungs' dispersive functions and thus abruptly aggravates the existing *yin* edema. In this case, treatment should be directed firstly to the primary disorder, namely *yang*-type edema. If the patient experiences an aversion to cold, fever or the aggravation of edematous conditions of the *yin* type after exposure to external factors, this does not signal an alleviation. It can only be explained as deficiencies of the body's anti-pathogenic *qi* complicated by hyperactive pathogenic factors, exhibiting even more complicated pathological conditions.

In terms of pathogenesis, the lungs, spleen and kidneys are interrelated. To this effect, *A Complete Collection of Jingyue's Treatise* says, "Diseases such as edema are caused by disorders of the lungs, spleen and kidneys. Since water is extreme *yin*, the primary cause of edema is related to the kidneys. Since water comes from *qi*, the secondary cause can be attributed to the lungs. Since water is checked only by earth, the spleen is responsible for the overflow of water. In cases of pulmonary deficiency, *qi* produces water instead of essence. Splenic deficiency means an inability of earth to restrain water; on the contrary, water restrains earth. In cases of renal deficiency, water moves recklessly as it fails to be dominated." This statement shows that if kidney water overflows the Lung Meridian, lung *qi* will not descend. Thus the lungs' ability to regulate the water passages will be impaired, and kidney *qi* will become even weaker, while pathogenic water will become even more hyperactive. Transmission of pathogenic factors from the Lung Meridian to the Kidney Meridian produces the same result. This statement also shows the mutual restriction and promotion that takes place between the spleen and kidneys. In cases of splenic deficiency, the spleen fails to check water. Excess water and dampness inevitably damage *yang*; thus splenic deficiency further develops into a deficiency of kidney *yang*. Likewise, a deficiency of kidney *yang* deprives the spleen of nourishment and warmth, thus aggravating the disease.

Differentiation and Treatment

Edema begins from the eyelids and then spreads to the head, face, limbs, or the whole body. There are also cases in which edema begins in the lower limbs, followed by systemic edema. In severe cases, abdominal fullness, stuffiness in the chest, asthmatic breathing and orthopnea are also present. When diagnosing edema, whether the complaint can be classified as *yang*-type edema or *yin*-type edema should be clarified first. The *yang* type has symptoms like chills, fever, possible coughing and a sore throat, edema starting from the the face, small amounts of dark yellow urine, possible fullness and abdominal distention, constipation, a sticky white or yellow tongue coating and a superficial, smooth and rapid, or deep and rapid pulse. *Yang* edema is caused by acute heat and excesses. *Yin* edema is characterized by pitted edema on the face and body, small amounts of urine, loose stools, soreness and coldness in the lumbar region, epigastric distress, abdominal distention, a heavy sensation in the body, a pale and swollen tongue with a white coating, a deep, slow pulse, and a pale or sallow complexion. This is a chronic cold syndrome caused by deficiencies.

The Inner Canon of the Yellow Emperor puts forward the principles of treatment, saying, "The treatment should start with taking the pulse to determine if it is a deep pulse or a superficial pulse. Then treatment should be directed at removing accumulated water, as if getting rid of rotten grass... The physician should then open up the patient's pores by causing perspiration in cases where the pulse is superficial and diuresis in cases where the pulse is deep." *Synopsis of Prescriptions of the Golden Chamber* states explicitly, "Edema is treated by diuresis if it is located below the loin, or by perspiration if above the loin." These principles are still significant as a guide to clinical practice. Methods of treatment mainly include causing perspiration, promoting diuresis, dispelling water, invigorating the spleen and replenishing *qi*, warming the kidneys and moving the turbid *qi* downwards. These methods are applied separately or in combination according to the actual conditions.

1. *Yang*-Type Edema

(1) Invasion by wind and overflow of water

Clinical manifestations: Edema starts from the eyelids and then spreads to the limbs and whole body. Its onset is acute. Other clinical manifestations are soreness and heaviness of the limbs and joints, dysuria, chills, an aversion to wind, and fever in most cases. The patient may also suffer from a cough, dyspnea, a thin white tongue coating, and a superficial and smooth or tense pulse. It is possible that the patient may show redness, swelling and pain in the throat, a red tongue, and a superficial, smooth and rapid pulse. A deep pulse appears if the edema is due to the overflow of water.

Analysis: Invasion by pathogenic wind impairs the lungs' regulation of the water passages. Failure of fluid to be sent to the urinary bladder leads to dysuria and general edema. Wind, a *yang* factor, occurs in gusts, and is characterized by upward dispersion and rapid change. It combines with water retained in the body to produce edema that starts from the face and head and then quickly spreads to the whole body. When the pathogenic factors reach the body surface, this hinders defensive *yang-qi*, resulting in chills, fever, soreness and heaviness of the limbs and joints. Invasion of the lungs by pathogenic water impairs dispersion and descent, thus causing coughing fits and dyspnea. A thin white tongue coating, and a superficial and smooth or tense pulse are signs of wind and water mixed with cold. A red tongue and a rapid, superficial pulse are signs of wind and water mixed with heat. Severe edema hinders *yang-qi* and thus a deep pulse results.

Treatment: To disperse wind, dissipate heat, promote dispersion and circulate water.

Prescription: Modified Decoction for Relieving Edema with Atractylodis Macrocephalae (295). Herba Ephedrae disperses wind, promotes dispersion and diuresis, and relieves edema; Gypsum Fibrosum disperses heat in the lungs; Rhizoma Atractylodis Macrocephalae invigorates the spleen and promotes diuresis; and Radix Glycyrrhizae, Rhizoma Zingiberis Recens and Fructus Jujubae harmonize the nutrient and defensive *qi*. To strengthen the diuretic effects, add Herba Plantaginis, Folium Pyrrosiae and Rhizoma Imperatae. In cases of redness, swelling and pain in the throat, remove Rhizoma Zingiberis Recens and Fructus Jujubae from the prescription, and add Radix Isatidis, Herba Taraxaci and Herba Houttuyniae to dissipate heat and eliminate toxins. If excess heat consumes *yin*, with symptoms of thirst and a red tongue, add Radix Rehmanniae and Radix Scrophulariae to nourish *yin* and disperse heat. If the external syndrome is pronounced, add Folium Perillae and Radix Ledebouriellae to eliminate wind-cold and relieve the external syndrome. If the patient is suffering from eczema, add Fructus Kochiae, Cortex Dictamni Radicis, and Radix Sophorae Flavescentis to eliminate wind, heat and dampness. If hematuria is present, add Herba Cirsii, Herba Capsellae and Rhizoma Imperatae to disperse heat and check bleeding. In cases of coughing and asthmatic breathing, add Semen Armeniacae Amarum and Radix Peucedani in mild cases, and Cortex Mori and Semen Lepidii seu Descurainiae in severe ones; these disperse heat in the lungs, relieve dyspnea and circulate water.

(2) Retained water and dampness

Clinical manifestations: Generalized massive edema, small amounts of urine, heaviness of the body, lassitude, stuffiness in the chest, a poor appetite, nausea, a sticky white tongue coating, and a deep and retarded pulse. Generally, there is no external syndrome. The onset of this disease is slow and its duration is long.

Analysis: Water and dampness retained in the muscles and the skin lead to edema of the limbs and body. They also impair the ability of the triple *jiao* to drain the water passages, as well as the ability of the urinary bladder to control urination, so the patient will only pass small amounts of urine. The retained water and dampness aggravate edema, and this causes generalized massive edema. When pathogenic dampness invades the spleen, the body's *yang-qi* will be hindered, resulting in heaviness, lassitude, stuffiness in the chest, and a poor appetite. A sticky white tongue coating and a deep and retarded pulse are signs of excess dampness and splenic deficiency.

Treatment: To invigorate the spleen, dry dampness, invigorate *yang* and promote diuresis.

Prescription: Modified Powder of Five Drugs Containing Poria (51) and Decoction Containing Five Kinds of Peel (50). Rhizoma Atractylodis Macrocephalae, Poria, and Pericarpium Citri Reticulatae invigorate the spleen and relieve dampness; and Ramulus Cinnamomi, Rhizoma Zingiberis Recens, Polyporus, Rhizoma Alismatis, Cortex Mori and Pericarpium Arecae invigorate *yang*, promote diuresis, move *qi*, and relax the middle *jiao*. If swelling is more pronounced in the upper half of the body and dyspnea is present, add Herba Ephedrae and Semen Armeniacae Amarum to promote pulmonary dispersion and relieve dyspnea. In cases of a thick, white, sticky tongue coating, an inability to taste anything, lassitude and epigastric distention, add Cortex Magnoliae Officinalis and Rhizoma Atractylodis to dry dampness, invigorate the spleen, circulate *qi* and relieve fullness.

(3) Excess dampness-heat

Clinical manifestations: Generalized edema, lustrous skin, distress in the chest and abdomen, restlessness, thirst, a hot sensation in the chest, small amounts of dark yellow urine, constipation, a sticky yellow tongue coating, and a deep, rapid pulse.

Analysis: If pathogenic water and dampness turn into heat, and spread to the muscles and skin, generalized edema with lustrous skin results. Retained dampness-heat blocks *qi* circulation, which causes thoracic and abdominal distress. The consumption of the body fluid due to excess heat results in restlessness, thirst, a hot sensation, small amounts of deep yellow urine, and constipation. A sticky yellow tongue coating and a deep, rapid pulse are signs of excess dampness-heat.

Treatment: To disperse heat and eliminate dampness both inside and outside the body.

Prescription: Modified *Shuzao* Decoction for Promoting Urination and Defecation (309). Radix Phytolaccae promotes diuresis and increases bowel movements; Semen Arecae and Pericarpium Arecae circulate *qi* and promote the movement of water; Poria, Rhizoma Alismatis, Caulis Aristolochiae Manshuriensis, Semen Zanthoxyli, and Semen Phaseoli eliminate retained water through urination and defecation; and Rhizoma seu Radix Notopterygii and Radix Gentianae Macrophyllae eliminate wind and relieve exterior symptoms by discharging surface water through sweating. If abdominal fullness persists and constipation is present, add Pill of Stephaniae Tetrandrae, Zanthoxyli, Lepidii seu Descurainiae, and Rhei (31) to strengthen the purgative effects. If the lungs are affected by the overflow of pathogenic water, and lung *qi* fails to descend, with symptoms of noisy breathing, orthopnea and a taut, rapid and strong pulse, eliminate water in the lungs by prescribing Decoction of Lepidii seu Descurainiae and Jujubae for Purging Lung-Heat (294).

2. *Yin*-Type Edema
(1) Spleen *yang*-deficiency

Clinical manifestations: Pitted edema below the loin is more pronounced than above it. Other clinical manifestations include epigastric distress, abdominal distention, a poor appetite, loose stools, a sallow complexion, lassitude, cold limbs, small amounts of urine, a pale tongue with a slippery white coating, and a deep, retarded pulse.

Analysis: This syndrome develops gradually over a long period of time. Deficient *yang-qi* of the middle *jiao* leads to the inability of *qi* to transform water. This causes an overflow of pathogenic water in the lower *jiao*; edema is thus more pronounced below the loin than above it, and pitted edema is seen. A deficiency of spleen-*yang* impairs transportation and transformation, thus causing epigastric distress, abdominal distention, a poor appetite, and loose stools. A deficiency of spleen *qi* implies that the sources for *qi* and blood are lacking. Shortage of nourishment and warmth gives rise to a sallow complexion, lassitude and cold limbs. When *yang* fails to produce *qi*, water and dampness are kept in the body, causing only small quantities of urine to be passed. A pale tongue with a slippery white coating, and a deep and retarded pulse are signs of splenic deficiency, water retention and hindrance of *yang-qi*.

Treatment: To warm and invigorate spleen *yang*, promote diuresis and dry dampness.

Prescription: Modified Decoction for Invigorating Spleen (180). Rhizoma Atractylodis Macrocephalae, Radix Glycyrrhizae and Fructus Jujubae replenish spleen *qi* to check water; Rhizoma Zingiberis, Radix Aconiti Lateralis Preparata and Fructus Tsaoko invigorate spleen *yang* to transport water and dampness; and Pericarpium Arecae, Poria, Cortex Magnoliae Officinalis, Radix Aucklandiae, Fructus Chaenomelis and Rhizoma Zingiberis Recens circulate *qi* and move water. The main function of this prescription is to warm *yang* and invigorate the spleen. If water and dampness are severe and the patient is only passing small quantities of urine, add Ramulus Cinnamomi, Polyporus and Rhizoma Alismatis to assist the bladder in promoting diuresis. In cases of splenic deficiency accompanied by shortness of breath, add Radix Astragali and Radix Codonopsis to replenish spleen *qi*.

There is another kind of edema caused by a bad diet, weak spleen and stomach, and the inability to fully absorb nutrition. This can be seen if the symptoms are general edema which is more pronounced on the head and face in the morning and in the lower limbs after physical labor, a good appetite, lassitude, normal stools, no reduction or even an increase in the quantity of urine passed, a sticky yellow tongue coating, and a weak pulse.

Splenic deficiency produces dampness, which leads to edema when retained. It also means impaired astringency, resulting in an increased volume of urine. Treatment aims to invigorate the spleen, replenish *qi*, and relieve dampness. It is not advisable simply to promote diuresis. In this case, Powder of Ginseng, Poria and Atractylodis Macrocephalae (190) can be prescribed. In this prescription, Radix Ginseng, Rhizoma Atractylodis Macrocephalae, Poria, Radix Glycyrrhizae, Rhizoma Dioscoreae, Semen Lablab Album and Semen Nelumbinis replenish *qi* and invigorate the spleen, Fructus Amomi regulates *qi* and harmonizes the stomach, Semen Coicis invigorates the spleen and resolves dampness, and Radix Platycodi conducts the action of the medicine upwards. To replenish *qi* and invigorate *yang*, add Radix Astragali and Ramulus Cinnamomi; to warm the kidneys and assist *yang*, add Radix Aconiti Lateralis Preparata and Fructus Psoraleae. Nutritious foods such as soybeans or peanuts are recommended.

(2) Kidney *yang*-deficiency

Clinical manifestations: Massive generalized and pitted edema which is more pronounced below the loin, and enlargement of the abdomen and swelling of the umbilicus in severe cases. Other manifestations include moisture of the external genitalia, palpitations, shortness of breath, pain, soreness, heaviness and a cold sensation in the lumbar region, reduced quantities of urine, cold limbs, lassitude, an aversion to cold, a grayish or pale complexion, a pale and swollen tongue with a white coating, and a deep and thready pulse or a deep and slow one.

Analysis: Kidney *yang*-deficiency means excess *yin* in the lower part of the body, so pitted edema is more pronounced below the loin. Water in the abdomen causes it to become enlarged and the umbilicus to become swollen. When this water spreads to the genitalia, it causes the scrotum to swell and produce moisture. Disturbance of the heart and lungs by water leads to palpitations and shortness of breath. Since the kidneys are located in the lumbar region, in cases where renal deficiencies are complicated by excess water, the patient will feel pain, soreness, heaviness, and a cold sensation in the lumbar region. Kidney *yang*-deficiency reduces the fire of the life gate, which deprives the limbs and body of nourishment, and leads to cold limbs, an aversion to cold and lassitude. It impairs bladder function; this explains the reduced quantities of urine and generalized massive edema. Failure of *yang-qi* to nourish in an upward direction causes a grayish or pale complexion. A pale and swollen tongue with a white coating, and a deep and thready or deep and slow pulse are signs of kidney *yang*-deficiency combined with excess water and dampness.

Treatment: To warm the kidneys, assist *yang*, promote *qi* and circulate water.

Prescription: Modified *Zhenwu* Decoction (223). Radix Aconiti Lateralis Preparata warms kidney *yang* and eliminates pathogenic water and dampness (*yin* and cold); Rhizoma Atractylodis Macrocephalae and Poria invigorate the spleen and conduct water downwards; Rhizoma Zingiberis Recens disperses water with its warmth; and Radix Paeoniae Alba harmonizes the nutrient and defensive *qi*, enters *yin* and relieves stagnation when used together with Radix Aconiti Lateralis Preparata. If cold caused by deficiencies is severe, add Semen Trigonellae, Radix Morindae Officinalis and Cortex Cinnamomi to warm kidney *yang* in order to assist transformation. In cases of obstruction to lung *qi* and dyspnea due to the invasion of lung *qi* by pathogenic water, add Semen Lepidii seu Descurainiae to promote smooth circulation, relieve dyspnea, circulate water and relieve edema. In cases where heart *yang* is blocked and the blood becomes stagnant as a result of water invading heart, the patient will show signs of palpitations, cyanosis of the lips and tongue, and a rapid feeble pulse. Then a large dose of Radix Aconiti Lateralis Preparata should be prescribed, with Ramulus Cinnamomi, Radix Glycyrrhizae Preparata, Radix Salviae Miltiorrhizze, Semen Persicae, and Flos Carthami to warm *yang* and resolve blood stasis. In cases of somnolence, nausea, or a smell of urine in the mouth, combine Radix Aconiti Lateralis Preparata with Radix et Rhizoma Rhei, Rhizoma Coptidis and Rhizoma Pinelliae to warm *yang*, eliminate toxins and relieve the turbid *qi*. If edema worsens and the patient shows an aversion to cold but an absence of sweating after exposure to external pathogenic cold, remove Radix Paeoniae Alba and add Herba Ephedrae, Herba Asari and Radix Glycyrrhizae to warm the meridians and disperse cold.

If *yang* deficiency in a prolonged case is complicated by *yin* deficiency, exhibiting repeated attacks of edema, lassitude, dizziness, tinnitus, lumbar soreness, nocturnal emissions, and bleeding of the gums, this suggests the failure of *yin* to preserve *yang*. Methods of counteracting this are to warm kidney *yang* and nourish *yin* fluid with diuresis by prescribing Decoction for Potently Invigorating *Qi* and Blood (21) and *Jisheng* Pill for Invigorating Kidney-*Qi* (206).

Remarks

In the treatment of edema, drastic purgatives for dispelling water should be used carefully. Clinical practice shows that if drastic purgatives are used recklessly, spleen *yang* will be seriously damaged and the body's anti-pathogenic *qi* will become even weaker, followed by symptoms of abdominal pain, diarrhea, nausea and vomiting, even though edema and abdominal distention are relieved temporarily. Especially when the lungs, spleen and kidneys are all deficient and triple *jiao* is impaired, temporary relief is soon followed by even more severe edema. If these drugs are used repeatedly, the body's anti-pathogenic *qi* will be destroyed, the amount of urine remain unchanged and edema will still exist. Therefore, the main methods of relieving edema are to promote pulmonary dispersion, cause sweating, invigorate *yang*, circulate water, invigorate the spleen, and warm the kidneys. In this way, edema subsides more slowly, but a faster recovery is expected. If edema is recent but severe, the anti-pathogenic *qi* is still strong, and the disease does not respond to the above methods of treatment, then a proper amount of drastic purgatives should be applied. When edema does subside, administer mild herbs. To dispel water without damaging the anti-pathogenic *qi*, and to strengthen resistance without retaining pathogenic factors, drastic purgatives for dispelling water can be combined with tonics.

The patient should be on a salt-free diet during the initial stages of treatment and a low-salt diet when edema gradually subsides. When the patient is cured, they can finally resume a normal diet. Pungent food, cigarettes, and alcohol should be avoided. If edema is caused by dystrophy, slightly less salty food is recommended although the patient does not have to be on a salt-free diet:

Case Studies

Name: Zhang XX; Sex: Female; Age: 35.
First visit: March 26, 1966.

The patient had suffered from edema of the face, eyes and lower limbs for over six months. Other clinical manifestations included epigastric and abdominal distention after eating, coughing fits, chest pain, shortness of breath, tinnitus, shallow sleep, palpitations, depression, red spots on the tongue, a thin, sticky tongue coating, and a thready and rapid pulse. She was suffering from tuberculosis of the right lung on the upper side, which was currently at the stage of absorption. The pathogenesis was deficient pulmonary and splenic *qi*, and deficient *yin*-blood. Treatment aimed to replenish the lung and spleen, nourish *yin* and calm the mind. The following herbs were prescribed:

Radix Astragali	12 g;
Rhizoma Atractylodis Macrocephalae (stir-baked)	9 g;
Poria	15 g;
Radix Glycyrrhizae Preparata	3 g;
Radix Aucklandiae	4.5 g;

Radix Salviae Miltiorrhizae	9 g;
Radix Paeoniae Rubra	12 g;
Herba Dendrobii	12 g.

Seven doses were prescribed.

This patient was hospitalized for tuberculosis. The prescription continued for over a month.

Second visit: May 7.

Edema of the face, eyes and lower limbs had subsided after the patient had taken over 30 doses. Other symptoms had also improved. The same herbs were prescribed to consolidate the results.

Discussion: Coughing, shortness of breath, edema and abdominal distention were all due to deficient pulmonary and splenic *qi*. In spite of the fact that signs of deficient *yin*-blood were present, such as a red tongue and a thready and rapid pulse, the key to the treatment was replenishing *qi* and nourishing *yin*. In the prescription, Radix Astragali, Rhizoma Atractylodis Macrocephalae, Poria and Radix Glycyrrhizae nourish the lung and spleen; Radix Aucklandiae regulates *qi* and invigorates transport and transformation; and Radix Salviae Miltiorrhizae, Radix Paeoniae Rubra and Herba Dendrobii nourish *yin* and calm the mind.

Name: Qin XX; Sex: Female; Age: 49; Occupation: Worker.

First visit: June 21, 1975.

She had suffered from general edema for nine years, with abdominal distention which was more pronounced after eating. The symptoms, which were aggravated in the summer, included a weighted sensation in the body, lassitude, loose stools and large quantities of urine. She had asked for help from both Chinese and Western doctors, but in vain. Her tongue was pale with a thick, gray, sticky coating and her pulse was soft and thready. Edema was caused by excess dampness following splenic deficiency. The principal method of treatment was to invigorate the spleen and relieve dampness. Modified *Weiling* Decoction (204) was prescribed.

Rhizoma Atractylodis	9 g;
Rhizoma Atractylodis Macrocephalae	9 g;
Cortex Magnoliae Officinalis	4.5 g;
Poria	12 g;
Radix Glycyrrhizae Preparata	4.5 g;
Ramulus Cinnamomi	4.5 g;
Radix Stephaniae Tetrandrae	12 g;
Radix Paeoniae Rubra	12 g;
Semen Arecae	4.5 g;
Massa Medicata Fermentata (charred)	12 g.

Fourteen doses were prescribed.

Second visit: July 5.

Abdominal distention and edema had improved, and urination and defecation had become normal. Nevertheless, the condition of the tongue remained unchanged. The same treatment was adopted. Nine grams of Herba Agastachis and nine grams of Herba Eupatorii were added to the previous prescription; another seven doses were prescribed.

Third visit: August 2.

She had not taken medicine for some time, so her condition was not stable, though edema had improved and both urination and defecation were normal. The tongue coating was thin and yellow, and the pulse was soft and thready. The same treatment was adopted. Cortex Magnoliae Officinalis was removed. Fourteen doses were prescribed.

Fourth visit: August 30.

The edema had almost completely subsided, but slight abdominal distention still existed. The patient's spirit was good, but her appetite was poor at times. Her tongue coating was thin and sticky, and yellow in the middle. Her pulse was soft and thready, but stronger than before. All this showed that splenic and gastric function were gradually being restored, but that residual dampness still remained. Since the disease responded to treatment with Chinese herbs, the same methods were adopted. Semen Arecae was removed from the prescription formulated at the first visit, and nine grams of Pericarpium Citri Reticulatae were added.

Discussion: This is a prolonged case of edema. Since the patient passed large quantities of urine, it is different from edema with dysuria. The pathogenesis was deficiency of the spleen leading to stagnant *qi*, which was even more pronounced when she was ill. Thus treatment aimed primarily at regulating *qi* and relieving distention. However, a pale tongue with a thick, gray, sticky coating suggested excess dampness due to splenic deficiency and the presence of heat; dampness therefore had to be dried, and the spleen invigorated. Once dampness had been eliminated, the heat was dispersed and *qi* circulated smoothly.

XXXVI. Stranguria

Stranguria refers to frequent urination and painful urination (possibly with dripping and pain in the lumbar region and abdomen) accompanied by contractions in the lower abdomen.

The term "stranguria" first appeared in *The Inner Canon of the Yellow Emperor*, but without a detailed description of its symptoms, etiology or pathology. The *Synopsis of Prescriptions of the Golden Chamber* was the first book to deal with its symptoms. It says, "One of symptoms of stranguria is dripping urination with pain in the lower abdomen and umbilicus."

There are five types of stranguria, stranguria due to urolithiasis, *qi* disorders, hematuria, chyluria, and stress. It can also be caused by heat. Clinical manifestations show that during their initial stages all five types are closely related to heat, especially stranguria due to urolithiasis, hematuria, and chyluria.

Urinary tract infections, stones in the urinary system, prostatitis, and chyluria in Western medicine may be diagnosed and treated according to the following descriptions.

Etiology and Pathogenesis

Synopsis of Prescriptions of the Golden Chamber holds that stranguria is due to "heat in the lower *jiao*." *The Pathogenesis and Manifestations of Diseases* says, "All types of stranguria are caused by renal deficiency and complicated by heat in the bladder." *A Complete Collection of Jingyue's Treatise* says, "There is no doubt that in its initial stages stranguria is caused by excess heat.... A prolonged case of stranguria manifesting the persistent discharge of white and cloudy urine, but the absence of pain or difficult urination, results from the sinking *qi* of the middle *jiao* and the weakness of the life gate."

All this shows that the downward movement of dampness-heat to the lower *jiao* causes stranguria in its initial stages, when it is characterized by painful, frequent, and urgent urination with deep yellow urine. In prolonged cases, the syndrome is transformed from one caused by excesses to one caused by deficiencies, or a combination of the two.

1. Retained Dampness-Heat

Dampness-heat comes from external invasion of pathogenic factors, excessive greasy, sweet or pungent food or an excessive intake of alcohol. Once produced, dampness-heat moves downwards to the lower *jiao*, impairing the bladder's ability to control urination, and leading to frequent, difficult and painful urination with dripping urine and a contracting feeling in the lower abdomen. If dampness-heat is retained over a long period of time, this causes the urine to solidify into stones, and stranguria with urolithiasis then appears. The impaired division of the clear and turbid *qi* due to retained dampness-heat in the lower *jiao* gives rise to milky urine, which is known as stranguria with chyluria. When heart fire moves down to the small intestine, it damages the blood vessels and causes extravasation of blood, and stranguria with hematuria occurs.

2. Splenic and Renal Deficiencies

In prolonged cases, these are caused by the consumption of the body's anti-pathogenic *qi* by dampness-heat, the weakness of the body in elderly patients, fatigue or excessive sexual activity. Deficient kidney *qi* of the middle *jiao* and the sinking of *qi* combine to produce stranguria due to disorders of *qi*. Deficient kidney *qi* means an inability to check greasy fluid; the result is cloudy urine or urination with greasy clots, which is referred to as stranguria with chyluria. Deficient kidney *yin* produces hyperactive fire, which causes extravasation of blood; stranguria with hematuria thus results. These three types of stranguria are recurrent. Since fatigue induces this complaint, the condition is known as stranguria caused by stress.

3. Stagnant Liver *Qi*

Depression and anger both damage the liver and cause stagnant liver *qi*, which turns into fire in prolonged cases. Stagnant *qi* in the lower *jiao* may be complicated by fire. In either case, the functions of the bladder are impaired, resulting in symptoms such as difficult and painful urination with dripping urine and a weighted distention of the lower abdomen. This condition is referred to as stranguria due to disorders of *qi*. *An Essential Medical Manual* states, "Stranguria due to *qi* disorders is of the two types, one caused by deficiencies and the other by excesses." In other words, this kind of stranguria is attributed to deficient or stagnant *qi*.

Differentiation and Treatment

Whether the condition is caused by deficiencies and excesses should be diagnosed. For example, stranguria due to stagnant liver *qi* is caused by excesses, while that due to deficient and sinking *qi* is caused by deficiencies. Stranguria with hematuria due to the downward movement of dampness-heat is caused by excesses, while that due to *yin* deficiency leading to hyperactive fire is caused by deficiencies. Stranguria with chyluria complicated by dampness-heat may develop into kidney deficiency, thus producing a combined syndrome of deficiency and excess.

In summary, stranguria's main manifestation in its initial stages is as a hot syndrome caused by excesses. The primary method of treatment is to disperse heat and promote diuresis. A prolonged case or the excessive oral administration of herbs that disperse heat and promote diuresis may lead to a deficiency syndrome. Treatment then aims primarily to replenish the spleen and kidneys. Replenishment and elimination should be used together in the treatment of syndromes combining deficiency and excess.

1. Stranguria due to Urolithiasis

Clinical manifestations: Sandy stones in the urine, difficult urination, or an abrupt discontinuation of the stream of urine, pain in the urethra, contractive feeling in the lower abdomen, or cramping pain in the lumbar and abdominal regions, blood-tinged urine occurs in severe cases only, a red tongue with a thin, yellow coating, and a taut or rapid pulse.

Analysis: The downward movement of dampness-heat solidifies urine into stones, resulting in difficult and painful urination. Big stones block the urethra, causing the abrupt discontinuation of the stream of urine and painful urination. Damage to the blood vessels by the stones leads to blood-tinged urine. A red tongue with a thin yellow coating and a rapid pulse are signs of excess dampness-heat. Pain in the urethra causes a taut pulse.

Treatment: To disperse heat, eliminate dampness, relieve stranguria and dispel stones.

Prescription: Powder of Pyrrosiae (76) is the main formula, in which Folium Pyrrosiae, Talcum, and Fructus Malvae relieve stranguria and dispel stones; Herba Dianthi and Semen Plantaginis disperse heat and promote diuresis. To help dispel stones, add Herba Lysimachiae, Spora Lygodii, and Endothelium Corneum Gigeriae Galli. In cases when the patient suffers from constipation, as well as a dry mouth and throat and the desire to drink cold drinks, add Powder for Dispersing Heat and Promoting Urination (12). In the recipe, Caulis Aristolochiae Manshuriensis, Semen Plantaginis, Herba Dianthi, Herba Polygoni Avicularis and Talcum relieve stranguria and eliminate dampness; and Radix et Rhizoma Rhei, Fructus Gardeniae and Radix Glycyrrhizae dissipate heat and fire. In cases of fever, add Herba Taraxaci and Cortex Phellodendri. In cases of hematuria, add Herba Cirsii, Pollen Typhae and Rhizoma Imperatae. In cases where there are no symptoms most of the time, 30-60 grams of Herba Lysimachiae can be prepared as a beverage to promote diuresis and dispel stones.

2. Stranguria due to *Qi* Disorders

Clinical manifestations: In cases of stagnant liver *qi*, clinical manifestations include difficult urination, distensive pain in the lower abdomen, a bluish tongue, and a deep and taut pulse. In cases of deficient *qi* in the middle *jiao*, symptoms include a weighted sensation and distending pain in the lower abdomen, dripping of urine after urination, a pale complexion, a pale, swollen tongue, and a weak pulse.

Analysis: The lower abdomen is traversed by the Liver Meridian of Foot-*Jueyin*. Depression leads to stagnant liver *qi*, and in extreme cases it can lead to the impaired control of urination. Thus symptoms such as difficult urination and distending pain appear. Stagnant liver *qi* also causes a bluish tongue and a deep and taut pulse. The sinking of *qi* in the middle *jiao* explains the weighted sensation and the abdominal pain. Deficient *qi* leads to an inability to control urination, and so the dripping of urine occurs. A pale complexion, a pale tongue and a weak pulse are signs of deficient *qi* and blood.

Treatment: To promote smooth circulation of *qi* in cases of stagnant liver *qi*, to replenish the middle *jiao* and benefit *qi* in cases when it is deficient in the middle *jiao*.

Prescription: Powder of Lignum Aquilariae Resinatum (149) should be prescribed for a syndrome caused by excesses; and modified Decoction for Strengthening Middle *Jiao* and Benefiting *Qi* (154) can be used for deficiency syndromes. In the former, Lignum Aquilariae Resinatum and Pericarpium Citri Reticulatae promote the smooth circulation of *qi*; Radix Paeoniae Alba nourishes the blood and the liver; and Folium Pyrrosiae, Talcum, Fructus Malvae, Radix Glycyrrhizae and Semen Vaccariae disperse heat and promote diuresis. In cases of distensive lower abdominal pain, add Pericarpium Citri Reticulatae Viride and Fructus Foeniculi to promote the circulation of liver *qi*. In cases where *qi* and blood are stagnant for prolonged periods of time, add Flos Carthami and Radix Paeoniae Rubra to activate blood circulation and relieve the stasis. The latter replenishes *qi* in the middle *jiao*. If signs of blood deficiency are also present, herbs that replenish blood should be used.

3. Stranguria with Hematuria

Clinical manifestations: Difficult and painful urination with hot purplish-red urine, which contains blood clots in serious cases. The pain is urgent and violent. The patient may also feel restless. The patient will have a yellow tongue coating and a smooth and rapid pulse. In prolonged cases, urine becomes pale red, and the pain less severe. The accompanying symptoms include lassitude, lumbar soreness, a slightly red tongue and a thready and rapid pulse, all of which suggest a deficiency syndrome.

Analysis: Retained dampness-heat in the lower *jiao* impairs the patient's control over urination, causing difficult and painful urination with hot urine. Heat damages the blood vessels and extravasates blood, thus resulting in purplish-red urine. Stagnant blood and heat block the urinary tract, causing blood clots in the urine and an urgent, violent pain. If heart fire is hyperactive, restlessness follows. A yellow tongue coating and a smooth and rapid pulse are signs of heat. In prolonged cases, the consumption of kidney *yin* is the reason for the slightly red urine, lassitude and lumbar soreness. A slightly red tongue and a thready and rapid pulse suggest heat caused by deficiencies.

Treatment: To dissipate heat, eliminate dampness, cool the blood and check bleeding in syndromes caused by excesses, and to nourish *yin*, disperse heat, reinforce resistance and check bleeding in syndromes caused by deficiencies.

Prescription: Decoction of Cirsii (38) should be prescribed for an excess syndrome; Bolus of Anemarrhenae, Phellodendri and Rehmanniae Preparata (181) can be used for syndromes caused by deficiencies. In the former, Herba Cirsii, Radix Rehmanniae, Pollen Typhae and Nodus Nelumbinis Rhizomatis cool the blood and check bleeding; Herba Lophatheri, Caulis Aristolochiae Manshuriensis, Fructus Gardeniae and Talcum disperse heat, eliminate dampness and relieve restlessness by clearing heat in the heart; Radix Angelicae Sinensis and Radix Glycyrrhizae harmonize the nutrient *qi* and check pain. The latter prescription nourishes *yin* and disperses heat. To reinforce resistance and check bleeding, add Herba Ecliptae, Herba Agrimoniae and Colla Corii Asini. In cases of lumbar pain, add Radix Dipsaci and Herba Taxilli.

4. Stranguria with Chyluria

Clinical manifestations: Urine is cloudy and white, like milk or rice water. It can be pinkish in cases where bleeding occurs or mixed with blood clots. The patient will feel a hot sensation and pain in the urethra during urination. Other signs include a red tongue with a sticky coating and a rapid pulse. In prolonged cases where relapses are repeated, urination will be difficult, but less painful. The patient's urine will be milky and the patient may experience lassitude, soreness and weakness in the lumbar region and knees, dizziness, tinnitus, emaciation, a pale tongue with a sticky coating, and a thready and weak pulse.

Analysis: The downward movement of dampness-heat to the bladder impairs its function, and thus the clear and turbid *qi* mix together, causing milky urine and heat and pain in the urethra during urination. Heat damages the blood vessels and causes extravasation. Thus pinkish urine results, showing that this syndrome is caused by excesses. In prolonged cases, renal deficiency implies the inability to control greasy fluid, resulting in greasy urine; it also causes soreness and weakness in the lumbar region and knees, dizziness, lassitude and emaciation, all of which suggest a syndrome caused by deficiencies.

Treatment: To clear dampness-heat and divide the clear and the turbid *qi* in a syndrome caused by excesses, and to replenish the kidneys and promote astringency in a syndrome caused by deficiencies.

Prescription: Modified Cheng's Decoction of Dioscoreae Septemlobae for Clearing Turbid Urine (305) can be used to treat syndromes caused by excesses; modified Pill of Six Drugs Containing Rehmanniae Preparata (56) can be used to treat syndromes caused by deficiencies. In the former, Rhizoma Dioscoreae Septemlobae and Rhizoma Acori Tatarinowii divide the clear and the turbid *qi*; Cortex Phellodendri, Poria and Semen Plantaginis disperse heat and eliminate dampness; Semen Nelumbinis and Radix Salviae Miltiorrhizae disperse cardiac heat and relieve restlessness; and Rhizoma Atractylodis Macrocephalae invigorates the spleen and relieves dampness. The latter prescription replenishes the kidneys, dissipates heat and relieves dampness. To replenish the kidneys and promote astringency, add Semen Cuscutae, Semen Euryales, Fructus Rosae Laevigatae, Os Draconis and Concha Ostreae. To disperse heat and relieve dampness, add Herba Capsellae, and Stigma Maydis, or 240 grams of Radix Oryzae Glutinosae which should be decocted as a beverage.

5. Stranguria Caused by Strain

Clinical manifestations: Red urine and difficult urination are less pronounced, but dripping urination is protracted and is often induced by strain. Other clinical manifestations include lassitude, soreness of the lumbar region and knees or a weighted sensation in the lower abdomen, dripping of urine after urination, a pale tongue, and a weak and feeble pulse.

Analysis: Prolonged cases of stranguria, excess oral administration of cold and cool herbs, weakness of the body following a prolonged illness, or stress may all lead to splenic and renal deficiencies complicated by turbid dampness. Exertion therefore induces attacks in which red urine and difficult urination are not pronounced. Deficient *qi* in the middle *jiao* and the impaired control of urine lead to lassitude, soreness and weakness, a weighted sensation, and dripping of urine. A pale tongue and a weak and feeble pulse are both signs of splenic and renal deficiency.

Treatment: To invigorate the spleen and replenish the kidneys.

Prescription: Modified Pill of Dioscoreae for Nourishing Kidney (41). Rhizoma Dioscoreae, Poria and Rhizoma Alismatis invigorate the spleen and eliminate dampness and Radix Rehmanniae Preparata, Fructus Corni, Radix Morindae Officinalis, Semen Cuscutae, Cortex Eucommiae, Radix Achyranthis Bidentatae, Herba Cistanches, Fructus Schisandrae and Halloysitum Rubrum replenish the kidneys and promote astringency. In cases of splenic deficiency and sinking *qi*, with a weighted lower abdominal sensation and dripping of urine at the end of the stream, Decoction for Strengthening Middle *Jiao* and Benefiting *Qi* (154) can also be used. In cases of kidney *yin*-deficiency when the patient's face is flushed, and the patient experiences restlessness, a hot sensation in the palms, soles and chest, a red tongue and a thready and rapid pulse, remove Radix Morindae Officinalis, Semen Cuscutae and Herba Cistanches and add Rhizoma Anemarrhenae and Cortex Phellodendri to nourish *yin* and subdue fire. In cases of kidney *yang*-deficiency, add powder of Cornu Cervi to warm the kidneys and assist *yang*.

In ancient times, some doctors held that replenishing and diaphoretic therapies should be avoided in the treatment of stranguria. For instance, *A Supplement to Diagnosis and Treatment* says, "Tonics cause the stagnation of *qi* to become even more intense, making the blood flow less smoothly and the heat becomes more excessive." *Synopsis of Prescriptions of the Golden Chamber* holds, "Inducing sweating is prohibited in the treatment of stranguria." Clinical experience shows that chills and fever often occur together with difficult and painful urination. Since these are caused by excess dampness-heat struggling with the body's anti-pathogenic *qi*, they are different from fever caused by external syndrome. It is unnecessary to prescribe acrid herbs that induce sweating for this condition. Fever in stranguria is mostly caused by heat in the bladder; *yin* fluid is insufficient in such cases. If sweating is induced in an incorrect fashion, this cannot lower the body temperature, but will consume *yin* fluid, thus aggravating hematuria. If external syndromes such as fever, chilliness, coughing and rhinorrhea are present, a proper quantity of herbs that eliminate wind and relieve external symptoms should be used. Both internal and external symptoms should be treated simultaneously. In cases where the illness is caused by excess heat, tonics are contraindicated. If stranguria is caused by the sinking *qi* of the middle *jiao* and renal deficiency with impaired astringent functioning, then *qi* of the middle *jiao* should be replenished, the kidneys should be invigorated and astringency promoted.

Appendix: Cloudy Urine

Cloudy urine, as white as rice water, is not accompanied by painful urination. It is closely related to the spleen and kidneys. There are four conditions which cause cloudy urine.

Cloudy urine, accompanied by fullness in the chest, thirst, a sticky yellow tongue coating and a soft pulse, is due to the downward movement of dampness-heat from the spleen and stomach to the bladder after excessive greasy or sweet food. Decoction of Dioscoreae Septemlobae for Clearing Turbid Urine (288) is then prescribed. Rhizoma Dioscoreae Septemlobae dispels turbid dampness; Fructus Alpiniae Oxyphyllae warms and replenishes the spleen and kidneys; Radix Linderae warms kidney *qi* and Rhizoma Acori Tatarinowii promotes diuresis. To help disperse heat and relieve dampness, add Herba Lysimachiae, Cortex Phellodendri, and Spora Lygodii.

If the patient has had cloudy urine for prolonged periods accompanied by a pale complexion, lassitude, a pale tongue and a weak and feeble pulse, this is due to the deficient and sinking *qi* of the spleen complicated by the downward movement of essence. Decoction for Strengthening Middle *Jiao* and Benefiting *Qi* (154) can be prescribed to replenish *qi* and send the clear *qi* upward.

Cloudy urine accompanied by restlessness, a hot sensation in the chest, thirst, a red tongue, and a thready and slightly rapid pulse is due to a deficiency of kidney *yin* complicated by the transmission of heat to the bladder. *Yin* can be nourished and the heat can be dispersed with Bolus of Anemarrhenae, Phellodendri and Rehmanniae Preparata (181).

Cloudy urine accompanied by a pale complexion, cold limbs, lassitude, a pale tongue and a deep and thready pulse can stem from renal deficiency, stagnant cold, and impaired control of urine. The kidneys are warmed and astringency promoted by prescribing *Yougui* Pill (82).

Case Studies

Name: Yao XX; Sex: Female; Age: 30.
First visit: August 15, 1963.

The patient came down with acute cystitis in 1960, and after taking furadantin and sintomycin, she became much better. However, she had relapses four or five times from March to July this year. Now, she micturated frequently and experienced a burning sensation in the urethra and lumbar pain. Her appetite was normal, her pulse taut and feeble at the right *cun* and *guan* positions, and deep and rapid at the left *cun* and *chi* positions, and her tongue was dark red with a sticky yellow coating. The pathogenesis was accumulated dampness-heat in the lower *jiao* and an inability to divide the clear and the turbid *qi*. The clear *qi* was sent upwards and the turbid *qi* downwards by prescribing the following herbs:

Rhizoma Dioscoreae Septemlobae	9 g;
Fructus Alpiniae Oxyphyllae	4.5 g;
Rhizoma Acori Tatarinowii	6 g;
Poria	6 g;
Herba Artemisiae Scopariae	6 g;
Rhizoma Alismatis	4.5 g;
Cortex Phellodendri (stir-baked with salty water)	3 g;
Rhizoma Alismatis	4.5 g;
Cortex Cinnamomi (ground to powder with coarse bark removed, and taken separately)	0.6 g;
Medulla Tetrapanacis	3 g.

Three doses were prescribed.
Second visit: August 27.

The burning sensation and hot urine had improved after six doses and Six-to-One Powder (54) was being taken as a beverage. The patient's pulse was deep, thready, and slightly rapid, and taut and rapid on the left *guan* position. Her tongue was pale with a sticky white coating. Treatment aimed at harmonizing the spleen and eliminating dampness. Rhizoma Acori Tatarinowii was removed from the prescription, and nine grams of Talcum, one and a half grams of Radix Glycyrrhizae and three grams of Rhizoma Atractylodis Macrocephalae were added. Another five doses were prescribed. All symptoms disappeared after these herbs were finished.

Discussion: Both the pulse and symptoms suggest stranguria due to heat. Thus Decoction of Dioscoreae Septemlobae for Clearing Turbid Urine (288) and Pill for Nourishing Kidney and Promoting Urination (304) were prescribed to clear dampness-heat and send the clear *qi* upwards and the turbid *qi* downwards.

Name: Huang XX; Sex: Female; Age: 28.
First visit: April 6, 1975.

The day before, the patient began to experience frequent, difficult and painful urination with hot urine, lumbar soreness, lower abdominal distention, restlessness and insomnia. Her tongue was red with a sticky coating. Her pulse was thready and rapid. The urinalysis showed protein ++, red blood cells ++++, and white blood cells 0-1. Thus the disease was due to the accumulation of dampness-heat in the lower *jiao*, which impaired the control of urine and caused a downward flow of blood. It was obviously a case of stranguria with hematuria. Treatment aimed to cool the blood, nourish *yin* and disperse dampness-heat. The following herbs were prescribed:

Radix Rehmanniae	15 g;
Herba Lophatheri	9 g;
Radix Glycyrrhizae	4.5 g;
Caulis Aristolochiae Manshuriensis	3 g;
Radix Scutellariae	15 g;
Herba Cirsii	30 g;
Radix Linderae	9 g.

Two doses were prescribed.

Second visit: April 8.

All symptoms had improved the day before, but frequent, difficult, and painful urination, lumbar soreness, and distending pain recurred this morning. The tongue coating was sticky, and the pulse was thready and rapid. The urinalysis showed a trace of protein, and red blood cells ++++. The same treatment was adopted. Fifteen grams of Rhizoma Dioscoreae Septemlobae were added to the previous prescription. Two doses were prescribed.

Third visit: April 10.

Frequent urination had improved markedly, the patient's urine had become clear, and the distending pain generally no longer bothered the patient, but she still suffered from lumbar soreness and lassitude. Her pulse was thready and rapid. The urinalysis showed red blood cells 0-1, and white blood cells 0-1. The same treatment was adopted. Caulis Aristolochiae Manshuriensis was removed. Four doses were prescribed.

Discussion: The initial stage of stranguria was marked by excess dampness and heat. Thus dampness-heat was dispersed and diuresis promoted. Since the patient exhibited restlessness, insomnia, a red tongue and a thready pulse, suggesting hyperactive heart-fire, Powder for Promoting Diuresis with additional herbs was prescribed. In the recipe, Radix Rehmanniae cools the blood and nourishes *yin* and Herba Lophatheri disperses cardiac heat and reduces fire. The use of fresh herbs here is preferable. Caulis Aristolochiae Manshuriensis and Radix Glycyrrhizae disperse heat, promote urination and relieve pain in the urethra; Herba Cirsii, used in large dosages, cools the blood and checks bleeding; Rhizoma Dioscoreae Septemlobae eliminates dampness and divides the clear and the turbid *qi*; and Radix Linderae circulates *qi* and eases pain in the urinary tract. All herbs combine to check bleeding and relieve stranguria.

XXXVII. Retention of Urine

In Chinese, retention of urine is known as *long-bi*. *Long* refers to mild dysuria when the patient only passes small amounts of urine and experiences dripping urination, while *bi* is more acute, when urine is completely retained. In either condition, the patient feels some difficulty in urination.

The term *long-bi* first appeared in *The Inner Canon of the Yellow Emperor*. According to this, the disease is located in the bladder and its pathogenesis is impaired control of urine and body fluid by the bladder and triple *jiao*. This name for this disease could not be used during the reign of Emperor Shang Di in the Eastern Han Dynasty because the emperor was called Liu Long, and it was considered graceless to use the same word for a disease. *Long-bi* then fell out of use in the medical classics written in the several years that followed until the time of the Ming Dynasty. This complaint should be discussed together with other urinary difficulties.

The causes for this disease have been discussed by medical scholars throughout the ages. Chao Yuanfang, a physician of the Sui Dynasty, held that it was caused by heat in the kidneys and the urinary bladder. Zhu Danxi thought that retention of urine could be caused by factors such as deficient *qi* and blood as well as phlegm, wind and heat caused by excesses. Zhang Jingyue attributed urine retention to the following four reasons: accumulation of pathogenic fire in the small intestine and bladder, blockage of the water passages by stale essence and stagnant blood, deficiency of kidney *yang* with impaired control of urine, and stagnant liver *qi* affecting the urinary bladder.

Experience has accumulated in the treatment of urine retention. Clinically, treatment is determined on the basis of causes. Apart from oral administration of Chinese herbal decoctions, Sun Simiao of the Tang Dynasty applied urethral catheterization with the tubal leaf of the spring onion; Zhang Jingyue mentioned urethral catheterization with a goose feather tube and Zhu Danxi adopted the method of induced vomiting*.

Retained urine from varying causes and anuria due to kidney failure in Western medicine can be differentiated and treated according to the following descriptions.

Etiology and Pathogenesis

The urinary bladder is primarily responsible for retained urine. Unobstructed urination relies on the normal functioning of the triple *jiao* in regulating body fluid, which is further guaranteed by the lungs, spleen and kidneys. Therefore, this disease is closely related to the kidneys, lungs, spleen and the triple *jiao*. In addition, stagnant liver *qi* and blockage by stagnant blood may also account for this illness.

1. Accumulation of Dampness-Heat

The downward movement of dampness-heat of the middle *jiao* to the urinary bladder, or the transmission of heat there from the kidneys to the urinary bladder may impair control of urination.

2. Lung Heat and Stagnant Lung *Qi*

The lung is the upper source of water, and regulates the body's water passages. If heat is retained in the lungs, it does not allow lung *qi* to descend and impairs regulation. The downward movement of excess heat to the urinary bladder produces a blockage of *qi* in both the upper and lower *jiao*.

3. Failure of Spleen *Qi* to Ascend

Stress, an improper diet, or a weakened system following prolonged illness may all lead to renal deficiency. The clear *qi* is unable to ascend, while the turbid *yin* cannot descend, resulting in dysuria.

4. Kidney Deficiency

Weak resistance due to old age or following prolonged illness causes kidney *yang*-deficiency and the declining of fire at life gate. Here the control of urination is impaired, and retention of urine then occurs. Accumulation of heat in the lower *jiao* over a long period of time consumes fluid, and causes deficient kidney *yin*. In this case, *yang-qi* fails to be produced, resulting in retained urine.

5. Stagnant Liver *Qi*

Emotional trauma leads to stagnant liver *qi*. If the free flow of *qi* is impaired, this affects the ability of the triple *jiao* to transport, transform and regulate body fluid. On the other hand, the Liver Meridian curves around the external genitalia and passes through the lower abdomen; this explains why disorders of the Liver Meridian can lead to retained urine.

6. Blockage of the Urinary Tract

Blockage by stagnant blood, stale essence, lumps or stones makes it difficult to urinate.

Diagnosis

The symptoms of both stranguria and urine retention are difficulty in micturation and passing only small quantities of urine. But in stranguria, there is frequent and painful urination, and the total amount of urine passed every day is normal. Things are different in urine retention as no pain is felt when urinating, and the total amount of urine passed is less than normal or even none at all.

Differentiation and Treatment

First of all, it should be distinguished whether the condition is caused by deficiencies or excesses. If the retained urine is due to accumulated dampness-heat, stagnant liver *qi*, heat retained in the lungs and stagnant lung *qi*, or stagnant blood blocking the urethra, then it is caused by excesses. However, deficiencies cause the retention of urine when the spleen *qi* fails to ascend and when there is a deficiency in kidney *yang*. Emphasis should be laid on removing any obstructions, because the *fu* organs function better when unobstructed. The method of removing obstructions when the syndrome is caused by excesses is different from that used when the syndrome is caused by deficiencies. Obstructions of the water passages can be removed in the former case by dispersing dampness-heat and stagnant blood and promoting the smooth circulation of *qi*. Urinary obstruction can be removed in the latter by replenishing the spleen and kidneys and assisting the regulation of body fluid. In the meantime, treatment should also be based on the causes and on which organs are diseased. Herbs that promote diuresis should not be used indiscriminately.

1. Dampness-Heat in the Urinary Bladder

Clinical manifestations: Retention of urine or discharge of small quantities of hot, dark yellow urine, distention and fullness in the lower abdomen, a bitter taste and stickiness in the mouth, or dryness of the mouth with no desire to drink, constipation, a red tongue with a sticky yellow coating at the root, and a rapid pulse.

Analysis: Accumulation of dampness-heat in the urinary bladder impairs control over urination, thus causing dysuria with hot, dark yellow urine, or retention of urine in severe cases. Stagnant *qi* due to retained dampness-heat leads to distention and fullness. Excess dampness-heat inside the body gives rise to a bitter taste and stickiness in the mouth. The inability to distribute fluid causes a dry mouth but with no desire to drink. A red tongue with a sticky yellow coating at the root, a rapid pulse and constipation are signs of dampness-heat in the lower *jiao*.

Treatment: To disperse heat, eliminate dampness and promote diuresis.

Prescription: Modified Powder for Dispersing Heat and Promoting Urination (12). Caulis Aristolochiae Manshuriensis, Semen Plantaginis, Herba Polygoni Avicularis, and Herba Dianthi promote diuresis; Fructus Gardeniae clears dampness-heat of the triple *jiao*; Talcum and Radix Glycyrrhizae clear dampness-heat in the lower *jiao*; and Radix et Rhizoma Rhei relieves constipation and reduces fire. Long-retained dampness-heat in the lower *jiao* consumes kidney *yin*, giving rise to thirst, a dry throat, hectic fever, night sweating, a hot sensation in the palms and soles, and a glossy red tongue. In this case, prescribe Pill for Nourishing Kidneys and Promoting Urination (304) and add Radix Rehmanniae, Semen Plantaginis, and Radix Achyranthis Bidentatae to nourish kidney *yin*, clear dampness-heat and regulate body fluid.

2. Excess Heat in the Lung

Clinical manifestations: Difficulty in urination or retention of urine, a dry throat, restlessness, thirst, shortness of breath or coughing, a thin yellow tongue coating, and a rapid pulse.

Analysis: Excess heat in the lungs prevents them from sending fluid down to the urinary bladder, resulting in the retention of urine. Excess heat in the lungs also causes the upward movement of lung *qi* coupled with a shortness of breath and coughing. A dry throat, restlessness, thirst, a yellow tongue coating and a rapid pulse are manifestations of heat retained inside the body.

Treatment: To disperse heat in the lungs and regulate the water passages.

Prescription: Modified Decoction for Clearing Away Lung-Heat (280). Radix Scutellariae, Cortex Mori and Radix Ophiopogonis disperse heat in the lungs and nourish lung *yin*; Semen Plantaginis, Caulis Aristolochiae Manshuriensis, Poria, and Fructus Gardeniae dissipate heat and promote urination. In cases of hyperactive heart fire with symptoms of restlessness and red tongue tip, add Rhizoma Coptidis and Herba Lophatheri to clear heart fire. In cases of lung *yin*-deficiency as shown by a dry, red tongue, add Radix Adenophorae, and Bulbus Lilii to nourish lung *yin*.

3. Stagnant Liver *Qi*

Clinical manifestations: Depression or irritability, retention of urine or difficulty in passing urine, distention and fullness of the hypochondrium and abdomen, a red tongue with a thin coating or a yellow coating, and a taut pulse.

Analysis: Stagnant liver *qi* due to emotional trauma impairs the ability of the triple *jiao* to produce *qi* and regulate fluid, resulting in the retention of urine or difficulty in passing urine, along with distention and fullness. A taut pulse suggests a hyperactive liver, and a red tongue with a thin coating or a yellow coating implies that stagnant liver *qi* has turned into fire.

Treatment: To regulate *qi* circulation and promote diuresis.

Prescription: Modified Powder of Lignum Aquilariae Resinatum (149). Lignum Aquilariae Resinatum and Pericarpium Citri Reticulatae promote the smooth circulation of liver *qi*; Radix Angelicae Sinensis, and Semen Vaccariae circulate *qi* and blood in the lower *jiao*; and Folium Pyrrosiae, Radix Semiaquilegiae and Talcum regulate the water passages. Since this prescription is not strong enough to regulate *qi*, Rhizoma Cyperi, Radix Curcumae, and Radix Linderae should be added to promote the smooth circulation of liver *qi*. If stagnant *qi* turns into fire, add Cortex Moutan, Radix Gentianae, and Fructus Gardeniae to disperse heat in the liver and reduce fire.

4. Blockage of the Urinary Tract

Clinical manifestations: Dripping urine, urinating with a stream as fine as a thread, or retention of urine in severe cases, distention, fullness and pain in the lower abdomen, a dark purplish tongue or a tongue with purple spots, and an unsmooth pulse.

Analysis: Blockage of the urethra by stagnant blood or stale essence leads to dripping, threadlike or retained urination, and lower abdominal distention, fullness and pain. A dark purplish tongue or a tongue with purple spots, and an unsmooth pulse are signs of stagnant *qi* and blood.

Treatment: To remove stagnant blood, disperse stagnation and regulate water passages.

Prescription: *Daididang* Pill (99). Radix Angelicae Sinensis Squama Manitis, Semen Persicae, Radix et Rhizoma Rhei and Natrii Sulfas remove blood stasis and resolve stagnation. To help activate blood circulation and remove stasis, add Flos Carthami and Radix Achyranthis Bidentatae. In prolonged cases which exhibit deficiencies of both *qi* and blood so that the patient has a pale complexion, add Radix Astragali, Radix Salviae Miltiorrhizae, and Radix Angelicae Sinensis to replenish *qi* and blood. In cases of temporary retention of urine which causes an unbearable feeling of distention, administer a small dose of Moschus as well. In cases of urolithiasis, add Herba Lysimachiae, Spora Lygodii, Fructus Malvae Verticillatae, Herba Dianthi and Herba Polygoni Avicularis to dispel stones and promote diuresis. In cases of hematuria, administer Radix Notoginseng and Succinum.

5. Deficiency of *Qi* of the Middle *Jiao*

Clinical manifestations: A weighted sensation in the lower abdomen, retention of urine, or dysuria with only small quantities of urine. Other manifestations include lassitude, shortness of breath, a feeble voice, a pale tongue with a thin coating, and a thready and weak pulse.

Analysis: The clear *qi* fails to ascend, and thus the turbid *yin* fails to descend; the result is dysuria. Deficient *qi* of the middle *jiao* causes the feeble voice and its sinking produces a weighted sensation. Deficient spleen *qi* means that its transporting and transforming functions are weak, causing lassitude and a poor appetite. A pale tongue and a thready and weak pulse are signs of deficient *qi*.

Treatment: To send the clear *qi* upwards and the turbid *yin* downwards, produce *qi*, and circulate water.

Prescription: Modified Decoction for Strengthening Middle *Jiao* and Benefiting *Qi* (154) and *Chunze* Decoction (194). The former replenishes the *qi* of the middle *jiao* and raises the clear *qi*. When spleen *qi* ascends, the turbid *yin* will descend. The latter produces *qi* and circulates water.

6. Deficient Kidney *Yang*

Clinical manifestations: Retained or dripping urine, a weak stream of urine, a pale complexion, lassitude, aversion to cold, a cold sensation, soreness and weakness of the lumbar region and knees, a pale tongue with a white coating, and a deep, thready and weak pulse.

Analysis: Deficient kidney *yang* means poor urinary regulation, thus retained or dripping urine occurs. A weak urinary stream, a pale complexion, and lassitude are signs of deficient kidney *qi*. An aversion to cold, soreness and weakness of the lumbar region and knees, a deep, thready and weak pulse, and a pale tongue with a white coating all suggest deficient kidney *yang*.

Treatment: To warm *yang*, replenish *qi*, reinforce the kidneys, and promote diuresis.

Prescription: *Jisheng* Pill for Invigorating Kidney-*Qi* (206) is the main formula. Cortex Cinnamomi and Radix Aconiti Lateralis Preparata replenish *yang* of the lower *jiao* and invigorate kidney *qi*; Pill of Six Drugs Containing Rehmanniae Preparata (56) replenishes the kidneys and nourishes *yin*; and Radix Achyranthis Bidentatae and Semen Plantaginis promote diuresis. In cases of *qi* deficiency due to old age, add Radix Ginseng, Cornu Cervi, Rhizoma Curculiginis and Herba Epimedii.

The following are methods of treatment:

(1) External application of drugs

A piece of Bulbus Allii, three pieces of Fructus Gardeniae, and a small amount of salt are pounded and placed on the umbilicus with a piece of paper in between. Another method is to stir-bake 250 grams of salt and wrap it in a cloth parcel to be placed on the abdomen and umbilicus while still hot.

(2) Acupuncture and massage

Zusanli (ST 36), *Zhongji* (RN 3), *Sanyinjiao* (SP 6) and *Yinlingquan* (SP 9) needles should be used, and strong stimulation should be provided by lifting, thrusting and rotating the needle vigorously. Moxibustion to *Guanyuan* (RN 4) and *Qihai* (RN 6) can also be used in cases of weak resistance.

Massage the lower abdomen over the urinary bladder.

(3) Catheterization

If drugs and acupuncture are not effective and the lower abdomen is extremely distended and full, with a dull resonance sounding after percussion over the urinary bladder, catheterization should be applied to relieve acute symptoms.

These methods of treatment for urine retention are not effective in the treatment of oliguria or anuria due to renal failure.

Case Studies

Name: Wu XX; Sex: Female; Age: 29.

The patient was admitted for difficult labor due to the premature rupture of the amniotic membrane. Retention of urine was relieved by catheterization, and then labor succeeded with the help of ventolise eutocique. For seven days after labor, the patient could not urinate on her own, so catheterization was applied every day. Acupuncture treatment was not effective.

The patient now exhibited retention of urine, a weighted sensation in the lower abdomen, foul-smelling lochia, an absence of milk secretion, a mild fever, sweating, pale lips and tongue, and a rapid and feeble pulse. Both appetite and defecation were normal. The disease was due to the deficiency and sinking of *qi* following labor complicated by impaired bladder function. The mild fever was the result of a common cold. *Qi* was replenished and sent upward by prescribing modified Decoction for Strengthening Middle *Jiao* and Benefiting *Qi* (154).

Radix Astragali	18 g;
Radix Codonopsis	12 g;
Rhizoma Cimicifugae	9 g;
Radix Bupleuri	6 g;
Radix Angelicae Sinensis	9 g;
Rhizoma Atractylodis Macrocephalae	9 g;
Radix Glycyrrhizae	3 g;
Pericarpium Citri Reticulatae	3 g;
Rhizoma Chuanxiong	6 g;
Rhizoma Zingiberis Recens	3 slices;
Fructus Jujubae	5 pieces.

The patient took one dose for three days. Milk began to flow on the second day, and she could urinate on her own on the third day. Her cold was also relieved.

Discussion: The deficiency and sinking of *qi* following labor does not allow the turbid *yin* to descend, resulting in urine retention, while the failure of the clear *qi* to ascend prevents milk secretion. The patient's weak resistance due to deficient *qi* resulted in her catching a common cold. Thus Decoction for Strengthening Middle *Jiao* and Benefiting *Qi* was prescribed. Rhizoma Chuanxiong, Rhizoma Zingiberis Recens and Fructus Jujubae activate blood circulation, remove stasis and regulate the nutrient and defensive *qi*.

Name: Li XX; Sex: Female; Age: 50.

The patient suffered from gastric perforation complicated by peritonitis. The perforation was sutured and gastrojejunostomy took place, the operation for which proceeded smoothly. Afterwards her blood pressure became very low, and oliguria or even anuria was present for several days. Gradually, she fell into a state of semicoma with muscular spasms. Nonprotein nitrogen determination showed 150 mg%. Since Western drugs were not effective, treatment with traditional Chinese medicine was requested.

The patient now had anuria, cold limbs and a thready pulse. She was in a state of semiconsciousness and her hands twitched from time to time. Modified *Zhenwu* Decoction (223) was prescribed to restore *yang* and promote diuresis. Herbs used included Radix Panacis Quinquefolii, Radix Paeoniae Alba, Poria, Radix Aconiti Lateralis Preparata (stir-baked at high temperature) and Semen Coicis. Following the first dose, the patient could urinate by herself, her limbs became warmer, and her muscular spasms were relieved. But she was still too weak to talk.

At her second visit, she was given herbs such as Radix Ginseng, Rhizoma Atractylodis Macrocephalae, Poria, Semen Plantaginis, Radix Achyranthis Bidentatae, Rhizoma Alismatis, and Semen Coicis. After two doses, she became completely conscious and felt much better. Furthermore, she was passing urine quite smoothly. Nevertheless, she complained of thirst. Therefore, Radix Codonopsis, Radix Adenophorae, Radix Ophiopogonis, Radix Trichosanthis, Semen Coicis and Rhizoma Polygonati Odorati were prescribed. After three visits, all symptoms improved, her blood pressure became normal, and nonprotein nitrogen dropped to 37.5 mg%. She was then allowed to leave hospital.

Discussion: Postoperative anuria in this case led to uremia. Chinese medicine holds that the kidneys are in charge of opening and closing the gate of urination. When kidney *yang* is sufficient, this gate opens; when the turbid *yin* is hyperactive, it closes. The patient exhibited cold limbs and a thready pulse at her first visit, suggesting deficient *yang*. Thus the gate was unable to open, and anuria occurred. To invigorate *yang* and promote diuresis, *Zhenwu* Decoction (223) was prescribed. Once this gate opened, uremia was resolved. After the first dose, the limbs became warm, and she could urinate by herself. Since the body's anti-pathogenic *qi* was still weak, she felt tired and did not want to talk. Herbs that invigorate the spleen, replenish *qi* and promote diuresis were prescribed at her second visit. Her condition then improve.

* This method is induced: "In case of *qi* deficiency, administer Radix Ginseng, Radix Astragali and Rhizoma Cimicifugae, and then induce vomiting. In case of blood deficiency, administer Four Drugs Decoction (93), and then induce vomiting artificially. In case of excessive phlegm, administer *Erchen* Decoction (3), then induce vomiting. In case of retained phlegm and stagnant *qi*, administer *Erchen* Decoction (3) added with Rhizoma Cyperi, and then induce vomiting." Zhu Danxi compared this with an apparatus which drips water; water drips from the bottom of the apparatus when the top is open, but stops dripping when the top is closed.

XXXVIII. Lumbago

Lumbago, on one or both sides, is a subjective symptom with pain in the area between the twelfth rib and iliac crest on the back of the body.

Lumbago is dealt with in several of the medical classics. According to *The Inner Canon of the Yellow Emperor*, the kidneys are located in the lumbar region. An inability to move the back is due to kidney deficiencies. The book also explains the relation between lumbago and the body's meridians; since all the meridians pass through the lumbar region, disorders of these meridians will give rise to lumbago. It says, "The Urinary Bladder Meridian of the Foot-*Taiyang* travels downwards to the lumbar region along the spinal column. Invasion of this meridian by external pathogenic factors will cause such pain in the spine and lower back that it will feel as if the back were being broken." *A Complete Collection of Jingyue's Treatise* outlines the types of back pain and their causes, saying, "Repeated attacks of prolonged lower back pain is due to renal deficiency. On rainy days, the dampness makes the back ache, as it does after sitting for a long time. Cold makes the patient like warmth and hate the cold, while heat makes the patient like the cold and hate the heat. Stagnant *qi* makes the patient feel depressed or angry, deficient *qi* makes the patient feel worried, and hepatic and renal deficiencies aggravate the symptoms when the patient indulges in light labor. Therefore, treatment should be given based on the diagnosis of the complaint."

Regarding treatment, *A Supplement to Diagnosis and Treatment* says, "The kidneys should be nourished before the invading pathogenic factors are eliminated and resistance strengthened. Then what to do next will all depend on the actual condition of the patient. If the pathogenic factors are acute, eliminate them first; if the patient's resistance is weak, strengthen it as soon as possible. New cases can be treated by eliminating pathogenic factors and regulating the meridians, while prolonged cases can be cured by replenishing the kidneys and nourishing the *qi* and blood."

Lumbago may appear in a great number of diseases. When treating lumbago in kidney disease, rheumatism, rheumatoid diseases, psoatic strain, and diseases of the vertebrae and spinal cord, please refer to the following descriptions.

Etiology and Pathogenesis
1. Exposure to Cold-Dampness

This may result from living in cold and damp places, wading through rivers, being caught in the rain, sweating after heavy physical work, or wearing cold and wet clothes. Blockage of the meridians by pathogenic cold-dampness leads to unsmooth *qi* and blood circulation, which then gives rise to lumbago.

2. Exposure to Dampness-Heat

This may come from the accumulation of internal dampness-heat, from exposure to dampness-heat, or from a long-term accumulation of cold-dampness. Blockage of the meridians also causes lumbago.

3. Renal Deficiency

Weak resistance, coupled with stress, prolonged illness, old age or excessive sexual activity, may cause deficient kidney *yang* or a deficiency of kidney essence and blood. In the former, the meridians are deprived of warmth, while in the latter, the tendons are deprived of nourishment. Either condition may lead to lumbago.

4. Stagnant *Qi* and Blood

This takes place when the meridians become obstructed after long-term lumbar pain, caused by doing physical work which requires the patient to bend over often or from renal impairment following trauma. The resultant stagnation, which can also be a result of contusions or sprains, leads to lumbago.

Pathogenic dampness is often one of the external factors involve in lumbago. This is because dampness is characterized by heaviness and turbidity, and thus is likely to stay in the lumbar region. Renal deficiency is often one of internal causes, because the kidneys are located in the lumbar region. These two types of lumbago, as well as lumbago due to stagnant *qi* and blood, often transform themselves into one another. For instance, lumbago due to the invasion of pathogenic dampness may lead to renal deficiency over a long period. Lumbago due to renal deficiency may become complicated by exposure to pathogenic dampness. Prolonged cases of lumbago due to stagnant *qi* and blood may produce renal deficiency.

To conclude, lumbago is most closely related to the kidneys, and external pathogenic factors take the opportunity to invade when the kidneys are deficient. Thus *Standard for Diagnosis and Treatment* says, "Lumbago is usually caused by wind, dampness, cold, heat, contusions, stagnant blood and *qi*, and retained phlegm. Yet renal deficiency also plays a key role."

Differentiation and Treatment

Since lumbago is caused by various diseases, it is necessary to find out the patient's case history and give them a medical checkup before diagnosis. First of all, it should be distinguished whether the syndrome is an external and internal syndrome, cold or hot in nature, and caused by deficiencies or excesses. Lumbago due to the invasion of external factors is generally an external syndrome caused by excesses, which has an acute onset characterized by pronounced pain. Lumbago caused by cold-dampness is accompanied by a cold and heavy sensation in the lumbar region. Lumbago from dampness-heat is accompanied by a burning sensation in the lumbar region or small quantities of deep yellow urine. Lumbago from stagnant blood causes pain that bores and has a fixed position; the patient has difficulty in turning around and probably has a history of trauma. In the case of lumbago due to invasion by external factors, treatment aims at eliminating pathogenic factors and removing any obstructions from the meridians.

Lumbago due to renal deficiency is an internal syndrome caused by deficiencies, with a slow onset characterized by mild recurrent pain. The pain is alleviated by pressure, and possibly accompanied by soreness and weakness in the lumbar region. Replenishing and warming the kidneys should be adopted as a primary method of treatment. Since renal deficiency is likely to be complicated with exposure to external pathogenic factors, and the prolonged retention of pathogenic factors is likely to damage the kidneys, attention should be paid to whether the condition is caused by deficiencies or excesses.

1. Cold-Dampness Lumbago

Clinical manifestations: Lumbar pain accompanied by a cold and heavy sensation, alleviated by warmth and aggravated on rainy days. Lying down does not alleviate the pain; instead, it may become even worse. The patient has difficulty turning round. The patient's tongue has a sticky, white coating and the pulse is deep and slow.

Analysis: Cold is characterized by contractions, and dampness by heaviness. Invasion of the lumbar region by cold-dampness therefore produces pain accompanied by a cold and heavy sensation, making it difficult to turn round. Dampness, a pathogenic factor of the *yin* type, is also characterized by stagnation and viscosity, and tends to stagnate when the patient lies down. Thus lumbago is not relieved in this position, but can become worse. On rainy days, cold-dampness becomes more hyperactive so the pain is more violent than before. A sticky white tongue coating and a deep and slow pulse are signs of retained cold-dampness. When pathogenic cold is predominant, lumbar pain is primarily accompanied by a cold sensation; when pathogenic dampness predominates, it is accompanied by a numb, heavy sensation.

Treatment: To eliminate cold-dampness, warm the meridians and remove any obstructions.

Prescription: Decoction of Glycyrrhizae, Zingiberis, Poria and Atractylodis Macrocephalae (85). Rhizoma Zingiberis and Radix Glycyrrhizae disperse cold and warm the middle *jiao*; and Poria and Rhizoma Atractylodis Macrocephalae invigorate the spleen and eliminate dampness. You Zaijing, a physician of the Qing Dynasty, says, "Radix Glycyrrhizae, Rhizoma Zingiberis, Poria and Rhizoma Atractylodis Macrocephalae do not treat kidney diseases. They are prescribed as treatment because cold-dampness is not located in the kidneys, but in the muscles of the lumbar region. Cold-dampness is not eliminated by warming the kidneys, but by warming and invigorating the spleen." Ramulus Cinnamomi and Radix Achyranthis Bidentatae can be added to remove obstructions from the meridians by providing warmth. Cortex Eucommiae, Herba Taxilli and Radix Dipsaci should be added to replenish the kidneys and strengthen the loin. If pain is severe and the limbs are cold, Radix Aconiti Lateralis Preparata can be added to warm the kidneys and eliminate cold. In cases of a thick, sticky tongue coating, Rhizoma Atractylodis should be added to relieve dampness. If signs of pathogenic wind are present, such as wandering pain or painful joints, Decoction of Angelicae Pubescentis and Taxilli (219) can be used to eliminate wind, remove obstructions from the meridians, and tonify the liver and kidneys.

2. Dampness-Heat Lumbago

Clinical manifestations: Lumbar pain accompanied by a hot sensation, aggravated on hot or rainy days, and possibly alleviated after physical exercise. This kind of pain often occurs in late summer. The patient only passes small quantities of deep yellow urine. The patient's tongue coating is yellow and sticky, the pulse soft and rapid.

Analysis: Dampness-heat retained in the lumbar region gives rise to lumbar pain accompanied by a hot sensation. Dampness-heat becomes more pronounced on hot rainy days, or in late summer, and thus the pain is aggravated. Physical exercise may help improve *qi* circulation and reduce stagnant dampness thus alleviating pain. The downward movement of dampness-heat to the bladder leads to the passage of only small amounts of deep yellow urine. A sticky, yellow tongue coating and a soft and rapid pulse are signs of dampness-heat.

Treatment: To clear dampness-heat, relax the tendons and relieve pain.

Prescription: Powder of Phellodendri and Atractylodis with Additional Drugs (111). Cortex Phellodendri and Rhizoma Atractylodis relieve dampness and disperse heat; Radix Stephaniae Tetrandrae and Rhizoma Dioscoreae Septemlobae eliminate dampness; Radix Angelicae Sinensis and Radix Achyranthis Bidentatae activate blood circulation and resolving blood stasis; and Carapax et Plastrum Testudinis replenishes the kidneys and nourishes *yin*. To disperse heat, eliminate wind and remove any obstructions in the meridians, Caulis Lonicerae and Cortex Erythrinae can be prescribed. If the pain is severe, add Olibanum and Myrrha to activate blood circulation and relieve pain.

If this syndrome is accompanied by urgent, frequent and painful urination, stranguria is suggested; if serious lumbar pain appears all of a sudden and spreads to the groin, accompanied by abdominal pain and nausea, this indicates that the complaint may be urinary calculi.

3. Renal Deficiency

Clinical manifestations: Lumbar pain occurs repeatedly and makes the patient feel sore and weak all over. The symptoms can be alleviated when the patient lies down or is given a massage. If kidney *yang* deficiency is pronounced, other symptoms will appear such as an aversion to cold, cold limbs, a cramping feeling in the lower abdomen, a pale complexion, a pale tongue, and a deep and thready pulse; if kidney *yin*-deficiency is pronounced, the accompanying symptoms are restlessness, insomnia, a dry mouth and throat, a facial flush, hot sensations in the palms, soles and chest, a red tongue, and a thready and rapid pulse.

Analysis: Deficient kidney essence leads to weak bones and insufficient marrow, making the patient feel sore and weak all over, including the lumbar region and knees. Since pain is caused by deficiencies, it can be alleviated by massage. As physical work consumes *qi*, pain is aggravated by physical movement and alleviated by lying down. Since the Kidney Meridian enters the abdomen, a cramping feeling is prevalent in cases of deficient kidney *yang*, which means that the body is failing to nourish the tendons and muscles. The failure of *yang* to warm the body surface and limbs gives rise to an aversion to cold and cold limbs. A pale complexion, a pale tongue and a deep and thready pulse are signs of cold due to *yang* deficiency. *Yin* deficiency implies insufficient body fluid, which allows fire caused by deficiencies to flare up, exhibiting symptoms of restlessness, insomnia, a dry mouth and throat, and hot sensations in the palms, soles and chest. A red tongue, and a thready and rapid pulse are signs of heat due *yin* deficiency.

Treatment: To replenish the kidneys and assist *yang* in cases of *yang* deficiency; to replenish the kidneys and nourish *yin* in cases of *yin* deficiency.

Prescription: *Yougui* Pill (82) in cases of *yang* deficiency. In this prescription, Cortex Cinnamomi, Radix Aconiti Lateralis Preparata, and Colla Cornus Cervi warm and nourish kidney *yang*; Radix Rehmanniae Preparata, Rhizoma Dioscoreae, Fructus Corni and Fructus Lycii nourish kidney *yin*; Cortex Eucommiae strengthens the loin and benefits essence; Semen Cuscutae replenishes the liver and kidneys; and Radix Angelicae Sinensis replenishes and circulates blood.

Zuogui Pill (79) is prescribed in cases of deficient *yin*. In this prescription, Radix Rehmanniae, Fructus Lycii, Fructus Corni, and Colla Carapax et Plastrum Testudinis nourish *yin* and replenish the kidneys; Semen Cuscutae, Colla Cornus Cervi and Radix Achyranthis Bidentatae warm the kidneys and strengthen the loin. If a case without any obvious signs of either *yin* or *yang* deficiency is prolonged, it is generally attributed to renal deficiency, and Pill for Warming Kidney-*Yang* and Relieving Abdominal Pain (167) is given to replenish the kidneys and strengthen the loin.

4. Stagnant Blood

Clinical manifestations: A persistent and acute lumbar pain in a fixed position. When the pain is mild, the patient has difficulty bending or straightening up; when the pain is severe, the patient will have problems turning around. The tongue is dark purple, or has purple spots. The pulse is unsmooth.

This syndrome often appears in cases of trauma. But stagnation of both *qi* and blood may follow a prolonged illness. The former is acute but the latter chronic.

Analysis: Blockage of the meridians by stagnant blood hinders *qi* and blood circulation, which causes the fixed lumbar pain aggravated by pressure. A dark purple tongue or a tongue with purple spots and an unsmooth pulse, are signs of stagnant blood.

Treatment: To activate blood circulation, remove blood stasis, regulate *qi* and relieve pain.

Prescription: Decoction for Relieving Pain and Removing Blood Stasis (162). In the formula, Radix Angelicae Sinensis, Rhizoma Chuanxiong, Semen Persicae and Flos Carthami activate blood circulation and remove blood stasis; Radix Achyranthis Bidentatae, Lumbricus, Myrrha, and Faces Trogopterori activate blood circulation, remove stasis, remove any obstructions from the meridians and relieve pain; Rhizoma Cyperi regulates *qi* and relieves pain; Radix Glycyrrhizae relieves acute symptoms and pain; and Rhizoma seu Radix Notopterygii and Radix Gentianae Macrophyllae eliminate wind and dampness. If signs of renal deficiency are also present, add Radix Dipsaci, Cortex Eucommiae and Herba Taxilli to replenish the liver and kidneys, and strengthen the tendons and bones. Medicines from animal substances that can help remove obstructions from the vessels such as Zaocys and Squama Manitis, can also be added to the treatment. Acupuncture, massage, steaming and washing with hot decoctions can also be used to gain better results.

Case Studies

Name: Lu XX; Sex: Male.

The kidneys dominate the bones, and any kidney deficiency will lead to lumbago. The patient often had lumbago in the afternoon and found that he was easily tired. He also had tinnitus and insomnia, and when he slept, his sleep was often disturbed by dreams. This indicates that nourishment should be given to the patient. Thus the following herbs were prescribed:

Radix Rehmanniae Preparata	18 g;
Fructus Amomi	1.8 g;
Cortex Eucommiae	12 g;
Rhizoma Cibotii	12 g;
Radix Dipsaci	9 g;
Semen Cuscutae	9 g;
Fructus Corni	9 g;
Carapax et Plastrum Testudinis	18 g;
Radix Achyranthis Bidentatae	12 g;
Cornu Cervi Degelatinatum	12 g;
Herba Taxilli	12 g.

Six grams of *Zuogui* Pill (79) and six grams of Pill for Replenishing *Yin* (22) were taken, the former in the morning and the latter in the evening.

Discussion: Lumbago due to renal deficiency has the following features: soreness is more pronounced than pain and lumbar soreness becomes serious when the patient undertakes physical work, but alleviated when the patient rests. Deficient kidney *yang* and kidney *yin* exhibit different symptoms, with signs of cold in the former and signs of heat in the latter. This case was due to kidney *yin*-deficiency. The herbs prescribed were based on *Zuogui* Pill (79), aimed at replenishing the liver and kidneys. The patent medicines *Zuogui* Pill (79) and Pill for Replenishing *Yin* (22) aim at replenishing the kidneys and reducing fire.

Name: Liu XX; Sex: Male: Age: 20.

The patient had had an operation to remove ureter stones in 1958. Afterwards, he experienced discomfort in the lower right abdomen (the operative area), an aching back, a cold and heavy sensation below the loins, constipation, yellow and cloudy urine, an absence of thirst, a poor appetite, insomnia, a sticky white tongue coating with coarse granules, and a deep, thready and unsmooth pulse. The urinalysis showed protein +++, red blood cells ++, white blood cells ++, and epithelial cells +. The patient had been admitted into hospital many times for this problem, and had been treated unsuccessfully with antibiotics. A number of doctors were called together to study the disease on December 14, 1960. According to the above symptoms, a diagnosis of invasion of the lumbar region and kidneys by dampness was established. Decoction of Glycyrrhizae, Zingiberis, Poria and Atractylodis Macrocephalae (85) was prescribed with additional ingredients:

Radix Glycyrrhizae Preparata	6 g;

Rhizoma Zingiberis (stir-baked at a high temperature)	6 g;
Poria	9 g;
Radix Angelicae Sinensis	9 g;
Rhizoma Atractylodis Macrocephalae	9 g;
Cortex Eucommiae	9 g.

One dose of this was taken every day.

The patient took 24 doses, one dose a day. The uncomfortable feeling in the lower right abdomen and the lumbar soreness were relieved, the lower limbs became warmer and freedom of movement was restored, bowel movements returned to normal, the deep and unsmooth pulse disappeared, and the patient's appetite and sleeping habits showed a great improvement. Urinalysis showed no abnormalities.

Discussion: Lumbar soreness, a cold and heavy sensation below the loins, an absence of thirst, and a white and sticky tongue coating with coarse granules all suggest the invasion of the lumbar region and kidneys by dampness, as described in *Synopsis of Prescriptions of the Golden Chamber*. Good results were achieved by administering Decoction of Glycyrrhizae, Zingiberis, Poria and Atractylodis Macrocephalae (85). Since this was a prolonged illness and lumbar soreness and a deep, thready and unsmooth pulse were present, Cortex Eucommia and Radix Angelicae Sinensis were added to replenish the kidneys, strengthen the loins, nourish blood and activate blood circulation. Constipation was not due to heat, but to cold. Although the urinalysis was positive, and urine was cloudy and yellow, these were not as important as the other symptoms. Generally, both the syndrome and the disease should be diagnosed at the same time, but if they are not consistent with each other, only one factor (either syndrome or disease) should be taken into account. In this case, the syndrome was taken into account, while the disease itself was neglected.

XXXIX. Diabetes

Diabetes is a disease characterized by polydipsia, polyphagia, polyuria, weight loss, and a sweet taste to the urine.

The earliest description of diabetes can be found in *The Inner Canon of the Yellow Emperor*. Different names have been given to this disease according to its causes and clinical manifestations such as diabetes due to the consumption of the body fluid by heat, diabetes marked by polydipsia, diabetes marked by polyphagia, etc. As to etiology, this book holds that excessive greasy or sweet food, emotional trauma, and the weakness of the five *zang* organs are closely related. The medical classic *Synopsis of Prescriptions of the Golden Chamber* details clearly how to diagnose and treat diabetes. Medical scholars of later generations have made further progress in the study of the disease. For instance, in his book *Clandestine Essentials from Imperial Library*, Wang Tao of the Tang Dynasty was the first doctor to describe the sweet taste of the urine of diabetic patients. Other scholars discovered possible complications of this disease, such as carbuncles, boils, edema, cataracts, night blindness, deafness, consumptive lung diseases marked by coughing, numbness of the limbs, prostration, etc.

The first classification of diabetes in history is seen in the book *Pathogenesis and Manifestations of Diseases* published in the Sui Dynasty. Eight syndromes are differentiated. However, it was not until the Song Dynasty that medical scholars started to classify the disease into upper, middle and lower types on the basis of the predominant symptoms. The upper type is marked by polydipsia, the middle type by polyphagia and the lower type by thirst and polyuria, or even milky urine.

Diabetes mellitus and diabetes insipidus in Western medicine can be diagnosed and treated according to the following descriptions.

Etiology and Pathogenesis

1. Improper Diet

Excessive consumption of sweet and fatty foods over a long period of time and an excessive intake of alcohol impair the ability of the spleen and stomach to transport and transform. Retained food and dryness-heat combine to consume body fluid and this can lead to diabetes.

2. Emotional Trauma

Protracted mental irritation, such as depression or anger, impairs the liver and causes stagnant liver *qi*. Over time stagnant *qi* turns into fire which then consumes fluid in the lungs and stomach, causing pulmonary dryness and gastric heat, and finally diabetes.

3. Excessive Sexual Activity

Deficient *yin* complicated by excessive sexual activity damages renal *yin* essence and causes hyperactive fire, which dries pulmonary and gastric fluid, leading to diabetes.

In summary, the pathogenesis of diabetes lies in an excess of dryness-heat and fluid consumption. It also has the following features:

(1) Deficient *yin* as a primary cause and dryness-heat as a secondary cause

These interact, becoming both cause and effect. The more excessive dryness-heat is, the more deficient *yin* will be; the more deficient *yin* is, the more excessive dryness-heat will be. Pathological changes mainly take place in the lungs, stomach and kidneys. Although only one out of these three organs may be affected gravely, this will of course affect the other two. For instance, in cases of pulmonary dryness with deficient *yin*, body fluid will fail to be distributed normally. As a result, the stomach will be deprived of moisture, and the kidneys will be deprived of nourishment. In cases of excess heat in the stomach, lung fluid will be consumed, and kidney *yin* damaged. In cases of deficient kidney *yin*, fire will become hyperactive, inevitably affecting both the lungs and the stomach.

(2) Damage to both *qi* and *yin* and *yin* and *yang* deficiencies

A prolonged case of diabetes allows *yin* to affect *yang*, damaging *qi* and *yin*, or sometimes causing deficiencies of both *yin* and *yang*. In severe cases, this causes an extreme deficiency of kidney *yang*. Signs of deficient *qi* or *yang* rarely appear during the initial stages of the disease.

(3) Various complications when deficient *yin* is combined with dryness-heat

Prolonged lack of moisture in the lungs may lead to pulmonary tuberculosis. If essence and blood from the liver and kidneys fail to nourish the ears and eyes due to deficient kidney *yin*, this may cause cataracts, night blindness and deafness. Retained dryness-heat damages the nutrient *yin* and blocks vessels. The accumulation of toxins forms pus, producing carbuncles, furuncles, boils and ulcers. Deficient spleen and kidney *yang* following *yin* deficiency causes an overflow of water and dampness that spreads to the muscles and skin, giving rise to edema. If *yin* fluid is consumed at a drastic rate, deficient *yin* cannot control *yang-qi*. A deficiency of floating *yang* results in a flushed face, headaches, restlessness, irritability, nausea, vomiting, sunken eyes, dry and red lips and tongue, and heavy breathing. Critical signs such as coma, cold limbs, and a feeble, thready and fainting pulse may subsequently occur due to the collapse of *yin* and *yang*.

Diagnosis

1. Thirst

Thirst with the desire to drink is a common symptom of febrile diseases resulting from invasion by external factors. This symptom is called the same name as diabetes in Chinese in the medical classic *Treatise on Cold Diseases*. This kind of thirst is different from diabetes in that it is not accompanied by polyphagia or polyuria.

2. Hyperthyroidism

The symptoms of hyperthyroidism are irritability, hunger, weight loss, palpitations, bulging eyeballs, and swellings on one or both sides of the neck. Hunger and weight loss both occur, as they do in middle diabetes. However, the patient does not suffer from bulging eyeballs or swellings in the neck in diabetes.

Differentiation and Treatment

Polydipsia, polyphagia and polyuria often appear at the same time in diabetes, though one may predominate. Treatment should start with the nourishment of *yin* no matter which body part is affected. If dryness-heat is hyperactive, add herbs that disperse heat; if *yin* affects *yang*, both *yin* and *yang* must be replenished.

1. Upper Type (Heat in the lungs which consumes body fluid)

Clinical manifestations: Restlessness, extreme thirst, polydipsia, a dry tongue, frequent and copious urination, a tongue with a red tip, red sides and a thin yellow coating, and a rapid pulse.

Analysis: Excessive pulmonary heat consumes body fluid, giving rise to a dry tongue, extreme thirst, polydipsia and restlessness. This dryness impairs the ability of the lungs to distribute fluid evenly throughout the body, thus the fluid only flows to the bladder, resulting in frequent and copious urination. Excess internal heat accounts for the color of the tongue and its coating, as well as for the rapidity of the pulse.

Treatment: To disperse heat, moisten the lungs, produce body fluid, and relieve thirst.

Prescription: Formula for Diabetes (244) with additional ingredients. In this formula, Radix Trichosanthis, Radix Rehmanniae, and Succus Nelumbinis Rhizomatis disperse heat, moisten the lungs, produce fluid and relieve thirst; cow's milk moistens dryness, and Rhizoma Coptidis reduces fire. In cases of *qi* and *yin* deficiency in the lungs and kidneys with symptoms of polydipsia, lassitude, and frequent urination, Decoction of Asparagi and Ophiopogonis (2) should be prescribed. Radix Ginseng, Radix Asparagi, Radix Ophiopogonis, and Radix Trichosanthis benefit *qi* and produce body fluid, and Radix Scutellariae, and Rhizoma Anemarrhenae produce body fluid and relieve restlessness. If *qi* and *yin* are being consumed by excess heat in the lungs and stomach with symptoms of polydipsia, a coarse yellow tongue coating, and a bounding and full pulse, White Tiger Decoction with Ginseng (103) can be prescribed to disperse heat in the lungs and stomach, produce body fluid and relieve thirst.

2. Middle Type (Excess heat in the stomach)

Clinical manifestations: Polyphagia, hunger, weight loss, constipation, a yellow tongue coating, and a smooth and forceful pulse.

Analysis: When stomach fire flares up, this strengthens digestion, increases the appetite, and results in hunger. However, fluid and blood are consumed and the muscles are deprived of nourishment, causing weight loss. The deficiency of essence in the lungs deprives the large intestine of moisture, which is the cause of constipation. A yellow tongue coating, and a smooth and forceful pulse are signs of excess heat in the stomach.

Treatment: To disperse heat in the stomach, reduce fire, nourish *yin*, and produce fluid.

Prescription: Jade Maid Decoction (71) with additional ingredients. Rhizoma Anemarrhenae and Gypsum Fibrosum disperse heat in the lungs and stomach, Radix Rehmanniae and Radix Ophiopogonis nourish *yin* in the lungs and stomach, and Radix Achyranthis Bidentatae sends fire downwards. To help disperse heat and reduce fire, add Radix Scutellariae and Fructus Gardeniae.

3. Lower Type

(1) Deficiency of kidney *yin*

Clinical manifestations: Polyuria with milky or sweet urine, thirst, a red, dry tongue, and a thready and rapid pulse.

Analysis: Renal deficiency means impaired control of urination, which causes polyuria. Impaired astringency causes the essence to flow downwards, and the result is milky or sweet urine. Thirst, a dry tongue and a thready and rapid pulse are signs of hyperactive fire due to deficient kidney *yin*.

Treatment: To nourish *yin* and strengthen the kidneys.

Prescription: Pill of Six Drugs Containing Rehmanniae Preparata (56). Large dosages of Radix Rehmanniae Preparata, Rhizoma Dioscoreae and Fructus Corni should be used to nourish *yin*, boost the essence and strengthen the kidneys. In cases of deficient kidney *yin* and hyperactive fire with symptoms of irritability, insomnia, and nocturnal emissions, add Rhizoma Anemarrhenae, Cortex Phellodendri and Concha Ostreae to nourish *yin*, disperse heat, boost the essence and subdue hyperactive *yang*.

(2) Deficiency of both *yin* and *yang*

Clinical manifestations: Polyuria with large quantities of milky urine (sometimes equaling the amount drunk by the patient), a dark complexion, dry and withered helixes, soreness and weakness of the lumbar region and knees, impotence, a pale tongue with a white coating, and a deep, thready and weak pulse.

Analysis: Impaired renal promotion in astringency leads to the frequent urination of large quantities of milky urine. The loss of food essence through urination causes malnutrition, giving the patient a dark complexion. Since the kidneys dominate the bones, open into the ears, and reside in the lumbar region, this deficiency also leads to the patient suffering from dry and withered helixes, and soreness and weakness of the lumbar region and knees. The decline of fire of the life gate leads to impotence. A pale tongue with a white coating and a deep, thready and weak pulse are signs of deficiency of both *yin* and *yang*.

Treatment: To warm *yang*, nourish the kidneys and promote astringency.

Prescription: Modified Pill for Invigorating Kidney-*Qi* (182) or modified *Yougui* Pill (82). In the former, Radix Aconiti Lateralis Preparata and Cortex Cinnamomi warm and replenish kidney *yang*, and Pill of Six Drugs Containing Rehmanniae Preparata (56) replenishes kidney *yin*. The latter is based on the former with Rhizoma Alismatis, Poria and Cortex Moutan removed, and Colla Cornu Cervi, Semen Cuscutae, Cortex Eucommiae, Fructus Lycii and Radix Angelicae Sinensis added. The first herbs warm *yang* and replenish the kidneys, and Radix Angelicae Sinensis replenishes blood. To promote astringency, herbs such as Fructus Rosae Laevigatae, Ootheca Mantidis and Semen Euryales can be used.

Treatment of accompanying diseases:

Night blindness and deafness both result from deficiencies of hepatic and renal essence and blood. Thus the liver and kidneys can be replenished by prescribing Bolus of Lycii, Chrysanthemi and Rehmanniae Preparata (144), which can be prescribed by itself or together with Goat Liver Pill (125).

Carbuncles, furuncles, boils and ulcer stem from damage done to the nutrient system by toxin-heat. Toxins can be eliminated and blood can be cooled by prescribing Decoction of Five Ingredients for Detoxification (52). A prolonged case exhibits damage to both the *qi* and *ying* systems, shown by festering skin eruptions. *Qi* can be replenished, toxins eliminated and pus drained if Decoction of Astragali and Glycyrrhizae (265) and Bolus of Calculus Bovis for Clearing Heat and Detoxification (308) with Caulis Lonicerae are prescribed.

Complications of pulmonary tuberculosis, edema and wind stroke can be treated according to descriptions in the relevant chapters.

In addition, the patient is advised to avoid mental stress and excessive sexual activity. Simple food containing little salt is recommended, for example, rice, vegetables, bean products, lean meat, and eggs. Overeating, or eating pungent or irritant food should be avoided.

Case Studies

Name: Chen XX; Sex: Female; Age: 32.
First visit: July 14, 1964.

The patient had been sick for two years. The symptoms included dizziness, gastric distress, a poor appetite, extreme thirst which forced her to drink four thermos bottles of water a day, frequent urination with profuse milky urine, a shortened menstrual cycle with decreased flow, lassitude, palpitations, somnolence, emaciation, a sallow complexion, a facial flush, red lips, shortness of breath, a feeble voice, a glossy tongue, and a deep, thready and rapid pulse. A urine test revealed glucose and so the diagnosis of diabetes was established. This was caused by emotional trauma, which led to the stagnation of *qi* and the production of fire, which consumed fluid and gave rise to deficient *yin* and hyperactive *yang*. Treatment sought to produce body fluid, relieve thirst, nourish *yin* and subdue hyperactive *yang*. The following herbs were prescribed:

Rhizoma Dioscoreae	30 g;
Os Draconis	30 g;
Concha Ostreae	30 g;
Radix Codonopsis	24 g;
Radix Ophiopogonis	12 g;

Radix Trichosanthis	15 g;
Radix Scrophulariae	24 g;
Rhizoma Anemarrhenae	21 g.

These were decocted in water to be taken in the morning and at night.

Second visit: After the tenth dose, the patient's pulse had become taut and rapid, the amount of water she drank every day was reduced by 3/4, and her urine test revealed glucose ++. All this showed that *qi* and *yin* were being gradually restored, as was the production of body fluid. But the nature of the pulse suggested that the liver and the gallbladder were still hyperactive. Thus 15 grams of Radix Paeoniae Alba were added to the previous prescription to calm the liver and nourish *yin*.

Third visit: After another ten doses, the patient's pulse had become smooth and retarded, her thirst was relieved, urination was normal and glucose + was revealed in urinalysis. But now she showed epigastric distention and a poor appetite. This proved that the ability of the spleen and stomach to transport and transform was still impaired, though by now *yin* and *yang* were in a state of balance. Thus herbs that help digestion were prescribed:

Radix Codonopsis	15 g;
Rhizoma Atractylodis Macrocephalae	12 g;
Poria	12 g;
Massa Medicata Fermentata	12 g;
Fructus Hordei Germinatus	12 g;
Pericarpium Citri Reticulatae	9 g;
Caulis Bambusae in Taeniam	12 g;
Fructus Amomi	3 g;
Endothelium Corneum Gigeriae Galli	12 g.

Fourth visit: After five doses, the patient's appetite increased, epigastric distention subsided and all symptoms disappeared. To further consolidate results, five doses of the following herbs were prescribed:

Rhizoma Dioscoreae	30 g;
Folium Mori	12 g;
Rhizoma Atractylodis Macrocephalae	12 g;
Radix Codonopsis	30 g;
Endothelium Corneum Gigeriae Galli	12 g;
Rhizoma Anemarrhenae	12 g;
Radix Trichosanthis	15 g.

The disease was cured after she had finished these doses.

Discussion: *A Guide to Clinical Practice* says, "Although diabetes is divided into three types, its pathogenesis falls into two categories; *yin* deficiency and *yang* hyperactivity, and fluid consumption and excess heat." Taking this case as an example, a thready and rapid pulse suggests deficient *yin* and hyperactive *yang*, as do the sallow complexion, malar flush, red lips and tongue. Symptoms such as dizziness, emaciation and reduced menstrual flow imply that *yin* essence and blood are deficient, while somnolence and palpitations result from the failure of the blood to nourish the heart. The patient's extreme thirst and the large quantities of milky urine passed are due to impaired renal control of urination and astringency following fluid consumption and deficient kidney *yin*.

Thus treatment aimed to produce fluid, relieve thirst, nourish *yin* and subdue hyperactive *yang*.

Rhizoma Dioscoreae invigorates the spleen and stomach, nourishes *yin* and consolidates kidney *yin*. Os Draconis, which is sweet and mild in nature, calms liver *yang* and consolidates kidney *yin*. Concha Ostreae, salty and cold in nature, replenishes *yin*, subdues *yang* and consolidates kidney *yin*. Radix Codonopsis replenishes *qi* and produces fluid since in this case both *qi* and *yin* have been damaged. Radix Ophiopogonis, Rhizoma Anemarrhenae and Radix Trichosanthis relieve thirst and produce fluid. Radix Scrophulariae nourishes *yin* and checks floating *yang*. The patient was cured of this disease after 20 consecutive doses.

XXXX. Spermatorrhea

The involuntary discharge of seminal fluid outside sexual intercourse is referred to as spermatorrhea.

Two types of spermatorrhea exist: nocturnal emissions and spontaneous emissions. The former take place while the patient is dreaming and constitute a relatively mild pathological condition, while the latter occur when the patient is awake or in a dreamless sleep and this condition is very severe. Although these conditions differ in severity, they share a common cause. Generally speaking, nocturnal emissions often signal the initial stages of the disease, while spontaneous emissions is a further development in protracted cases.

The kidneys store essence. *The Inner Canon of the Yellow Emperor* says, "At the age of 16, kidney *qi* is vigorous, kidney essence begins to multiply, and soon sufficient quantities are produced to allow the flow of seminal fluid...." Therefore, it is a physiological phenomenon that an unmarried man experiences spermatorrhea once or twice a month. To this effect, *A Complete Collection of Jingyue's Treatise* states, "A healthy young man who has not had sexual intercourse for a long time experiences spermatorrhea, because there is too much seminal fluid in his body." But it is a pathological phenomenon if spermatorrhea occurs too frequently, for example, once every three to five days, or even every day or every other day, or if spontaneous emissions are accompanied by symptoms such as dizziness, soreness and weakness of the lumbar region and knees, lassitude, a poor memory, palpitations, and insomnia. It is also possible for healthy men to develop symptoms including dizziness, lassitude and palpitations after normal seminal emissions, solely because they lack knowledge and seminal emissions make them nervous.

Pathological spermatorrhea is present in neurosis, prostatitis, and certain chronic diseases in Western medicine.

Etiology and Pathogenesis
1. Deficient *Yin* and Hyperactive Fire

Excess mental strain consumes heart *yin* and produces hyperactive heart fire, which further induces ministerial fire, disturbing the seminal chamber; as a result, spontaneous emissions occur. The heart controls the whole body, including the mind and the essence. When the heart and mind are calm, the essence is well stored, but an impaired cardiac ability to dominate essence leads to spermatorrhea.

Excessive sexual activity consumes kidney *yin* and causes hyperactive fire, also producing spermatorrhea. *Thorough Interpretation of Medicine* says, "Deficient kidney *yin* does not allow the kidneys to store essence, and excess liver *yang* causes hyperactive fire. These combine to produce nocturnal emissions."

2. Inability to Store Kidney Essence due to Renal Deficiencies

This occurs in men who marry too young, or who indulge in excessive sexual activity. The inability to store kidney essence and the weakness of the seminal gate lead to nocturnal or spontaneous emissions.

These may also be caused by congenital renal deficiency, which does not allow the kidneys to store essence.

3. Retained Dampness-Heat

Excessive alcohol intake or excessive greasy or sweet food damages the spleen and stomach, and produces dampness-heat. The downward movement of the dampness-heat disturbs the seminal chamber and causes spermatorrhea. *Collection of Experiences of Famous Physicians in the Ming Dynasty* says, "Nocturnal emissions and spontaneous emissions are conventionally treated on the basis of renal deficiency. Herbs that replenish the kidneys and prevent emissions have proved ineffective. This is because many men who suffer from phlegm-fire and dampness-heat after excess alcohol or too much highly-flavored food develop this disease. The kidneys store essence, which is derived from the passage of food through the spleen and stomach. If the latter are damaged by excessive intake of highly-flavored food, dampness-heat is produced, the *qi* of the middle *jiao* becomes turbid, and the essence produced by the spleen and stomach is mixed with turbid *qi*. When the kidneys are functioning normally, they have no problems storing essence but when the essence is mixed with turbid *qi*, fire disturbs the kidneys and spermatorrhea occurs."

In short, spermatorrhea mainly involves the heart, liver and kidneys. In addition to renal deficiency and weakness of the seminal gate, hyperactive fire in the liver also impairs renal functions. *Diagnosis and Treatment of Classified Syndromes* says, "The essence of *zang-fu* organs is transmitted to the kidneys. The disturbance of the kidneys by fire impairs their ability to store essence. The heart produces monarch or primary fire, while the kidneys and liver produce ministerial or secondary fire. Once monarch fire becomes hyperactive, ministerial fire follows closely. Spermatorrhea then occurs."

Differentiation and Treatment

First of all, nocturnal emissions and spontaneous emissions should be distinguished from each other. They can be diagnosed based on the patient's general state of health, the duration of the disease and the quality of the pulse. There is a saying, "Spermatorrhea which occurs with dreams is a disorder of the heart; without dreams, it is a kidney disorder." As a matter of fact, whether spermatorrhea occurs in conjunction with dreams cannot be used as a ground for diagnosis.

Clinically, nocturnal emissions are generally caused by deficient *yin* and hyperactive fire, while spontaneous emissions are for the most part due to renal deficiency combined with a lack of essence, cardiac and splenic deficiency following stress or congenital renal deficiency. Thus, nourishing the kidneys and preventing emissions should not be the only methods used for dealing with spermatorrhea regardless of its nature. The general principles to be followed are that the kidneys should be replenished and essence consolidated when dealing with a deficiency syndrome without any signs of heat; *yin* should be nourished and fire dispersed when the patient is suffering from a deficiency syndrome with signs of heat; finally, if dampness-heat has been retained, it should be dispersed. In the last condition, astringency should not be promoted, because eliminating dampness-heat will relieve the spermatorrhea.

1. Deficient *Yin* and Hyperactive Fire

Clinical manifestations: Nocturnal emissions, restlessness, insomnia, dizziness, blurred vision, palpitations, lassitude, possible lumbar soreness and tinnitus, small amounts of yellow urine, a hot sensation when passing urine, a red tongue, and a thready and rapid pulse.

Analysis: Excess mental stress consumes heart *yin* and causes hyperactive heart fire, which induces ministerial fire, disturbing the seminal chamber. Deficient kidney *yin* produces hyperactive ministerial fire, which disturbs the seminal chamber. In either case, spermatorrhea results. Hyperactive heart fire consumes nutrient blood, thus depriving the heart and body of nourishment, with ensuing symptoms including palpitations and lassitude. The depletion of nourishment in the brain causes dizziness and blurred vision. Hyperactive ministerial fire due to deficient kidney *yin* leads to lumbar soreness and tinnitus. The patient experiences a hot sensation when passing urine and passes only small quantities of yellow urine because of the downward movement of heart fire to the small intestine, and the transmission of heat to the urinary bladder. A red tongue and a thready and rapid pulse are signs of *yin* deficiency.

Treatment: To nourish *yin*, disperse fire, calm the mind and consolidate essence.

Prescription: Bolus of Anemarrhenae, Phellodendri and Rehmanniae Preparata (181) or modified Pill for Relieving Nocturnal Emissions (14). Both formulas nourish kidney *yin* and dissipate ministerial fire. The former is stronger, and thus should be used in cases when *yin* is deficient and fire hyperactive. The latter replenishes *qi*, and can be used for both *qi* and *yin* deficiencies. To disperse heat in the lungs, calm the mind and consolidate essence, add Rhizoma Coptidis, Semen Ziziphi Spinosae, Fructus Schisandrae, Os Draconis and Concha Ostreae.

If spermatorrhea is caused by hyperactive monarch and ministerial fire after excess stress, nourish the heart and calm the mind by prescribing Pill for Tranquilizing (128). The patient should not only be treated with medication; it is more important that the patient should get rid of any distracting thoughts.

2. Renal Deficiency with Impaired Storage Function

Clinical manifestations: Increased frequency of nocturnal emissions or even spontaneous emissions, dizziness, blurred vision, tinnitus, lumbar soreness, a pale complexion, an aversion to cold, cold limbs, a pale tongue and a deep and thready pulse, or a red tongue and a thready and rapid pulse.

Analysis: Prolonged spermatorrhea consumes *yin* essence and affects *yang*. The resultant weakness of the seminal gate causes the increased frequency of spermatorrhea. Deficient kidney *yin* deprives the head and face of nourishment, thus producing dizziness, a blurred vision and a pale complexion. Deficient kidney essence deprives the lumbar region and ears of nourishment so that lumbar soreness and tinnitus occur. If *yang* deficiency is more pronounced, a pale tongue and a deep and thready pulse appear; if *yin* deficiency is more pronounced, a red tongue and a thready and rapid pulse are present.

Treatment: To replenish the kidneys and nourish essence.

Prescription: In cases of deficient *yang*, prescribe modified *Yougui* Pill (82); and in cases of deficient *yin*, use modified Pill of Six Drugs Containing Rehmanniae Preparata (56). At the same time, Golden Lock Bolus for Keeping Kidney-Essence (184) or Pill Containing Two Drugs (70) can be taken with water. In the formula of *Yougui* Pill (82), Radix Aconiti Lateralis Preparata, Cortex Cinnamomi, Semen Cuscutae, Cortex Eucommiae and Colla Cornus Cervi warm and tonify kidney *yang*, and Radix Rehmanniae Preparata, Rhizoma Dioscoreae, Fructus Lycii and Radix Angelicae Sinensis replenish essence and blood. Pill of Six Drugs Containing Rehmanniae Preparata (56) replenishes kidney *yin*.

3. Retained Dampness-Heat

Clinical manifestations: Increased frequency of spermatorrhea or discharge of seminal fluid while urinating, restlessness, insomnia, a bitter taste in the mouth or thirst, hot yellow urine or difficult urination, a sticky yellow tongue coating, and a soft and rapid pulse.

Analysis: The downward movement of dampness-heat disturbs the seminal chamber, causing spermatorrhea or urinary discharge of semen in a severe case. Its upward disturbance leads to restlessness, insomnia, a bitter taste in the mouth or thirst, while its downward movement to the bladder gives rise to hot yellow urine or difficult urination. A sticky yellow tongue coating and a soft and rapid pulse are signs of retained dampness-heat.

Treatment: To dissipate heat and relieve dampness.

Prescription: Modified Cheng's Decoction of Dioscoreae Septemlobae for Clearing Turbid Urine (305). Rhizoma Dioscoreae Septemlobae, Cortex Phellodendri, Poria and Semen Plantaginis disperse heat and resolve dampness, Radix Salviae Miltiorrhizae and Semen Nelumbinis dissipate heat in the heart and calm the mind, and Rhizoma Atractylodis Macrocephalae invigorates the spleen and resolves dampness. It is not advisable to administer herbs that promote astringency for this type of spermatorrhea. In cases of difficult urination accompanied by distending sensations in the lower abdomen, add Herba

Patriniae, Radix Paeoniae Rubra and Caulis Sargentodoxae to recirculate stagnant blood and disperse heat, because a prolonged illness often affects the blood vessels and produces heat.

Appendix: Impotence

Impotence refers to the inability to maintain a satisfactory penile erection.

Impotence often occurs together with spermatorrhea and premature ejaculation. Throughout the ages, medical scholars have always believed that this disease is closely related to hepatic and renal ailments. *The Inner Canon of the Yellow Emperor* says, "When the tendon branch of Foot-*Jueyin* Meridian suffers from a disorder, it will give rise to a dysfunction of the penis, which will cause the patient to have difficulties in maintaining an erection in cases where he suffers from internal disorders. It may also cause the penis to shrink when attacked by the cold." The kidney stores essence, on which reproduction is based, and it opens into the external genitalia and anus. Thus, renal deficiency causes a weak erection, and the extreme decline of renal fire leads to an inability to achieve a satisfactory erection. The external genitalia is the confluence of the tendon branch of the three *yin* and *yang* meridians of the foot, which are nourished and moistened by the *Yangming* meridians. Thus dampness-heat retained in the *Yangming* meridians causes penile weakness.

1. Declining of Fire of the Life Gate

Excessive sexual activity or masturbation since childhood causes a deficiency of essence and the decline of fire at the life gate, exhibiting symptoms such as impotence, a pale complexion, dizziness, blurred vision, lassitude, soreness and weakness of the lumbar region and knees, a pale tongue with a white coating, and a deep and thready pulse. Treatment aims at replenishing the kidneys and strengthening *yang*. Modified Pill of Five Kinds of Seed for Reproduction (47) or Pill for Impotence (320) should be prescribed.

2. Damage to the Heart and Spleen

Anxiety damages the heart and spleen, and gives rise to deficiencies of both *qi* and blood, followed by impotence, lassitude, insomnia, a pale complexion, a pale tongue with a thin, sticky coating, and a thready pulse. Treatment aims at replenishing the heart and spleen by prescribing modified Decoction for Invigorating Spleen and Nourishing Heart (110).

3. Damage to the Kidneys

Fear damages the kidneys, giving rise to impotence, depression, palpitations, insomnia, a taut and thready pulse, and a sticky yellow tongue coating, or a pale-green tongue. Treatment aims at replenishing the kidneys and calming the mind by prescribing Powerful Decoction for Potently Invigorating *Qi* and Blood (21) with a proper amount of Semen Ziziphi Spinosae and Radix Polygalae.

4. Downward Movement of Dampness-Heat

The medical classic *Diagnosis and Treatment of Classified Syndromes* says, "Dampness-heat moves downwards and causes a weakness of the penis and impotence." The clinical manifestations are impotence, small amounts of dark yellow urine, soreness of the lower limbs, a yellow tongue coating, and a deep and smooth or a soft, smooth and rapid pulse. Treatment aims at dissipating heat and relieving dampness by prescribing modified Bolus of Anemarrhenae, Phellodendri and Rehmanniae Preparata (181).

Clinical practice has shown that impotence is much more likely to be caused by the decline of fire at the life gate than by dampness-heat. In the course of treatment, the doctor should ensure that the patient builds up his self-confidence and takes enough exercise.

Case Studies

If kidney *qi* is sufficient, then the essence can be safely stored in the body. However, if it is weak, its ability to store essence will be impaired, and spermatorrhea will ensue. Other symptoms are soreness of the lower legs, lassitude, a bitter taste in the mouth, tinnitus, and constipation with dry stools. At the left *chi* position, the pulse is superficial and rough due to deficiency of kidney *qi*; at the *guan* position it is taut, full and rapid. The tongue coating is yellow and dry. Dampness-heat assists ministerial fire and disturbs the seminal chamber. The basic principle of treatment remains to nourish that which is deficient, and reduce that which is in excess. The prescription consists of Radix Asparagi, Radix Rehmanniae, Radix Codonopsis, Cortex Phellodendri, Radix Glycyrrhizae Preparata, Fructus Amomi, Radix Gentianae, Fructus Gardeniae and Radix Bupleuri.

Discussion: Pill for Relieving Nocturnal Emissions (14) can be prescribed together with additional medication to treat spermatorrhea due to deficiency of kidney *yin* and hyperactive ministerial fire. The addition of Radix Gentianae, Fructus Gardeniae and Radix Bupleuri disperse heat in the liver. This example shows that there is no need to use astringents in the treatment of this type of spermatorrhea otherwise fire will become more hyperactive and dampness more severe.

Deficiency of kidney *yin* means an impaired ability to store essence. Hyperactivity of liver *yang* implies a deficiency of *qi*. In a prolonged illness, both *qi* and *yin* are deficient and the leakage of essence leads to spontaneous emissions. The kidneys dominate the bones; empty marrow leads to lumbar soreness and a weakness of the lower limbs. Constipation is due to the dryness of the large intestine caused by this deficiency. The patient's pulse will be feeble. Treatment begins by nourishing essence with a prescription consisting of Radix Rehmanniae Preparata (stir-baked), Concha Ostreae (calcined), Semen Cuscutae, Semen Astragali Complanati, Cortex Eucommiae, Os Draconis (calcined), Fructus Psoraleae, Rhizoma Dioscoreae, Radix Codonopsis, Semen Euryales, Fructus Lycii and Semen Nelumbinis.

Discussion: This case exhibits a deficiency of *yin* and a weakness of the renal seminal gate. The symptoms and pulse both suggest a deficiency syndrome. Thus, Radix Rehmanniae Preparata, Semen Cuscutae, Semen Astragali Complanati, Fructus Lycii, Cortex Eucommiae and Fructus Psoraleae should be prescribed to replenish kidney essence; and Radix Codonopsis and Semen Euryales to replenish *qi* and nourish the essence.

XXXXI. Tinnitus and Deafness

Tinnitus refers to ringing noises in the ears which resemble the chirping of cicadas or the sound of the tides rising and falling. Deafness refers to a condition where partial or complete loss of hearing occurs. These two conditions may occur separately or in combination, as deafness can be a further development of tinnitus. They share a common pathogenesis, and thus can be discussed together.

Tinnitus and deafness as discussed in this chapter are caused by internal disorders. If these complaints are caused by violent explosions, drugs or skin ulcers, they can also be dealt with according to the following principles. For symptoms such as dizziness, insomnia and memory loss which appear in conjunction with tinnitus, refer to the relevant chapters.

Etiology and Pathogenesis

Tinnitus and deafness are most closely related to the kidneys, because the kidneys are linked to the body opening in the ears. To this effect, *The Inner Canon of the Yellow Emperor* notes, "Kidney *qi* communicates with the ear. When the kidneys are functioning well, five types of sound can be heard with the naked ear." Since the 12 regular meridians travel all the way to the ears, either the disturbance of the *qi* of these meridians or failure of the clear *yang-qi* to ascend may result in tinnitus and deafness.

1. Weak Constitution
(1) Deficient kidney essence

This may be the result of prolonged illness or excessive sexual activity. The ear, which is the external orifice of the kidneys, is linked to the brain. The kidneys store essence and dominate both the bones and the marrow, while the brain is the sea of marrow. Thus, sufficient essence nourishes the sea of marrow, and normal hearing is ensured. On the contrary, if essence is consumed, the sea of marrow will become empty, and tinnitus will ensue.

(2) Deficient spleen *qi*

This takes place after stress or prolonged illness, which causes insufficient *qi* and blood and the depletion of the meridians and vessels. Lack of nourishment of the ears leads to tinnitus and deafness.

Deficient spleen *yang* does not allow *yang-qi* to ascend, which is another cause of tinnitus and deafness.

2. Emotional Trauma

Depression leads to stagnant liver *qi*, which over time becomes fire. Excess anger also damages the liver and displaces liver and gallbladder fire upwards along the meridians. When the clear cavity is clouded, tinnitus and deafness occur.

3. Improper Diet

An excessive intake of alcohol or highly-flavored food over a long period of time produces dampness-heat, which forms phlegm and turns into fire. Ascending phlegm-fire blocks the clear cavity, resulting in frequent attacks of tinnitus, or even deafness in severe cases.

To summarize, in this case splenic and renal deficiencies are the primary causes of deafness and tinnitus, with retained phlegm-fire as a secondary cause. Of course, these causes of illness are all interrelated as the upward displacement of liver fire may result from deficient kidney water, and in turn damage kidney *yin*. In this condition, tinnitus and deafness will be aggravated. The spleen distributes essential substance throughout the body and when *qi* can ascend, it functions well. However, when the spleen is deficient, the clear *qi* will fail to ascend to nourish the ear and the ear orifice will then be clouded by turbid *qi*. Splenic deficiency also means impaired transportation and transformation. As a result, phlegm-dampness is produced, which turns into fire over time, forming phlegm-fire. Therefore, tinnitus and deafness resulting from phlegm-fire are mostly related to complaints of the spleen and stomach.

Differentiation and Treatment

It is necessary to clarify whether tinnitus and deafness are recent complaints or long-term conditions, and whether they are caused by deficiencies or excesses. Generally when tinnitus or deafness have an abrupt onset, they are caused by excesses, often of hyperactive fire or retained phlegm-fire. Treatment aims to disperse this fire, relieve phlegm and send the turbid *qi* downwards. Tinnitus and deafness with a gradual onset usually indicate splenic and renal deficiencies. Treatment involves invigorating the spleen, sending the clear *qi* upwards, replenishing the kidneys and benefiting the essence.

1. Excess Syndromes

(1) Hyperactive liver and gallbladder fire

Clinical manifestations: Sudden onset of tinnitus or deafness, headaches, a flushed face, a bitter taste in the mouth, a dry throat, restlessness, irritability which aggravates the symptoms, insomnia, constipation, a red tongue with a yellow coating, and a taut and rapid pulse.

Analysis: Excess anger damages the liver, and liver and gallbladder fire are displaced upwards, blocking the ears. This results in tinnitus, deafness, headaches, a flushed face, a bitter taste and a dry throat. Hyperactive fire in these organs induces emotional irritation. Disturbance of the heart and mind by liver fire brings about restlessness and insomnia. Anger causes unhealthy *qi*, aggravating tinnitus and deafness. Constipation is the consequence of fluid consumption in the intestines due to retained liver fire. A red tongue with a yellow coating and a taut and rapid pulse are signs of hyperactive liver fire.

Treatment: To disperse heat in the liver and gallbladder.

Prescription: Modified Decoction of Gentianae for Purging Liver-Fire (78). Radix Gentianae and Fructus Gardeniae, both bitter in nature, disperse gallbladder fire; Radix Bupleuri and Radix Scutellariae soothe the liver and dissipate heat; Caulis Aristolochiae Manshuriensis, Semen Plantaginis and Rhizoma Alismatis conduct heat downward; Radix Rehmanniae and Radix Angelicae Sinensis nourish liver *yin*. In cases of constipation, add Radix et Rhizoma Rhei. If liver fire flares up, it is likely to consume renal water; if signs of renal deficiency are pronounced and a syndrome combining deficiency and excess appears, add a proper amount of Cortex Moutan, Fructus Ligustri Lucidi and Herba Ecliptae to nourish renal water.

(2) Retained phlegm-fire

Clinical manifestations: Intermittent ringing in the ears like the chirping of cicadas. This gives rise to a sensation that the ears are blocked, thus impairing hearing. Other symptoms are stuffiness in the chest, excess sputum, a bitter taste in the mouth, dizziness, nausea, difficulty in urination and defecation, a thin, sticky, yellow tongue coating, and a taut and smooth pulse.

Analysis: Phlegm-fire blocks the clear cavity, causing ringing noises and blockages of the ears, thus impairing hearing. Retained turbid phlegm in the middle *jiao* hinders the circulation of *qi*, which causes stuffiness, excess sputum and nausea. The transformation of phlegm into fire leads to a bitter taste in the mouth and difficulty in urination and defecation. A thin, yellow, sticky tongue coating and a taut and smooth pulse are signs of retained phlegm-fire.

Treatment: To relieve phlegm, dissipate fire, harmonize the stomach, and send the turbid *qi* downwards.

Prescription: Decoction of Coptidis for Clearing Away Gallbladder-Heat (264). Here, *Erchen* Decoction (3) combined with Fructus Aurantii Immaturus and Caulis Bambusae in Taeniam relieve phlegm, harmonize the stomach and send the turbid *qi* downwards and Rhizoma Coptidis disperses fire. In cases of rising liver *yang* with dizziness, add Concha Margaritifera Usta, Ramulus Uncariae cum Uncis and Concha Haliotidis to calm the liver and suppress hyperactive *yang*. In cases of excess sputum, stuffiness in the chest and difficulty in defecating, prescribe Pill of Lapis Chloriti Usta for Expelling Phlegm (323) to subdue fire and eliminate phlegm.

2. Deficiency Syndromes

(1) Deficient kidney essence

Clinical manifestations: Tinnitus or deafness is often accompanied by dizziness, lumbar soreness and weak knees, a facial flush, thirst, hot sensations in the palms and soles, spermatorrhea, a red tongue, and a thready and weak pulse.

Analysis: Deficient kidney essence deprives the clear cavity of nourishment, resulting in tinnitus and deafness. The upward movement of deficiency fire due to deficient kidney *yin* leads to dizziness, a facial flush, thirst and hot sensations. Disturbance of the seminal chamber by deficiency fire is the cause of spermatorrhea. Deficient kidney essence also means deficient marrow, thus the lower back may feel sore and the patient may suffer from weak knees. A red tongue, and a thready and weak pulse are both signs of deficient kidney essence.

Treatment: To replenish the kidneys and benefit essence.

Prescription: Modified *Zuoci* Pill for Relieving Deafness (123). In this formula, Pill of Six Drugs Containing Rehmanniae Preparata replenishes kidney *yin*, magnetitum tranquilizes and promotes astringency, and Fructus Schisandrae consolidates essence. To nourish *yin* and produce essence, add Carapax et Plastrum Testudinis, Colla Corii Asini, Os Sepiellae seu Sepiae Draconis, Concha Ostreae, Fructus Ligustri Lucidi and Fructus Mori. To strengthen the lumbar region and knees, use Radix Achyranthis Bidentatae and Cortex Eucommiae. In cases of deficient kidney *yang* when the patient has a sore lower back, cold limbs, impotence, a pale tongue and a weak and feeble pulse, Pill of Cistanches (137) can be prescribed to warm and replenish kidney *yang*.

Deafness during old age is usually caused by deficiencies of kidneys and essence. Long-standing oral administration of Bolus of Placenta Hominis (172) tonifies *yin*, *yang*, *qi* and blood. But recovery is not easy.

(2) Failure of clear *qi* to ascend

Clinical manifestations: Tinnitus and deafness occur intermittently, and are alleviated by rest and aggravated by stress. Other symptoms include lassitude, a poor appetite, loose stools, a thready and weak pulse, and a thin, sticky, white tongue coating.

Analysis: Deficient spleen *qi* does not allow *yang-qi* to nourish the clear cavity, resulting in tinnitus and deafness. Splenic deficiency means that transportation is impaired, and gastric deficiency implies impaired reception; these both explain the lack of appetite and loose stools experienced by the patient. A lack of nourishment of the limbs due to deficient spleen *yang* produces lassitude. Stress damages the *qi* of the middle *jiao*, aggravating tinnitus. A thready and weak pulse, and a thin, sticky, white tongue coating are signs of deficient spleen *qi*.

Treatment: To replenish *qi* and send the clear *qi* upwards.

Prescription: Modified Decoction for Benefiting *Qi* and Improving Hearing (245). Radix Ginseng and Radix Astragali benefit the *qi* of the middle *jiao*; Rhizoma Cimicifugae and Radix Puerariae send the clear *qi* upwards; Fructus Viticis sends the clear *qi* upwards and soothes the ears; and Cortex Phellodendri and Radix Paeoniae Alba assist in harmonizing the *qi* of the spleen and stomach. To disperse cardiac heat, add Rhizoma Acori Tatarinowii and Folium Allii Fistulosi.

In cases of the upward displacement of phlegm-dampness due to excess alcohol, symptoms include dizziness, a heavy sensation in the head as if it were tightly wrapped with a towel, stuffiness in the chest, nausea, a soft and smooth pulse and a sticky tongue coating. To treat this condition, remove Cortex Phellodendri and Radix Paeoniae Alba and add Rhizoma Atractylodis Macrocephalae, Poria, Rhizoma Pinelliae and Rhizoma Alismatis which invigorate the spleen, relieve phlegm, and eliminate dampness.

Case Studies

Name: Qin XX; Sex: Male; Age: 30; Occupation: Worker.

Case history: Since October last year, the patient had suffered from impaired hearing. The disease was diagnosed as hysterical deafness, but the treatment given to him was not effective. He went to Shanghai for treatment early this year, and his condition improved greatly. On February 26, he accidentally fell from a height and lost consciousness. When he came to, he found that he once again suffered from impaired hearing, and that he had difficulties sleeping at night. During hospitalization following the accident, the diagnosis of sequelae of cerebral concussion, neurasthenia and hysterical deafness was established. The patient suffered greatly over the next eight months, and so decided to return to Shanghai.

First visit: June 12, 1964.

It had been eight months since the patient lost hearing in both ears. Other clinical symptoms were headaches, dizziness, an inability to use his brain, insomnia (with only two or three hours of sleep every night), lassitude, constipation, a thorny red tongue, and a taut pulse. The patient's appetite was fairly good. All this was due to phlegm-fire retained in the clear passages. Treatment aimed to clear heat in the liver and soothe the ears. The following herbs were prescribed:

Concha Haliotidis	12 g;
Rhizoma Acori Tatarinowii	9 g;
Radix Polygalae Preparata	3 g;
Radix Glycyrrhizae	3 g;
Flos Chrysanthemi	9 g;
Radix Paeoniae Rubra	9 g;
Fructus Gardeniae	9 g;
Fructus Forsythiae	12 g;
Radix Scutellariae	6 g;
Folium Ilicis Latifolia	9 g.

Six doses were prescribed.

Second visit: June 19.

The patient still suffered from deafness, headaches, dizziness and insomnia, although he could sometimes hear things by chance. The tip of his tongue was red and his pulse was slightly taut. The same method of treatment was adopted. Nine grams of Radix Astragali, nine grams of Radix Rehmanniae and 15 grams of Fructus Forsythiae were added; another seven doses were prescribed.

Third visit: June 26.

The patient's hearing had been restored to a certain extent but he still suffered from headaches, insomnia and emaciation. His tongue was cracked and the tip was red, and he had a thready and taut pulse. This was due to deficient *yin* and hyperactive *yang*. The previous treatment was adopted with modified ingredients:

Concha Haliotidis	12 g;
Rhizoma Acori Tatarinowii	9 g;
Radix Polygalae Preparata	4.5 g;
Radix Astragali	9 g;
Radix Rehmanniae	9 g;
Radix Glycyrrhizae	3 g;
Radix Platycodi	3 g;
Flos Chrysanthemi	9 g;
Fructus Tribuli	9 g;
Fructus Forsythiae	12 g;
Folium Ilicis Latifolia	9 g.

Seven doses were prescribed.

Fourth visit: July 3.

The patient's hearing was further restored, and dizziness and insomnia had improved. However, his tongue was still red, and his pulse taut and thready, The same treatment was adopted. Fructus Tribuli was removed and 15 grams of Caulis polygoni Multiflori were added. Another seven doses were prescribed.

Discussion: Deafness is most often due to hepatic and renal deficiencies and rising liver *yang*. This case was followed by cerebral concussion, which further aggravated the problem. In addition to herbs that disperse hepatic heat and suppress hyperactive *yang*, Rhizoma Acori Tatarinowii and Radix Polygalae could be used to subdue liver fire and remove obstructions of the otic collateral; Radix Rehmanniae and Radix Astragali were also prescribed to nourish *yin*, benefit *qi* and assist hearing. After less than a month of treatment, the patient's condition had improved markedly.

A patient named Ding had tinnitus and a blocked sensation in his ears due to both cardiac and renal deficiencies, combined with hyperactive liver *yang*. The kidneys open into the ears, as well as being connected to the heart. Thus deficient kidneys or a deficient heart means that the *yin* essence is depleted, which allows *yang* to be detached and rising liver *yang* causes gallbladder fire to flare up. A pill made of the following ingredients was prescribed to be taken in the morning to replenish the heart and kidneys, and the following decoction was prescribed to be taken in the afternoon to disperse heat in the *Shaoyang* meridians, which travel around the ears.

Pill:

Radix Rehmanniae Preparata	120 g;
Radix Ophiopogonis	45 g;
Carapax et Plastrum Testudinis	60 g;
Concha Ostreae	45 g;
Radix Paeoniae Alba	45 g;
Fructus Schisandrae	30 g;
Herba Ecliptae	45 g;
Magnetitum	30 g;
Lignum Pini Poriaferum	45 g;
Lignum Aquilariae Resinatum	15 g;
Cinnabaris (used as coating)	15 g.

Decoction:

Spica Prunellae	6 g;
Cortex Moutan	3 g;
Radix Rehmanniae	9 g;
Fructus Gardeniae	3 g;
Fructus Ligustri Lucidi	9 g;
Poria	1.5 g;
Radix Glycyrrhizae	1.2 g.

Discussion: Radix Rehmanniae Preparata, Carapax et Plastrum Testudinis and Radix Paeoniae Alba replenish kidney *yin*, and Spica Prunellae, Magnetitum and Concha Ostreae calm the liver and suppress hyperactive *yang*. This method is known as "strengthening water to check hyperactive *yang*."

XXXXII. *Bi*-Syndrome

The Chinese character *bi* literally means obstruction. The symptoms of *bi*-syndrome are pain, soreness, heaviness and numbness of the tendons, muscles and joints, sometimes even redness, swelling, a burning sensation or pain in the joints and limited motion. This is caused by retarded *qi* and blood circulation following invasion of the surface and the meridians by external pathogenic wind, cold, dampness and heat.

As a common disease, *bi*-syndrome may occur in people of either sex and at any age. It is more common in damp and cold places where the weather is changeable. Mild cases may only show soreness and pain in a certain part of the body or certain joints, which becomes aggravated when the weather changes. In severe cases, marked pain, soreness and swelling are recurrent. This may lead to deformities of the joints, affecting the flexibility of the limbs.

The earliest description of *bi*-syndrome can be found in *The Inner Canon of the Yellow Emperor*, which explains its etiology, pathogenesis, classification and clinical manifestations. It says, "Wind, cold and dampness combine to cause *bi*-syndrome. If wind predominates, wandering *bi* will result; if cold predominates, painful *bi* will result; and if dampness predominates, fixed *bi* will result." *Synopsis of Prescriptions of the Golden Chamber* recommends Decoction of Aconiti Preparata (64) for *bi*-syndrome marked by cold-dampness with symptoms of pain and limited motion of joints, and Decoction of Cinnamomi, Paeoniae and Anemarrhenae (227) for *bi*-syndrome of the wind-dampness type. These two formulae are still used today.

Rheumatic arthritis, hypertrophic arthritis, rheumatoid arthritis, and rheumatic fever in Western medicine may be diagnosed and treated according to the following descriptions.

Etiology and Pathogenesis

The external cause of *bi*-syndrome is the invasion of the muscles, joints and meridians by pathogenic wind, cold and dampness. The internal cause of this is weak resistance and deficiencies of the nutrient and defensive *qi*. The pathogenesis is *qi* and blood stagnation.

External pathogenic factors invade when the body is weak.

The medical classic *Prescriptions for Life Saving* explains it thus: "*Bi*-syndrome is produced by weak resistance and deficiencies of the nutrient and defensive *qi* complicated by the invasion of pathogenic wind, cold and dampness." Invasion of the muscles, joints and meridians by pathogenic wind, cold and dampness can be a result of prolonged residence in a damp place, wading through water, being caught by the rain and abnormal weather changes.

Retained heat due to excess *yang-qi* and deficient *yin* and hyperactive *yang* make it possible for the invading pathogenic cold to turn into heat. When heat spreads along the meridians to the joints, a series of heat-related signs can be seen, thus this type of *bi*-syndrome is a heat-related syndrome.

In a prolonged case of *bi*-syndrome, pathogenic factors in the meridians turn into heat, giving rise to symptoms similar to those of a heat-related *bi*-syndrome.

If a *bi*-syndrome caused by wind, cold, dampness or heat becomes lingering, *qi* and blood stagnation will result, and ecchymosis and nodules may form around the joints.

This development allows pathogenic factors to travel from the meridians to the *zang-fu* organs. At this stage, *bi*-syndrome is quite serious, with deficiencies and excesses co-existing in many parts of the body. The symptoms of this are usually muscular atrophy and deformity or rigidity of joints as well as palpitations, coughing, asthmatic breathing, and edema.

Differentiation and Treatment

From the point of view of pathogenesis, *bi*-syndrome is usually classified into two types, one caused by wind-cold-dampness and the other by heat. Their common symptoms are arthralgia and the inflexibility of limbs and joints. Since wind, cold and dampness often occur in combination, it must be determined which is the predominant factor. It is also necessary to clarify whether excess pathogenic factors or deficient anti-pathogenic *qi* is more pronounced. *Bi*-syndrome during its initial stage is caused by excesses, so treatment aims primarily to eliminate pathogenic factors. Prolonged cases exhibit deficient anti-pathogenic *qi* complicated by excess pathogenic factors. As treatment, the *qi* should be promoted and the pathogenic factors should be eliminated. In cases where phlegm and blood are stagnant, both problems should be resolved.

1. *Bi*-Syndrome of the Wind-Cold-Dampness Type

(1) Wandering *bi*-syndrome

Clinical manifestations: Wandering pain in the joints, limited flexibility, external symptoms such as aversion to wind and fever may be present, a thin white tongue coating, and a superficial pulse.

Analysis: These are common symptoms of the *bi*-syndrome caused by wind, cold and dampness. These symptoms block the meridians and retard the circulation of *qi* and blood, causing pain. When the muscles and joints are deprived of nourishment, their flexibility is limited. Wandering *bi*-syndrome is characterized by pain which spreads from the upper limbs to the lower limbs, and vice versa. This is because pathogenic wind occurs in gusts marked by rapid change. The invasion of pathogenic wind causes a struggle between the anti-pathogenic *qi* and the pathogenic factors, producing external symptoms. A thin white tongue coating and a superficial pulse are also external signs of the *bi*-syndrome caused by pathogenic factors.

Treatment: To eliminate wind, remove obstructions from the meridians, and disperse cold and dampness.

Prescription: Decoction of Ledebouriellae (139) is the main formula. Its chief function is to eliminate wind and dampness. In the formula, Radix Ledebouriellae, Radix Gentianae Macrophyllae, Radix Angelicae Pubescentis and Poria eliminate wind and dampness; Ramulus Cinnamomi, Herba Ephedrae and Radix Puerariae relieve symptoms in the muscles and disperse cold; Radix Angelicae Sinensis nourishes the blood, harmonizes the nutrient *qi*, and removes obstructions from the meridians; Semen Armeniacae Amarum promotes pulmonary dispersal and circulates *qi*. Radix Scutellariae can be removed if there are no signs of heat.

If pain in the joints is accompanied by signs of heat such as a dry, sore throat or a sticky white tongue coating with a yellow tinge, then cold and hot herbs can be combined, and modified Decoction of Cinnamomi, Paeoniae, and Anemarrhenae (227) should be prescribed.

(2) *Bi*-syndrome marked by severe pain

Clinical manifestations: Arthralgia is severe with a fixed location. It is aggravated by cold and alleviated by warmth. The affected joints are inflexible, but the skin there is not red or hot. The tongue coating is thin and white, the pulse taut and tense.

Analysis: Cold, a *yin* factor, may cause stagnation; thus arthralgia caused by cold has a fixed location. The circulation of *qi* and blood becomes further retarded on exposure to cold; thus arthralgia is severe, and is aggravated by cold and alleviated by warmth. Contractions caused by the cold make the joints less flexible. Because of pathogenic cold, the skin of the painful areas is not red or hot, the tongue coating is white and the pulse is taut.

Treatment: To disperse cold, relieve pain, eliminate wind and remove dampness.

Prescription: Decoction of Aconiti Preparata (64) is the main formula. This focuses on eliminating the cold. In this formula, Rhizoma Aconiti Preparata warms the meridians, disperses cold, eliminates wind and dampness and relieves pain; Herba Ephedrae warms the meridians and disperses the cold; Radix Astragali replenishes *qi* and nourishes the body surface so as to prevent perspiration; and Radix Paeoniae Rubra activates blood circulation and disperses pathogenic factors. Since Rhizoma Aconiti Preparata is toxic, it is not advisable to use large dosages; however, it becomes less toxic after boiling for a long time. If pain is more pronounced in the shoulders or elbows, add Radix seu Rhizoma Notopterygii and Rhizoma Curcumae Longae to eliminate wind, remove obstructions from the meridians and relieve pain. If pain is more pronounced in the knee and ankle joints, add Radix Achyranthis Bidentatae, Radix Angelicae Pubescentis and Fructus Chaenomelis to remove obstructions from the meridians, eliminate dampness and relieve pain. For pain in the lumbar region, add Cortex Eucommiae, Herba Taxilli, Radix Dipsaci and Herba Erodii seu Geranii to strengthen the lumbar region, eliminate wind and relieve pain. In all these conditions, herbs that activate blood circulation and remove vascular obstruction can be added, such as Caulis Spatholobi, Radix Angelicae Sinensis and Caulis Trachelospermi.

(3) *Bi*-syndrome marked by localized pain

Clinical manifestations: Arthralgia is accompanied by heaviness or swelling of the joints with fixed pain. Other clinical manifestations are a heavy sensation in the hands and feet, limited flexibility, numbness of the muscles and skin, a sticky white tongue coating, and a soft and retarded pulse.

Analysis: Dampness, a *yin* factor, may cause viscosity and heaviness resulting in a heavy sensation with a fixed location. Invasion by pathogenic dampness blocks *qi* and blood circulation and produces a dysfunction of the meridians, resulting in numbness of the muscles and skin and limited flexibility. A sticky white tongue coating and a soft, retarded pulse are signs of dampness-syndrome.

Treatment: To eliminate dampness, remove obstructions from the meridians, dispel wind and disperse cold.

Prescription: Modified Decoction of Coicis (319). This primarily eliminates dampness, and secondarily dispels wind and cold. Semen Coicis and Rhizoma Atractylodis invigorate the spleen and eliminate dampness; Herba Ephedrae, Ramulus Cinnamomi and Radix Aconiti Preparata eliminate both internal and external cold and dampness so as to invigorate *yang*; Rhizoma seu Radix Notopterygii, Radix Angelicae Pubescentis and Radix Ledebouriellae eliminate wind and dampness; Rhizoma Chuanxiong and Radix Angelicae Sinensis activate blood circulation and remove vascular obstructions; and Radix Glycyrrhizae harmonizes the middle *jiao*. In cases of numbness of the muscles and skin, add Ramulus Mori, Caulis Spatholobi and Herba Siegesbeckiae to eliminate wind and remove obstructions from the meridians.

In cases where it is difficult to clarify which pathogenic factor predominates, for example, when the condition is complex and the patient is suffering from violent pain, prescribe a general formula named Decoction for Relieving *Bi*-Syndromes (329). In this, Rhizoma seu Radix Notopterygii, Radix Angelicae Pubescentis, Radix Gentianae Macrophyllae, Caulis Piperis Kadsurae and Ramulus Mori eliminate wind and dampness and remove obstructions from the meridians; Radix Angelicae Sinensis, Olibanum and Rhizoma Chuanxiong activate blood circulation and relieve pain; Cortex Cinnamomi disperses cold; and Radix Aucklandiae and Radix Glycyrrhizae regulate *qi* and relieve acute pain. If it is possible to recognize wind as the predominant factor in a complicated condition, prescribe large doses of Rhizoma seu Radix Notopterygii, Radix Angelicae Pubescentis and Radix Ledebouriellae. If cold predominates, Radix Aconiti Preparata and Herba Asari can be added; whilst Semen Coicis and Radix Stephaniae Tetrandrae can be used if dampness is the predominant pathogenic factor.

Symptoms resulting from deficient *qi* and blood or hepatic and renal deficiency may appear in prolonged cases. These include lassitude, an aversion to cold, a preference for warmth, pain or a cold sensation in the lumbar region and knees, a pale tongue, and a thready pulse. In these cases, use herbs that replenish *qi* and blood, or replenish the liver and kidneys, or modified Decoction for Replenishing *Qi* and Blood to Relieve Wind *Bi*-Syndrome (19). In this formula, Radix Ginseng, Radix Astragali, Radix Rehmanniae Preparata, Radix Paeoniae Alba, Radix Angelicae Sinensis and Rhizoma Chuanxiong replenish *qi* and blood; Cortex Eucommiae, Radix Achyranthis Bidentatae and Radix Dipsaci replenish the kidneys and strengthen the lumbar region; and Cortex Cinnamomi, Herba Asari, Radix Ledebouriellae, Radix Angelicae Pubescentis, Radix Gentianae Macrophyllae and Poria warm *yang*, disperse cold and eliminate wind and dampness. This formula not only eliminates wind, cold and dampness, but also tonifies *qi* and blood and nourishes the liver and kidneys.

2. *Bi*-Syndrome due to Heat

Clinical manifestations: The onset of the disease is acute, with the joints swelling, becoming red and hot to touch. The pain is aggravated by touching and alleviated by coldness. At the same time, one or several joints may lose their flexibility. Some cases exhibit wandering pains. The systemic symptoms include fever, sweating, an aversion to wind, thirst, restlessness, a dry yellow tongue coating, and a smooth, rapid pulse.

Analysis: Fire is the most severe form of heat, which is a *yang* factor. Heat is characterized by the speed of its onset, which explains why *bi*-syndrome caused by heat breaks out all of a sudden. Invasion of the joints by pathogenic heat blocks *qi* and blood circulation, giving rise to redness, swelling, a hot sensation, and pain in the joints. This redness, swelling and pain make the joints less flexible. If there are wandering pains, these are caused by invasion of pathogenic wind. Fever, thirst, a dry yellow tongue coating, and a smooth and rapid pulse are caused by excess heat.

Treatment: To disperse heat, remove obstructions from the meridians and eliminate wind and dampness.

Prescription: Modified White Tiger Decoction with Cinnamomi (104). Gypsum Fibrosum and Radix Glycyrrhizae disperse heat; Rhizoma Anemarrhenae dissipates heat and nourishes *yin*; Ramulus Cinnamomi eliminates wind and removes obstructions from the meridians; and Radix Glycyrrhizae and Fructus Oryzae Sativae nourish the stomach and harmonize the middle *jiao* in order to protect the body's anti-pathogenic *qi* when heat is being dispersed. Herbs that disperse heat, activate blood circulation and remove vascular obstruction can be added, such as Fructus Forsythiae, Cortex Moutan, Cortex Phellodendri, Radix Paeoniae Rubra, Caulis Lonicerae and Radix Stephaniae Tetrandrae.

If heat is not as pronounced as dampness and is marked by a headache or a heavy sensation in the head, stuffiness in the chest, a sticky yellow tongue coating and a soft, rapid pulse, then add Semen Coicis, Radix Stephaniae Tetrandrae and Talcum to disperse heat and relieve dampness.

If the *bi*-syndrome is caused by heat, heat may turn into fire and consume fluid, making the joints red, swollen and painful, and causing muscle contractions, a high fever, thirst, restlessness, a red tongue with little moisture, and a taut, rapid pulse. All this suggests the penetration of the bones and muscles by toxin-heat. Treatment then aims to disperse heat, eliminate toxins, nourish *yin* and cool blood by prescribing Powder of Cornu Rhinocerotis (307) and adding herbs that nourish *yin* and produce fluid, such as Radix Rehmanniae, Radix Scrophulariae and Radix Ophiopogonis. In cases where the patient experiences a downward movement of dampness-heat causing swelling and pain in the lower limbs, urine which is dark yellow and hot, a sticky yellow tongue coating, and a soft and rapid pulse, prescribe Pill of Phellodendri, Atractylodis and Cyathulae (16) along with herbs that disperse heat and relieve dampness, such as Cortex Erythrinae, Radix Stephaniae Tetrandrae, Rhizoma Dioscoreae Septemlobae and Caulis Aristolochiae Manshuriensis.

If the above symptoms cannot be eliminated over time, *qi* and blood may stagnate, followed by swelling and deformities, pain and limited flexibility. When the internal organs are affected, clinical manifestations will include palpitations, stuffiness in the chest, shortness of breath, ecchymosis, a bluish-purple tongue, and a deep, unsmooth pulse. Treatment primarily activates blood circulation and resolves stasis. This can be done by prescribing Decoction for Relieving *Bi*-Syndrome (231) along with herbs that replenish *qi* and invigorate *yang* such as Radix Astragali and Ramulus Cinnamomi, or medication made from animal substances such as Zaocys, Scorpio, Squama Manitis, Lumbricus and Eupolyphaga seu Steleophaga.

Acupuncture and moxibustion, massage, steaming and washing with hot decoctions, and physical therapy are also effective, and can be used by themselves or in combination with each other.

Remarks

When methods of dispersing cold, dispelling dampness and dissipating heat are adopted in the treatment of various *bi*-syndromes, attention should be paid to eliminating wind. For the treatment of the wandering *bi*-syndrome, in addition to herbs that eliminate wind, herbs that activate blood circulation and replenish blood should be used, such as Radix Angelicae Sinensis, Radix Paeoniae Rubra, Flos Carthami, Rhizoma Chuanxiong, Rhizoma Curcumae Longae, Olibanum and Myrrha. The reason is that if the blood circulates around the body smoothly, this facilitates the elimination of wind. An old saying in the medical world is that "blood should be treated before wind, and wind will be eliminated when the blood circulates smoothly."

In the treatment of localized *bi*-syndrome, herbs that invigorate the spleen and replenish *qi* should be added to those that eliminate dampness. This is because the normal functioning of the spleen in transportation and transformation ensures the spontaneous elimination of dampness. In treating prolonged cases, attention should also be paid to activating blood circulation, resolving stasis and replenishing the liver and kidneys.

Case Studies

This female patient was thin and weak, with deficiencies of both *qi* and blood. As she worked too hard, her body had been invaded by pathogenic wind and dampness, and she felt pain in her joints. Her pulse was rapid, unsmooth and irregular, skipping a beat every ten or 20 beats. She had suffered from these problems over a long period of time. Now her symptoms included emaciation, dull skin, rigidity and swelling of the elbows, wrists, ankles and knees, as well as in the small joints of the hands and feet. The skin around these joints was slightly red, and the severe pain she felt was aggravated by massage. All this was due to the fact that cold had turned into heat, dampness into dryness, and wind-dryness was combined with wind-heat. Treatment sought to nourish the blood, produce fluid, eliminate dryness and heat and remove obstructions from the meridians by dispelling heat instead of by offering warmth. Herbs that are bitter and cold in nature were used. The following herbs were prescribed:

Radix Angelicae Sinensis (fibrous roots)	9 g;
Herba Taxilli	9 g;
Radix Achyranthis Bidentatae	12 g;
Lumbricus	9 g;
Radix Aucklandiae	9 g;
Rhizoma Acori Tatarinowii	3 g;
Fructus Corni	9 g;

Cortex Lycii	9 g;
Carapax Trionycis	12 g;
Rhizoma Picrorrhizae	2.4 g.

The patient felt slightly better after one week of treatment, much better after two weeks and even better after four weeks. After two months, she had regained her health completely.

Discussion: A weakened resistance made the patient's joints and muscles more liable to be invaded by pathogenic factors, thus the resulting *bi*-syndrome was stubborn. The pathogenic factors penetrated deeply, reaching the heart and thus causing an irregular pulse with missing beats and swollen joints due to stagnant blood. A prolonged illness damaged the liver and kidneys, producing fire due to a deficiency of *yin*. Fire and wind-dampness combined to cause pain in the joints which became slightly reddish. This pain was aggravated by pressure. Since the condition was complex, exhibiting signs of both deficiency and excess, a simple method was not believed to be effective. So the doctor adopted a flexible method, nourishing the blood, eliminating wind, activating blood circulation, removing obstructions from the meridians, replenishing the liver and kidneys and dispersing heat. In this prescription, Radix Angelicae Sinensis nourishes the blood and activates blood circulation; Lumbricus, Radix Achyranthis Bidentatae and Radix Aucklandiae eliminate wind and remove obstructions from the meridians; Fructus Corni, Carapax Trionycis and Herba Taxilli replenish the liver and kidneys; Rhizoma Picrorrhizae and Cortex Lycii disperse heat caused by deficiencies. In spite of the fact that this patient had suffered from a prolonged illness, complicated symptoms and an abnormal pulse, she recovered fully. Thus it is possible for patients to recover fully as long as the syndrome is diagnosed correctly, herbs are used properly and treatment is given at the correct rate.

Name: Yang XX; Sex: Female; Age: 16; Occupation: Student.
First visit: June 6, 1963.

The patient had had a high fever for a whole week, and her joints were red, swollen and painful. According to the patient, she often had a sore throat in the past. During the past week, she caught a cold and ran a high fever. She was afraid of wind and did not sweat. In the meantime, she had a sore throat and her left ankle joint became red, swollen, painful, losing much of its flexibility. Then her right ankle and both her wrists also became red, swollen and painful. The condition was so bad that she could hardly sleep at night, and it was aggravated by pressure. She gradually lost her appetite. After her body temperature rose to 39°C, she received penicillin injections of 40 units for four consecutive days. As a result, her fever subsided and her sore throat improved. On June 4, she came down with abdominal pain and diarrhea, having bowel movements twice a day. The stool examination showed no mucus or blood in the stools. The side and tip of the patient's tongue were red, and the coating was white and sticky at the root. Her pulse was rapid.

Physical examination: The patient's tonsils were congested and swollen, her throat was slightly red. Blowing systolic murmur II° was heard at the apex. Blood test showed white blood cells 10,900, acidophils 2%, neutrophils 78%, lymphocytes 20%, ESR 110 mm, antistreptolysin-0 test 2,500 units per ml, and reactive protein C+++.

Diagnosis: Retained heat complicated by cold gave rise to the patient's aversion to wind and her high fever. If the patient has excessive heat affecting the lungs and stomach added to the sudden invasion of wind-cold, then heat tends to be retained in the meridians, blocking *qi* and blood circulation. The consequences of this are redness, swelling and pain in the joints, limiting their flexibility. Invasion of the body surface by cold resulted in arthralgia that grew worse at night. A red tongue with a sticky coating and a rapid pulse were signs of retained dampness-heat. Abdominal pain and diarrhea were not caused by the invasion of the *Taiyin* meridians by cold-dampness, but by the downward movement of heat to the large intestine. Because heat was retained in the *Yangming* meridians, treatment aimed at eliminating wind and dissipating heat in those meridians with modified White Tiger Decoction with Cinnamomi (104):

Ramulus Cinnamomi	3 g;
Herba Ephedrae (preparata)	3 g;
Rhizoma seu Radix Notopterygii	9 g;
Radix Angelicae Pubescentis	9 g;
Radix Ledebouriellae	9 g;
Rhizoma Atractylodis Macrocephalae	12 g;
Rhizoma Anemarrhenae	6 g;
Gypsum Fibrosum	15 g;
Caulis Lonicerae	15 g;
Semen Coicis	12 g;
Semen Coicis Preparata	12 g;
Radix Paeoniae Alba	9 g;
Radix Paeoniae Rubra	9 g;
Radix Salviae Miltiorrhizae	15 g;
Ramulus Mori (stir-baked in wine)	30 g.

The patient took one dose, and the following day returned to the clinic. The pain was less violent at night so she was able to sleep well. Redness and swelling of the joints on the right side had subsided, but redness, swelling, and a burning sensation still existed on the left side. The patient's throat was no longer sore, but she was still slightly thirsty. She was sent to hospital because her condition had not undergone a marked improvement. The six doses she took in the hospital were all based on the previous prescription. On her last visit, her body temperature was normal, all her joints were free of pain and swelling, both urination and defecation were normal, sleep was good, and the pulse was thready and retarded. A blood test showed antistreptolysin-0 2,500 units per ml, and reactive protein C++. Since her recovery from this disease, she was allowed to leave hospital on June 14. A follow-up visit showed that she had not suffered from a relapse.

Discussion: This is a case of *bi*-syndrome caused by heat. Wind, cold and dampness had turned into heat, but cold and dampness had not yet been completely eliminated. Thus treatment included dispelling heat, eliminating dampness, removing obstructions from the meridians and dispersing cold. In the prescription, Rhizoma Anemarrhenae and Gypsum Fibrosum, which are sweet and cold in nature, clear heat caused by excesses from the *qi* system; Herba Ephedrae, Ramulus Cinnamomi and Radix Ledebouriellae eliminate wind and disperse cold; Rhizoma seu Radix Notopterygii, Radix Angelicae Pubescentis, Semen Coicis, Caulis Lonicerae and Ramulus Mori eliminate wind and dampness, and remove obstructions from the meridians; and Radix Salviae Miltiorrhizae and Radix Paeoniae Rubra activate blood circulation and remove stasis to eliminate pathogenic wind.

XXXXIII. *Wei*-Syndrome

Wei-syndrome refers to a condition when the muscles are weak and flaccid or when muscles have atrophied after prolonged immobility. This disease most commonly affects the lower limbs.

The Inner Canon of the Yellow Emperor describes this disease in great detail, pointing out that its main pathogenesis is heat in the lungs. Pulmonary dryness and heat prevent body fluid from reaching the five *zang* organs, giving rise to weak and flaccid muscles in the lower limbs and motor impairment. This book also classifies the *wei*-syndrome into five categories according to the relationship between the five *zang* organs and the five tissues (skin, vessel, tendon, bone, and muscle). As a matter of fact, this classification is inappropriate. But it is true that the pathological conditions of *wei*-syndrome differ in depth and intensity. This book also states, "The *wei*-syndrome can only be treated through the *Yangming* meridians." The theory of "dampness-heat producing *wei*-syndrome" was also put forward for the first time in this book. Later medical scholars contributed further to the recognition and treatment of this disease. For instance, *A Complete Collection of Jingyue's Treatise* says, "It is sometimes the case that *wei*-syndrome is caused by the exhaustion of the body's primordial *qi*. A deficiency of essence means an inability to irrigate, while blood deficiency implies an inability to nourish." *A Guide to Clinical Practice with Case Records* attributes this disease to "disorders of the liver, kidney, lung and stomach meridians."

Polyneuritis, acute myelitis, progressive myotrophy, myasthenia gravis, periodic paralysis, myodystrophy, hysterical paralysis, and sequelae following infection of the central nervous system manifesting flaccid paralysis may be diagnosed and treated according to the following descriptions.

Etiology and Pathogenesis

The causes of *wei*-syndrome can be both external and internal. The external causes refer to exposure to pathogenic warmth and heat, and invasion by dampness-heat; the syndrome they cause is of the excess type. The internal ones include deficient *qi*, blood, *yin* and essence; this syndrome is of the deficiency type. The pathogenesis of the disease is malnutrition of the muscles and tendons, and the changes affect the lungs, stomach, liver and kidneys.

1. Consumption of Fluid due to Heat in the Lungs

Muscles and tendons rely on the warmth and nourishment of *qi*, blood and fluid in order to function normally and the distribution of *qi*, blood and fluid in the body is guaranteed by normal pulmonary functioning. Exposure to pathogenic warmth and heat produces a high fever. Residual pathogenic factors following an illness produce a low fever. In either case, pulmonary fluid is consumed, depriving muscles and tendons of nourishment and subsequently *wei*-syndrome occurs. Ding Ganren (1866-1926 A.D.) said, "Weeds and trees rely on the nourishment and moisture of the rain and dew in order to grow. To avoid paralysis of the lower limbs, the body fluid in the lungs should be distributed normally." He added, "In the late stages of a febrile disease, the *yin* fluid is damaged. Hyperactive fire caused by deficiencies and heat in the lungs cause paralysis in the lower limbs."

2. Invasion by Dampness-Heat

If the patient lives in a damp place or is caught in the rain, this allows dampness to remain inside the body. Over a long period of time, the dampness turns into heat. If the spleen and stomach are damaged as a result of an improper diet, such as excess greasy or spicy food or excess alcohol, then dampness is produced, which may also turn into heat over a long period of time. Once produced, dampness-heat invades the muscles and tendons, and impairs *qi* and blood circulation. If the patient has lost the use of their muscles and tendons, then this leads to *wei*-syndrome.

3. Splenic and Gastric Deficiency

The spleen and stomach are the sources of *qi*, blood and body fluid. If the patient suffers from constitutional deficiencies or has suffered from a prolonged illness, then this means that the sources are insufficient. Malnutrition of the muscles and tendons leads to *wei*-syndrome.

4. Hepatic and Renal Deficiency

The kidneys store essence, while the liver stores blood. The essence and blood constitute the material basis of physiological functioning. Weakness following a prolonged illness or excessive sexual activity damages these organs and causes deficiencies of essence and blood. Malnutrition of the muscles and tendons leads to *wei*-syndrome.

Diagnosis

Some diseases at certain stages exhibit symptoms similar to those of the *wei*-syndrome. Attention should be paid to the differences.

1. *Bi*-Syndrome

Some patients with *bi*-syndrome may lack flexibility in their limbs and when *bi*-syndrome is in its later stages, they may suffer from muscular atrophy. The former is caused by pain, swelling, or rigidity in the joints. *Wei*-syndrome is characterized by flaccid and weak muscles. Patients lose control of their limbs, as if their joints have been detached from their bodies.

Some patients with *wei*-syndrome may also feel pain in the muscles and tendons. This is completely different from the type of pain felt by patients suffering from *bi*-syndrome, who will feel pain in their joints.

2. Apoplexy

Patients suffering from apoplexy may also lose the use of their muscles. However, in this case paralysis affects upper and lower limbs on the same side of the body simultaneously, and the accompanying symptoms include contortions of the facial muscles and around the eyes, slurred speech, and even the loss of consciousness.

In *wei*-syndrome, paralysis often occurs in the lower limbs. In a very few cases, the upper and lower limbs on the same side become paralyzed at the same time, but this is not accompanied by any of the symptoms of apoplexy.

Differentiation and Treatment

In *wei*-syndrome, paralysis most often affects the lower limbs, although there are also cases where both upper and lower limbs are affected. A patient with severe *wei*-syndrome cannot walk unaided or hold anything in their hands. Muscular atrophy and paralysis occur in prolonged cases.

It should be diagnosed whether the syndrome is caused by deficiencies or excesses. *Wei*-syndrome caused by fluid consumption due to heat in the lungs or by the invasion of dampness-heat has an acute onset and develops rapidly; it is usually caused by excesses. Treatment aims to disperse heat, moisten dryness and eliminate dampness. *Wei*-syndrome caused by a weak spleen and stomach or hepatic and renal deficiency develops gradually over a long time; this is usually caused by deficiencies. Treatment aims to replenish *qi*, invigorate the spleen and nourish the liver and kidneys. Attention should also be paid to complicated conditions, such as those caused by deficiencies complicated by excesses or excesses complicated by deficiencies. To promote the production of body fluid, *qi*, blood and essence, the principle of getting rid of *wei*-syndrome by treating the *Yangming* meridians should be taken into account. This is because body fluid in the lungs originates in the spleen and stomach, and likewise essence and blood in the liver and kidneys are produced there. Weakness of the spleen and stomach affects their sources and deprives the muscles and tendons of nourishment, with the result that flaccidity is hard to cure.

Therefore, efforts should be made to replenish the stomach and nourish *yin* in cases of deficient body fluid in the stomach but invigorate the spleen and benefit *qi* in cases of deficient spleen-*qi*. When the tendons and muscles are supplied with sufficient *qi*, blood and body fluid and once organic functions have been restored, the *wei*-syndrome will go away. However, the principle of treating the *Yangming* meridians cannot be used for all kinds of *wei*-syndrome. In order to treat the *wei*-syndrome correctly, its cause must first be correctly determined.

1. Consumption of Fluid due to Pulmonary Heat

Clinical manifestations: Weakness and flaccidity of the limbs occur suddenly during or after an illness. The accompanying symptoms include fever, restlessness, thirst, coughing, a dry throat, dark yellow urine, constipation, a red tongue with a yellow coating, and a thready and rapid pulse.

Analysis: Consumption of fluid prevents it from being distributed around the body. Malnutrition of the muscles and tendons leads to weak and flaccid limbs. If lung *qi* does not descend, a cough will occur; if fluid does not go upwards to provide nourishment, the patient will suffer from thirst and a dry throat; if fluid is not distributed around the large intestine, the patient will experience constipation and dark yellow urine. A red tongue with a yellow coating and a thready and rapid pulse are signs of fluid consumption by internal heat.

Treatment: To disperse heat, moisten dryness, nourish the lungs and produce body fluid.

Prescription: Modified Decoction for Clearing Away Dryness and Treating Lung Disorders (285). Folium Mori, which is light in nature, promotes pulmonary dispersal and dissipates dryness in the lungs; Gypsum Fibrosum dispels dryness and heat in the lungs and stomach; Colla Corii Asini, Radix Ophiopogonis and Fructus Cannabis moisten the lung and produce body fluid; Radix Ginseng and Radix Glycyrrhizae tonify *qi* and produce fluid; and Semen Armeniacae Amarum and Folium Eriobotryae, both bitter in nature, promote the smooth circulation of lung *qi*. In cases of excess phlegm, add Bulbus Fritillariae Cirrhosae and Fructus Trichosanthis to disperse heat in the lungs and relieve phlegm. In cases of high fever, thirst and sweating, remove Radix Ginseng and Colla Corii Asini from the prescription, use large doses of Gypsum Fibrosum and add Rhizoma Anemarrhenae, Fructus Forsythiae and Flos Lonicerae to disperse heat and other pathogenic factors.

If the patient is suffering from a poor appetite and a dry mouth and throat after fever has subsided, this suggests that pulmonary and gastric *yin* have been damaged. Decoction for Benefiting Stomach (246) should be prescribed with Semen Coicis, Rhizoma Dioscoreae and Fructus Setariae Germinatus added to benefit the stomach and produce body fluid.

2. Invasion by Dampness-Heat

Clinical manifestations: Heaviness, flaccidity, weakness, or slight swelling and numbness of the limbs, particularly the lower limbs. Other clinical manifestations are fever, distress in the chest and epigastrium, difficult urination with dark yellow urine and a burning sensation on passing urine, a sticky yellow tongue coating, and a soft and rapid pulse.

Analysis: Invasion of the muscles and skin by dampness produces heaviness and slight swelling. Invasion of the meridians by dampness-heat blocks *qi* and blood circulation, causing the muscles and tendons to become flaccid, weak and numb. Dampness-heat retained in the chest and diaphragm leads to distress and stuffiness there. Its downward movement gives rise to difficult and painful urination with dark yellow urine and a burning sensation on passing urine. Fever, a sticky yellow tongue coating and a soft and rapid pulse are signs of retained dampness-heat.

Treatment: To disperse heat and eliminate dampness.

Prescription: Modified Powder of Phellodendri and Atractylodis with Additional Drugs (111). Cortex Phellodendri disperses heat: Rhizoma Atractylodis dispels dampness; and Rhizoma Dioscoreae Septemlobae and Radix Stephaniae Tetrandrae dissipate heat and eliminate dampness. To eliminate dampness and remove obstructions from the meridians, add Semen Coicis, Excrementum Bombycis and Fructus Chaenomelis. In cases of excess dampness when the tongue coating is sticky and white, add Cortex Magnoliae Officinalis, Poria and Gypsum Fibrosum to regulate *qi* and eliminate dampness. Aromatics such as Herba Agastachis and Herba Eupatorii can be added to resolve dampness in the summer. If *yin* is damaged by dampness-heat with signs including emaciation, a hot sensation in the lower limbs, restlessness, a thready and rapid pulse and a tongue with a red tip and border or a tongue with exfoliated coating in the center, remove Rhizoma Atractylodis and add Radix Rehmanniae, Radix Ophiopogonis and Radix Trichosanthis to disperse heat and produce fluid. In cases where the limbs are numb and there is only limited flexibility of the joints complicated by signs of stagnant blood such as a purple tongue and an unsmooth pulse, add Semen Persicae, Flos Carthami, Radix Paeoniae Rubra and Ramulus Mori to activate blood circulation and remove obstructions from the meridians.

3. Splenic and Gastric Deficiency

Clinical manifestations: The disease develops gradually and persists for a long time as the weakness and flaccidity of the limbs become more serious. Muscular atrophy is pronounced. Other clinical manifestations include lassitude, a poor appetite, loose stools, a pale complexion and puffy face, a thin white tongue coating, and a thready pulse.

Analysis: Deficiency of these organs means that the sources of *qi* and blood are insufficient, thus the limbs are deprived of nourishment and become flaccid and weak, with pronounced muscular atrophy. The sinking of clear *qi* due to impaired transport causes a poor appetite and loose stools. Lassitude, a puffy face, a pale complexion and a thready pulse are caused by deficiencies of the *qi* and blood following weaknesses of the spleen and stomach.

Treatment: To invigorate the spleen and benefit *qi*.

Prescription: Modified Powder of Ginseng, Poria, and Atractylodis Macrorecphalae (190). Radix Ginseng, Rhizoma Atractylodis Macrocephalae, Rhizoma Dioscoreae, Semen Lablab Album and Semen Nelumbinis invigorate the spleen and benefit *qi*; and Poria, Semen Coicis, Pericarpium Citri Reticulatae and Fructus Amomi invigorate the spleen, eliminate dampness, harmonize the stomach and regulate *qi*. In cases where the patient has an aversion to cold and cold limbs, add Radix Aconiti Lateralis Preparata and Rhizoma Zingiberis to warm spleen *yang*. In cases where both *qi* and blood are deficient, add Radix Astragali in large doses, along with Radix Angelicae Sinensis to help replenish *qi* and blood.

4. Hepatic and Renal Deficiency

Clinical manifestations: This disease develops gradually. Weakness, flaccidity, and immobility occur in the upper and lower limbs. Other clinical manifestations are soreness and weakness of the lumbar region, dizziness, tinnitus, spermatorrhea, nocturnal enuresis, irregular menstruation, a red tongue with only a small amount of tongue coating, and a thready and rapid pulse.

Analysis: Malnutrition of the muscles and tendons due to deficiencies of hepatic and renal essence and blood leads to weak and flaccid limbs. A deficiency of *yin*-fluid in the liver and kidneys causes the ministerial and monarch fire to become hyperactive. This burns the lungs, making the disease even more serious. Renal deficiency deprives the lumbar region of nourishment, causing soreness and weakness. A red tongue with only small amounts of tongue coating and a thready and rapid pulse are signs of deficient *yin* and hyperactive fire. Disturbance of the seminal chamber by ministerial fire produces spermatorrhea. The upward movement of deficiency fire leads to dizziness and tinnitus. The failure of kidney water to check heart fire causes insomnia and palpitations. In prolonged cases, deficient *yin* affects *yang* and thus a condition where there are deficiencies of both *yin* and *yang* develops, exhibiting symptoms of lassitude, an aversion to cold, frequent urination, impotence, a slightly red tongue and a deep and thready pulse.

Treatment: To replenish the liver and kidneys, nourish *yin* and disperse heat.

Prescription: Modified *Huqian* Bolus (171) should be prescribed. Radix Rehmanniae Preparata, Carapax et Plastrum Testudinis, Rhizoma Anemarrhenae and Cortex Phellodendri nourish *yin* and suppress fire; Radix Paeoniae Alba soothes the liver and nourishes the tendons; Os Tigris strengthens the tendons and bones; Herba Cynomorii strengthens *yang* and benefits essence in order to relieve the possible side effects of *yin* tonics; Rhizoma Zingiberis warms the middle *jiao*; and Pericarpium Citri Reticulatae regulates *qi* and invigorates the spleen. This formula is commonly used in the treatment of *wei*-syndrome caused by *yin* deficiencies of the liver and kidneys complicated by heat. *Huqian* Bolus, as recorded in the *Variorum of Prescriptions*, contains three extra drugs than the original prescription. These are Radix Angelicae Sinensis, Radix Achyranthis Bidentatae and mutton, all of which supplement the kidneys and aid the *yang*.

In cases where the patient suffers from a sallow complexion, palpitations, anxiety, a slightly red tongue and a thready and weak pulse, add Radix Astragali, Radix Codonopsis, Radix Angelicae Sinensis and Caulis Spatholobi to replenish *qi* and blood. In cases of *yin* deficiency affecting *yang* with symptoms of aversion to cold, impotence, large quantities of clear urine, a pale tongue and a deep, thready and weak pulse, remove Rhizoma Anemarrhenae and Cortex Phellodendri and add proper amounts of herbs that replenish the kidneys and assist *yang*, such as Cornu Cervi, Fructus Psoraleae, Radix Morindae Officinalis and Cortex Cinnamomi.

Powder of Placenta Hominis or powder made from the dried marrow of pigs and cows mixed with rice powder can be taken with white sugar and water. If the patient's appetite is good, then he can eat cooked marrow and soybean.

Improved results will be gained if medication is used along with acupuncture, massage and physical therapy. It is not advisable to prescribe herbs that make the patient sweat or to give acupuncture using red-hot needles or moxibustion without taking into account the patient's actual condition. This is because these methods may consume body fluid and aggravate the disease. The patient should avoid highly-flavored food, refrain from sexual activity, keep away from damp places, and take care not to get tired.

Case Studies

A patient named Feng You suffered from flaccidity of the lower limbs after a febrile disease, and could not walk by himself. Other clinical manifestations were that he suffered from a painful cough and expectorated sputum. He had a poor appetite, a dry throat, a soft, smooth and rapid pulse, and a red tongue with a yellow coating. It was a couple of months since flaccidity had occurred, and so treatment was aimed at nourishing *yin* and dispersing heat from the *Yangming* meridians. The prescription consisted of the following herbs:

Radix Adenophorae	9 g;
Herba Dendrobii	9 g;
Radix Trichosanthis	9 g;
Radix Glycyrrhizae	4.5 g;
Bulbus Fritillariae Cirrhosae	9 g;

Rhizoma Anemarrhenae	4.5 g;
Pericarpium Trichosanthis	9 g;
Semen Armeniacae Amarum	9 g;
Caulis Trachelospermi	9 g;
Radix Achyranthis Bidentatae	6 g;
Ramulus Mori	9 g;
Semen Benincasae	9 g;
Fresh Rhizoma Phragmitis (with joints removed)	30 cm.

Second visit: The patient's cough and the signs of internal heat had been alleviated after ten doses, but the flaccidity of the lower limbs remained unchanged. To relieve paralysis, fluid in the lungs should be distributed normally in the body. When the liver is well-nourished with blood, the tendons will become relaxed and likewise when the kidneys have sufficient nourishment, the bones will become strong. When *yin* blood is sufficient, heat will be spontaneously dispersed from the meridians. Thus if only the *Yangming* meridians are treated, the *wei*-syndrome will disappear. This is because the *Yangming* meridians are in charge of moistening the muscles and tendons and making the joints flexible.

Radix Ophiopogonis	6 g;
Radix Glehniae	9 g;
Lignum Pini Poriaferum	9 g;
Rhizoma Dioscoreae	9 g;
Radix Rehmanniae	12 g;
Rhizoma Anemarrhenae	4.5 g;
Bulbus Fritillariae Cirrhosae	6 g;
Radix Trichosanthis	9 g;
Caulis Trachelospermi	6 g;
Radix Achyranthis Bidentatae	9 g;
Ramulus Mori	9 g.

Third visit: Heat in the five *zang* organs may lead to *wei*-syndrome. According to the medical classics, there are five kinds of *wei*-syndrome, but these can be grouped in two major types — one caused by heat and the other caused by dampness. Trees wither if it does not rain for a long time; they also wither if surrounded by dampness. Flaccidity of the lower limbs can be explained in the same way. This patient had a soft and rapid pulse and a crimson tongue, which suggested that *wei*-syndrome was due to heat. When the heat in the *Yangming* meridians was dispersed and lung *yin* was nourished, the patient could move his lower limbs by himself, in spite of the fact that he could not yet walk. So the treatment was basically correct. Herbs that replenish essence and blood were added in the hope that good effects would gradually be achieved.

Radix Glehniae	9 g;
Radix Ophiopogonis	6 g;
Lignum Pini Poriaferum	9 g;
Rhizoma Dioscoreae	9 g;
Herba Dendrobii	9 g;
Radix Rehmanniae	9 g;
Rhizoma Anemarrhenae	4.5 g;
Radix Achyranthis Bidentatae	6 g;

Caulis Trachelospermi	9 g;
Fructus Leonuri	9 g;
Ramulus Mori	9 g;
Spinal cord of pigs (washed in wine, to be decocted with the other ingredients)	2 pieces;
Huqian Bolus (to be taken early in the morning with diluted salt water)	9 g.

Discussion: This case was caused by the malnutrition of the tendons and muscles due to the consumption of their fluid by pulmonary heat following a febrile disease. The method of treatment adopted was treating the upper part of the body for a disease in the lower part.

Another patient named Cheng Zuo had swollen legs, which were so flaccid and weak that he could not walk any distance, even after the swelling had subsided. Other signs included a pale tongue with a white coating, a soft and retarded pulse and a poor appetite. These were all caused by the invasion of pathogenic dampness-heat, which infiltrated the tendons and vessels from the muscles, causing stagnant *qi* and blood. It has been said that dampness-heat shortens the large tendons and prolongs the small ones, causing spasms in the former, and flaccidity in the latter. Treatment aimed at invigorating the spleen, eliminating dampness, removing blood stasis and promoting the smooth circulation of *qi* and blood in the meridians:

Poria	12 g;
Rhizoma Alismatis	4.5 g;
Radix Stephaniae Tetrandrae	9 g;
Radix Angelicae Sinensis	6 g;
Rhizoma Atractylodis Macrocephalae	4.5 g;
Rhizoma Atractylodis	3 g;
Pericarpium Citri Reticulatae	3 g;
Radix Achyranthis Bidentatae	6 g;
Flos Carthami	2.4 g;
Semen Coicis	12 g;
Fructus Chaenomelis	9 g;
Radix Gentianae Macrophyllae	4.5 g;
Radix Salviae Miltiorrhizae	6 g;
Ramulus Mori	9 g.

Five hundred grams of Rhizoma Atractylodis were soaked in rice water for seven days, steamed nine times in a cooking pot, then dried in the sun and ground to powder. This was then decocted with 250 g of Semen Coicis and 250 g of Ramulus Mori (stir-baked in wine) to make pills, three grams of which were taken a time on an empty stomach with boiled water.

The disease gradually subsided after 50-odd doses of the decoction and two of the pills.

Discussion: This *wei*-syndrome was due to the invasion of dampness-heat, which spread from the muscles to the tendons and vessels, causing *qi* and blood stagnation. Thus the main ingredients of the prescription included Rhizoma Atractylodis, Radix Achyranthis Bidentatae, Radix Angelicae Sinensis and Flos Carthami. The patient took both the decoction and the pills for some time, then gradually recovered. The treatment adopted in this case was entirely different from the previous one, which was due to fluid consumption by heat in the lungs.

Name: Wang XX; Sex: Male; Age: 41; Occupation: Worker.
First visit: December 8, 1972.

The patient had suffered from the atrophy of the thenar muscle on both sides of the body for two years. He also noted twitching and atrophy of the muscles in his arms and weakness in his lower limbs. The disease began in July 1968 after he was caught in the rain while sweating and feeling very tired after work. Since then, his condition had steadily deteriorated. It was diagnosed in the department of neurology of a medical college as amyotrophic lateral sclerosis. He had received both Western and Chinese medicine, but in vain. The accompanying symptoms included lower back pain, cold limbs, spermatorrhea, insomnia, lassitude, a poor appetite, a red tongue with a purple border and a thin yellow coating, and a thready and weak pulse. The pathogenesis was deficiencies of the liver, spleen and kidneys, consumption of essence and blood, and malnutrition of the muscles and tendons. The diagnosis proposed using traditional Chinese medicine as *wei*-syndrome. Treatment replenished *qi* and blood, invigorated the spleen and kidneys, relaxed the tendons and activated blood circulation. The following herbs were prescribed to control the pathological conditions:

Radix Polygoni Multiflori Preparata	12 g;
Radix Rehmanniae Preparata	12 g;
Rhizoma Cibotii Preparata	15 g;
Radix Dipsaci	12 g;
Radix Codonopsis	9 g;
Radix Angelicae Sinensis	9 g;
Radix Paeoniae Rubra	9 g;
Fructus Chaenomelis	6 g;
Radix Achyranthis Bidentatae	9 g;
Herba Taxilli	15 g;
Flos Carthami	4.5 g;
Radix Aucklandiae	4.5 g.

The patient returned to his home town with the prescription, and was advised to take these herbs for two months.

On April 8, 1973, the patient wrote to the doctor that he had done as directed and that his condition had improved. His lower limbs were stronger and felt more stable when walking. The cramps which he used to feel in his legs had disappeared. He had more energy and a normal appetite but he still had trouble lifting his arms and muscular twitching was not improved. Early in the morning when he woke up, his throat felt dry. He woke easily at night, and occasionally experienced spermatorrhea. Muscular atrophy remained unchanged. The same treatment was adopted, adding herbs that replenish *qi* and nourish *yin*.

Nine grams of Radix Astragali, nine grams of Radix Scrophulariae and three grams of Radix Glycyrrhizae were added to the previous prescription, and Radix Aucklandiae was removed.

This prescription was used for two months in a row.

During the hot summer of 1973, the patient had a hot sensation in his palms, soles and chest, as well as experiencing thirst and a dry throat. Radix Asparagi, Radix Ophiopogonis and Cortex Moutan were thus added to nourish *yin* and disperse heat. In winter, an extract of those herbs was produced together with herbs that produce essence, in the hope that good results could be achieved by strengthening resistance.

The extract for use during the winter was composed of the following ingredients:

Radix Rehmanniae	90 g;
Radix Rehmanniae Preparata	90 g;
Rhizoma Dioscoreae	90 g;
Cortex Moutan	45 g;
Radix Polygoni Multiflori Preparata	90 g;
Rhizoma Cibotii Preparata	90 g;
Herba Taxilli	90 g;
Radix Dipsaci	90 g;
Radix Asparagi	90 g;
Radix Ophiopogonis	90 g;
Radix Codonopsis	90 g;
Radix Astragali	90 g;
Radix Angelicae Sinensis	90 g;
Fructus Lycii	90 g;
Semen Ziziphi Spinosae	90 g;
Semen Platycladi	90 g;
Radix Polygalae Preparata	30 g;
Rhizoma Anemarrhenae	45 g;
Cortex Phellodendri	45 g;
Colla Corii Asini	120 g;
Colla Carapax et Plastrum Testudinis	120 g;
Fructus Jujubae	120 g.

All these herbs were soaked in water overnight and then decocted three times until a thick broth was made. Colla Corii Asini and Colla Carapax et Plastrum Testudinis were melted in preserved wine, then mixed into the broth. Finally, 500 grams of crystal sugar was added and an extract was made. This was taken twice daily, one spoon a time with boiled water. Each dose lasted for two months.

In March 1974, after two months of oral administration, the patient became more lively and began to be able to sleep well; spermatorrhea improved, and the muscular twitching of his upper limbs ceased. However, muscular atrophy and the weakness he felt in lifting his arms remained unchanged. He could walk fairly steadily. Muscular atrophy of the lower limbs was not severe.

After one year of treatment with Chinese herbal medicine, his conditions had been kept under control, and his symptoms were slightly improved. It was therefore not deemed necessary to change the treatment or the prescription. It was suggested that pills should be taken during the period between March and November, and the extract should be taken between December and March. The patient was advised to eat more nutritious food and do proper exercises to improve his general health.

Colla Corii Asini, Colla Carapax et Plastrum Testudinis, and crystal sugar were removed, and 500 grams of Fructus Jujubae were added to make pills. These were taken twice daily, three grams a time with boiled water.

A recent letter reported that his condition was stable and that he was taking pills continuously. His blood and urine was tested on April 28, 1975, revealing hemochrome 14.5 g; WBC 7,200, platelets 106,000, and normal urinalysis.

XXXXIV. Fever due to Internal Disorders

Fever due to internal disorders refers to fever caused by deficient *qi* and blood in the *zang-fu* organs and by the imbalance of *yin* and *yang*. Its main symptom is fever, a low fever in most cases, without any external syndromes. This fever will be hard to bring down even after sweating. Other symptoms may also appear sometimes such as restlessness and hot sensations in the palms, soles and chest, but in most circumstances the patient's temperature will not be very high.

The Inner Canon of the Yellow Emperor attributes this disease to the loss of balance between *yin* and *yang*, saying that deficient *yin* produces internal heat. According to this book, the principal treatment should be to nourish *yin* and suppress fire. In treating fever due to deficient *yang*, or cold syndrome with pseudo-heat symptoms as it was called by medical scholars of later generations, *Treatise on Cold Diseases* by Zhang Zhongjing recommends warm and hot herbs such as Decoction for Treating *Yang* Exhaustion (90) to restore *yang* and alleviate fever. This method is not only applicable to patients with deficient *yang-qi* at the later stage of disease due to the invasion by cold, but also to those with deficient *yang-qi* and fever caused by internal disorders. In his other book *Synopsis of Prescriptions of the Golden Chamber*, Zhang Zhongjing prescribes Decoction for Mildly Warming Middle *Jiao* (34), which is sweet and warm in nature, for consumptive diseases with symptoms of restlessness, hot sensations in the palms and soles, a dry throat and thirst. This prescription has made a notable impact on the treatment of such diseases. Li Dongyuan, the author of *Comments on the Spleen and Stomach*, pointed out that fever can be produced by a weak spleen and a stomach with insufficient primordial *qi*. He put forward the principle of getting rid of high fever by using sweet and warm herbs, and he prescribed the Decoction for Strengthening Middle *Jiao* and Benefiting *Qi*. In his book *Supplementary Discourses on Investigating Medical Problems*, Zhu Danxi says, "Excess *yang* leads to a deficiency of *yin*. There is likely to be an excess of *qi* and a deficiency of blood." He recommends Pill for Replenishing *Yin* (22) for the treatment of fire disturbance due to a deficiency of *yin*. *A Complete Collection of Jingyue's Treatise* analyses the causes of fever due to internal disorders, concluding that internal heat is produced by an improper diet, stress, excessive alcohol intake, excessive sexual activity, emotional trauma, the administration of certain herbs and deficient *yin*. Since then, the theories about this disease and its treatment have all been developed on the basis of Zhang Jingyue's book.

Fever due to internal disorders also covers functional low fever, fever that occurs with tumors, hematopathy, desmosis, tuberculosis, endocrinopathy and certain chronic infectious diseases, and fever that is produced from unknown causes.

Etiology and Pathogenesis

Fever due to internal damage is often caused by the impairment of the *zang-fu* organs as a result of weak resistance, stress, emotional trauma, and hemorrhage. Since this kind of fever comes from deficiencies, it can also be called fever caused by deficiencies, fire caused by deficiencies or fever due to stress. As for its pathogenesis, deficiency or excess should be taken into account. If the *qi*, blood, *yin* and *yang* are deficient, then the condition is attributable to deficiencies; if the patient experience emotional traumas or stagnant blood, then the condition is based on excesses.

1. Fever due to Deficient *Yin*

This can either be caused by a weak resistance or by a prolonged febrile disease, long-term diarrhea, or excessive oral administration of warm and dry herbs. In all conditions, depleted *yin*-fluid fails to check fire, thus giving rise to hyperactive *yang-qi* and fever.

2. Fever due to Deficient *Qi*

Stress, coupled with a bad diet, is liable to cause fever and deficiencies of spleen and stomach *qi*. The pathogenesis is complicated and still a matter of some controversy. Medical scholars of different schools have agreed only to discuss the question centered on the so-called *yin* fire, a doctrine put forward by Li Dongyuan. The existence of *yin* fire depends on that of *yang* fire, which is usually regarded as another name of primordial *qi*. Stress and an improper diet damage the primordial *qi* (*yang* fire) of the spleen and stomach and impair the production of digestion and essence. Damage to *yang* affects *yin* and turns *yang* fire into *yin* fire. Therefore, fever caused by deficient *qi* is produced by the loss of balance between *yin* and *yang*. Nevertheless, the root cause of the disease should be found in *yang*, with *yin* being only the secondary reason. This kind of fever is completely different from that caused by a simple deficiency of *yin*.

3. Fever due to Deficient *Yang*

This can be brought about by deficient *yang*, a prolonged cold syndrome or the excessive use of cold or cool herbs. All these result in deficient kidney *yang* and cold produced in the middle *jiao*. *Yang* therefore encounters resistance outside the body, resulting in a condition called cold syndrome with pseudo-hot symptoms. Fever occurs when *yang* floats to the surface.

4. Fever due to Deficient Blood

A prolonged illness can lead to deficient heart blood and liver blood. Splenic deficiency means an inability to produce blood. Loss of blood due to hemorrhage, childbirth, or surgery may cause blood deficiency. Blood is related to *yin*. Deficient *yin* and blood do not allow *yin* to check *yang* and thus give rise to floating *yang* accompanied by fever.

5. Fever due to Stagnant Fire

This refers to fever caused by heat in the *zang-fu* organs following stagnation of *yang-qi*. Depression impairs the liver's ability to regulate the free flow of *qi*, and the stagnant *qi* thus formed turns into fire and produces fever. Excess anger leads to hyperactive liver fire along with fever. This kind of fever is related to emotional changes.

In addition, retained food or prolonged pain can also lead to stagnant *qi*, which then turns into fire and produces fever.

6. Fever due to Stagnant Blood

This is the result of stagnant *qi*, trauma or hemorrhage. The stagnation of both *qi* and blood causes fever.

Diagnosis

1. Internal Disorders and External Pathogenic Factors

External factors first invade the external part of the body and then travel inside to its internal part. The disease they produce develops quickly and does not last long. The external syndrome will take the form of a high fever or chills which cannot be relieved, even by wearing thick clothes. The dorsum of the hand is hotter than the palm. The accompanying symptoms include nasal stuffiness with discharge, a headache and a sore throat. Fever is generally reduced after sweating. The pulse is superficial, rapid and tense, and the tongue coating is thin and white, or yellow.

Fever due to internal disorders is the result of emotional upsets or stress. It develops gradually and lasts for a long time. There is no external syndrome, and the disease is located inside the body. A low fever will not be accompanied by chills. It is possible that a cold sensation may be present, but this can be reduced by wearing thick clothes. The palm is hotter than the dorsum. Accompanying symptoms include dizziness, lassitude, unwillingness to speak and sweating, as well as night sweats. Generally the fever does not subside after sweating. The patient has a weak pulse or a taut and unsmooth pulse and a tongue with no or little coating.

2. Dampness-Heat and Deficient *Yin*

In fever due to dampness-heat, the skin is moist. Since heat is retained inside the body, the skin is slightly hot at the first touch, and becomes hotter and even scorching later. The patient has a dry mouth, but no desire to drink. The patient has a thick, sticky, yellow tongue coating and a soft, smooth and rapid pulse.

In fever due to a deficiency of *yin*, the fever is as if the patient had been steamed. The patient has dry skin, thirst coupled with a desire to drink, a red tongue with a thin coating and little moisture, and a thready and rapid pulse.

3. Dampness-Heat and Deficient *Qi*

The first is often accompanied by fullness and distress in the chest and hypochondrium, a heavy sensation in the body and limbs, a bitter taste and stickiness in the mouth, and a thick, sticky, yellow tongue coating.

Fever due to a deficiency of *qi* is not accompanied by fullness or distress. Its symptoms include unwillingness to speak, lassitude, and a thin white tongue coating which is not sticky.

Differentiation and Treatment

Fever due to internal disorders is a complicated condition which is very common. It is very important to determine the cause. It is wrong to regard persistent fever as always being due to internal disorders. It is easy to diagnose fever due to external pathogenic factors, but fever due to external dampness-heat tends to be mistakenly attributed to internal disorders. This is because fever from dampness-heat is recessive and lingering, so it persists for a long time. Dampness is a *yin* factor, and the fever caused by it usually occurs in the afternoon; pathogenic dampness prevents body fluid from moving upwards and thus causes a dry mouth and tongue. If herbs that nourish *yin* are administered, the pathogenic dampness will become even more stubborn, the condition will be aggravated, and fever will persist. Blockage of *qi* circulation by pathogenic dampness often produces stuffiness in the chest, a heavy sensation, and lassitude, all of which can be incorrectly attributed to *qi*. If warm and sweet herbs that replenish *qi* are taken, *qi* circulation will be retarded even more, it will be impossible to eliminate dampness-heat, and the pathological condition of the patient will further deteriorate.

The treatment of fever caused by internal disorders can be determined on the basis of its causes. The methods of treatment include nourishing *yin* and producing body fluid, replenishing *qi* and blood, warming *yang* and replenishing the kidneys, soothing the liver and relieving stagnation, activating blood circulation and removing blood stasis. It will not do to arbitrarily prescribe herbs that cause sweating or herbs that are bitter or cold in nature if the patient suffers from fever. Since *yin*, *yang*, *qi* and blood tend to be impaired in these cases, the administration of acrid and dispersive herbs will produce dryness and further damage *yin*, making *yin* blood even more depleted, fire even more hyperactive, and fever even more pronounced. Herbs that are bitter and cold tend to damage spleen *yang* and impair its ability to produce *qi* and blood, thus aggravating the condition. They also produce dryness and damage *yin*, which is harmful to patients who are already suffering from a deficiency of *yin*. However, their proper usage consolidates *yin*. For instance, Cortex Phellodendri in Bolus of Anemarrhenae, Phellodendri and Rehmanniae Preparata (181) calms ministerial fire and consolidates kidney essence and *yin*. Since the spleen and stomach are weak when fever is due to internal disorders, they cannot accept excessive tonics, and their functions will be further impaired if too many *yin* tonics are taken. To protect the spleen and stomach, it is advisable to take herbs in small doses at regular intervals; large doses should be avoided.

1. Production of Heat due to Deficient *Yin*

Clinical manifestations: Hectic fever in the afternoon or at night, or a hot sensation in the palms, soles and chest, and a facial flush, restlessness, night sweating, insomnia, sleep which is disturbed by dreams, thirst, a dry throat, constipation, small amounts of yellow urine, a dry, red tongue with little or no coating or a cracked tongue, and a thready and rapid pulse.

Analysis: Deficient *yin* is either caused by a weak resistance or by a prolonged febrile disease, long-term diarrhea, or excessive administration of aromatic and dry herbs. It produces internal heat and causes the *ying* system to become diseased. This explains the occurrence of hectic fever in the afternoon or at night and the hot sensations. The displacement of heart fire leads to a facial flush, restlessness and insomnia. Internal heat forces the body fluid outward, and as a result, the patient will sweat profusely at night. A dry red tongue and a thready and rapid pulse are signs of internal heat due to deficient *yin*.

Treatment: To nourish *yin* and disperse heat.

Prescription: Modified Powder for Relieving Deficiency-Heat Syndrome (282). Carapax Trionycis and Rhizoma Anemarrhenae nourish *yin* and moisten dryness, and Cortex Lycii Radix Stellariae, Rhizoma Picrorrhizae, Herba Artemisiae Annuae and Radix Gentianae Macrophyllae disperse heat caused by deficiencies and relieve hectic fever. To help nourish *yin*, add Radix Rehmanniae, Radix Scrophulariae and Radix Polygoni Multiflori. In cases of insomnia, add Semen Ziziphi, Spinosae, Semen Platycladi and Caulis Polygoni Multiflori to nourish the heart and calm the mind. If there is night sweating, add Os Draconis, Concha Ostreae and Fructus Tritici Levis (light) to constrict the body surface and check sweating. In cases of constipation, add Fructus Cannabis to moisten the large intestine.

If signs of *yin* deficiency are pronounced, with symptoms such as thirst, restlessness, a red tongue and a malar flush, prescribe Pill for Replenishing *Yin* (22) or Bolus of Anemarrhenae, Phellodendri and Rehmanniae Preparata (181) to nourish *yin* and suppress fire. If signs of *qi* deficiency also appear, such as lassitude, dizziness and shortness of breath, add Radix Codonopsis, Radix Glehniae, Radix Ophiopogonis and Fructus Schisandrae to nourish *qi* and *yin*.

2. Deficient *Qi* and Blood

Clinical manifestations: Fever which is induced or aggravated by overwork, dizziness, lassitude, spontaneous sweating, shortness of breath, susceptibility to common colds, unwillingness to speak, a poor appetite, loose stools, a pale tongue with a thin white coating, and a thready and weak pulse. If blood deficiencies are more pronounced, the patient's complexion, lips and nails will be pale and they may suffer from palpitations.

Analysis: This fever comes from deficiencies of spleen and stomach *qi* following stress as a result of overwork. A weak spleen and stomach mean that the source of *qi* and blood is lacking, so dizziness, lassitude and shortness of breath occur. Deficient *qi* implies that the body surface is weak, resulting in spontaneous sweating and a susceptibility to common colds. Impaired transportation and transformation cause the patient's appetite to be poor and their stools to be loose. A pale tongue and a thready and weak pulse are signs of *qi* and blood deficiency after prolonged fever. Blood deficiency is caused by prolonged illness, splenic deficiency which does not allow it to produce blood, or excessive blood loss. Since *qi* and blood have the same origin, deficiencies of both *qi* and blood often occur concurrently.

Treatment: To replenish *qi*, produce blood and dissipate heat with sweet and warm herbs.

Prescription: Modified Decoction for Strengthening Middle *Jiao* and Benefiting *Qi* (154). Radix Astragali and Radix Codonopsis invigorate the middle *jiao* and benefit *qi*; Rhizoma Atractylodis Macrocephalae, Pericarpium Citri Reticulatae and Radix Glycyrrhizae invigorate the spleen and harmonize the middle *jiao*, Radix Angelicae Sinensis nourishes blood, and Rhizoma Cimicifugae and Radix

Bupleuri elevate the clear *qi* of the spleen and stomach. In cases of profuse spontaneous sweating, add Os Draconis and Concha Ostreae to constrict the body surface and check sweating. In cases when chills and fever occur alternately, combined with sweating and an aversion to wind, add Ramulus Cinnamomi and Radix Paeoniae Alba to harmonize the nutrient and defensive *qi*. If the patient feels an aversion to cold, add Cortex Cinnamomi to warm *yang*. If signs of dampness appear, such as a sticky white tongue coating and stuffiness and distress in the chest and abdomen, add Rhizoma Atractylodis, Cortex Magnoliae Officinalis and Poria to invigorate the spleen and dry dampness. If splenic deficiency is complicated by dampness-heat, with the patient exhibiting a sticky yellow tongue coating and a bitter taste in the mouth, Decoction for Lifting *Yang* and Benefiting Stomach (53) is prescribed to replenish *qi*, invigorate the spleen, disperse heat and resolve dampness.

In cases of blood deficiency, prescribe Decoction for Invigorating Spleen and Nourishing Heart (110) or Decoction of Angelicae Sinensis for Enriching Blood (131).

Fever due to deficient *yang* is caused by delaying treatment of a cold syndrome or treating it incorrectly, or by constitutional weakness or by a deficiency of *qi*. Its clinical manifestations include fever accompanied by an aversion to cold, cold limbs or cold lower limbs, a pale complexion, dizziness, somnolence, soreness of the lumbar region and knees, a moist and swollen tongue with tooth prints and a white coating, and a deep, thready and weak pulse or a superficial, large and weak pulse. Treatment seeks to warm the kidneys and replenish *yang*. This can be done by prescribing modified Pill for Invigorating Kidney-*Qi* (182). A special form of fever caused by *yang* deficiency is a cold syndrome combined with a pseudo-hot syndrome caused by excess *yin* that resists *yang*. Modified Decoction for Treating *Yang* Exhaustion (90) is used to treat this.

3. Retention of Heat in the Liver Meridian

Clinical manifestations: Fever fluctuates along with the emotions. Other clinical manifestations include irritability, restlessness, a hot sensation in the body, stuffiness in the chest, distention of the hypochondriac region, sighing, a bitter taste in the mouth, a yellow tongue coating, a taut and rapid pulse, irregular menstruation, dysmenorrhea, and a distending sensation in the breasts.

Analysis: Emotional irritation causes stagnant liver *qi*, which then turns into fire and brings on fever; this explains the fluctuation of fever, the hot sensations and the restlessness. Stagnant *qi* also gives rise to stuffiness, distention and irritability, while sighing temporarily relaxes the stagnant *qi*. A bitter taste, a yellow tongue coating and a taut and rapid pulse are signs of stagnant *qi* turning into fire. The liver stores blood, and thus stagnant liver *qi* retards blood circulation. The results are irregular menstruation, dysmenorrhea and a distending sensation in the breasts.

Treatment: To promote the smooth circulation of liver *qi*, and disperse heat.

Prescription: Modified *Xiaoyao* Powder with Moutan and Gardeniae (63). Cortex Moutan and Fructus Gardeniae disperse heat which has been retained in the Liver Meridian; Radix Bupleuri promotes the smooth circulation of liver *qi*; Herba Menthae in small doses helps relieve stagnation; Radix Angelicae Sinensis and Radix Paeoniae Alba nourish blood and soothe the liver; and Rhizoma Atractylodis Macrocephalae, Poria and Radix Glycyrrhizae invigorate the spleen. In cases of pain in the hypochondriac region, add Fructus Toosendan, Rhizoma Corydalis and Radix Curcumae to regulate *qi* and relieve pain. In cases of abdominal distention, add Rhizoma Cyperi and Fructus Liquidambaris to promote the smooth circulation of *qi*. In cases where the patient feels a hot sensation on the face and has blurred vision, add Semen Celosiae and Semen Cassiae to disperse heat in the liver and improve sight.

In prolonged cases of heat retention in the Liver Meridian complicated by *yin* consumption or in cases of *yin* deficiency complicated by heat retained in the Liver Meridian, Decoction for Nourishing Fluid and Clearing Away Liver-Heat (303) can be prescribed. Pill of Six Drugs Containing Rehmanniae Preparata (56) nourishes kidney *yin*; Radix Angelicae Sinensis and Radix Paeoniae Alba nourish blood and soothe the liver; Radix Bupleuri promotes the smooth circulation of liver *qi*; and Fructus Gardenia disperses heat which has been retained in the Liver Meridian. If stagnant liver *qi* becomes fire, a hot syndrome caused by excesses can be seen in the Liver Meridian. Symptoms of this are a red face and eyes, restlessness, irritability, dark yellow urine, constipation, a crimson tongue, and a taut and rapid pulse. In these cases, Decoction of Gentianae for Purging Liver-Fire (78) should be prescribed to disperse heat in the liver and reduce fire.

4. Stagnant Blood

Clinical manifestations: Fever in the afternoon or at night, thirst, a dry throat coupled with the desire to drink small quantities, pain in the limbs at a fixed location, palpable masses, squarrose and dry skin, a dark or sallow complexion, bluish-purple lips and tongue or a tongue with purple spots, and a thready and unsmooth pulse.

Analysis: Stagnant blood can be caused by stagnant *qi*, traumas or hemorrhaging. Since the *xue* system is diseased, and blood is related to *yin*, fever usually occurs in the afternoon or at night. Heat retained inside the body leads to thirst and dryness; since it is held in the *ying* system, only a small quantity of liquid is needed. Stagnant blood blocks *qi* and blood circulation, and thus produces a fixed pain or palpable masses. Stagnant blood prevents the production of new blood, and the head, face and skin fail to be nourished by sufficient *qi* and blood. The consequences are therefore the dark complexion and squarrose and dry skin. Bluish-purple lips and tongue and an unsmooth pulse are further signs of blood stagnation.

Treatment: To activate blood circulation and remove blood stasis.

Prescription: Modified Decoction for Removing Blood Stasis in the Chest (135). Semen Persicae, Flos Carthami and Radix Paeoniae Rubra activate blood circulation and remove blood stasis; Radix Angelicae Sinensis, Rhizoma Chuanxiong and Radix Rehmanniae nourish blood and activate blood circulation; Radix Bupleuri and Fructus Aurantii promote the smooth circulation of *qi*; and Radix Platycodi and Radix Achyranthis Bidentatae help the movement of the drugs upwards and downwards. To disperse heat in the *xue* system, add a proper amount of Cortex Moutan and Radix et Rhizoma Rhei. In cases of aversion to cold and cold limbs, add Ramulus Cinnamomi to remove vascular obstructions by warmth. In cases of deficient *qi*, add Radix Astragali to replenish *qi* and circulate blood. In cases where the patient complains of a headache, add Scolopendra and Nidus Vespae to eliminate wind and remove obstructions from the meridians. If there are palpable masses in the hypochondrium, add Bolus of Carapax Trionycis (325) to soften hard masses.

In addition to these four major syndromes of fever due to internal damage, there is also fever due to the retention of food, which often occurs in children. Fever due to the disharmony of the nutrient and defensive *qi* is principally caused by the invasion of external pathogenic factors, although it is also related to internal disorders.

Remarks

The fevers described above are interrelated, and one may become another or they may occur concurrently, complicating each other. For instance, prolonged fever due to external factors can develop into fever due to internal disorders, while fever due to stagnant *qi* consumes *yin* fluid and then gradually turns into fever caused by *yin* deficiency. *Qi* and blood deficiency often occur together as liver *qi* produces fire which consumes *yin* on the one hand and causes blood stagnation on the other.

Case Studies

Name: X XX; Sex: Female; Age: 40.

The patient had suffered a low fever every afternoon for three years, and her temperature often reached 37.7-37.8°C. She felt numb in the lower limbs and listless at night. She had received many examinations, but the cause was still unknown. The pulse was thready, slightly rapid, and slightly taut at the left *guan* position. Her tongue was slightly red with no coating. All this suggested *yin* deficiency. The following herbs were prescribed to nourish the kidneys and lower fever:

Radix Rehmanniae	24 g;
Fructus Corni	12 g;
Rhizoma Dioscoreae	12 g;
Cortex Moutan	12 g;
Poria	9 g;
Rhizoma Alismatis	9 g;
Radix Bupleuri	9 g;
Radix Paeoniae Alba	9 g;
Fructus Schisandrae	6 g;
Cortex Cinnamomi (decocted later)	6 g.

In this prescription, Pill of Six Drugs Containing Rehmanniae Preparata (56) nourishes kidney *yin*; Fructus Schisandrae replenishes *qi* and strengthens *yin*; Radix Bupleuri promotes the smooth circulation of *qi* and disperses fire; Radix Paeoniae Alba disperses heat caused by deficiencies and protects nutrient *yin*; and Cortex Cinnamomi conducts fire back to its origin in order to reduce the fever. After seven doses taken over ten days, the patient's temperature had decreased to 37°C. To achieve better results, another ten doses were prescribed.

Discussion: The medical classic *Thorough Interpretation of Medicine* says, "I successfully treated a case of malaria when the patient had a flushed face and felt thirsty on the basis of kidney *yin*-deficiency. If a patient experiences chills, a high fever, a flushed face and thirst, one dose of Pill of Six Drugs Containing Rehmanniae Preparata (56) and Radix Bupleuri, Radix Paeoniae Alba, Cortex Cinnamomi, and Fructus Schisandrae will cure the disease." Later medical scholars pointed out that this prescription was also effective in the treatment of fever without chills, intermittent and persistent fever, and that it did not necessarily have to be reserved for cases with chills and high fever.

Name: Jia XX; Sex: Male; Age: 37.

The patient suddenly felt chilly two months ago. Then fever developed, with slight sweating, nausea, vomiting, a mild headache and general aching. Vomiting ceased three days later, but was followed by a poor appetite, loose stools, and a dull pain in the abdomen. The patient's pathological condition was deteriorating and fever had persisted over the past month.

Since the patient had fever without chills but with spontaneous sweating, weight loss, unwillingness to speak, thirst, a poor appetite, lassitude, loose stools, passing only small amounts of urine, a deep, weak and rapid pulse, and a pale tongue with a sticky white coating, the diagnosis of fever due to *yang* deficiency was established, and Decoction for Strengthening the Middle *Jiao* was prescribed:

Radix Astragali	12 g;
Rhizoma Atractylodis Macrocephalae	12 g;
Pericarpium Citri Reticulatae	6 g;
Rhizoma Cimicifugae	3 g;
Radix Bupleuri	3 g;
Radix Codonopsis	9 g;

Radix Angelicae Sinensis	12 g;
Rhizoma Zingiberis Recens	3 g;
Fructus Jujubae	5 pieces;
Mel	15 g.

After four doses, the patient's appetite had improved and his stools had become more solid, but he still had a mild fever. He then developed night sweats, a dry skin, thirst with a desire to drink small quantities, fever which became worse in the afternoon, a deep and soft pulse, and a red tongue. All this suggested that in his case, the *yang* deficiency had become a *yin* deficiency. Since his condition had changed, treatment changed accordingly. Modified Decoction of Astragali and Carapax Trionycis (268) was then prescribed:

Radix Astragali	12 g;
Carapax Trionycis	12 g;
Cortex Lycii	15 g;
Radix Gentianae Macrophyllae	12 g;
Poria	12 g;
Radix Stellariae	12 g;
Rhizoma Anemarrhenae	9 g;
Rhizoma Picrorrhizae	4.5 g;
Cortex Moutan	9 g;
Radix Scrophulariae	9 g;
Radix Rehmanniae	12 g;
Radix Glycyrrhizae	6 g.

His body temperature became normal after four doses but began to fluctuate again a week later. For this reason, the previous prescription was combined with Powder for Relieving Deficiency-Heat Syndrome (282). After four weeks, his temperature was restored to normal levels. Then Decoction of Six Mild Drugs (55) was administered to achieve still better results. He left hospital with an improved appetite, a rosy face and normal urination and defecation.

Discussion: Fever was not accompanied by external syndrome or excess internal syndrome. Symptoms of deficient spleen *qi*, such as lassitude, a weak pulse, a poor appetite and loose stools, were pronounced. Thus it was actually a case of fever due to *qi* deficiency. Conditions improved when the Decoction for Strengthening Middle *Jiao* and Benefiting *Qi* (154) was administered. The reason for the persistence of afternoon fever and night sweating was deficient *yin*-fluid in the *zang-fu* organs following impaired transportation and transformation. When herbs that nourish *yin* and disperse heat were administered, they rendered good therapeutic results.

Name: Gan XX; Sex: Male; Age: 47.

The patient's condition was characterized by *yang* deficiency. Accidental exposure to external pathogenic factors gave rise to chills, fever (that was more pronounced in the afternoon), dizziness and a poor appetite. Acrid and cool herbs for relieving external syndrome, herbs that are bland for inducing diuresis, and herbs that nourish *yin* and disperse heat were administered in succession, but in vain. On the contrary, the patient's condition was deteriorating.

He now had a hot sensation in the lower abdomen, a fever in the afternoon that was burning hot (although the skin was not hot on palpation), an aversion to cold on his back, and dizziness, which was more pronounced in the afternoon and accompanied by palpitations and restlessness. Other clinical manifestations were abdominal distention and fullness, a poor appetite, a dry mouth with no desire to drink, the regurgitation of clear fluid after drinking, clear urine, one bowel movement every few days with moist stools, weight loss, a pale complexion, a moist white tongue coating, and a superficial pulse with no root. *Zhenwu* Decoction (223) was modified in the treatment:

Radix Aconiti Lateralis Preparata (decocted 50 minutes earlier)	30 g;
Rhizoma Atractylodis Macrocephalae	15 g;
Poria	18 g;
Radix Paeoniae Alba	24 g;
Cortex Cinnamomi	9 g;
Carapax et Plastrum Testudinis	15 g;
Os Draconis	30 g;
Concha Ostreae	30 g;
Radix Glycyrrhizae Preparata	15 g;
Rhizoma Zingiberis Recens	15 g.

Each dose was decocted three times. The first cup was taken all at once, and the second and third cups were taken bit by bit at short intervals, one dose a day. After the second dose, the chills disappeared, the fever improved, and the patient could do certain outdoor exercises. Then Rhizoma Zingiberis Recens was removed, and Radix Aconiti Lateralis Preparata was reduced to 15 g.

After another four doses, all the symptoms had vanished. To achieve still better results, Pill of Aconiti Lateralis Preparata, Cinnamomi and Rehmanniae was taken.

Discussion: This was a case of *yang* deficiency complicated by exposure to external pathogenic factors and excessive administration of acrid and cool herbs, bland herbs for promoting diuresis and herbs that nourish *yin*. These damaged kidney *qi* and made *yang-qi* float to the surface, resulting in fever. Cold water retained in the middle *jiao* prevented the body fluid from nourishing upwards, and the results were abdominal distention and fullness, and a dry mouth with no desire to drink. The failure of the clear *yang-qi* to ascend gave rise to dizziness and palpitations. *Zhenwu* Decoction was prescribed to warm *yang* and circulate water. For fear that the floating *yang* might get out of control, Os Draconis and Concha Ostreae were added to suppress it. Cortex Cinnamomi and Radix Glycyrrhizae Preparata conducted fire back to its origin and invigorated the middle *jiao*. Carapax et Plastrum Testudinis was added to nourish the source of *qi* and blood. The correct diagnosis and a proper combination of herbs ensured good results.

Name: Chen XX; Sex: Female; Age: 32.

The patient fell sick because of depression over her mother's illness. Clinical manifestations were fever in the afternoon that could be alleviated by lying close to a brick wall, dizziness, insomnia, restlessness, a bitter taste in the mouth, fullness and stuffiness in the costal and hypochondriac region, sighing, irregular menstruation with a small amount of purple flow, and pain and distention in the lumbar and abdominal regions. She had taken such herbs as Rhizoma Coptidis and Four Drugs Decoction (93), but in vain.

The patient's pulse now felt taut, thready and straight. She was thin and her cheeks were flushed. She had red lips and a red tongue with a small amount of coating. All these were due to stagnant *qi* that had become fire and deficient blood that failed to nourish the liver. Prolonged oral administration of bitter and cold herbs stopped the spleen *yang* from ascending. The following herbs were prescribed first:

Radix Puerariae	3 g;
Rhizoma Cimicifugae	1.5 g;
Rhizoma seu Radix Notopterygii	1.5 g;
Radix Angelicae Pubescentis	1.5 g;
Radix Ledebouriellae	3 g;
Radix Paeoniae Alba	9 g;
Radix Glycyrrhizae	6 g;
Radix Glycyrrhizae Preparata	6 g;
Radix Ginseng	3 g;
Rhizoma Zingiberis Recens and Fructus Jujubae	a proper amount.

Two doses were administered in succession. The fever gradually subsided, but other symptoms remained unchanged. The following herbs were then prescribed:

Radix Bupleuri	12 g;
Radix Paeoniae Alba	12 g;
Radix Angelicae Sinensis	12 g;
Poria	9 g;
Rhizoma Atractylodis Macrocephalae	9 g;
Radix Glycyrrhizae Preparata	9 g;
Cortex Moutan	6 g;
Fructus Gardeniae	3 g;
Rhizoma Zingiberis (roasted)	1.5 g;
Herba Menthae	1.5 g;
Rhizoma Cyperi	3 g;
Radix Curcumae	3 g;
Carapax Trionycis	9 g;
Concha Ostreae	9 g.

After one dose, she slept well and, in addition, felt relaxed and comfortable in the chest with an improved appetite. Nevertheless, she still felt tired. Decoction for Invigorating Spleen and Nourishing Heart (110) and *Xiaoyao* Pill (250) were used alternately for seven days until the fever had subsided and she had recovered her energy. Then Powder of Ginseng, Poria and Atractylodis Macrocephalae (190) and *Xiaoyao* Pill (250) were administered alternately. The patient's menstruation then became normal.

Discussion: This is a case of stagnant liver *qi*; thus the smooth circulation of liver *qi* should be promoted first. Since pathogenic heat was prevented from reaching the surface due to the prior administration of bitter and cold herbs, *Dongyuan* Decoction for Eliminating Retained Fire was used temporarily instead; *Xiaoyao* Pill (250) was prescribed to treat the disease directly. The addition of Rhizoma Cyperi and Radix Curcumae helped regulate *qi* and relieve stagnation. Carapax Trionycis and Concha Ostreae were added to nourish *yin* and soothe the liver. The treatment concluded by adding herbs that regulate the spleen and stomach.

Name: Wang XX; Sex: Male; Age: 11.

The patient had run a persistently high fever for over a month, with body temperature reaching 42°C at the highest. However, antibiotics and antipyretics proved ineffective. His temperature rose by two degrees in the afternoon every day, then dropped slightly early the next morning. In spite of this, the patient did not feel hot at all. His pulse was taut and unsmooth, his tongue was dark and he had a fixed pain in the right hypochondrium. He was not thirsty, and he was urinating and defecating normally.

The fact that the patient did not feel hot when he had a high fever showed that there was no external heat. In addition, the absence of thirst and normal defecation implied an absence of internal heat. A taut and unsmooth pulse, a pain with a fixed location in the hypochondrium and a dark tongue were signs of stagnant blood. Thus treatment aimed at activating blood circulation and removing blood stasis by prescribing modified Decoction for Removing Blood Stasis in the Chest (135).

Radix Angelicae Sinensis	4.5 g;
Radix Paeoniae Rubra	4.5 g;
Rhizoma Chuanxiong	4.5 g;
Stigma Croci	4.5 g;
Fructus Aurantii (stir-baked)	4.5 g;
Radix Bupleuri	4.5 g;
Myrrhae Preparata	4.5 g;
Semen Persicae	6 g;
Radix Achyranthis Bidentatae	6 g;
Lumbricus	6 g;
Radix Rehmanniae	9 g;
Radix Platycodi	3 g;
Radix Glycyrrhizae	3 g.

The patient took the decoction for a whole week, with either Carapax Trionycis and Concha Ostreae or Rhizoma Corydalis and Resina Draconis added to the above prescription, and as a result the afternoon fever subsided slightly. *Xiaojin* Pill was then added and taken twice daily, one bolus a time. Two weeks later, the fever began to subside and the pain was reduced. Another week later; the afternoon fever was mild; hypochondriac pain had gone away; melena was seen only occasionally; the dark color on the tongue had faded; and a thready pulse still existed. The decoction was reduced to one dose every two days in order to protect the body's anti-pathogenic *qi* while eliminating blood stasis. When the patient came back for a check-up 20 days later, he told the doctor that he had not had any fever for more than two weeks, so he had stopped taking the medication a week ago. During this period, his body weight had increased from 29.5 to 31 kg, his tongue had become bright red and his pulse smooth. He had become vigorous both mentally and physically.

The disease was initially diagnosed as bronchial lymphoid tuberculosis and high fever pending further examination, then as chronic proliferative lymphadenitis, and finally as kidney abscesses.

Discussion: This case helps illustrate fever due to stagnant blood in internal medicine, although the disease occurred in a child. The doctor excluded the possibility of external and internal heat syndromes on the basis of clinical manifestations, and then established the diagnosis of fever due to stagnant blood. The initial therapeutic results were achieved by using Decoction for Removing Blood Stasis in the Chest (135). To resolve stagnant blood and reduce fever, *Xiaojin* Bolus was added.

XXXXV. Consumptive Disease

Consumptive disease is a general term covering various chronic diseases caused by the impairment of the *zang-fu* organs and the exhaustion of the body's primordial *qi*. It includes various deficiency syndromes resulting from congenital defects, lack of proper care in infancy or during prolonged illness, internal disorders due to stress, and the exhaustion of primordial *qi*.

There are many descriptions of consumptive diseases in the medical classics. *The Inner Canon of the Yellow Emperor* states, "Deprivation of essence and *qi* leads to deficiencies." This shows that when the body's *yin* blood and *yang-qi* are exhausted, this can cause consumptive disease. When differentiating *yin* and *yang* deficiencies, the book says, "*Yang* deficiencies produce external cold, and *yin* deficiencies lead to internal heat." The same book summarizes five kinds of damage: "eye strain damages the blood; lying down for long periods of time damages the *qi*; sitting down for long periods of time damages the muscles; standing for long periods of time damages the bones; and walking for long periods of time damages the tendons." This classic also explains a serious condition called the deficiency of all five *zang* organs.

Classic on Medical Problems was the first to propose the theory of "impairment of the five *zang* organs." On the basis of the symptoms shown, it predicts the severity and changes of internal disorders, and according to the characteristics of the five *zang* organs, it proposes the main therapeutic principles: "In cases where the functioning of the lungs is impaired, *qi* should be replenished; in cases where the functioning of the heart is impaired, the nutrient and defensive *qi* should be regulated; in cases where the functioning of the spleen is impaired, a proper diet is recommended; in cases where the functioning of the liver is impaired, the middle *jiao* should be relaxed; and in cases where the functioning of the kidneys is impaired, the essence should be nourished."

Synopsis of Prescriptions of the Golden Chamber discusses consumptive diseases systematically in a special essay. It advocates using the pulse to differentiate between syndromes. For instance, "a large pulse suggests a consumptive disease, and an extremely feeble pulse also suggests a consumptive disease." As treatment, this book recommends Decoction for Potently Warming the Middle *Jiao* (25) and Pill for Invigorating Kidney-*Qi* (182) in cases of *yang* deficiency, Pill of Dioscoreae (327) to promote the anti-pathogenic *qi* and eliminate pathogenic factors, Pill of Rhei and Eupolyphaga seu Steleophaga (334) to remove blood stasis and promote tissue growth, and Decoction of Ziziphi Spinosae (315) in cases of *yin* deficiency with insomnia. Thus this book not only makes up for the shortcomings of the two previous classics, but also puts forward new suggestions regarding treatment.

Pathogenesis and Manifestations of Diseases specifically describes the pathological changes that occur in five kinds of consumption, six kinds of exhaustion, and seven kinds of impairment, and summarizes the corresponding syndromes in detail.

Comments on the Spleen and Stomach and *Danxi's Experience on Medicine* both further expound upon descriptions of consumptive disease. The former recommends replenishing the middle *jiao* by using sweet and warm herbs, with an emphasis on the spleen and stomach. The latter focuses on nourishing *yin* and suppressing fire, with an emphasis on the liver and kidneys.

A Complete Collection of Jingyue's Treatise of the Ming Dynasty holds that *yang* is more important than *yin* in the body; more attention should thus be paid to replenishing kidney *yang* with warm herbs.

Treatise on Phthisis says, "The lungs, spleen and kidneys are the three organs responsible for consumptive diseases. The lungs are located at the top of the five *zang* organs; the spleen is the mother of the body; and the kidneys are the root of life. Treating the lungs, spleen and kidneys is the way to deal with consumptive disease."

All these medical classics have made great contributions to discussions on the theory of consumptive diseases and the therapeutic principles to be applied in their treatment.

Various chronic and consumptive diseases in Western medicine are included in the following discussion.

Etiology and Pathogenesis

The causes of consumptive disease include congenital defects and undernourishment, resulting from weak resistance and various diseases. Consumption of *yin*, *yang*, *qi* and blood are responsible for its pathogenesis, and all the five *zang* organs are involved.

1. Congenital Defects Leading to Weak Constitution

This is a result of the old age of the parents, which means they have insufficient essence and blood, or of a lack of proper care during pregnancy; either may lead to malnutrition of the fetus. If the mother suffers from oligogalactia or constitutional deficiencies of essence and blood, these often retard the growth of teeth and hair in the infant, also causing weak bones and muscles, emaciation, and listlessness; this results in maldevelopment and then consumptive disease. Adults with congenital defects are susceptible to disease and find it difficult to recover, once they have contracted a disease. As a result, *qi* and blood become exhausted, both *yin* and *yang* are impaired and the five *zang* organs are affected. Consumptive disease will then occur.

2. Lack of Proper Care After Birth Impairing the Five *Zang* Organs

(1) Excess physical and mental strain, premature marriage, bearing many children and excessive sexual activity all consume primordial *qi* and essence and damage the *zang* organs, thus gradually causing consumptive disease.

(2) An improper diet or stress may damage the spleen and stomach, impairing the production of *qi* and blood. This results in a lack of nourishment for the internal organs and the meridians, and deficiencies both inside and outside the body. If an improper diet with impaired splenic and gastric functions is complicated by repeated exposure to external pathogenic factors, conditions will be aggravated and consumptive disease will occur.

(3) The following conditions can all develop into consumptive diseases: slow recuperation following a severe illness, consumption of *yin* blood in a prolonged febrile disease, damage to *yang-qi* in a prolonged cold disease, the inability to nourish fresh blood due to the stagnation of the blood inside the body, overfatigue soon after childbirth, failure of essence and *qi* to be restored after a chronic disease, and the consumption of the anti-pathogenic *qi* due to persistent invasion by external factors.

The kidneys are involved in congenital defects, and the spleen may be damaged due to lack of proper care in infancy. The spleen and kidneys are closely related because splenic digestion and absorption need the warmth provided by the kidneys and the kidneys need the nourishment of *yin* blood, which is produced by the spleen. Problems with either the spleen or the kidneys can lead to consumptive disease.

Differentiation and Treatment

However complex the clinical manifestations of consumptive disease may be, they are all related to the five *zang* organs, and any deficiencies in these organs never go beyond *yin*, *yang*, *qi*, and blood.

Thus, in differentiating consumptive diseases, *yin*, *yang*, *qi*, and blood should be thought of as a rope that holds a net, and the deficiency of the five *zang* organs as the mesh. Once the rope is pulled up, the mesh opens automatically.

Traditional Chinese medicine holds that the five *zang* organs are related to one another, *qi* and blood are of the same origin, and *yin* and *yang* have the same root. Therefore mutual influences and mutual transformations exist among the *zang* organs, between *qi* and blood, and between *yin* and *yang*. For instance, disorders of the spleen can affect the lungs, disorders of the lungs can affect the kidneys — in fact disorders of any one organ can affect the other organs. If *qi* is deficient, no blood can be produced; if blood is deficient, no *qi*; if *qi* is deficient, so is *yang*. Deficiency of *yin* affects *yang*, and deficiency of *yang* affects *yin*. It is also possible that the pathological changes of one or two organs are always more pronounced than those of the others. Thus it is necessary to have a good understanding of the development of pathological conditions in the process of consumptive disease in order to determine the correct method of treatment.

The basic principle of treatment in cases where the patient is suffering from a deficiency syndrome is reinforcement. Since *qi* and blood of the *zang-fu* organs are innate and receive further nourishment after birth, to replenish the spleen and kidneys is a key point in the treatment of such diseases. Through many years of clinical practice, medical scholars have found that it is more difficult to recover from *yin* deficiency than *yang* deficiency. Since *yin* and *yang* have the same origin, it is advisable to add a proper amount of *yin* tonics to formulae that reinforce *yang* when treating a *yang* deficiency, and vice versa. Although consumptive diseases are predominantly caused by deficiencies, signs of excesses often exist, such as *yin* deficiency complicated by hyperactive fire, *yang* deficiency complicated by retained water and fluid, blood deficiency complicated by blood stagnation, and *qi* deficiency complicated by the invasion of external factors. Consequently, both the primary and secondary disorders are often treated at the same time, though the primary method adopted is reinforcement. If complications are pronounced, the elimination of pathogenic factors will then become the primary method of treatment. For example, in cases of splenic deficiency complicated by phlegm-dampness retained in the middle *jiao*, and renal deficiency complicated by the invasion of pathogenic factors, elimination should precede reinforcement. The following are four categories of common syndromes of consumptive disease:

1. Deficient *Qi*

(1) Deficient lung *qi*

Clinical manifestations: Shortness of breath, spontaneous sweating, an aversion to wind, lassitude, dislike of speaking, a low voice or cough, an increased susceptibility to common colds, a pale complexion, a pale tongue, and a weak pulse.

Analysis: Deficient lung *qi* gives rise to shortness of breath, lassitude, a dislike of speaking and a low voice. Since the lungs dominate the skin and hair, deficient lung *qi* means a weak resistance, which explains the increased susceptibility to common colds and the coughing fits. The weakness of the body surface causes an aversion to wind and spontaneous sweating. In cases of *qi* deficiency, *qi* fails to allow the blood to nourish upwards and fill the vessels, resulting in a pale complexion, a pale tongue, and a weak pulse.

Treatment: To replenish the lungs and benefit *qi*.

Prescription: Modified Decoction for Invigorating Lungs (158). Radix Ginseng, and Radix Astragali replenish lung *qi*; Cortex Mori and Radix Asteris moisten the lungs and relieve the cough; and Radix Rehmanniae Preparata, and Fructus Schisandrae replenish the kidneys and receive *qi*. In cases of inability to dominate or receive *qi*, with the symptom of asthmatic breathing on slight exertion, add Gecko to replenish the lungs and kidneys and soothe asthma. If there is persistent spontaneous sweating, add Jade Screen Powder (73) to benefit *qi*, constrict the body surface and make the sweating cease.

In cases of deficient *qi* and *yin* with hectic fever, a malar flush, a dry throat and a red tongue, prescribe Powder of Astragali and Carapax Trionycis (268) to benefit *qi*, harmonize the nutrient *qi* and disperse heat caused by deficiencies.

(2) Deficient spleen *qi*

Clinical manifestations: A poor appetite, epigastric discomfort after eating, lassitude, loose stools, a sallow complexion, a pale tongue with a thin coating, and a weak pulse.

Analysis: Deficient spleen *qi* means that the ability of the gastrointestinal tract to transport and transform is impaired, causing a poor appetite, epigastric discomfort after eating and loose stools. Splenic deficiencies also implies that the sources of *qi* and blood are not sufficient to nourish the body. The consequences are lassitude, a sallow complexion and a weak pulse. In severe cases, a prolonged deficiency of *qi* can lead to the *qi* of the middle *jiao* becoming exhausted or deficient spleen *yang*, as shown by a weighted sensation in the epigastrium and abdomen and persistent diarrhea.

Treatment: To invigorate the spleen and benefit *qi*.

Prescription: Modified Powder of Ginseng, Poria and Atractylodis Macrocephalae (190). Radix Ginseng and Rhizoma Atractylodis Macrocephalae invigorate the spleen and benefit *qi*; Poria and Radix Glycyrrhizae harmonize the middle *jiao* and regulate the stomach; and Rhizoma Dioscoreae, Semen Lablab Album, Semen Nelumbinis and Semen Coicis invigorate the spleen, remove dampness through urination and check diarrhea. If epigastric fullness and distention, vomiting and belching are also present, add Pericarpium Citri Reticulatae and Rhizoma Pinelliae to harmonize the stomach and send the unhealthy *qi* downwards. In cases of food retention, add Massa Medicata Fermentata, Fructus Hordei Germinatus and Endothelium Corneum Gigeriae Galli to harmonize the stomach and assist digestion. In cases of *yang* deficiency of the middle *jiao* and *qi* deficiency with cold signs, exhibiting epigastric and abdominal pain, add Radix Paeoniae Alba, Ramulus Cinnamomi, Saccharum Granorum and Rhizoma Zingiberis to soothe the middle *jiao* and relieve pain. For the prostration of *qi* in the middle *jiao* with persistent diarrhea and a weighted sensation in the epigastrium and abdomen, prescribe Decoction for Strengthening Middle *Jiao* and Benefiting *Qi* (154) to lift *yang* and benefit *qi*. In cases of deficient spleen *yang* with diarrhea, add Cortex Cinnamomi and Rhizoma Zingiberis (stir-baked at a high temperature) to warm the middle *jiao*, disperse cold, and check diarrhea.

If both lung and spleen *qi* are deficient, the patient will be susceptible to common colds. The continuous invasion of external pathogenic factors damages the body's anti-pathogenic *qi*, thus making this deficiency impossible to cure. The medical classic *Synopsis of Prescriptions of the Golden Chamber* recommends Pill of Dioscoreae (327) for such a condition to promote the anti-pathogenic *qi* and eliminate pathogenic factors. In this formula, Rhizoma Dioscoreae, Decoction of Four Mild Drugs (91), Four Drugs Decoction (93) and Colla Corii Asini all replenish *qi* and blood, and Radix Ledebouriellae, Semen Sojae Germinatum, Ramulus Cinnamomi and Radix Bupleuri eliminate pathogenic factors. These should be taken in the form of pills to facilitate long-term oral administration.

Qi deficiency involves not only the lungs and spleen, but the other *zang* organs as well. Both the heart and the lungs are located in the upper *jiao*, and pectoral *qi* circulates in these two organs. Thus in cases of deficient lung *qi*, heart *qi* is also likely to be insufficient, and this will show itself in palpitations, shortness of breath, spontaneous sweating and a weak pulse. In the meantime, the lungs dominate *qi*, which has its origin in the kidneys, the spleen determines the condition of the acquired constitution, and the kidneys are the origin of the congenital constitution. Consequently, deficient lung *qi* and spleen *qi* give rise to deficient kidney *qi* with impaired reception of *qi*, as shown by asthmatic breathing, incontinence, loose stools and deficient *yang* with signs of cold limbs and a feeble pulse.

Qi deficiency thus primarily affects the spleen and lungs at the initial stages, and moves to the heart and kidneys in the later stages of the disease. Methods for treating heart *yang* and kidney *yang* deficiency should then be adopted accordingly. If the stagnant *qi* seen in liver disorders affects the spleen, causing lassitude, a poor appetite and loose stools, then treatment for deficient spleen *qi* should be adopted.

2. Deficient Blood

(1) Deficient heart blood

Clinical manifestations: Palpitations, poor memory, insomnia, sleep disturbed by dreams, a pale complexion, a pale tongue, and a thready pulse or a knotted and intermittent pulse.

Analysis: The heart controls the mind. Deficient heart blood impairs the functioning of the mind, leading to palpitations, poor memory, insomnia and poor sleep disturbed by dreams. The heart dominates the blood and the vessels, so the patient's complexion reflects the condition of the heart. If the patient is suffering from a blood deficiency, this does not allow the blood to nourish the face or fill up the vessels, and so a pale complexion, a pale tongue and a thready pulse ensue. Obstructed circulation gives rise to a knotted and intermittent pulse.

Treatment: To nourish the blood and calm the mind.

Prescription: Modified Decoction for Nourishing Heart (208). Radix Astragali, Radix Ginseng, Lignum Pini Poriaferum and Radix Glycyrrhizae benefit *qi* and invigorate the spleen to produce blood; and Radix Angelicae Sinensis, Rhizoma Chuanxiong, Fructus Schisandrae, Radix Polygalae, Semen Platycladi and Radix Ophiopogonis nourish the heart blood and calm the mind. In cases of palpitations or a knotted and intermittent pulse, prescribe Decoction of Glycyrrhizae Preparata (186) to restore normal pulse and relieve palpitations.

(2) Deficient liver blood

Clinical manifestations: Dizziness, blurred vision, tinnitus, pain in the hypochondrium, restlessness, irregular menstruation, amenorrhea, squarrose and dry skin, a pale complexion, a pale or bluish-purple tongue, and a taut and thready, or a thready and unsmooth pulse.

Analysis: Blood deficiency means a lack of nourishment for the liver. This makes liver *yang* rise, causing dizziness, blurred vision, tinnitus and restlessness. Deficient liver blood deprives the liver meridians of nourishment, and the resultant stagnation of *qi* in the meridians causes hypochondriac pain. A pale tongue, a pale complexion and a thready, taut pulse are signs of deficient liver blood. Blood deficiency also explains why the patient may suffer from irregular menstruation or amenorrhea. Stagnant blood inside the body prevents the production of fresh blood, resulting in squarrose and dry skin, a bluish-purple tongue and a thready and unsmooth pulse. Since the liver opens into the eyes and dominates the tendons, deficient liver blood reduces nourishment to these parts of the body and produces dry eyes, contracture of the hands and feet and numb limbs with limited movement.

Treatment: To nourish liver blood, activate blood circulation and remove stasis in cases of blood stagnation.

Prescription: Four Drugs Decoction (93) with additional ingredients. In this formula, Radix Angelicae Sinensis and Radix Rehmanniae nourish *yin* blood; Radix Paeoniae Alba enters the liver and harmonizes the nutrient *qi*; and Rhizoma Chuanxiong regulates *qi* and activates blood circulation. For dizziness and tinnitus, add Fructus Ligustri Lucidi, Magnetitum, and Concha Ostreae to nourish *yin* and suppress hyperactive *yang*. If there is restlessness, add Semen Ziziphi Spinosae, Radix Polygalae and Dens Draconis to soothe the heart and calm the mind. In cases of hypochondriac pain, add Radix Bupleuri, Radix Curcumae and Rhizoma Corydalis to promote the smooth circulation of *qi*. In cases of stagnant blood following a prolonged liver disorder or amenorrhea, add Semen Persicae and Folium Lycopi to activate blood circulation, remove stasis and produce fresh blood. If the hands and feet are numb, add Caulis Spatholobi, Fructus Chaenomelis and Herba Lycopodii to ease the tendons and meridians. For impaired vision and dry eyes, use the above formula together with Bolus of Lycii, Chrysanthemi and

Rehmanniae Preparata (144). In a prolonged case of *qi* and blood deficiency, herbs that replenish both *qi* and blood should also be prescribed.

Blood deficiency actually involves all five *zang* organs. Blood deficiency in the lungs and kidneys is a factor in *yin* deficiency. It must be pointed out that blood deficiency is closely related to the spleen, since it is either the result of an insufficient source of blood or an excessive loss of blood. The production of blood relies on the normal functioning of spleen *qi* to transport and transform. Excessive blood loss is often caused by the impaired ability of the liver to store blood and the impaired ability of the spleen to control blood. Persistent hemorrhaging in particular is mostly due to impaired splenic control of blood. Thus herbs that invigorate the spleen and benefit *qi* should be added to the formulae for treating deficiencies of heart blood or liver blood; an example is the addition of Decoction for Invigorating Spleen and Nourishing Heart (110). If excessive blood loss leads to deficient *qi*, or the latter condition fails to control the blood properly, prescribe Decoction of Angelicae Sinensis for Enriching Blood (131). A large dose of Radix Astragali is used in this prescription to benefit *qi* in cases of blood loss. If *qi* and blood fail to recover after blood loss, and deficiency cold syndromes such as lassitude and aversion to cold appear, prescribe Decoction of Ginseng for Nourishing *Qi* and *Ying* (11) to warm up and replenish *qi* and blood. Since *qi* and blood deficiencies often appear at the same time, replenishing *qi* and blood is one of the common treatments for consumptive diseases.

3. Deficient *Yang*

(1) Deficient heart *yang*

Clinical manifestations: Palpitations, shortness of breath, spontaneous sweating, lassitude, somnolence, cold limbs, stuffiness and pain in the heart and chest, a pale complexion, a pale or dark purple tongue, and a thready and weak or knotted and intermittent pulse.

Analysis: Deficiencies of heart *yang* and *qi* are basically the same, and so they exhibit common symptoms. The difference is that cold signs are not pronounced when heart *qi* is deficient, but are pronounced when heart *yang* is deficient, and the latter condition often develops from the former. When both are deficient, the heart and mind fail to be nourished, and palpitations, shortness of breath, lassitude and somnolence ensue. Deficient heart *yang* also impedes the distribution of *yang-qi* to the limbs and body surface, explaining why the limbs feel cold to the touch. Sweat is the fluid of the heart. When heart *qi* is deficient, it is unable to check its fluid, and spontaneous sweating follows. Deficient heart *yang* also causes *qi* and blood stagnation, with stuffiness and pain in the heart and chest and a dark purple tongue. A pale complexion, a pale tongue and a thready and weak pulse or a knotted and intermittent one, are also signs of deficient heart *yang*.

Treatment: To warm and invigorate heart *yang*.

Prescription: Decoction of Cinnamomi and Glycyrrhizae (228) with additional ingredients. In this formula, Ramulus Cinnamomi enters the heart and assists heart *yang*, and Radix Glycyrrhizae invigorates the middle *jiao* and benefits *qi*. For stuffiness and pain in the heart and chest, add Flos Inulae, Radix Notoginseng, Flos Carthami and Radix Curcumae to activate blood circulation, remove blood stasis, regulate *qi* and relieve pain. Another method of treating this is to suck one piece of Bolus of Styrax (143) to regulate *qi* and restore consciousness. In severe cases, heart *yang*-deficiency may exhibits signs that the *yang-qi* has been exhausted such as palpitations, coughing, asthmatic breathing, profuse sweating, cold limbs and a feeble and thready pulse. In this condition, Decoction of Ginseng, Aconiti Lateralis Preparata, Os Draconis and Concha Ostreae (193) are used to benefit *qi*, activate the pulse, restore *yang*, prevent it from being exhausted and check sweating.

(2) Deficient spleen *yang*

Clinical manifestations: A sallow complexion, a poor appetite, a cold sensation, lassitude, unwillingness to speak, a feeling of coldness in the abdomen or pain, borborygmus and diarrhea (all of which are induced by exposure to cold or a bad diet), a pale tongue with a white coating, and a weak and feeble pulse.

Analysis: Deficient spleen-*yang* is a further development of deficient spleen *qi*. Deficient *qi* in the middle *jiao* may be complicated by cold, as well as by impaired transportation and transformation which cause the patient to have a poor appetite, feel cold and experience lassitude, and unwillingness to speak. In cases of deficient *yang* and excess *yin*, *yang-qi* cannot be distributed normally, and retained cold and stagnant *qi* will follow, with symptoms of abdominal pain, borborygmus and loose stools containing undigested food. Exposure to cold or an improper diet causes the *yang* of the middle *jiao* to become even more deficient, thus inducing new attacks or aggravating pathological conditions. A sallow complexion, a pale tongue with a white coating, and a weak and feeble pulse are signs of deficient spleen *yang*.

Treatment: To warm the middle *jiao* and invigorate the spleen.

Prescription: Modified Bolus of Aconiti Lateralis Preparata for Regulating Middle *Jiao* (163). Radix Aconiti Lateralis Preparata, acrid and warm in nature, assists *yang*; Rhizoma Zingiberis warms the middle *jiao* and disperses cold; Radix Codonopsis, Rhizoma Atractylodis Macrocephalae and Radix Glycyrrhizae benefit *qi* and invigorate the spleen. In cases of abdominal coldness, pain and persistent diarrhea, replace Rhizoma Zingiberis with Rhizoma Zingiberis (stir-baked at a high temperature), and add Pericarpium Zanthoxyli and Semen Myristicae to warm the middle *jiao*, disperse cold, strengthen the intestines and check diarrhea. If vomiting occurs after eating, add Rhizoma Pinelliae and Pericarpium Citri Reticulatae to harmonize the middle *jiao* and send the unhealthy *qi* downwards.

(3) Deficient kidney *yang*

Clinical manifestations: An aversion to cold, cold limbs, diarrhea in the mornings with undigested food in the stools, backache, lumbago, spermatorrhea, impotence, polyuria or incontinence, oliguria, a pale complexion, a pale and swollen tongue with tooth prints and a white coating, and a deep and slow pulse.

Analysis: In cases of deficient kidney *yang* and declining fire at the life gate, the spleen fails to be warmed by kidney *yang* and its digestive functions are impaired, leading to diarrhea in the morning with undigested food in the stools. A deficiency of *yang* also deprives the limbs and bones of warmth, causing an aversion to cold and cold limbs. The lumbar region is the residence of the kidneys, and the *Du Meridian* (Governor Vessel) which travels along the spinal column is connected to the kidneys and dominates all the *yang* meridians. This explains the backache and lumbago in cases of deficient kidney *yang*. The kidneys store essence, and its function will be impaired if *yang-qi* is deficient, resulting in spermatorrhea and impotence. Weak kidney *qi* causes polyuria or incontinence. The impaired control of urine due to deficient kidney *yang* results in oliguria. A pale complexion, a pale and swollen tongue with tooth prints and white coating, and a deep, slow pulse are signs of deficient *yang-qi* and excess *yin* cold.

Treatment: To warm and replenish kidney *yang*, and nourish essence and blood.

Prescription: Modified *Yougui* Pill (82). Radix Aconiti Lateralis Preparata and Cortex Cinnamomi warm and replenish kidney *yang*; Semen Cuscutae and Colla Cornus Cervi warm kidney *yang* and replenish kidney essence when combined with Radix Rehmanniae Preparata, Rhizoma Dioscoreae, Fructus Corni, Cortex Eucommiae and Fructus Lycii; and Radix Angelicae Sinensis warms and nourishes the blood. For persistent diarrhea, assist *yang* and benefit *qi* by reducing the herbs that nourish essence and blood and adding Radix Ginseng, Rhizoma Atractylodis Macrocephalae and Radix Glycyrrhizae to invigorate the spleen and check diarrhea. In cases when diarrhea occurs in the morning, combine this formula with Pill of Four Miraculous Drugs (94) to warm the kidneys, strengthen the intestines and check diarrhea. In cases of deficient *yang* and retained fluid with symptoms of marked edema, reduced urine, abdominal distention, and sometimes even a swollen scrotum and palpitations, add Poria, Semen Plantaginis, Rhizoma Alismatis and Rhizoma Atractylodis Macrocephalae, or *Zhenwu* Decoction (223) to warm *yang*, promote diuresis and relieve edema. In cases of spermatorrhea, add Fructus Rosae Laevigatae, Oötheca Mantidis and Stamen Nelumbinis, or prescribe Golden Lock Bolus for Keeping Kidney-Essence (184) to promote astringency and guard essence. In cases where the kidneys fail to receive *qi*, and the patient suffers from asthmatic breathing and shortness of breath, both of which are aggravated by exertion, add Fructus Psoraleae and Fructus Schisandrae to help the kidneys to receive *qi* and soothe the asthma.

The syndrome of deficient *yang* as mentioned above is a further development of *qi* deficiency. The heart, spleen and kidneys are interrelated. Prolonged deficiency of spleen *yang* can lead to deficient kidney *yang*, and vice versa. The production of essence and *qi* relies on the kidneys, which also are responsible for maintaining the metabolic rate of the fluid. However, these are also related to the normal transporting and transforming functions of the spleen, thus spleen and kidney *yang*-deficiencies sometimes exist concurrently. The formula to treat this condition is Decoction of Cinnamomi and Aconiti Lateralis Preparata for Regulating Middle *Jiao* (229). Deficiencies of heart and kidney *yang* are also interrelated. The former often originates from declining fire at the life gate, and it is clinically possible for both to be present at the same time.

Deficient kidney essence shares some of the symptoms of kidney deficiency, such as dizziness, tinnitus, soreness and weakness in the lumbar region and knees, sexual hypofunction, excessive loss of hair, loose teeth, impaired intelligence and premature senility. But there are no marked signs of deficiencies of either heat or cold. Herbs that replenish the kidneys are used in the treatment, for example, Placenta Hominis, Cornu Cervi, Carapax et Plastrum Testudinis, Cortex Eucommiae, Fructus Lycii, Radix Polygoni Multiflori, Fructus Corni and Radix Rehmanniae Preparata.

4. Deficient *Yin*

(1) Deficient lung *yin*

Clinical manifestations: A dry cough, a dry throat, loss of voice in severe cases, fever in the afternoon, night sweats, a facial flush, a red tongue with little moisture, no tongue coating or very little coating, and a thready and rapid pulse.

Analysis: Deficient lung *yin* does not allow the lungs to stay clean and moist, giving rise to a nonproductive cough. The damage done to the lung vessels by coughing causes hemoptysis. When body fluid is consumed, it fails to nourish upwards and thereby produces a dry throat which may even cause the patient to lose their voice. Fever in the afternoon is a result of the displacement of fire due to *yin* deficiency. Night sweats is the result of internal heat caused by the same deficiency, which compels body fluid outward. A facial flush, a red tongue with little moisture, no coating or little coating, and a thready and rapid pulse are signs of internal heat due to deficient *yin*.

Treatment: To nourish *yin* and moisten the lungs.

Prescription: Modified Decoction of Lilii for Strengthening Lungs (116). Bulbus Lilii and Radix Ophiopogonis nourish *yin* and moisten the lungs; Radix Scrophulariae, Radix Rehmanniae and Radix Rehmanniae Preparata nourish *yin* and disperse heat; Radix Angelicae Sinensis replenishes *yin* blood; and Radix Platycodi, Bulbus Fritillariae Cirrhosae and Radix Glycyrrhizae dispel heat from the lungs, relieve phlegm and check coughing. To treat the fever, add Cortex Lycii, Radix Stellariae and Carapax Trionycis which nourish *yin* and disperse heat caused by deficiencies. If the the patient sweats at night, add Fructus Tritici Levis (light), Concha Ostreae and Radix Ephedrae to stop the sweating. If there is hemoptysis, add Colla Corii Asini, Rhizoma Bletillae and Herba Agrimoniae to nourish the blood and stop hemorrhaging. If signs of liver fire appear, use Powder of Indigo Naturalis and Concha Meretricis seu Cyclinae (321) together with the above formula.

(2) Deficient heart *yin*

Clinical manifestations: Palpitations, insomnia, restlessness, irritability, fever in the afternoon, night sweats, a facial flush, ulcers on the tongue, a red tongue with little moisture, and a thready and rapid pulse.

Analysis: Deficient *yin* blood deprives the heart of nourishment, causing palpitations and insomnia. Internal heat due to *yin* deficiencies produces hyperactive heart fire along with restlessness, irritability and a facial flush. Since the tongue is the mirror of the heart, this hyperactivity gives rise to ulcers on the tongue. Sweat is the fluid of the heart and hyperactive fire forces the body fluid outward, causing night sweating and fever in the afternoon. A red tongue with little moisture and a thready and rapid pulse are signs of hyperactive fire due to *yin* deficiency.

Treatment: To nourish *yin* and replenish the heart.

Prescription: Modified King of Heaven Tonic Pill for Mental Discomfort (39). Radix Rehmanniae, Radix Asparagi, Radix Ophiopogonis and Radix Scrophulariae nourish *yin* fluid; Radix Salviae Miltiorrhizae, Radix Angelicae Sinensis, Radix Polygalae, Semen Ziziphi Spinosae, Semen Platycladi and Poria soothe the heart and calm the mind; Radix Ginseng replenishes heart *qi*, Fructus Schisandrae strengthens heart fluid; and Radix Platycodi forces the action of the medication upwards. This formula principally nourishes *yin*. For hyperactive fire with symptoms of restlessness, irritability, and tongue ulcers, add Rhizoma Coptidis, Caulis Aristolochiae Manshuriensis and Herba Lophatheri to reduce heart fire and conduct the heat downwards.

(3) Deficient spleen *yin*

Clinical manifestations: Dry mouth and lips, a poor appetite, constipation with dry stools, retching in severe cases, hiccups, a facial flush, a glossy dry tongue or a dry mouth, and a thready and rapid pulse.

Analysis: Deficient *yin* leads to hyperactive fire, which further consumes splenic and gastric *yin* fluid, thus leading to a dry mouth and lips, a facial flush, and a poor appetite. The lack of fluid in the gastrointestinal tract causes constipation with dry stools. Deficient stomach *yin* in its later stages exhibits a dry crimson tongue, or a glossy tongue, dryness of the mouth and hiccups, all of which suggest that stomach *yin* has been completely exhausted.

Treatment: To nourish *yin* and harmonize the stomach.

Prescription: Decoction for Benefiting Stomach (246) with additional ingredients. In this formula, Radix Adenophorae, Radix Ophiopogonis, Radix Rehmanniae and Rhizoma Polygonati Odorati nourish *yin* fluid. They are nutritious but not sticky, so they do not impair the functions of the spleen and stomach. The addition of crystal sugar nourishes the stomach and harmonizes the middle *jiao*. To treat constipation with dry stools, drink the above decoction with honey. In cases where the mouth is dry and the patient is suffering from hiccups, add Radix Ginseng and Herba Dendrobii to replenish *qi* and *yin*, and Semen Canavaliae and Calyx Kaki to conduct the unhealthy *qi* downwards and relieve the hiccups. If the patient experiences restlessness and thirst, add Radix Trichosanthis and Succus Saccharum to produce body fluid and relieve the thirst. To treat the patient's lack of appetite, add Fructus Setariae Germinatus and Fructus Hordei Germinatus to nourish the stomach and harmonize the middle *jiao*.

(4) Deficient liver *yin*

Clinical manifestations: Headache, dizziness, tinnitus, dry eyes, photophobia, blurred or impaired vision, irritability, numb limbs and body, muscular twitching and cramps, a facial flush, a dry red tongue and a taut, thready and rapid pulse.

Analysis: A deficiency of *yin* blood in the liver fails to check *yang*, and disturbance of the clear cavity by a deficiency of hyperactive *yang* causes headaches, tinnitus, and even dizziness in severe cases. The inability of *yin* blood to nourish the eyes explains their dryness, photophobia, and blurred or impaired vision. Deficient liver *yin* causes hyperactive liver fire, making the patient irritable. Since the liver dominates the tendons, deficient *yin* blood results in their malnutrition, and causes numb limbs and body, muscular twitching and cramps. A facial flush, a dry red tongue and a taut, thready and rapid pulse are signs of hyperactive fire due to *yin* deficiency.

Treatment: To nourish liver *yin*.

Prescription: Modified Decoction for Replenishing Liver (157). Four Drugs Decoction (93) nourishes the blood and soothes the liver, and Semen Ziziphi Spinosae, Fructus Chaenomelis, Radix Ophiopogonis and Radix Glycyrrhizae nourish liver *yin*. If headaches, dizziness and tinnitus are severe or muscular twitching and cramps appear, add Concha Haliotidis, Flos Chrysanthemi and Ramulus Uncariae cum Uncis to calm liver *yang*. For dry eyes, photophobia and impaired vision, add Fructus Lycii, Fructus Ligustri Lucidi and Semen Cassiae to nourish the liver and improve sight. In cases where the patient feels numbness of the limbs and body, add Caulis Spatholobi and Retinervus Luffae Fructus to nourish the blood and remove obstructions from the meridians. If there is hyperactive liver fire accompanied by irritability, dark yellow urine and constipation, add Radix Gentianae, Radix Scutellariae and Fructus Gardeniae to disperse heat from the liver and reduce fire. For hypochondriac pain, add Fructus Toosendan and Rhizoma Corydalis to regulate *qi* and relieve pain.

(5) Deficient kidney *yin*

Clinical manifestations: Excessive hair loss, loose teeth, dizziness, tinnitus, deafness in severe cases, a dry mouth, a sore throat, fever in the afternoon, a facial flush, spermatorrhea, lumbar soreness, muscular atrophy and motor impairment of the legs, a red tongue with little moisture, and a deep and thready pulse.

Analysis: The kidneys are related to the hair and the teeth are related to the bones which are dominated by the kidneys. Thus deficient kidney *yin* causes hair loss and loose teeth. It also means insufficient marrow and malnutrition of the brain, resulting in dizziness and tinnitus. If fire caused by deficiencies flares up, then this causes a dry mouth, a sore throat, fever in the afternoon and a facial flush. If the seminal gate is disturbed by the same fire, this results in spermatorrhea and lumbar soreness. Exhaustion of essence leads to deafness, while exhaustion of marrow produces muscular atrophy and motor impairment. A red tongue with little moisture, and a deep and thready pulse are signs of depleted kidney *yin*.

Treatment: To nourish kidney *yin*.

Prescription: Modified *Zuogui* Pill (79). Radix Rehmanniae Preparata, Fructus Corni, Semen Cuscutae, Radix Achyranthis Bidentatae and Colla Carapax et Plastri Testudinis nourish kidney *yin*, and Colla Cornus Cervi produces essence and marrow. For spermatorrhea or polyuria, add Os Draconis, Concha Ostreae, Fructus Rosae Laevigatae and Stamen Nelumbinis to promote astringency. In cases of deafness, muscular atrophy and motor impairment of the legs, prescribe Bolus of Placenta Hominis (172) and *Huqian* Bolus (171) to produce essence and blood, and strengthen the tendons and bones.

Deficient *yin* may involve all five *zang* organs. Deficient kidney *yin* often leads to deficient *yin* blood in the spleen, lungs, heart and liver, and vice versa. Since the kidneys store essence, the liver stores blood, and essence and blood nourish each other, the liver and kidneys have common sources and are closely related. *Yin* deficiency can affect both organs at the same time, and common examples involve the lungs, kidneys and liver.

Deficiencies of *yin* and *yang* can change from one into the other. A prolonged deficiency of one can lead to a deficiency of the other, and either can lead to deficiencies of both *yin* and *yang*. That is why *yin* tonics should be added to the formula for deficient *yang*, and vice versa. Doctors in ancient times said, "Those who are good at *yang* replenishment can draw *yang* from *yin*; when assisted by *yin*, *yang* has no limit. Those who are good at *yin* replenishment can absorb *yin* from *yang*; when assisted by *yang*, the sources of *yin* can never be exhausted." For instance, *Zuogui* Pill (79) for kidney *yin*-deficiency not only consists of *yin* tonics, but also of *yang* tonics such as Colla Cornus Cervi and Semen Cuscutae. The *Yougui* Pill (82) for kidney *yang*-deficiency is made up of *yang* tonics as well as *yin* tonics such as Radix Rehmanniae Preparata and Fructus Lycii. It must be pointed out that this principle does not mean *yin* and *yang* tonics can be used interchangeably in every situation. As a matter of fact, they should mainly be prescribed depending upon the predominant pathogenesis of the disease.

Consumptive disease is likely to be complicated by invading external pathogenic factors. The presence of external syndromes further weakens the body's anti-pathogenic *qi*. Thus eliminating pathogenic factors should be combined with replenishment. Only when the pathogenic factors are eliminated can replenishment be most effective. According to a medical book published in the Qing Dynasty, pathogenic factors should be expelled by means of replenishment when internal disorders are more pronounced than invasion by pathogenic factors, but pathogenic factors should be expelled through elimination when the opposite applies. The formula called Powder for Benefiting Nutrient System and Expelling Pathogenic Factors (247) and that called Decoction of Bupleuri and Citri Reticulatae for Expelling Pathogenic Factors (240) can be used in these cases respectively.

Prolonged consumptive diseases can be complicated by stagnant *qi* and blood with symptoms of weight loss, abdominal fullness, an inability to eat, squarrose and dry skin and dark eyes. All this suggests stagnant dry blood. Treatment then involves removing blood stasis and promoting tissue regeneration.

There are a variety of therapeutic approaches that can be taken for consumptive disease, such as *qigong* exercises, acupuncture, moxibustion and massage, all of which can be used in combination with herbs.

The prognosis of consumptive disease depends on the strength of the *qi* of the middle *jiao*. If this *qi* has been exhausted, the prognosis is poor. If deficiencies cause the patient to suffer from coughing, a hoarse voice, shortness of breath, asthmatic breathing, swelling in the lower legs, loose stools, a poor appetite and weight loss, then the condition will prove difficult to cure. A smooth pulse indicates that there is a possibility of recovery; a marked taut and large pulse suggests that the condition has been aggravated; and a very rapid pulse implies a critical condition. A dry red tongue and frequent hiccups are signs that stomach *qi* has been depleted.

Remarks

The four categories of consumptive disease often complicate each other. In their earlier stages, consumptive diseases generally affect both *qi* and blood, combining with deficiencies of *qi* or blood or both. Long-term consumptive diseases or those with severe pathological conditions mostly affect *yin* and *yang*, causing deficiencies of *yin*, or *yang*, or both. Nevertheless, *qi* and blood, and *yin* and *yang* are closely related. Since body fluid, essence and blood all fall into the category of *yin* fluid, deficient *yin* can include deficient blood, as well as deficiency fire. Deficient *yang* includes deficient *qi*, and the former is more serious than the latter. Such conditions when two or more organs are diseased at the same time are usually found in protracted cases, and therefore are even more difficult to cure. Nevertheless the clinical manifestations of consumptive disease never go beyond these four categories of syndrome. Their diagnosis in relation to the five *zang* organs is very significant when considering clinical treatment.

Case Studies

Name: Liang XX; Sex: Female; Age: 30.

Chief complaint: Hectic fever, spontaneous sweating, dizziness, headache, insomnia, palpitations, nausea, a poor appetite, inability to taste, lumbar soreness and lassitude developed after excessive loss of blood during labor. These symptoms had become worse over the past month.

Examination: The patient's body temperature was normal. She looked pale, and was short of breath when talking. Her pulse was deep, thready and weak. Her tongue was red with no coating.

Pathogenesis: Heart and spleen deficiency complicated by an excessive loss of blood during labor.

Treatment: To replenish the heart and spleen, and benefit *qi* and blood.

Prescription: Modified Decoction for Invigorating Spleen and Nourishing Heart (110). The prescription consisted of the following herbs:

Radix Astragali	15 g;
Radix Codonopsis	9 g;
Rhizoma Atractylodis Macrocephalae	9 g;
Lignum Pini Poriaferum	9 g;
Semen Ziziphi Spinosae (stir-baked)	12 g;
Radix Polygalae	4.5 g;
Arillus Longan	9 g;
Pericarpium Citri Reticulatae	4.5 g;
Caulis Spatholobi (as a substitute for Radix Angelicae Sinensis)	9 g;
Semen Cuscutae	9 g;
Flos Chrysanthemi	9 g;
Radix Glycyrrhizae Preparata	3 g.

After six doses, hectic fever, spontaneous sweating, dizziness, headache, palpitations and insomnia had all disappeared. Lumbar soreness and lassitude had improved. The patient's pulse had become stronger and her tongue was slightly red with no coating. Pericarpium Citri Reticulatae and Flos Chrysanthemi were removed from the previous prescription and nine grams of Radix Dipsaci and nine grams of Rhizoma Cibotii were added. Another three doses were prescribed. The patient was advised to stop taking medication after three doses.

Discussion: This consumptive disease resulted from cardiac and splenic deficiencies following excessive loss of blood during labor. Deficient heart blood caused the patient's pale complexion, palpitations, insomnia, dizziness, headache and hectic fever. Deficient spleen *qi* caused her shortness of breath, lassitude and poor appetite. Thus Decoction for Invigorating Spleen and Nourishing Heart (110) was prescribed to replenish the heart and spleen, and nourish *qi* and blood. Since the kidneys are the basis of the congenital constitution, herbs that replenish the kidneys, such as Radix Dipsaci and Rhizoma Cibotii, were added when the functions of the heart and spleen were restored.

Name: Li XX; Sex: Female; Age: 28; Occupation: Worker.

Since March 1965, the patient had noted dizziness, lassitude, a poor appetite, weight loss, petechia, bleeding gums and menorrhagia. In August that year, she was admitted to hospital for aplastic anemia. After receiving treatment such as a blood transfusion and hormone therapy, her pathological condition became stable and she left hospital three months later. In late February this year, she entered hospital once again when she suffered a relapse. During this two months at hospital, she received 3,800 ml of blood transfusion, 300 ml every five to seven days, and prednisone treatment. The bleeding had now improved, but she still suffered from dizziness, lassitude, palpitations, shortness of breath, a sallow complexion, excessive hair growth and a change of temperament. The patient wanted to have traditional treatment, and so she was referred to our hospital.

The examination she received on May 7, 1966 showed that she was obese. She had a sallow complexion and the number of red blood cells reaching 2,240,000, hemochrome only 7 g, white blood cells 4,900, reticulocytes 0.3% and platelets 34,000. The diagnosis was aplastic anemia.

The patient had taken 15 mg of prednisone daily in the previous hospital. Since it was not advisable to stop this suddenly, the same dosage was used for some time before it was gradually decreased.

First visit (May 7, 1966): Clinical manifestations were dizziness, lassitude, palpitations, shortness of breath, weight loss, a poor appetite, a pale tongue with a thin coating, and a thready and deep pulse. The pathogenesis was deficiencies of both *qi* and blood. Treatment aimed to benefit *qi* and nourish blood. The prescription consisted of the following herbs:

Radix Angelicae Sinensis	12 g;
Radix Rehmanniae Preparata	12 g;
Radix Paeoniae Alba (stir-baked)	9 g;
Radix Codonopsis	9 g;
Cortex Cinnamomi	2.4 g;
Pericarpium Citri Reticulatae	6 g.

Two doses were prescribed.

During the period between May 9 and May 27, Radix Codonopsis and Cortex Cinnamomi were removed, and Radix Astragali and Herba Agrimoniae added.

Second visit (May 28): The patient exhibited weight loss, profuse menstrual flow, epistaxis, the continuous appearance of bleeding spots on the skin, lassitude, palpitations, insomnia and a poor appetite. The blood test given to her on May 23 showed hemochrome of 5 g; and red blood cells 1,820,000. The patient's dizziness had improved slightly following a transfusion of 300 ml of blood the previous day. Her tongue coating was thin, and her pulse was soft and smooth. The method of treatment sought to invigorate the spleen, warm the kidneys, benefit *qi* and replenish blood. The following herbs were prescribed:

Cornu Cervi Degelatinatum	12 g;
Radix Angelicae Sinensis	9 g;
Radix Astragali	15 g;
Radix Rehmanniae Preparata	2 g;
Pericarpium Citri Reticulatae	6 g;
Radix Morindae Officinalis	15 g.

Three doses were prescribed.

Then treatment continued like this until she left hospital on October 5. Radix Rehmanniae Preparata was replaced by Radix Rehmanniae, and at the same time hemostatics (such as Flos Sophorae Immaturus or Herba Agrimoniae) and herbs that resolve dampness and assist digestion (such as Herba Agastachis, Massa Medicata Fermentata, Fructus Setariae Germinatus and Fructus Hordei Germinatus) were added. The blood test before she left hospital showed that hemochrome had increased to 9.5 g, red blood cells to 3,090,000 and platelets to 120,000. Myelogram was normal. The follow-up visit six years later revealed that the patient's condition was stable.

Discussion: This is a case of consumptive disease due to blood deficiency. At the beginning, the patient was given treatment according to the prescription Powerful Tonic Decoction of Ten Drugs (5) to replenish both *qi* and blood, but with little effect. This is because only one symptom — the patient's deep and thready pulse — reflected the deficiency of kidney *yang*. Since the disease had been contracted a long time ago, the kidneys must have been damaged and therefore treating the kidneys became the key factor when curing the disease. Herbs that replenish kidney essence, such as Cornu Cervi Degelatinatum and Radix Morindae Officinalis, were added to the formula to replenish *qi* and blood. Once *yang-qi* and *yin* blood both increased, the pathological conditions were relieved.

Chen XX was a young man who liked alcohol and was excessively active sexually. He exhibited renal deficiency in the lower part of the body and *qi* deficiency in the upper part, with symptoms of lassitude, unwillingness to speak, shortness of breath at the slightest exertion, weight loss, a cold sensation in the bones, night sweats and a cough with sputum. He had to wear thick clothes and a cotton-padded hat on hot summer days. However, his appetite was good, and he slept well. His shortness of breath and aversion to cold both suggested deficiencies of the lung *qi* and kidneys. *The Inner Canon of the Yellow Emperor* says, "Aversion to cold cannot be relieved by drinking hot soup, warming oneself by a fire or wearing thick clothes.... The kidneys (water) dominate the bones and produce marrow. Renal deficiency means insufficient marrow, which causes a cold sensation in the bones." It is very difficult to treat a syndrome like this which shows deficiencies of both *yin* and *yang*. Nevertheless, the patient was still young and his sleeping habits, appetite and bowel movements were all normal. All this suggested that the spleen and stomach were functioning well, which ensured a supply of essence to all *zang-fu* organs. The doctor advised the patient, "Your disease cannot be cured by medication alone. It is important to rest both your body and mind as well. The best course of action is to find a quiet place far from home where you can rest properly, and at the same time take medication to regulate *yin*, *yang*, *qi* and blood."

Following the doctor's advice, Chen left home and went to a quiet place to recuperate. An examination showed that his pulse was thready and feeble in all six positions, but especially at the *chi* position on both sides. All other symptoms remained the same. Moxibustion was then applied to *Zusanli* (ST 36), *Shenshu* (BL 23), *Guanyuan* (RN 4) and *Qihai* (RN 6). Decoction of Four Mild Drugs (91) was prescribed for replenishment along with Radix Astragali, Radix Polygalae and Fructus Lycii. The patient was told to remain sitting in the morning and afternoon and to keep his body and mind relaxed. Practising *taijiquan* was also recommended to produce harmony between *qi* and blood. The patient's doctor visited him once every three days, on order to monitor any developments in his condition.

One month later, the shortness of breath that the patient had experienced on exertion had improved greatly along with the other symptoms. Decoction for Relieving *Yin*-Deficiency Syndrome (335) was prescribed, with Fructus Tritici Levis (light) and Radix Rehmanniae Preparata added. This was taken in decocted form. Powder for Invigorating Heart-*Qi* (336) was also administered with boiled water every morning and evening. Moxibustion was discontinued.

Another month passed and the patient's physical and mental conditions both improved; his appetite was stronger and his mental state was more stable than before. The patient's cough gradually disappeared, the night sweats ceased and his muscles became much stronger but he still felt cold. This was because *yang* was still deficient, even though *yin* had already been restored, so the main task was to assist *yang*. Colla Carapax et Plastri Testudinis and Colla Cornus Cervi were added to the previous prescription.

Still another month passed before the patient began to feel vigorous. He now liked to speak and walked with firm steps. He did not feel the cold as much as he had several months before, and no longer wore thick clothes or a hat. The other symptoms had all disappeared. Then Decoction for Invigorating Spleen and Nourishing Heart (110) was prescribed, as well as Pill for Invigorating Kidney-*Qi* (182) which was taken twice a day with lightly salted water. After the fourth month, he did not feel cold any longer. Then *Zuogui* Decoction (80) and Pill for Debility were administered alternately to achieve better results.

His recovery was mainly attributed to proper rest and care, although medication also played a role.

Discussion: This was a case of consumptive disease due to deficiencies of *yin* and *yang*, and thus both were replenished in the treatment. While receiving treatment in the form of medication, the patient was told to remain cheerful, eat proper food, and do certain exercises. All this helped him recover in a short time. From this case, we can see that only when medical treatment is combined with emotional stability, a proper diet, and physical exercises can satisfactory results be achieved in dealing with consumptive diseases.

Index of Medical Formulae

(1) *Yiguan* Decoction (from *Liuzhou Medical Talks*):
Radix Adenophorae, Radix Ophiopogonis, Radix Angelicae Sinensis, Radix Rehmanniae, Fructus Lycii and Fructus Toosendan.

(2) Decoction of Asparagi and Ophiopogonis (from *Insight into Medicine*):
Radix Asparagi, Radix Ophiopogonis, Radix Trichosanthis, Radix Scutellariae, Rhizoma Anemarrhenae, Radix Glycyrrhizae, Radix Ginseng and Folium Nelumbinis.

(3) *Erchen* Decoction (from *Benevolent Prescriptions from the Pharmaceutical Bureau of Taiping Period*):
Rhizoma Pinelliae, Pericarpium Citri Reticulatae, Poria and Radix Glycyrrhizae Preparata.

(4) *Eryin* Decoction (from *A Complete Collection of Jingyue's Treatise*):
Radix Rehmanniae, Radix Ophiopogonis, Semen Ziziphi Spinosae, Radix Glycyrrhizae, Radix Scrophulariae, Poria, Rhizoma Coptidis, Caulis Aristolochiae Manshuriensis, Medulla Junci and Herba Lophatheri.

(5) Powerful Tonic Decoction of Ten Drugs (from *Benevolent Prescriptions from the Pharmaceutical Bureau of Taiping Period*):
Radix Rehmanniae Preparata, Radix Paeoniae Alba, Radix Angelicae Sinensis, Radix Chuanxiong, Radix Ginseng, Rhizoma Atractylodis Macrocephalae, Poria, Radix Glycyrrhizae Preparata, Radix Astragali and Cortex Cinnamomi.

(6) Powder of Ten Drugs' Ashes (from *Miraculous Books of Ten Effective Recipes*):
Herba seu Radix Cirsii Japanici, Herba Cirsii, Folium Nelumbinis, Cacumen Platycladi, Radix Rubiae, Fructus Gardeniae, Rhizoma Imperatae, Radix et Rhizoma Rhei, Cortex Moutan and Vagina Trachycarpi.

(7) Decoction of Jujubae (from *Treatise on Cold Diseases*):
Radix Euphorbiae Pekinensis, Flos Genkwa, Radix Kansui and Fructus Jujubae.

(8) Powder of Caryophylli for Relieving Regurgitation (from *Benevolent Prescriptions from the Pharmaceutical Bureau of Taiping Period*):
Rhizoma Atractylodis Macrocephalae, Rhizoma Cyperi, Radix Ginseng, Semen Amomi, Flos Caryophylli, Fructus Hordei Germinatus, Radix Aucklandiae, Semen Myristicae, Massa Medicata Fermentata, Radix Glycyrrhizae Preparata, Lignum Aquilariae Resinatum, Pericarpium Citri Reticulatae Viride, Cortex Magnoliae Officinalis, Herba Agastachis, Pericarpium Citri Reticulatae, Rhizoma Pinelliae and Fructus Tsaoko.

(9) Powder of Caryophylli (from *A Complete Collection of Ancient and Modern Medical Works*):
Flos Caryophylli, Calyx Kaki, Rhizoma Alpiniae Officinarum and Radix Glycyrrhizae Preparata.

(10) *Duqi* Pill of Seven Ingredients (from *Notes on Medical Works*):
Radix Rehmanniae, Fructus Corni, Rhizoma Dioscoreae, Poria, Cortex Moutan, Rhizoma Alismatis and Fructus Schisandrae.

(11) Decoction of Ginseng for Nourishing *Qi* and *Ying* (from *Benevolent Prescriptions from the Pharmaceutical Bureau of Taiping Period*):
Radix Ginseng, Radix Glycyrrhizae, Radix Angelicae Sinensis, Radix Paeoniae Alba, Radix Rehmanniae Preparata, Cortex Cinnamomi, Fructus Jujubae, Radix Astragali, Radix Atractylodis Macrocephalae, Poria, Fructus Schisandrae, Radix Polygalae, Pericarpium Citri Reticulatae and Rhizoma

Zingiberis Recens.

(12) Powder for Dispersing Heat and Promoting Urination (from *Benevolent Prescriptions from the Pharmaceutical Bureau of Taiping Period*):

Caulis Aristolochiae Manshuriensis, Semen Plantaginis, Herba Polygoni Avicularis, Herba Dianthi, Talcum, Radix Glycyrrhizae, Radix et Rhizoma Rhei, Fructus Gardeniae and Medulla Junci.

(13) Eight Precious Ingredients Decoction (from *Classification and Treatment of Traumatic Diseases*):

Radix Ginseng, Radix Atractylodis Macrocephalae, Poria, Radix Glycyrrhizae, Radix Angelicae Sinensis, Radix Paeoniae Alba, Radix Chuanxiong, Radix Rehmanniae Preparata, Rhizoma Zingiberis Recens and Fructus Jujubae.

(14) Pill for Relieving Nocturnal Emissions (from *Main Rules in Medical and Health Service*):

Radix Asparagi, Radix Rehmanniae Preparata, Radix Ginseng, Cortex Phellodendri, Fructus Amomi and Radix Glycyrrhizae.

(15) Decoction Containing Three Kinds of Seed for the Aged (from *Han's Medical Treatise*):

Fructus Perillae, Semen Sinapis Albae and Semen Raphani.

(16) Pill of Phellodendri, Atractylodis and Cyathulae (from *Orthodox Medical Record*):

Rhizoma Atractylodis, Cortex Phellodendri and Radix Cyathulae.

(17) Powder of Three Holy Ingredients (from *A Medical Text for Confucianists to Serve Family Members and Relatives*):

Pedicullus Melo, Radix Ledebouriellae and Rhizoma et Radix Veratri.

(18) Three Crude Drugs Decoction (from *Benevolent Prescriptions from the Pharmaceutical Bureau of Taiping Period*):

Herba Ephedrae, Semen Armeniacae Amarum and Radix Glycyrrhizae.

(19) Decoction for Replenishing *Qi* and Blood to Relieve Wind *Bi*-Syndrome (from *Useful Prescriptions for Women*):

Radix Rehmanniae Preparata, Radix Paeoniae Alba, Radix Angelicae Sinensis, Rhizoma Chuanxiong, Radix Ginseng, Radix Astragali, Poria, Radix Glycyrrhizae, Radix Angelicae Pubescentis, Cortex Eucommiae, Radix Achyranthis Bidentatae, Radix Dipsaci, Lignum Cinnamomi, Herba Asari, Radix Gentianae Macrophyllae, Rhizoma Zingiberis Recens and Radix Ledebouriellae.

(20) Decoction for Relieving Stagnation Syndrome (from *An Introduction to Medicine*):

Pericarpium Citri Reticulatae Viride, Pericarpium Citri Reticulatae, Radix Platycodi, Herba Agastachis, Cortex Cinnamomi, Radix Glycyrrhizae, Rhizoma Sparganii, Rhizoma Curcumae, Rhizoma Cyperi, Fructus Alpiniae Oxyphyllae, Rhizoma Zingiberis Recens and Fructus Jujubae.

(21) Decoction for Potently Invigorating *Qi* and Blood (from *A Complete Collection of Jingyue's Treatise*):

Radix Ginseng, Rhizoma Dioscoreae (stir-baked), Radix Rehmanniae Preparata, Cortex Eucommiae, Fructus Lycii, Radix Angelicae Sinensis, Fructus Corni and Radix Glycyrrhizae Preparata.

(22) Pill for Replenishing *Yin* (from *Danxi's Experience on Medicine*):

Rhizoma Anemarrhenae, Cortex Phellodendri, Radix Rehmanniae Preparata, Carapax et Plastrum Testudinis and pig's spine.

(23) Great Blue Dragon Decoction (from *Treatise on Cold Diseases*):

Herba Ephedrae, Semen Armeniacae Amarum, Ramulus Cinnamomi, Radix Glycyrrhizae, Gypsum Fibrosum, Rhizoma Zingiberis Recens and Fructus Jujubae.

(24) Bolus for Serious Endogenous Wind-Syndrome (from *Essentials of Seasonal Febrile Diseases*):

Radix Paeoniae Alba, Colla Corii Asini, Carapax et Plastrum Testudinis, Radix Rehmanniae, Fructus

Cannabis, Fructus Schisandrae, Concha Ostreae, Radix Ophiopogonis, Radix Glycyrrhizae Preparata, egg yolk and Carapax Trionycis.

(25) Decoction for Potently Warming Middle *Jiao* (from *Synopsis of Prescriptions of the Golden Chamber*):

Pericarpium Zanthoxyli, Rhizoma Zingiberis, Radix Ginseng and Saccharum Granorum.

(26) Decoction for Potent Purgation (from *Treatise on Cold Diseases*):

Radix et Rhizoma Rhei, Cortex Magnoliae Officinalis, Fructus Aurantii Immaturus and Natrii Sulfas.

(27) Decoction of Gentianae Macrophyllae (from *Basic Questions*: *Discourse on Mechanism for Preserving Life*):

Radix Gentianae Macrophyllae, Radix Angelicae Sinensis, Radix Glycyrrhizae, Rhizoma seu Radix Notopterygii, Radix Ledebouriellae, Radix Angelicae Dahuricae, Radix Rehmanniae Preparata, Poria Gypsum Fibrosum, Rhizoma Chuanxiong, Radix Paeoniae Alba, Radix Angelicae Pubescentis, Radix Scutellariae, Radix Rehmanniae, Radix Atractylodis Macrocephalae and Herba Asari.

(28) Decoction of Bupleuri for Regulating *Shaoyang* and *Yangming* Meridians (from *Treatise on Cold Diseases*):

Radix Bupleuri, Radix Scutellariae, Rhizoma Pinelliae, Fructus Aurantii Immaturus, Radix Paeoniae Alba. Radix et Rhizoma Rhei, Rhizoma Zingiberis Recens and Fructus Jujubae.

(29) Powder of Chuanxiong with Folium Camelliae Sinensis (from *Benevolent Prescriptions from the Pharmaceutical Bureau of Taiping Period*):

Rhizoma Chuanxiong, Herba Schizonepetae, Herba Menthae, Rhizoma seu Radix Notopterygii, Herba Asari or Rhizoma Cyperi, Radix Angelicae Dahuricae, Radix Glycyrrhizae and Radix Ledebouriellae.

(30) Decoction of Phragmitis (from *Essentially Treasured Prescriptions for Emergencies*):

Rhizoma Phragmitis (fresh), Semen Coicis, Semen Benincasae and Semen Persicae.

(31) Pill of Stephaniae Tetrandrae, Zanthoxyli, Lepidii seu Descurainiae and Rhei (from *Synopsis of Prescriptions of the Golden Chamber*):

Radix Stephaniae Tetrandrae, Pericarpium Zanthoxyli, Semen Lepidii seu Descurainiae and Radix et Rhizoma Rhei.

(32) Small Dose of Pinelliae Decoction (from *Synopsis of Prescriptions of the Golden Chamber*):
Rhizoma Pinelliae and Rhizoma Zingiberis Recens.

(33) Small Blue Dragon Decoction (from *Treatise on Cold Diseases*):

Herba Ephedrae, Ramulus Cinnamomi, Radix Paeoniae Alba, Radix Glycyrrhizae, Rhizoma Zingiberis, Herba Asari, Rhizoma Pinelliae and Fructus Schisandrae.

(34) Decoction for Mildly Warming Middle *Jiao* (from *Treatise on Cold Diseases*):

Ramulus Cinnamomi, Radix Paeoniae Alba, Radix Glycyrrhizae, Rhizoma Zingiberis Recens, Fructus Jujubae and Saccharum Granorum.

(35) Decoction for Mild Purgation (from *Treatise on Cold Diseases*):

Radix et Rhizoma Rhei, Cortex Magnoliae Officinalis and Fructus Aurantii Immaturus.

(36) Decoction of Bupleuri for Regulating *Shaoyang* Meridians (from *Treatise on Cold Diseases*):

Radix Bupleuri, Radix Scutellariae, Rhizoma Pinelliae, Radix Ginseng, Radix Glycyrrhizae, Rhizoma Zingiberis Recens and Fructus Jujubae.

(37) Decoction for Mild Phlegm-Heat Syndrome in the Chest (from *Treatise on Cold Diseases*):
Rhizoma Coptidis, Rhizoma Pinelliae and Fructus Trichosanthis.

(38) Decoction of Cirsii (from *Prescriptions for Life Saving*):

Radix Rehmanniae, Herba Cirsii, Talcum, Medulla Tetrapanacis, Pollen Typhae (stir-baked), Herba

Lophatheri, Nodus Nelumbinis Rhizomatis, Radix Angelicae Sinensis, Fructus Gardeniae and Radix Glycyrrhizae.

(39) King of Heaven Tonic Pill for Mental Discomfort (from *Secret Recipes for Longevity*):

Radix Ginseng, Radix Scrophulariae, Radix Salviae Miltiorrhizae, Poria, Fructus Schisandrae, Radix Polygalae, Radix Platycodi, Radix Angelicae Sinensis, Radix Asparagi, Radix Ophiopogonis, Semen Platycladi, Semen Ziziphi Spinosae, Radix Rehmanniae and Cinnabaris.

(40) Decoction of Gastrodiae and Uncariae cum Uncis (from *New Concept for Diagnosis and Treatment of Miscellaneous Diseases*):

Rhizoma Gastrodiae, Ramulus Uncariae cum Uncis, Concha Haliotidis, Radix Cyathulae, Herba Taxilli, Cortex Eucommiae, Fructus Gardeniae, Radix Scutellariae, Herba Leonuri, Lignum Pini Poriaferum (cinnabaris coated) and Caulis Polygoni Multiflori.

(41) Pill of Dioscoreae for Nourishing Kidney (from *Benevolent Prescriptions from the Pharmaceutical Bureau of Taiping Period*):

Rhizoma Dioscoreae, Herba Cistanches, Radix Rehmanniae Preparata, Fructus Corni, Lignum Pini Poriaferum, Semen Cuscutae, Fructus Schisandrae, Halloysitum Rubrum, Radix Morindae Officinalis, Rhizoma Alismatis, Cortex Eucommiae and Radix Achyranthis Bidentatae.

(42) Powder for Treating Food-Refusal Dysentery (from *Insight into Medicine*):

Radix Ginseng, Rhizoma Coptidis, Rhizoma Acori Tatarinowii, Radix Salviae Miltiorrhizae, Semen Caesalpiniae Minacis, Poria, Pericarpium Citri Reticulatae, Semen Benincasae, Fructus Oryzae Sativae and Petiolus Nelumbinis.

(43) Decoction of Cocculi Trilobi (from *Synopsis of Prescriptions of the Golden Chamber*):

Caulis Cocculi Trilobi, Gypsum Fibrosum, Ramulus Cinnamomi and Radix Ginseng.

(44) Powder of Aucklandiae for Promoting Smooth Circulation of *Qi* (from *Shen's Treatise on the Importance of Life Preservation*):

Radix Aucklandiae, Pericarpium Citri Reticulatae Viride, Pericarpium Citri Reticulatae, Radix Glycyrrhizae, Fructus Aurantii, Cortex Magnoliae Officinalis, Radix Linderae, Rhizoma Cyperi, Rhizoma Atractylodis, Fructus Amomi, Lignum Cinnamomi and Rhizoma Chuanxiong.

(45) Powder for Relieving Cough (from *Insight into Medicine*):

Herba Schizonepetae, Radix Platycodi, Radix Glycyrrhizae, Rhizoma Cynanchi Stauntonii, Pericarpium Citri Reticulatae, Radix Stemonae and Radix Asteris.

(46) Pill for Relieving Epigastric Fullness (from *Secret Records of the Cabinet of Orchids*):

Cortex Magnoliae Officinalis, Fructus Aurantii Immaturus, Rhizoma Coptidis, Radix Scutellariae, Rhizoma Anemarrhenae, Rhizoma Pinelliae, Pericarpium Citri Reticulatae, Poria, Polyporus, Rhizoma Alismatis, Fructus Amomi, Rhizoma Zingiberis, Rhizoma Curcumae Longae, Radix Ginseng, Rhizoma Atractylodis Macrocephalae and Radix Glycyrrhizae Preparata.

(47) Pill of Five Kinds of Seed for Reproduction (from *Danxi's Experience on Medicine*):

Fructus Lycii, Fructus Rubi, Semen Cuscutae, Fructus Schisandrae and Semen Plantaginis.

(48) Pill of Five Kinds of Seed (from *Effective Prescriptions from Physicians of Successive Generations*):

Semen Persicae, Semen Armeniacae Amarum, Semen Platycladi, Semen Pini, Semen Pruni and Pericarpium Citri Reticulatae (fresh).

(49) Decoction of Five Kinds of Juice for Relieving Dysphagia (from proved formula):

Succus Allii Tuberosi Herbae, Lactis Bovis, Succus Zingiberis Recens, Succus Pyri and Succus Nelumbinis Rhizomatis.

(50) Decoction Containing Five Kinds of Peel (from *The Treasured Classics*):

Cortex Mori, Pericarpium Citri Reticulatae, Rhizoma Zingiberis Recens, Pericarpium Arecae and

Poria.

(51) Powder of Five Drugs Containing Poria (from *Treatise on Cold Diseases*):

Ramulus Cinnamomi, Rhizoma Atractylodis Macrocephalae, Poria, Polyporus and Rhizoma Alismatis.

(52) Decoction of Five Ingredients for Detoxification (from *Golden Mirror of Orthodox Medical Lineage*):

Flos Lonicerae, Flos Chrysanthemi, Herba Taraxaci, Herba Violae and Herba Begoniae Fimbristipulatae.

(53) Decoction for Lifting *Yang* and Benefiting Stomach (from *Comments on the Spleen and Stomach*):

Radix Astragali, Rhizoma Pinelliae, Radix Ginseng, Radix Angelicae Pubescentis, Radix Ledebouriellae, Radix Paeoniae Alba, Rhizoma seu Radix Notopterygii, Pericarpium Citri Reticulatae (fresh), Poria, Radix Bupleuri, Rhizoma Alismatis, Rhizoma Atractylodis Macrocephalae, Rhizoma Coptidis, Radix Glycyrrhizae Preparata, Rhizoma Zingiberis Recens and Fructus Jujubae.

(54) Six-to-One Powder (from *Principles on Classification and Differentiation of Cold Diseases*):

Talcum and Radix Glycyrrhizae.

(55) Decoction of Six Mild Drugs (from *Orthodox Medical Record*):

Radix Ginseng, Radix Glycyrrhizae Preparata, Poria, Rhizoma Atractylodis Macrocephalae, Pericarpium Citri Reticulatae and Rhizoma Pinelliae Preparata.

(56) Pill of Six Drugs Containing Rehmanniae Preparata (from *Medical Elucidation of Pediatrics*):

Radix Rehmanniae Preparata, Rhizoma Dioscoreae, Poria, Cortex Moutan, Rhizoma Alismatis and Fructus Corni.

(57) Decoction of Six Ground Ingredients (from *Standard for Diagnosis and Treatment*):

Lignum Aquilariae Resinatum, Radix Aucklandiae, Semen Arecae, Radix Linderae, Fructus Aurantii Immaturus and Radix et Rhizoma Rhei.

(58) Pill for Killing Parasites (from *Variorum of Prescriptions*):

Semen Arecae, Fructus Carpesii, Radix Meliae, Alumen Exsiccatum, Pulvis Minium (stir-baked), Fructus Quisqualis and Fructus Ulmi.

(59) Decoction for Clearing Liver-Heat (from *A Complete Collection of Jingyue's Treatise*):

Pericarpium Citri Reticulatae Viride, Pericarpium Citri Reticulatae, Radix Paeoniae Alba, Cortex Moutan, Fructus Gardeniae, Rhizoma Alismatis and Bulbus Cirrhosae.

(60) Pill for Relieving Masses (from *Diagnosis and Treatment of Classified Syndromes*):

Rhizoma Sparganii, Rhizoma Curcumae, Resina Ferulae, Pamex, Rhizoma Cyperi, Realgar, Semen Arecae, Lignum Sappan, Concha Arcae and Faeces Trogopterori.

(61) Moon Brilliance Pill (from *Insight into Medicine*):

Radix Asparagi, Radix Ophiopogonis, Radix Rehmanniae, Radix Rehmanniae Preparata, Rhizoma Dioscoreae, Radix Stemonae, Radix Adenophorae, Bulbus Fritillariae Cirrhosae, Poria, Colla Corii Asini, Radix Notoginseng, Jecur Lutrae, Flos Chrysanthemi and Folium Mori.

(62) Decoction of Salviae Miltiorrhizae (from *Golden Mirror of Orthodox Medical Lineage*):

Radix Salviae Miltiorrhizae, Lignum Santali Albi and Fructus Amomi.

(63) *Xiaoyao* Powder with Moutan and Gardeniae (from *General Medicine*):

Radix Angelicae Sinensis, Radix Paeoniae Alba, Rhizoma Atractylodis Macrocephalae, Radix Bupleuri, Poria, Radix Glycyrrhizae, Rhizoma Zingiberis (roasted), Herba Menthae, Cortex Moutan and Fructus Gardeniae.

(64) Decoction of Aconiti Preparata (from *Synopsis of Prescriptions of the Golden Chamber*):

Radix Aconiti Preparata, Herba Ephedrae, Radix Paeoniae, Radix Astragali and Radix Glycyrrhizae.

(65) Pill of Aconiti Preparata and Halloysitum Rubrum (from *Synopsis of Prescriptions of the Golden Chamber*):

Pericarpium Zanthoxyli, Rhizoma Aconiti Preparata, Radix Aconiti Lateralis Preparata, Rhizoma Zingiberis and Halloysitum Rubrum.

(66) Bolus of Mume (from *Treatise on Cold Diseases*):

Fructus Mume, Rhizoma Coptidis, Cortex Phellodendri, Radix Ginseng, Radix Angelicae Sinensis, Radix Aconiti Lateralis Preparata, Ramulus Cinnamomi, Pericarpium Zanthoxyli, Rhizoma Zingiberis and Herba Asari.

(67) Bolus of Calculus Bovis for Clearing Heart-Heat (from *Experience on Treating Eruptive Diseases in Successive Generations*):

Rhizoma Coptidis, Radix Scutellariae, Fructus Gardeniae, Radix Curcumae, Calculus Bovis and Cinnabaris.

(68) Decoction for Removing Blood Stasis in the Lower Abdomen (from *Correction of Medical Classics*):

Fructus Foeniculi, Rhizoma Zingiberis, Rhizoma Corydalis, Myrrha, Rhizoma Chuanxiong, Cortex Cinnamomi, Radix Paeoniae Rubra, Pollen Typhae and Faeces Trogopterori.

(69) Plaster of Polygoni Orientalis (from *A Complete Collection of Jingyue's Treatise*):

Fructus Polygoni Orientalis, Radix et Rhizoma Rhei, Natrii Sulfas, Fructus Persicae, lime and distiller's yeast.

(70) Pill Containing Two Drugs (from *Standard for Diagnosis and Treatment*):

Fructus Rosae Laevigatae and Semen Euryales.

(71) Jade Maid Decoction (from *A Complete Collection of Jingyue's Treatise*):

Gypsum Fibrosum, Radix Rehmanniae Preparata, Radix Ophiopogonis, Rhizoma Anemarrhenae and Radix Achyranthis Bidentatae.

(72) *Yushu* Pill (from *Hundred and One Selected Prescriptions*):

Pseudobulbus Cremastrae Pleiones, Semen Euphorbiae Lathyridis, Radix Euphobriae Pekinensis, Moschus, Realgar, Cinnabaris and Galla Chinensis.

(73) Jade Screen Powder (from *Effective Prescriptions from Physicians of Successive Generations*):

Radix Astragali, Rhizoma Atractylodis Macrocephalae and Radix Ledebouriellae.

(74) Fragrant Powder for Strengthening Anti-Pathogenic *Qi* (from *Standard for Diagnosis and Treatment*):

Radix Linderae, Rhizoma Cyperi, Rhizoma Zingiberis, Fructus Perillae and Pericarpium Citri Reticulatae.

(75) Powder for Restoring Anti-Pathogenic *Qi* (from proved formula):

Cortex Magnolicae Officinalis, Rhizoma Atractylodis, Pericarpium Citri Reticulatae, Radix Glycyrrhizae, Herba Agastaches, Herba Eupatorii, Fructus Tsaoko, Rhizoma Pinelliae, Semen Arecae, Rhizoma Acori Tatarinowii and Folium Nelumbinis.

(76) Powder of Pyrrosiae (from *A Supplement to Diagnosis and Treatment*):

Folium Pyrrosiae, Fructus Malvae, Herba Dianthi, Talcum and Semen Plantaginis.

(77) *Longhu* Pill (from proved formula):

Calculus Bovis, Fructus Crotonis Degelatinatum, Cinnabaris and Arsenicum.

(78) Decoction of Gentianae for Purging Liver-Fire (from *Secret Records of the Cabinet of Orchids*):

Radix Gentianae, Rhizoma Alismatis, Caulis Aristolochiae Manshuriensis, Semen Plantaginis, Radix Angelicae Sinensis, Radix Bupleuri and Radix Rehmanniae, (Radix Scutellariae and Fructus Gardeniae are included in modern formula).

(79) *Zuogui* Pill (from *A Complete Collection of Jingyue's Treatise*):

Radix Rehmanniae Preparata, Rhizoma Dioscoreae, Fructus Corni, Semen Cuscutae, Fructus Lycii, Radix Cyathulae, Colla Cornus Cervi and Colla Carapax et Plastrum Testudinis.

(80) *Zuogui* Decoction (from *A Complete Collection of Jingyue's Treatise*):

Radix Rehmanniae Preparata, Fructus Corni, Fructus Lycii, Rhizoma Dioscoreae, Poria and Radix Glycyrrhizae Preparata.

(81) *Zuojin* Pill (from *Danxi's Experience on Medicine*):

Rhizoma Coptidis and Fructus Evodiae.

(82) *Yougui* Pill (from *A Complete Collection of Jingyue's Treatise*):

Radix Rehmanniae Preparata, Rhizoma Dioscoreae, Fructus Corni, Fructus Lycii, Cortex Eucommiae, Semen Cuscutae, Radix Aconiti Lateralis Preparata, Cortex Cinnamomi, Radix Angelicae Sinensis and Colla Cornus Cervi.

(83) *Yougui* Decoction (from *A Complete Collection of Jingyue's Treatise*):

Radix Rehmanniae Preparata, Fructus Corni, Fructus Lycii, Rhizoma Dioscoreae, Cortex Eucommiae, Cortex Cinnamomi, Radix Aconiti Lateralis Preparata and Radix Glycyrrhizae.

(84) Decoction of Glycyrrhizae, Tritici Levis and Jujubae (from *Synopsis of Prescriptions of the Golden Chamber*):

Radix Glycyrrhizae, Fructus Triticilevis and Fructus Jujubae.

(85) Decoction of Glycyrrhizae, Zingiberis, Poria, and Atractylodis Macrocephalae (from *Synopsis of Prescriptions of the Golden Chamber*):

Radix Glycyrrhizae, Rhizoma Zingiberis, Poria and Rhizoma Atractylodis Macrocephalae.

(86) Decoction of Kansui and Pinelliae (from *Synopsis of Prescriptions of the Golden Chamber*):

Radix Kansui, Rhizoma Pinelliae, Radix Paeoniae and Radix Glycyrrhizae.

(87) Decoction for Various Kinds of Malaria (from *A Complete Collection of Jingyue's Treatise*):

Radix Ginseng, Rhizoma Atractylodis Macrocephalae, Poria, Radix Glycyrrhizae Preparata, Pericarpium Citri Reticulatae, Rhizoma Pinelliae Preparata, Fructus Tsaoko, Fructus Mume, Rhizoma Zingiberis Recens and Fructus Jujubae.

(88) Decoction of Magnoliae Officinalis and Pinelliae (from *Benevolent Prescriptions from the Pharmaceutical Bureau of Taiping Period*):

Folium Perillae, Rhizoma Pinelliae Preparata, Cortex Magnolicae Officinalis, Poria, Rhizoma Zingiberis Recens and Fructus Jujubae.

(89) Pill of Four Wonderful Ingredients (from *Practical Set Prescriptions for Studying*):

Rhizoma Atractylodis, Cortex Phellodendri, Radix Achyranthis Bidentatae and Semen Coicis.

(90) Decoction for Treating *Yang* Exhaustion (from *Treatise on Cold Diseases*):

Radix Aconiti Lateralis Preparata, Rhizoma Zingiberis and Radix Glycyrrhizae.

(91) Decoction of Four Mild Drugs (from *Benevolent Prescriptions from the Pharmaceutical Bureau of Taiping Period*):

Radix Codonopsis, Rhizoma Atractylodis Macrocephalae, Poria and Radix Glycyrrhizae.

(92) Decoction of Four Ingredients for Recapturing *Yang* (from *A Complete Collection of Jingyue's Treatise*):

Radix Ginseng, Radix Aconiti Lateralis Preparata, Rhizoma Zingiberis (baked) and Radix Glycyrrhizae Preparata.

(93) Four Drugs Decoction (from *Benevolent Prescriptions from the Pharmaceutical Bureau of*

Taiping Period):

Radix Angelicae Sinensis, Radix Paeoniae Alba, Rhizoma Chuanxiong and Radix Rehmanniae Preparata.

(94) Pill of Four Miraculous Drugs (from *Standard for Diagnosis and Treatment*):

Fructus Psoraleae, Semen Myristicae, Fructus Evodiae, Fructus Schisandrae, Rhizoma Zingiberis Recens and Fructus Jujubae.

(95) Pill of Marine Drugs for Relieving Goiter (from *A Complete Collection for Treating Sores*):

Concha Meretricis seu Cyclinae, Thallus Laminariae, Sargassum, Os Sepiae, Thallus Eckloniae, Pericarpium Citri Reticulatae and Radix Aristolochiae.

(96) Powder for Restoring Pulse (from *Essentially Treasured Prescriptions for Emergencies*):

Radix Ginseng, Radix Ophiopogonis and Fructus Schisandrae.

(97) Decoction of Iron Scale (from *Insight into Medicine*):

Radix Asparagi, Radix Ophiopogonis, Bulbus Cirrhosae, Arisaema cum Bile, Exocarpium Citri Rubrum, Radix Polygalae, Rhizoma Acori Tatarinowii, Fructus Forsythiae, Poria, Lignum Pini Poriaferum, Radix Scrophulariae, Ramulus Uncariae cum Uncis, Radix Salviae Miltiorrhizae, Cinnabaris and Iron Scale.

(98) Powder for Dissipating Blood Stasis (from *Benevolent Prescriptions from the Pharmaceutical Bureau of Taiping Period*):

Faeces Trogopterori and Pollen Typhae.

(99) *Daididang* Pill (from *Standard for Diagnosis and Treatment*):

Radix et Rhizoma Rhei, Radix Angelicae Sinensis, Radix Rehmanniae, Squama Manitis, Natrii Sulfas, Semen Persicae and Cortex Cinnamomi.

(100) Decoction of Pulsatillae (from *Treatise on Cold Diseases*):

Radix Pulsatillae, Cortex Fraxini, Rhizoma Coptidis and Cortex Phellodendri.

(101) Extractum of Anas Domesticus (from *Miraculous Books of Ten Effective Recipes*):

Anas Domesticus, Fructus Jujubae, Radix Ginseng, Poria, Rhizoma Atractylodis, Cortex Magnoliae Officinalis, Pericarpium Citri Reticulatae, Rhizoma Zingiberis, all cooked in old wine.

(102) Pill of Alumen and Curcumae (from proved formula):

Alumen and Radix Curcumae.

(103) White Tiger Decoction with Ginseng (from *Treatise on Febrile Diseases*):

Rhizoma Anemarrhenae, Gypsum Fibrosum, Radix Glycyrrhizae, Fructus Oryzae Sativae and Radix Ginseng.

(104) White Tiger Decoction with Cinnamomi (from *Synopsis of Prescriptions of the Golden Chamber*):

Rhizoma Anemarrhenae, Gypsum Fibrosum, Radix Glycyrrhizae, Fructus Oryzae Sativae and Ramulus Cinnamomi.

(105) Semen Sinapis Albae Cake (from *Zhang's Medical Treatise*):

Pound 30 grams of Semen Sinapis Albae, 30 grams of Rhizoma Corydalis, 15 grams of Herba Asari into powder, then mix the powder with 1.5 grams of Moschus and ginger juice. Apply the mixture externally to such acupuncture points as *Feishu* (BL 13), *Gaohuang* (BL 43), and *Bailao* (Extra) during hot summer days. Numbness and pain may soon appear in these places. Do not remove the drug until three pieces of incense are burned up. Go through the same procedure after ten days. The disease will be cured after three courses of treatment.

(106) Decoction of Pinelliae, Atractylodis Macrocephalae and Gastrodiae (from *Insight into Medicine*):

Rhizoma Pinelliae, Rhizoma Atractylodis Macrocephalae, Rhizoma Gastrodiae, Pericarpium Citri

Reticulatae, Poria, Radix Glycyrrhizae, Rhizoma Zingiberis Recens and Fructus Jujubae.

(107) Decoction of Pinelliae and Magnoliae Officinalis (from *Synopsis of Prescriptions of the Golden Chamber*):

Rhizoma Pinelliae, Cortex Magnolicae Officinalis, Folium Perillae, Poria and Rhizoma Zingiberis Recens.

(108) Decoction of Pinelliae and Panicum (from *The Inner Canon of the Yellow Emperor*):

Rhizoma Pinelliae and Semen Panicum.

(109) Pill of Pinelliae and Sulfur (from *Benevolent Prescriptions from the Pharmaceutical Bureau of Taiping Period*):

Rhizoma Pinelliae and Sulfur.

(110) Decoction for Invigorating Spleen and Nourishing Heart (from *Prescriptions for Life Saving*):

Radix Codonopsis, Radix Astragali, Rhizoma Atractylodis Macrocephalae, Lignum Pini Poriaferum, Semen Ziziphi Spinosae, Arillus Longan, Radix Aucklandiae, Radix Glycyrrhizae Preparata, Radix Angelicae Sinensis, Radix Polygalae, Rhizoma Zingiberis Recens and Fructus Jujubae.

(111) Powder of Phellodendri and Atractylodis with Additional Drugs (from *Danxi's Experience on Medicine*):

Cortex Phellodendri, Rhizoma Atractylodis, Radix Angelicae Sinensis, Radix Achyranthis Bidentatae, Radix Stephaniae Tetrandrae, Rhizoma Dioscoreae Septemlobae and Carapax et Plastrum Testudinis.

(112) Four Drugs Decoction with Additional Drugs (from *Supplement to Synopsis of Prescriptions of the Golden Chamber*):

Radix Paeoniae Alba, Radix Angelicae Sinensis, Radix Rehmanniae, Rhizoma Chuanxiong, Fructus Viticis, Flos Chrysanthemi, Radix Scutellariae and Radix Glycyrrhizae.

(113) Decoction for Purgation with Modification (from proved formula):

Radix et Rhizoma Rhei, Natrii Sulfas Exsiccatus, Fructus Aurantii Immaturus, Lapis Chloriti Usta, Spina Gleditsiae, pig's bile, vinegar.

(114) Modified Decoction of Polygonati Odorati (from *Popular Treatise on Cold Diseases*):

Rhizoma Polygonati Odorati, Bulbus Allii Fistulosi, Radix Platycodi, Radix Cynanchi Atrati, Semen Sojae Preparatum, Herba Menthae, Radix Glycyrrhizae Preparata and Fructus Jujubae.

(115) Gemma Agrimoniae (from proved formula):

For adults, 50 grams of Gemma Agrimoniae Powder should be taken with warm water on an empty stomach early in the morning; for children, 25-35 grams should be taken accordingly. Since the herb has purgative effect, other purgatives are not necessary.

(116) Decoction of Lilii for Strengthening Lungs (from *Variorum of Prescriptions*):

Radix Rehmanniae, Radix Rehmanniae Preparata, Radix Ophiopogonis, Bulbus Fritillariae Cirrhosae, Bulbus Lilii, Radix Angelicae Sinensis, Radix Paeoniae (stir-baked), Radix Glycyrrhizae, Radix Scrophulariae and Radix Platycodi.

(117) Decoction of Stemonae (from proved formula):

Cut 30 grams of Radix Stemonae into small bits, then cook them in 200 ml of water for half an hour until 30 ml of medicinal broth is made. This is used for retention enema before sleep. One course of treatment lasts 10-12 days. The above dosage is for children. For adults, double the dosage.

(118) Decoction of Rehmanniae (from *Expounding Prescriptions*):

Radix Rehmanniae, Radix Morindae Officinalis, Fructus Corni, Herba Dendrobii, Herba Cistanches, Fructus Schisandrae, Cortex Cinnamomi, Poria, Radix Ophiopogonis, Radix Aconiti Lateralis Preparata, Rhizoma Acori Tatarinowii, Radix Polygalae, Rhizoma Zingiberis Recens, Fructus Jujubae and Herba

Menthae.

(119) Powder of Sanguisorbae (from proved formula):

Radix Sanguisorbae, Radix Rubiae, Radix Scutellariae, Rhizoma Coptidis, Fructus Gardeniae and Poria.

(120) Decoction of Chuanxiong, Angelicae Dahuricae, and Gypsum Fibrosum (from *Golden Mirror of Orthodox Medical Lineage*):

Rhizoma Chuanxiong, Radix Angelicae Dahuricae, Gypsum Fibrosum, Flos Chrysanthemi, Radix Ligustici and Rhizoma seu Radix Notopterygii.

(121) Decoction of Paeoniae (from *Basic Questions: Discourse on Mechanism for Preserving Life*):

Radix Scutellariae, Radix Paeoniae, Radix Glycyrrhizae Preparata, Rhizoma Coptidis, Radix et Rhizoma Rhei, Semen Arecae, Radix Angelicae Sinensis, Radix Aucklandiae and Cortex Cinnamomi.

(122) Decoction of Paeoniae Alba and Glycyrrhizae (from *Treatise on Cold Diseases*):

Radix Paeoniae Alba and Radix Glycyrrhizae Preparata.

(123) *Zuoci* Pill for Relieving Deafness (from *Medical Elucidation of Pediatrics*):

Radix Rehmanniae Preparata, Fructus Corni, Rhizoma Dioscoreae, Cortex Moutan, Poria, Rhizoma Alismatis, Fructus Schisandrae and Magnetitum.

(124) Pill of Precious Drugs (from *Benevolent Prescriptions from the Pharmaceutical Bureau of Taiping Period*):

Cinnabaris, Moschus, Benzoinum, gold and silver foil, Cornu Rhinocerotis, Calculus Bovis, Succinum, Realgar, Carapax Eretmochelydis and Borneolum Syntheticum.

(125) Goat Liver Pill (from *Leiyuan Prescriptions*):

Faeces Vespertilionis, Periostracum Cicadae, Herba Equiseti Hiemalis, Radix Angelicae Sinensis and Goat liver.

(126) Pill of Coptidis and Cinnamomi (from *Han's Medical Treatise*):

Rhizoma Coptidis and Cortex Cinnamomi.

(127) Bolus of Calculus Bovis for Resurrection (from *Essentials of Seasonal Febrile Diseases*):

Calculus Bovis, Radix Curcumae, Cornu Rhinocerotis, Rhizoma Coptidis, Cinnabaris, Borneolum Syntheticum, Margarita, Fructus Gardeniae, Realgar, Radix Scutellariae, Moschus and gold foil.

(128) Pill for Tranquilizing (from *Insight into Medicine*):

Poria, Lignum Pini Poriaferum, Radix Polygalae, Radix Ginseng, Rhizoma Acori Tatarinowii and Dens Draconis.

(129) Decoction of Angelicae Sinensis and Six Ingredients (from *Secret Records of the Cabinet of Orchids*):

Radix Angelicae Sinensis, Radix Rehmanniae, Radix Rehmanniae Preparata, Rhizoma Coptidis, Radix Scutellariae, Cortex Phellodendri and Radix Astragali.

(130) Pill of Angelicae Sinensis, Gentianae and Aloe (from *Expounding Prescriptions*):

Radix Angelicae Sinensis, Radix Gentianae, Fructus Gardeniae, Rhizoma Coptidis, Radix Scutellariae, Cortex Phellodendri, Radix et Rhizoma Rhei, Indigo Naturalis, Aloe, Radix Aucklandiae and Moschus.

(131) Decoction of Angelicae Sinensis for Enriching Blood (from *Differentiation of Endogenous and Exogenous Diseases*):

Radix Astragali and Radix Angelicae Sinensis.

(132) Decoction of Lophatheri and Gypsum Fibrosum (from *Treatise on Cold Diseases*):

Herba Lophatheri, Gypsum Fibrosum, Radix Ophiopogonis, Radix Ginseng, Rhizoma Pinelliae, Fructus Oryzae Sativae and Radix Glycyrrhizae Preparata.

(133) Pill of Succus Bambusae for Eliminating Phlegm (from *A Reference of the Ancient and Modern Medicine*):

Lapis Chloriti Usta, Lignum Aquilariae Resinatum, Radix et Rhizoma Rhei, Radix Scutellariae, Succus Bambusae, Rhizoma Pinelliae, Exocarpium Citri Rubrum, Radix Glycyrrhizae, Succus Zingiberis, Poria and Radix Ginseng.

(134) Pill of Cinnabaris for Tranquilizing (from *Invention of Medicine*):

Rhizoma Coptidis, Cinnabaris, Radix Rehmanniae, Radix Angelicae Sinensis and Radix Glycyrrhizae Preparata.

(135) Decoction for Removing Blood Stasis in the Chest (from *Correction of Medical Classics*):

Radix Angelicae Sinensis, Radix Rehmanniae, Semen Persicae, Flos Carthami, Fructus Aurantii, Radix Paeoniae Rubra, Radix Bupleuri, Radix Glycyrrhizae, Radix Platycodi, Rhizoma Chuanxiong and Radix Achyranthis Bidentatae.

(136) *Zhouju* Pill (from *A Complete Collection of Jingyue's Treatise*):

Radix Kansui, Flos Genkwa, Radix Euphorbiae Pekinensis, Radix et Rhizoma Rhei, Semen Pharbitidis, Radix Aucklandiae, Pericarpium Citri Reticulatae Viride, Pericarpium Citri Reticulatae, Calomelas and Semen Arecae.

(137) Pill of Cistanches (from *Standard for Diagnosis and Treatment*):

Herba Cistanches, Semen Cuscutae, Fructus Corni, Poria, Radix Ginseng, Cortex Cinnamomi, Radix Ledebouriellae, Radix Rehmanniae Preparata, Radix Astragali, Radix Aconiti Lateralis Preparata, Rhizoma seu Radix Notopterygii, Rhizoma Alismatis and goat's kidney.

(138) Decoction for Eliminating Phlegm (from *Prescriptions for Life Saving*):

Rhizoma Pinelliae, Pericarpium Citri Reticulatae, Fructus Aurantii Immaturus, Poria, Radix Glycyrrhizae and Rhizoma Arisaematis Preparata.

(139) Decoction of Ledebouriellae (from *Expounding Prescriptions*):

Radix Ledebouriellae, Radix Angelicae Sinensis, Poria, Semen Armeniacae Amarum, Radix Scutellariae, Radix Gentianae Macrophyllae, Radix Puerariae, Herba Ephedrae, Cortex Cinnamomi, Rhizoma Zingiberis Recens, Radix Glycyrrhizae and Fructus Jujubae.

(140) Decoction of Ophiopogonis (from *Synopsis of Prescriptions of the Golden Chamber*):

Radix Ophiopogonis, Radix Ginseng, Rhizoma Pinelliae, Radix Glycyrrhizae, Fructus Oryzae Sativae and Fructus Jujubae.

(141) Pill of Ophiopogonis, Schisandrae and Rehmanniae Preparata (from *Comprehensive Medical Collections*):

Radix Rehmanniae Preparata, Fructus Corni, Rhizoma Dioscoreae, Cortex Moutan, Rhizoma Alismatis, Poria, Radix Ophiopogonis and Fructus Schisandrae.

(142) Decoction of Perillae for Keeping *Qi* Downward (from *Benevolent Prescriptions from the Pharmaceutical Bureau of Taiping Period*):

Fructus Perillae, Pericarpium Citri Reticulatae, Rhizoma Pinelliae, Radix Angelicae Sinensis, Radix Peucedani, Cortex Magnoliae Officinalis, Cortex Cinnamomi, Radix Glycyrrhizae and Rhizoma Zingiberis Recens.

(143) Bolus of Styrax (from *Benevolent Prescriptions from the Pharmaceutical Bureau of Taiping Period*):

Rhizoma Atractylodis Macrocephalae, Radix Aristolochiae, Cornu Rhinocerotis, Rhizoma Cyperi, Cinnabaris, Fructus Chebulae, Lignum Santali Albi, Benzoinum, Lignum Aquilariae Resinatum, Moschus, Flos Caryophylli, Fructus Piperis Longi, Oleum Styrax, Olibanum and Borneolum Syntheticum.

(144) Bolus of Lycii, Chrysanthemi and Rehmanniae Preparata (from *Comprehensive Medical Collections*):

Fructus Lycii, Flos Chrysanthemi, Radix Rehmanniae Preparata, Fructus Corni, Rhizoma Dioscoreae, Rhizoma Alismatis, Cortex Moutan and Poria.

(145) Powder of Armeniacae Amarum and Perillae (from *Essentials of Seasonal Febrile Diseases*):

Semen Armeniacae Amarum, Folium Perillae, Pericarpium Citri Reticulatae, Rhizoma Pinelliae, Rhizoma Zingiberis Recens, Fructus Aurantii, Radix Peucedani, Radix Platycodi, Poria, Radix Glycyrrhizae and Fructus Jujubae.

(146) *Gengyi* Pill (from *Extensive Notes on Medicine*):

Aloe and Cinnabaris.

(147) Decoction of Coptidis for Regulating Middle *Jiao* (from *Zhang's Medical Treatise*):

Radix Ginseng, Rhizoma Atractylodis Macrocephalae, Rhizoma Zingiberis, Radix Glycyrrhizae Preparata, Rhizoma Coptidis and Poria.

(148) Decoction of Evodiae (from *Treatise on Cold Diseases*):

Fructus Evodiae, Radix Ginseng, Rhizoma Zingiberis Recens and Fructus Jujubae.

(149) Powder of Lignum Aquilariae Resinatum (from *Supplement to Synopsis of Prescriptions of the Golden Chamber*):

Lignum Aquilariae Resinatum, Folium Pyrrosiae, Talcum, Radix Angelicae Sinensis, Pericarpium Citri Reticulatae, Radix Paeoniae Alba, Fructus Malvae, Radix Glycyrrhizae and Semen Vaccariae.

(150) Decoction of Adenophorae and Ophiopogonis (from *Essentials of Seasonal Febrile Diseases*):

Radix Adenophorae, Radix Ophiopogonis, Rhizoma Polygonati Odorati, Folium Mori, Radix Glycyrrhizae, Radix Trichosanthis and Semen Lablab Album.

(151) Pill of Alpiniae Officinarum and Cyperi (from *A Collection of Effective Prescriptions*):

Rhizoma Alpiniae Officinarum and Rhizoma Cyperi.

(152) Powder for Easing Diaphragm (from *Insight into Medicine*):

Radix Adenophorae, Poria, Radix Salviae Miltiorrhizae, Bulbus Fritillariae Cirrhosae, Radix Curcumae, Pericarpium Amomi, Petillus Nelumbinis and Testa Oryzae Sativae.

(153) Decoction of Colla Corii Asini for Invigorating Lung (from *Medical Elucidation of Pediatrics*):

Colla Corii Asini, Fructus Aristolochiae, Fructus Arctii, Radix Glycyrrhizae Preparata, Semen Armeniacae Amarum and Fructus Oryzae Glutinous.

(154) Decoction for Strengthening Middle *Jiao* and Benefiting *Qi* (from *Comments on the Spleen and Stomach*):

Radix Ginseng, Radix Astragali, Rhizoma Atractylodis Macrocephalae, Radix Glycyrrhizae, Radix Angelicae Sinensis, Pericarpium Citri Reticulatae, Rhizoma Cimicifugae and Radix Bupleuri.

(155) Decoction for Replenishing *Qi* and Invigorating Spleen (from *The Medical Prescriptions of General Medicine*):

Radix Ginseng, Rhizoma Atractylodis Macrocephalae, Poria, Radix Glycyrrhizae, Radix Astragali, Pericarpium Citri Reticulatae, Fructus Amomi, Massa Pinelliae Rhizomatis, Rhizoma Zingiberis Recens and Fructus Jujubae.

(156) Decoction for Invigorating *Yang* (from *Correction of Medical Classics*):

Radix Angelicae Sinensis, Rhizoma Chuanxiong, Radix Astragali, Semen Persicae, Lumbricus, Radix Paeoniae Rubra and Flos Carthami.

(157) Decoction for Replenishing Liver (from *Golden Mirror of Orthodox Medical Lineage*):

Radix Angelicae Sinensis, Radix Paeoniae Alba, Rhizoma Chuanxiong, Radix Rehmanniae Preparata, Semen Ziziphi Spinosae, Fructus Chaenomelis and Radix Glycyrrhizae Preparata.

(158) Decoction for Invigorating Lungs (from *Perpetual Sealed Prescriptions*):
Radix Ginseng, Radix Astragali, Radix Rehmanniae Preparata, Fructus Schisandrae, Radix Asteris and Cortex Mori.

(159) Pill for Replenishing Marrow (from *Miraculous Books of Ten Effective Recipes*):
Cow's spine, goat's spine, soft-shelled turtle, black-bone chicken, Rhizoma Dioscoreae, Semen Nelumbinis, Fructus Jujubae, Fructus Kaki Pruina, Colla Corii Asini, beeswax, Powder for Harmonizing the Stomach (Rhizoma Atractylodis, Cortex Magnoliae Officinalis, Pericarpium Citri Reticulatae, Radix Glycyrrhizae, Rhizoma Zingiberis Recens and Fructus Jujubae), powder of Decoction of Four Mild Drugs (91), Rhizoma Anemarrhenae and Cortex Phellodendri.

(160) Decoction of Polygoni Multiflori and Ginseng for Malaria (from *A Complete Collection of Jingyue's Treatise*):
Radix Polygoni Multiflori, Radix Ginseng, Radix Angelicae Sinensis, Pericarpium Citri Reticulatae and Rhizoma Zingiberis Recens.

(161) Bolus of Gleditsiae (from *Synopsis of Prescriptions of the Golden Chamber*):
Fructus Gleditsiae and Fructus Jujubae.

(162) Decoction for Relieving Pain and Removing Blood Stasis (from *Correction of Medical Classics*):
Radix Gentianae Macrophyllae, Rhizoma Chuanxiong, Semen Persicae, Flos Carthami, Radix Glycyrrhizae, Rhizoma seu Radix Notopterygii, Myrrha, Rhizoma Cyperi, Faeces Trogopterori, Radix Achyranthis Bidentatae, Lumbricus and Radix Angelicae Sinensis.

(163) Decoction of Aconiti Lateralis Preparata for Regulating Middle *Jiao* (from *Benevolent Prescriptions from the Pharmaceutical Bureau of Taiping Period*):
Radix Aconiti Lateralis Preparata, Radix Ginseng, Rhizoma Atractylodis Macrocephalae, Rhizoma Zingiberis (baked) and Radix Glycyrrhizae Preparata.

(164) Powder of Phaseoli and Angelicae Sinensis (from *Synopsis of Prescriptions of the Golden Chamber*):
Semen Phaseoli and Radix Angelicae Sinensis.

(165) Plaster of Resina Ferulae (from *Synopsis of Prescriptions of the Golden Chamber*):
Rhizoma seu Radix Notopterygii, Radix Angelicae Pubescentis, Radix Scrophulariae, Cortex Cinnamomi, Radix Paeoniae Rubra, Squama Manitis, Oleum Styrax, Radix Rehmanniae, Rat Faeces, Radix et Rhizoma Rhei, Radix Angelicae Dahuricae, Rhizoma Gastrodiae, Flos Carthami, Moschus, Eupolyphaga seu Steleophaga, Minium, Natrii Sulfas, Resina Ferulae, Olibanum and Myrrha.

(166) Powder of Ophicalcitum (from *Miraculous Books of Ten Effective Recipes*):
Ophicalcitum (calcined).

(167) Pill for Warming Kidney-*Yang* and Relieving Abdominal Pain (from *Benevolent Prescriptions from the Pharmaceutical Bureau of Taiping Period*):
Fructus Psoraleae, Cortex Eucommiae, Semen Juglandis and Bulbus Allii.

(168) Decoction of Artemisiae Annuae and Carapax Trionycis (from *Essentials of Seasonal of Febrile Diseases*):
Herba Artemisiae Annuae, Carapax Tri-onycis, Radix Rehmanniae, Rhizoma Anemarrhenae and Cortex Moutan.

(169) Decoction of Alismatis (from *Synopsis of Prescriptions of the Golden Chamber*):
Rhizoma Alismatis and Rhizoma Atractylodis Macrocephalae.

(170) Decoction of Poria, Cinnamomi, Atractylodis Macrocephalae and Glycyrrhizae (from *Synopsis of Prescriptions of the Golden Chamber*):
Poria, Ramulus Cinnamomi, Rhizoma Atractylodis Macrocephalae and Radix Glycyrrhizae.

(171) *Huqian* Bolus (from *Danxi's Experience on Medicine*):

Carapax et Plastrum Testudinis, Cortex Phellodendri, Rhizoma Anemarrhenae, Radix Rehmanniae Preparata, Radix Paeoniae Alba, Herba Cynomorii, Pericarpium Citri Reticulatae, Os Tigris and Rhizoma Zingiberis.

(172) Bolus of Placenta Hominis (from *The Effective Prescriptions for Longevity*):

Placenta Hominis, Radix Rehmanniae Preparata, Cortex Eucommiae, Radix Asparagi, Radix Ophiopogonis, Carapax et Plastrum Testudinis, Cortex Phellodendri and Radix Achyranthis Bidentatae.

(173) Decoction for Purging Stomach-Fire (from *Synopsis of Prescriptions of the Golden Chamber*):

Radix et Rhizoma Rhei, Radix Scutellariae and Rhizoma Coptidis.

(174) Powder for Expelling Lung-Heat (from *Medical Elucidation of Pediatrics*):

Cortex Mori, Cortex lycii, Radix Glycyrrhizae and Fructus Oryzae Sativae.

(175) Decoction of Notopterygii for Eliminating Dampness (from *Differentiation of Endogenous and Exogenous Diseases*):

Rhizoma seu Radix Notopterygii, Radix Angelicae Pubescentis, Rhizoma Chuanxiong, Fructus Viticis, Radix Glycyrrhizae, Radix Ledebouriellae and Rhizoma Ligustici.

(176) Powder of Quisqualis (from *Standard for Diagnosis and Treatment*):

Fructus Quisqualis, Radix Glycyrrhizae (soaked in pig's bile), Fructus Ulmi and Fructus Toosendan.

(177) Pill for Stabilizing Emotion (from *Essentially Treasured Prescriptions for Emergencies*):

Radix Codonopsis, Lignum Pini Poriaferum, Rhizoma Acori Tatarinowii, Radix Polygalae, all of them are soaked in fluid of Radix Glycyrrhizae; The other formula consists of Poria, Rhizoma Atractylodis Macrocephalae and Radix Ophiopogonis.

(178) Pill for Relieving Epilepsy (from *Insight into Medicine*):

Rhizoma Gastrodiae, Bulbus Fritillariae Cirrhosae, Arisaema cum Bile, Rhizoma Pinelliae (ginger treated), Pericarpium Citri Reticulatae, Poria, Lignum Pini Poriaferum, Radix Salviae Miltiorrhizae, Rhizoma Acori Tatarinowii, Radix Polygalae, Scorpio, Bombyx Batryticatus, Succinum, Cinnabaris, Succus Bambusae, Succus Zingiberis and Radix Glycyrrhizae.

(179) Decoction for Relieving Asthma (from *Excellent Prescriptions for Longevity*):

Semen Ginkgo, Herba Ephedrae, Cortex Mori, Flos Farfarae, Rhizoma Pinelliae, Semen Armeniacae Amarum, Fructus Perillae, Radix Scutellariae and Radix Glycyrrhizae.

(180) Decoction for Invigorating Spleen (from *Prescriptions for Life Saving*):

Radix Aconiti Lateralis Preparata, Rhizoma Zingiberis, Rhizoma Atractylodis Macrocephalae, Radix Glycyrrhizae, Cortex Magnolicae Officinalis, Radix Aucklandiae, Fructus Tsaoko, Semen Arecae, Fructus Chaenomelis, Rhizoma Zingiberis Recens, Fructus Jujubae and Poria.

(181) Bolus of Anemarrhenae, Phellodendri and Rehmanniae Preparata (from *Golden Mirror of Orthodox Medical Lineage*):

Rhizoma Anemarrhenae, Cortex Phellodendri, Radix Rehmanniae Preparata, Fructus Corni, Rhizoma Dioscoreae, Poria, Cortex Moutan and Rhizoma Alismatis.

(182) Pill for Invigorating Kidney-*Qi* (from *Synopsis of Prescriptions of the Golden Chamber*):

Ramulus Cinnamomi, Radix Aconiti Lateralis Preparata, Radix Rehmanniae Preparata, Fructus Corni, Rhizoma Dioscoreae, Poria, Cortex Moutan and Rhizoma Alismatis.

(183) Powder of Toosendan (from *Basic Questions*: *Discourse on Mechanism for Preserving Life*):

Fructus Toosendan and Rhizoma Corydalis.

(184) Golden Lock Bolus for Keeping Kidney-Essence (from *Variorum of Prescriptions*):

Semen Astragali Complanati, Semen Euryales, Semen Nelumbinis, Os Draconis, Concha Ostreae and Semen Nelumbinis.

(185) Powder of Inulae (from *Benevolent Prescriptions from the Pharmaceutical Bureau of Taiping Period*):

Flos Inulae, Herba Ephedrae, Radix Peucedani, Herba Schizonepetae, Rhizoma Pinelliae (ginger treated), Radix Paeoniae Rubra, Radix Glycyrrhizae, Rhizoma Zingiberis Recens and Fructus Jujubae.

(186) Decoction of Glycyrrhizae Preparata (from *Treatise on Cold Diseases*):

Radix Glycyrrhizae Preparata, Radix Ginseng, Ramulus Cinnamomi, Rhizoma Zingiberis Recens, Colla Corii Asini, Radix Rehmanniae, Radix Ophiopogonis, Fructus Cannabis and Fructus Jujubae.

(187) *Zhuju* Pill (from *Essentially Treasured Prescriptions for Emergencies*):

Rhizoma Coptidis, Colla Corii Asini, Radix Angelicae Sinensis and Rhizoma Zingiberis.

(188) Decoction of Ginseng and Aconiti Lateralis Preparata (from *Useful Prescriptions for Women*):

Radix Ginseng, Radix Aconiti Lateralis Preparata, Rhizoma Zingiberis and Fructus Jujubae.

(189) Decoction of Ginseng and Perillae (from *Benevolent Prescriptions from the Pharmaceutical Bureau of Taiping Period*):

Radix Ginseng, Folium Perillae, Radix Puerariae, Radix Peucedani, Rhizoma Pinelliae (Alumen treated), Poria, Exocarpium Citri Rubrum, Radix Glycyrrhizae, Radix Platycodi, Fructus Aurantii, Radix Aucklandiae, Pericarpium Citri Reticulatae, Rhizoma Zingiberis and Fructus Jujubae.

(190) Powder of Ginseng, Poria and Atractylodis Macrocephalae (from *Benevolent Prescriptions from the Pharmaceutical Bureau of Taiping Period*):

Radix Ginseng, Poria, Rhizoma Atractylodis Macrocephalae, Radix Platycodi, Rhizoma Dioscoreae, Radix Glycyrrhizae, Semen Lablab Album, Semen Nelumbinis, Fructus Amomi and Semen Coicis.

(191) Powder of Ginseng and Gecko (from *Prescriptions for Life Saving*):

Radix Ginseng and Gecko.

(192) Pill of Ginseng and Aconiti Lateralis Preparata for Restoration (from *Popular Treatise on Cold Diseases*):

Radix Ginseng, Radix Aconiti Lateralis Preparata, Ramulus Cinnamomi, Rhizoma seu Radix Notopterygii, Radix Astragali, Herba Asari, Radix Glycyrrhizae Preparata and Radix Ledebouriellae.

(193) Decoction of Ginseng, Aconiti Lateralis Preparata, Os Draconis and Concha Ostreae (from *Effective Prescriptions from Physicians of Successive Generations*):

Radix Ginseng, Radix Aconiti Lateralis Preparata, Os Draconis and Concha Ostreae.

(194) *Chunze* Decoction (from *Variorum of Prescriptions*):

Rhizoma Atractylodis Macrocephalae, Ramulus Cinnamomi, Polyporus, Rhizoma Alismatis, Poria and Radix Ginseng.

(195) Decoction of Cacumen Platycladi (from *Synopsis of Prescriptions of the Golden Chamber*):

Cacumen Platycladi, Rhizoma Zingiberis, Folium Artemisiae Argyi and horse's urine.

(196) Pill of Aurantii Immaturus for Relieving Stagnation (from *Differentiation of Endogenous and Exogenous Diseases*):

Radix et Rhizoma Rhei, Fructus Aurantii Immaturus, Radix Scutellariae, Rhizoma Coptidis, Massa Medicata Fermentata, Rhizoma Atractylodis Macrocephalae, Poria and Rhizoma Alismatis.

(197) Antiphlogistic Powder of Schizonepetae and Ledebouriellae (from *Essential Points for Surgical Diseases*):

Herba Schizonepetae, Radix Ledebouriellae, Rhizoma seu Radix Notopterygii, Radix Angelicae Pubescentis, Radix Bupleuri, Radix Peucedani, Rhizoma Chuanxiong, Fructus Aurantii, Poria, Radix Platycodi and Radix Glycyrrhizae.

(198) Powder of Artemisiae Scopariae and Four Ingredients with Poria (from *Passing on Medical*

Experience):

Herba Artemisiae Scopariae, Poria, Rhizoma Atractylodis Macrocephalae, Rhizoma Alismatis, Polyporus and Ramulus Cinnamomi.

(199) Decoction of Artemisiae Scopariae, Atractylodis Macrocephalae and Aconiti Lateralis Preparata (from *Insight into Medicine*):

Herba Artemisiae Scopariae, Rhizoma Atractylodis Macrocephalae, Radix Aconiti Lateralis Preparata, Rhizoma Zingiberis, Radix Glycyrrhizae Preparata and Cortex Cinnamomi.

(200) Decoction of Artemisiae Scopariae (from *Treatise on Cold Diseases*):

Herba Artemisiae Scopariae Fructus Gardeniae and Radix et Rhizoma Rhei.

(201) Powder of Rubiae (from *A Complete Collection of Jingyue's Treatise*):

Radix Rubiae, Radix Scutellariae, Colla Corii Asini, Cacumen Platycladi, Radix Glycyrrhizae and Radix Rehmanniae.

(202) Powder for Treating Face Distortion (from *Yang's Family Prescriptions*):

Rhizoma Typhonii, Bombyx Batryticatus and Scorpio.

(203) Powder of Pharbitidis and Foeniculi (from *A Medical Text for Confucianists to Serve Family Members and Relatives*):

Semen Pharbitidis and Fructus Foeniculi.

(204) *Weiling* Decoction (from *Danxi's Experience on Medicine*):

Rhizoma Atractylodis, Cortex Magnoliae Officinalis, Pericarpium Citri Reticulatae, Radix Glycyrrhizae, Rhizoma Zingiberis Recens, Fructus Jujubae, Ramulus Cinnamomi, Rhizoma Atractylodis Macrocephalae, Rhizoma Alismatis, Poria and Polyporus.

(205) *Jichuan* Decoction (from *A Complete Collection of Jingyue's Treatise*):

Radix Angelicae Sinensis, Radix Achyranthis Bidentatae, Herba Cistanchis, Rhizoma Alismatis, Rhizoma Cimicifugae and Fructus Aurantii.

(206) *Jisheng* Pill for Invigorating Kidney-*Qi* (from *Prescriptions for Life Saving*):

Radix Rehmanniae, Rhizoma Dioscoreae, Fructus Corni, Cortex Moutan, Poria, Rhizoma Alismatis, Radix Aconiti Lateralis Preparata, Ramulus Cinnamomi, Radix Achyranthis Bidentatae and Semen Plantaginis.

(207) Decoction for Nourishing Stomach (from *Standard for Diagnosis and Treatment*):

Radix Adenophorae, Radix Ophiopogonis, Rhizoma Polygonati Odorati, Semen Lablab Album, Folium Mori and Radix Glycyrrhizae.

(208) Decoction for Nourishing Heart (from *Standard for Diagnosis and Treatment*):

Radix Astragali, Poria, Lignum Pini Poriaferum, Radix Angelicae Sinensis, Rhizoma Chuanxiong, Radix Glycyrrhizae Preparata, Massa Pinelliae Rhizomatis, Ginseng and Cortex Cinnamomi.

(209) Pill of Magnoliae Officinalis and Rhei (from *Synopsis of Prescriptions of the Golden Chamber*):

Cortex Magnoliae Officinalis, Radix et Rhizoma Rhei and Fructus Aurantii Immaturus.

(210) Magic Powder (from *Insight into Medicine*):

Rhizoma Atractylodis, Pericarpium Citri Reticulatae, Cortex Magnoliae Officinalis, Radix Glycyrrhizae, Herba Agastaches and Fructus Amomi.

(211) Pill of Six Mild Drugs with Aucklandiae and Amomi (from *Verses of Modern Prescription*):

Radix Aucklandiae, Fructus Amomi, Pericarpium Citri Reticulatae, Rhizoma Pinelliae, Radix Codonopsis, Rhizoma Atractylodis Macrocephalae, Poria and Radix Glycyrrhizae.

(212) Fructus Aristolochiae Compound Cake (from proved formula):

Grind 9 grams of Fructus Aristolochiae, 18 grams of Radix Glycyrrhizae, 18 grams of Semen Ginkgo, 45 grams of Fructus Oryzae Glutinous, 4.5 grams of Herba Ephedrae, and 90 grams of Folium

Ilicis Cornutae to powder and mix them well. Each time add 1/3 of the mixed powder to 100 ml of normal saline to make thick paste. Six medicinal cakes made from the thick paste are then applied to three pairs of Bailao (Extra), Feishu (BL 13), and Gaohuang (BL 43) acupoints.

(213) Decoction for Activating Blood Circulation and Dredging Meridian (from *Invention of Medicine*):

Radix Bupleuri, Radix Trichosanthis, Radix Angelicae Sinensis, Flos Carthami, Radix Glycyrrhizae, Squama Manitis, Radix et Rhizoma Rhei and Semen Persicae.

(214) Decoction for Promoting Smooth Circulation of *Qi* and Eliminating Phlegm (from proved formula):

Rhizoma Pinelliae, Retinervus Citri Reticulatae, Poria, Radix Glycyrrhizae, Rhizoma Zingiberis Recens, Arisaema cum Bile, Fructus Aurantii Immaturus, Radix Aucklandiae and Rhizoma Cyperi.

(215) Decoction for Promoting Smooth Circulation of *Qi* and Regulating the Middle *Jiao* (from *Standard for Diagnosis and Treatment*):

Radix Astragali, Radix Ginseng, Rhizoma Atractylodis Macrocephalae, Radix Paeoniae Alba, Radix Angelicae Sinensis, Pericarpium Citri Reticulatae, Radix Glycyrrhizae, Radix Bupleuri, Rhizoma Cimicifugae, Fructus Viticis, Rhizoma Chuanxiong and Herba Asari.

(216) Pill for Promoting Digestion (from *Danxi's Experience on Medicine*):

Massa Medicata Fermentata, Fructus Crataegi, Poria, Rhizoma Pinelliae, Pericarpium Citri Reticulatae, Fructus Forsythiae and Semen Raphani.

(217) Decoction for Deficiency Syndrome (from *Miraculous Books of Ten Effective Recipes*):

Radix Ginseng, Radix Astragali, Rhizoma Atractylodis Macrocephalae, Radix Glycyrrhizae, Poria, Fructus Schisandrae, Radix Angelicae Sinensis, Radix Rehmanniae, Radix Rehmanniae Preparata, Radix Asparagi, Radix Ophiopogonis, Radix Paeoniae Rubra, Radix Paeoniae Alba, Radix Bupleuri, Cortex Magnolicae Officinalis, Cortex Lycii, Cortex Phellodendri, Rhizoma Anemarrhenae, Petiolus Nelumbinis, Pericarpium Citri Reticulatae, Rhizoma Zingiberis and Fructus Jujubae.

(218) Decoction of Ginseng (from *A Complete Collection of Jingyue's Treatise*):

Radix Ginseng.

(219) Decoction of Angelicae Pubescentis and Taxilli (from *Essentially Treasured Prescriptions for Emergencies*):

Radix Angelicae Pubescentis, Herba Taxilli, Radix Gentianae Macrophyllae, Radix Ledebouriellae, Herba Asari, Radix Angelicae Sinensis, Radix Paeoniae, Rhizoma Chuanxiong, Radix Rehmanniae, Cortex Eucommiae, Radix Achyranthis Bidentatae, Radix Ginseng, Poria, Radix Glycyrrhizae and Lignum Cinnamomi.

(220) Pill for Pursuing Parasites (from *Standard for Diagnosis and Treatment*):

Semen Arecae, Omphalia, Radix Aucklandiae, Radix Meliae, Fructus Gleditsiae, Semen Pharbitidis and Herba Artemisiae Scopariae.

(221) Powder of Gentianae Macrophyllae and Carapax Trionycis (from *Main Rules in Medical and Health Service*):

Cortex Lycii, Radix Bupleuri, Radix Gentianae Macrophyllae, Rhizoma Anemarrhenae, Radix Angelicae Sinensis, Carapax Trionycis, Herba Artemisiae Annuae and Fructus Mume.

(222) *Zhenren* Decoction for Nourishing Viscera (from *Standard for Diagnosis and Treatment*):

Fructus Chebulae, Pericarpium Papaveris, Semen Myristicae, Rhizoma Atractylodis Macrocephalae, Radix Ginseng, Radix Aucklandiae, Cortex Cinnamomi, Radix Glycyrrhizae Preparata, Rhizoma Zingiberis Recens and Fructus Jujubae.

(223) *Zhenwu* Decoction (from *Treatise on Cold Diseases*):

Radix Aconiti Lateralis Preparata, Rhizoma Atractylodis Macrocephalae, Poria, Radix Paeoniae,

Rhizoma and Zingiberis Recens.

(224) Decoction of Cinnamomi (from *Treatise on Cold Diseases*):

Rhizoma Cimicifugae, Radix Paeoniae, Rhizoma Zingiberis Recens, Radix Glycyrrhizae Preparata and Fructus Jujubae.

(225) Decoction of Cinnamomi, Glycyrrhizae, Os Draconis and Concha Ostreae (from *Treatise on Cold Diseases*):

Rhizoma Cimicifugae, Radix Glycyrrhizae Preparata, Os Draconis and Concha Ostreae.

(226) Decoction of Cinnamomi, Magnoliae Officinalis, and Armeniacae Amarum (from *Treatise on Cold Diseases*):

Rhizoma Cimicifugae, Radix Paeoniae, Radix Glycyrrhizae Preparata, Rhizoma Zingiberis Recens, Fructus Jujubae, Cortex Magnolicae Officinalis and Semen Armeniacae Amarum.

(227) Decoction of Cinnamomi, Paeoniae and Anemarrhenae (from *Synopsis of Prescriptions of the Golden Chamber*):

Ramulus Cinnamomi, Radix Paeoniae, Radix Glycyrrhizae Preparata, Herba Ephedrae, Rhizoma Atractylodis Macrocephalae, Rhizoma Anemarrhenae, Radix Ledebouriellae, Radix Aconiti Lateralis Preparata and Rhizoma Zingiberis Recens.

(228) Decoction of Cinnamomi and Glycyrrhizae (from *Treatise on Cold Diseases*):

Ramulus Cinnamomi and Radix Glycyrrhizae Preparata.

(229) Decoction of Cinnamomi and Aconiti Lateralis Preparata for Regulating Middle *Jiao* (from proved formula):

Cortex Cinnamomi, Radix Aconiti Lateralis Preparata, Radix Codonopsis, Rhizoma Atractylodis Macrocephalae, Rhizoma Zingiberis Recens and Radix Glycyrrhizae.

(230) Decoction of Cinnamomi and Astragali (from *Synopsis of Prescriptions of the Golden Chamber*):

Ramulus Cinnamomi, Radix Astragali, Radix Paeoniae, Radix Glycyrrhizae, Rhizoma Zingiberis Recens and Fructus Jujubae.

(231) Decoction for Relieving *Bi*-Syndrome (from *Diagnosis and Treatment of Classified Syndromes*):

Semen Persicae, Flos Carthami, Rhizoma Chuanxiong, Radix Angelicae Sinensis and Radix Clematidis.

(232) *Taohua* Decoction (from *Treatise on Cold Diseases*):

Halloysitum Rubrum, Rhizoma Zingiberis and Fructus Oryzae Sativae.

(233) Decoction of Persicae and Carthami (from *Su'an Medical Records*):

Radix Salviae Miltiorrhizae, Radix Paeoniae Rubra, Semen Persicae, Flos Carthami, Radix Codonopsis Pilosulae, Rhizoma Corydalis, Pericarpium Citri Reticulatae Viride, Radix Angelicae Sinensis, Rhizoma Chuanxiong, and Radix Rehmanniae.

(234) Decoction of Platycodi, and Armeniacae Amarum (from *A Complete Collection of Jingyue's Treatise*):

Radix Platycodi, Semen Armeniacae Amarum, Radix Glycyrrhizae, Flos Lonicerae, Bulbus Fritillariae Cirrhosae, Fructus Aurantii, Caulis Sargentodoxae, Fructus Forsythiae, Spica Prunellae, Bulbus Lilii, Radix Ophiopogonis and Colla Corii Asini.

(235) Decoction of Platycodi (from *Treatise on Cold Diseases*):

Radix Platycodi and Radix Glycyrrhizae.

(236) Decoction of Trichosanthis, Allii Macrostemi and Pinelliae (from *Synopsis of Prescriptions of the Golden Chamber*):

Fructus Trichosanthis, Bulbus Allii Macrostemi, rice wine and Rhizoma Pinelliae.

(237) Decoction of Trichosanthis Allii Macrostemi and Wine (from *Synopsis of Prescriptions of the Golden Chamber*):

Fructus Trichosanthis, Bulbus Allii Macrostemi and rice wine.

(238) Decoction of Bupleuri, Cinnamomi and Zingiberis (from *Treatise on Cold Diseases*):

Radix Bupleuri, Rhizoma Zingiberis, Ramulus Cinnamomi, Radix Scutellariae, Radix Trichosanthis, Concha Ostreae and Radix Glycyrrhizae Preparata.

(239) Powder of Bupleuri for Releasing Stagnant Liver-*Qi* (from *A Complete Collection of Jingyue's Treatise*):

Radix Bupleuri, Fructus Aurantii, Radix Paeoniae, Radix Glycyrrhizae, Rhizoma Chuanxiong.

(240) Decoction of Bupleuri and Citri Reticulatae for Expelling Pathogenic Factors (from *Buju's Medical Works*):

Radix Bupleuri, Radix Puerariae, Rhizoma Pinelliae, Cortex Magnoliae Officinalis, Rhizoma Alismatis, Rhizoma Zingiberis Recens, Radix Glycyrrhizae, Radix Gentianae Macrophyllae, Herba Agastaches, Pericarpium Citri Reticulatae, Fructus Crataegi and Fructus Jujubae.

(241) Decoction of Sargassum for Goiter (from *Golden Mirror of Orthodox Medical Lineage*):

Sargassum, Thallus Laminariae seu Eckloniae, Rhizoma Pinelliae, Pericarpium Citri Reticulatae, Pericarpium Citri Reticulatae Viride, Fructus Forsythiae, Bulbus Fritillariae Thunbergii, Radix Angelicae Sinensis, Rhizoma Chuanxiong, Radix Angelicae Pubescentis and Radix Glycyrrhizae.

(242) Bolus for Lubricating Intestine (from *Shen's Treatise on the Importance of Life Preservation*):

Radix Angelicae Sinensis, Radix Rehmanniae, Fructus Cannabis, Semen Persicae and Fructus Aurantii.

(243) Decoction for Cleansing Phlegm (from *Prescriptions for Life Saving*):

Radix Pinelliae Praeparata, Rhizoma Arisaematis Preparata, Pericarpium Citri Reticulatae, Fructus Aurantii Immaturus, Poria, Radix Ginseng, Rhizoma Acori Tatarinowii, Caulis Bambusae in Taeniam, Radix Glycyrrhizae and Rhizoma Zingiberis Recens.

(244) Formula for Diabetes (from *Danxi's Experience on Medicine*):

Powder of Rhizoma Coptidis, Powder of Radix Trichosanthis, Succus Rehmanniae, Succus Nelumbinis Rhizomatis, human milk, Succus Zingiberis and Mel.

(245) Decoction for Benefiting *Qi* and Improving Hearing (from *Standard for Diagnosis and Treatment*):

Radix Astragali, Radix Ginseng, Rhizoma Cimicifugae, Radix Puerariae, Fructus Viticis, Radix Paeoniae, Cortex Phellodendri and Radix Glycyrrhizae Preparata.

(246) Decoction for Benefiting Stomach (from *Essentials of Seasonal Febrile Diseases*):

Radix Adenophorae, Radix Ophiopogonis, Radix Rehmanniae, Radix Polygonati Odorati and crystal sugar.

(247) Powder for Benefiting Nutrient System and Expelling Pathogenic Factors (from *Buju's Medical Works*):

Radix Bupleuri, Radix Puerariae, Radix Rehmanniae Preparata, Radix Angelicae Sinensis, Radix Ginseng, Radix Gentianae, Macrophyllae, Radix Dipsaci, Radix Glycyrrhizae, Rhizoma Zingiberis Recens and Fructus Jujubae.

(248) Decoction for Regulating Nutrient System (from *Standard for Diagnosis and Treatment*):

Rhizoma Curcumae, Rhizoma Chuanxiong, Radix Angelicae Sinensis, Rhizoma Corydalis, Radix Paeoniae Rubra, Herba Dianthi, Radix et Rhizoma Rhei, Semen Arecae, Pericarpium Citri Reticulatae, Pericarpium Arecae, Semen Lepidii seu Descurainiae, Poria, Cortex Mori, Herba Asari, Cortex Cinnamomi, Radix Glycyrrhizae Preparata, Rhizoma Zingiberis, Fructus Jujubae and Radix Angelicae

Dahuricae.

(249) Decoction of Belamcandae and Ephedrae (from *Synopsis of Prescriptions of the Golden Chamber*):

Rhizoma Belamcandae, Herba Ephedrae, Herba Asari, Radix Asteris, Flos Farfarae, Rhizoma Pinelliae, Fructus Schisandrae, Rhizoma Zingiberis Recens and Fructus Jujubae.

(250) *Xiaoyao* Powder (from *Benevolent Prescriptions from the Pharmaceutical Bureau of Taiping Period*):

Radix Bupleuri, Rhizoma Atractylodis Macrocephalae, Radix Paeoniae Alba, Radix Angelicae Sinensis, Poria, Radix Glycyrrhizae Preparata, Herba Menthae and Rhizoma Zingiberis, (roasted).

(251) Decoction for Relieving Stagnation (from *Secret Records of the Cabinet of Orchids*):

Radix Rehmanniae, Radix Rehmanniae Preparata, Semen Persicae, Flos Carthami, Radix Angelicae Sinensis, Radix Glycyrrhizae Preparata and Rhizoma Cimicifugae.

(252) Decoction for Dredging Meridian and Cold Extremities (from *Treatise on Cold Diseases*):

Radix Aconiti Lateralis Preparata, Rhizoma Zingiberis, Radix Glycyrrhizae Preparata and Bulbus Allii Fistulosi.

(253) Decoction for Opening Orifice and Activating Blood Circulation (from *Correction of Medical Classics*):

Radix Paeoniae Rubra, Rhizoma Chuanxiong, Semen Persicae, Flos Carthami, Moschus, Bulbus Allii Fistulosi, Rhizoma Zingiberis Recens, Fructus Jujubae and wine.

(254) Decoction for Removing Blood Stasis (from *A Complete Collection of Jingyue's Treatise*):

Radix Angelicae Sinensis, Fructus Crataegi, Rhizoma Cyperi, Flos Carthami, Radix Linderae, Pericarpium Citri Reticulatae Viride, Radix Aucklandiae and Rhizoma Alismatis.

(255) Decoction of Mori (from *A Complete Collection of Jingyue's Treatise*):

Cortex Mori, Rhizoma Pinelliae, Fructus Perillae, Semen Armeniacae Amarum, Bulbus Fritillariae Cirrhosae, Radix Scutellariae, Rhizoma Coptidis and Fructus Gardeniae.

(256) Decoction of Mori and Armeniacae Amarum (from *Essentials of Seasonal Febrile Diseases*):

Folium Mori, Semen Armeniacae Amarum, Bulbus Fritillariae Thunbergii, Radix Adenophorae, Semen Sojae Preparatum, Fructus Gardeniae and Exocarpium Pyri.

(257) Decoction of Mori and Chrysanthemi (from *Essentials of Seasonal Febrile Diseases*):

Folium Mori, Flos Chrysanthemi, Fructus Forsythiae, Herba Menthae, Radix Platycodi, Semen Armeniacae Amarum, Rhizoma Phragmitis and Radix Glycyrrhizae.

(258) Bolus for Regulating Middle *Jiao* (from *Treatise on Cold Diseases*):

Radix Ginseng, Rhizoma Atractylodis Macrocephalae, Rhizoma Zingiberis and Radix Glycyrrhizae Preparata.

(259) Decoction of Terra Flava Usta (from *Synopsis of Prescriptions of the Golden Chamber*):

Terra Flava Usta, Radix Glycyrrhizae, Radix Rehmanniae, Rhizoma Atractylodis Macrocephalae, Radix Aconiti Lateralis Preparata, Colla Corii Asini and Radix Scutellariae.

(260) Pill of Coptidis for Clearing Away Heat (from *A Collection of Ancient and Modern Prescriptions*):

Radix Scutellariae, Rhizoma Coptidis, Cortex Phellodendri, Fructus Gardeniae, Flos Chrysanthemi, Radix Platycodi, Herba Menthae, Rhizoma Chuanxiong, Radix et Rhizoma Rhei, Fructus Forsythiae, Radix Angelicae Sinensis, Radix Puerariae, Radix Scrophulariae, Radix Trichosanthis and Rhizoma Curcumae Longae.

(261) Decoction of Coptidis and Colla Corii Asini (from *Treatise on Cold Diseases*):

Rhizoma Coptidis, Colla Corii Asini, Radix Scutellariae, egg yolk and Radix Paeoniae.

(262) Decoction of Coptidis and Elsholtziae (from *Syndrome Differentiation for Life Saving*):
Rhizoma Coptidis, Herba Elsholtziae and Cortex Magnoliae Officinalis.

(263) Decoction of Coptidis for Detoxification (from *Clandestine Essentials from Imperial Library*):
Rhizoma Coptidis, Radix Scutellariae, Cortex Phellodendri and Fructus Gardeniae.

(264) Decoction of Coptidis for Clearing Away Gallbladder-Heat (from *Essentially Treasured Prescriptions*):
Rhizoma Pinelliae, Pericarpium Citri Reticulatae, Poria, Radix Glycyrrhizae, Fructus Aurantii Immaturus, Caulis Bambusae in Taeniam, Rhizoma Coptidis and Fructus Jujubae.

(265) Decoction of Astragali and Glycyrrhizae (from *Benevolent Prescriptions from the Pharmaceutical Bureau of Taiping Period*):
Radix Astragali and Radix Glycyrrhizae.

(266) Decoction of Astragali (from *Supplement to Synopsis of Prescriptions of the Golden Chamber*):
Radix Astragali, Pericarpium Citri Reticulatae, Fructus Cannabis and Mel.

(267) Decoction of Astragali for Strengthening Middle *Jiao* (from *Synopsis of Prescriptions of the Golden Chamber*):
Radix Astragali, Radix Paeoniae Alba, Ramulus Cinnamomi, Radix Glycyrrhizae Preparata, Rhizoma Zingiberis Recens, Fructus Jujubae and Saccharum Granorum.

(268) Decoction of Astragali and Carapax Trionycis (from *Main Rules in Medical and Health Service*):
Radix Astragali, Carapax Trionycis, Radix Asparagi, Cortex Lycii, Radix Gentianae Macrophyllae, Radix Bupleuri, Radix Asteris, Rhizoma Pinelliae, Poria, Rhizoma Anemarrhenae, Radix Rehmanniae, Radix Paeoniae Alba, Cortex Mori, Radix Ginseng, Cortex Cinnamomi, Radix Platycodi and Radix Glycyrrhizae.

(269) Decoction of Gardeniae for Clearing Liver-Fire (from *Diagnosis and Treatment of Classified Syndromes*):
Fructus Gardeniae, Cortex Moutan, Radix Bupleuri, Radix Angelicae Sinensis, Radix Paeoniae, Poria, Rhizoma Chuanxiong, Fructus Arctii and Radix Glycyrrhizae.

(270) Pill for Treating Phlegm-Syndrome (from *Treatise on the Tripartite Pathogenesis of Diseases*):
Radix Kansui, Radix Euphobriae Pekinensis and Semen Sinapis Albae.

(271) Bolus of Cannabis (from *Treatise on Cold Diseases*):
Fructus Cannabis, Radix Paeoniae, Fructus Aurantii Immaturus Preparata, Radix et Rhizoma Rhei, Cortex Magnoliae Officinalis Preparata and Semen Armeniacae Amarum.

(272) Decoction of Ephedrae, Armeniacae Amarum, Gypsum Fibrosum and Glycyrrhizae (from *Treatise on Cold Diseases*):
Herba Ephedrae, Semen Armeniacae Amarum, Gypsum Fibrosum and Radix Glycyrrhizae Preparata.

(273) Decoction of Ephedrae (from *Treatise on Cold Diseases*):
Herba Ephedrae, Ramulus Cinnamomi, Semen Armeniacae Amarum and Radix Glycyrrhizae Preparata.

(274) Decoction of Ephedrae, Aconiti Lateralis Preparata and Asari (from *Treatise on Cold Diseases*):
Herba Ephedrae, Radix Aconiti Lateralis Preparata and Herba Asari.

(275) Decoction of Inulae and Haematitum (from *Synopsis of Prescriptions of the Golden Cham-

ber):

Flos Inulae, Haematitum, Radix Ginseng, Rhizoma Pinelliae, Radix Glycyrrhizae Preparata, Rhizoma Zingiberis Recens and Fructus Jujubae.

(276) Decoction of Inulae (from *Synopsis of Prescriptions of the Golden Chamber*):

Flos Inulae, Xinjiang (dark reddish silk dyed with madder) and Bulbus Allii Fistulosi.

(277) Decoction of Cornu Saigae Tataricae (from *Supplementary Notions of Medical Experience*):

Cornu Saigae Tataricae, Carapax et Plastrum Testudinis, Radix Rehmanniae, Cortex Moutan, Radix Paeoniae Alba, Radix Bupleuri, Herba Menthae, Periostracum Cicadae, Flos Chrysanthemi, Spica Prunellae and Concha Haliotidis.

(278) Decoction of Cornu Saigae Tataricae and Ramulus Uncariae cum Uncis (from *Popular Treatise on Cold Diseases*):

Cornu Saigae Tataricae, Folium Mori, Bulbus Fritillariae Cirrhosae, Radix Rehmanniae (fresh), Ramulus Uncariae cum Uncis, Flos Chrysanthemi, Radix Paeoniae Alba, Radix Glycyrrhizae, Caulis Bambusae in Taeniam and Lignum Pini Poriaferum.

(279) Decoction for Clearing Away Heat in the Lung and Resolving Phlegm (from *The Medical Prescriptions of General Medicine*):

Radix Scutellariae, Fructus Gardeniae, Radix Platycodi, Radix Ophiopogonis, Cortex Mori, Bulbus Fritillariae Cirrhosae, Rhizoma Anemarrhenae, Semen Trichosanthis, Exocarpium Citri Rubrum, Poria and Radix Glycyrrhizae.

(280) Decoction for Clearing Away Lung-Heat (from *Supplement to Diagnosis and Treatment*):

Poria, Radix Scutellariae, Cortex Mori, Radix Ophiopogonis, Semen Plantaginis, Fructus Gardeniae and Caulis Aristolochiae Manshuriensis.

(281) Powder for Clearing Away Stomach-Heat (from *Secret Records of the Cabinet of Orchids*):

Radix Angelicae Sinensis, Radix Rehmanniae, Cortex Moutan, Rhizoma Cimicifugae and Rhizoma Coptidis.

(282) Powder for Relieving Deficiency-Heat Syndrome (from *Standard for Diagnosis and Treatment*):

Radix Stellariae, Rhizoma Picrorhizae, Radix Gentianae Macrophyllae, Carapax Trionycis, Cortex Lycii, Herba Artemisiae Annuae, Rhizoma Anemarrhenae and Radix Glycyrrhizae.

(283) Decoction for Clearing Away Heat in the *Ying* System (from *Essentials of Seasonal Febrile Diseases*):

Cornu Rhinocerotis, Radix Rehmanniae, Radix Scrophulariae, Gemma Bambusae, Flos Lonicerae, Fructus Forsythiae, Rhizoma Coptidis, Radix Salviae Miltiorrhizae and Radix Ophiopogonis.

(284) Decoction for Clearing Away Miasmic Toxins (from proved formula):

Herba Artemisiae Annuae, Radix Bupleuri, Poria, Rhizoma Anemarrhenae, Pericarpium Citri Reticulatae, Rhizoma Pinelliae, Radix Scutellariae, Rhizoma Coptidis, Fructus Aurantii Immaturus, Radix Dichroae, Caulis Bambusae in Taeniam and Six-to-One Powder (54).

(285) Decoction for Clearing Away Dryness and Treating Lung Disorders (from *Rules for Physicians*):

Folium Mori, Gypsum Fibrosum, Semen Armeniacae Amarum, Radix Glycyrrhizae, Radix Ophiopogonis, Radix Ginseng, Colla Corii Asini, Semen Sesami Nigrum (stir-baked) and Folium Eriobotryae Preparata.

(286) Decoction for Clearing Away Summer-Heat and Benefiting *Qi* (from *Compendium of Seasonal Febrile Diseases*):

Radix Panacis Quinquefolii, Herba Dendrobii, Radix Ophiopogonis, Rhizoma Coptidis, Herba

Lophatheri, Petiolus Nelumbinis, Radix Glycyrrhizae, Rhizoma Anemarrhenae, Fructus Oryzae Sativae and Exocarpium Citrulli.

(287) Powder of Lonicerae and Forsythiae (from *Essentials of Seasonal Febrile Diseases*):

Flos Lonicerae, Fructus Forsythiae, Semen Sojae Preparatum, Fructus Arctii, Herba Menthae, Spica Schizonepetae, Radix Platycodi, Radix Glycyrrhizae, Herba Lophatheri and Rhizoma Phragmitis.

(288) Decoction of Dioscoreae Septemlobae for Clearing Turbid Urine (from *Danxi's Experience on Medicine*):

Rhizoma Dioscoreae Septemlobae, Rhizoma Acori Tatarinowii, Radix Linderae, Fructus Alpiniae Oxyphyllae, Poria and Radix Glycyrrhizae.

(289) Decoction of Dichroae (from *Benevolent Prescriptions from the Pharmaceutical Bureau of Taiping Period*):

Rhizoma Alpiniae officinarum, Fructus Mume, Rhizoma Anemarrhenae, Radix Dichroae, Fructus Tsaoko and Radix Glycyrrhizae.

(290) Decoction of Allii Fistulosi and Sojae Preparatum (from *A Handbook of Prescriptions for Emergencies*):

Bulbus Allii Fistulosi and Semen Sojae Preparatum.

(291) Decoction of Seven Ingredients Containing Allii Fistulosi (from *Clandestine Essentials from Imperial Library*):

Bulbus and Radix Allii Fistulosi, Radix Puerariae, Semen Sojae Preparatum, Rhizoma Zingiberis Recens, Radix Ophiopogonis, Radix Rehmanniae and Fresh Water.

(292) Pill of Succinum for Relieving Insomnia (from proved formula):

Succinum, Radix Codonopsis, Poria, Radix Polygalae, Cornu Saigae Tataricae and Radix Glycyrrhizae.

(293) Decoction of Puerariae, Scutellariae and Coptidis (from *Treatise on Cold Diseases*):

Radix Puerariae, Radix Scutellariae, Rhizoma Coptidis and Radix Glycyrrhizae Preparata.

(294) Decoction of Lepidii seu Descurainiae and Jujubae for Purging Lung-Heat (from *Synopsis of Prescriptions of the Golden Chamber*):

Semen Lepidii seu Descurainiae and Fructus Jujubae.

(295) Decoction for Relieving Edema with Atractylodis Macrocephalae (from *Synopsis of Prescriptions of the Golden Chamber*):

Herba Ephedrae, Gypsum Fibrosum. Rhizoma Zingiberis Recens, Fructus Jujubae, Radix Glycyrrhizae and Rhizoma Atractylodis Macrocephalae.

(296) Decoction for Relieving Edema with Pinelliae (from *Synopsis of Prescriptions of the Golden Chamber*):

Herba Ephedrae, Gypsum Fibrosum, Rhizoma Zingiberis Recens, Fructus Jujubae, Radix Glycyrrhizae and Rhizoma Pinelliae.

(297) Pill for Relieving Edema (from *Danxi's Experience on Medicine*):

Rhizoma Chuanxiong, Rhizoma Atractylodis, Rhizoma Cyperi, Fructus Gardeniae (stir-baked) and Massa Medicata Fermentata.

(298) Powder of Nitrum and Alumen (from *Synopsis of Prescriptions of the Golden Chamber*):
Nitrum and Alumen.

(299) Purple-Snow Pellet (from *Benevolent Prescriptions from the Pharmaceutical Bureau of Taiping Period*):

Talcum, Gypsum Fibrosum, Calcitum, Magnetitum, Cornu Saigae Tataricae, Radix Aristolochiae, Cornu Rhinocerotis, Lignum Aquilariae Resinatum, Flos Caryophylli, Rhizoma Cimicifugae, Radix Scrophulariae, Radix Glycyrrhizae, Natrii Sulfas, Cinnabaris, Moschus, Gold and Nitrum.

(300) Pill of Stannum Nigrum (from *Benevolent Prescriptions from the Pharmaceutical Bureau of Taiping Period*):

Stannum Nigrum, Sulfur, Fructus Toosendan, Semen Trigonellae, Radix Aucklandiae, Radix Aconiti Lateralis Preparata, Semen Myristicae, Actinolitum, Lignum Aquilariae Resinatum, Fructus Foeniculi, Cortex Cinnamomi and Fructus Psoraleae.

(301) Powder for Treating Diarrhea with Abdominal Pain (from *A Complete Collection of Jingyue's Treatise*):

Rhizoma Atractylodis Macrocephalae, Radix Paeoniae Alba, Radix Ledebouriellae and Pericarpium Citri Reticulatae (stir-baked).

(302) Decoction for Clearing Away Gallbladder-Heat (from *Essentially Treasured Prescriptions for Emergencies*):

Rhizoma Pinelliae, Pericarpium Citri Reticulatae, Radix Glycyrrhizae, Fructus Aurantii Immaturus, Caulis Bambusae in Taeniam, Rhizoma Zingiberis Recens and Poria.

(303) Decoction for Nourishing Fluid and Clearing Away Liver-Heat (from *Notes on Medical Works*):

Radix Rehmanniae, Fructus Corni, Poria, Radix Angelicae Sinensis, Rhizoma Dioscoreae, Cortex Moutan, Rhizoma Alismatis, Radix Paeoniae Alba, Radix Bupleuri, Fructus Gardeniae and Semen Ziziphi Spinosae.

(304) Pill for Nourishing Kidney and Promoting Urination (from *Secret Records of the Cabinet of Orchids*):

Rhizoma Anemarrhenae, Cortex Phellodendri and Cortex Cinnamomi.

(305) Cheng's Decoction of Dioscoreae Septemlobae for Clearing Turbid Urine (from *Insight into Medicine*):

Rhizoma Dioscoreae Septemlobae, Semen Plantaginis, Poria, Plumula Nelumbinis, Rhizoma Acori Tatarinowii, Cortex Phellodendri, Radix Salviae Miltiorrhizae and Rhizoma Atractylodis Macrocephalae.

(306) Decoction of Cornu Rhinocerotis and Rehmanniae (from *Essentially Treasured Prescriptions for Emergencies*):

Cornu Rhinocerotis, Radix Rehmanniae, Cortex Moutan and Radix Paeoniae.

(307) Powder of Cornu Rhinocerotis (from *Essentially Treasured Prescriptions for Emergencies*):

Cornu Rhinocerotis, Rhizoma Coptidis, Rhizoma Cimicifugae, Fructus Gardeniae and Herba Artemisiae Scopariae.

(308) Bolus of Calculus Bovis for Clearing Heat and Detoxification (from *Treatise on Diagnosis and Treatment of External and Surgical Diseases*):

Calculus Bovis, Moschus, Myrrha and Olibanum.

(309) *Shuzao* Decoction for Promoting Urination and Defecation (from *Effective Prescriptions from Physicians of Successive Generations*):

Radix Phytolaccae, Rhizoma Alismatis, Semen Phaseoli, Semen Zanthoxyli, Caulis Aristolochiae Manshuriensis, Poria, Pericarpium Arecae, Semen Arecae, Rhizoma Zingiberis Recens, Rhizoma seu Radix Notopterygii and Radix Gentianae Macrophyllae.

(310) Powder for Causing Sneezing (from *Insight into Medicine*):

Herba Asari, Spina Gleditsiae and Rhizoma Pinelliae.

(311) Powder of Elsholtziae with Modification (from *Essentials of Seasonal Febrile Diseases*):

Herba Elsholtziae, Flos Lablab Album (fresh), Cortex Magnoliae Officinalis, Flos Lonicerae and Fructus Forsythiae.

(312) Pill for Relieving Slurred Speech (from *Insight into Medicine*):

Rhizoma Typhonii, Rhizoma Acori Tatarinowii, Radix Polygalae, Rhizoma Gastrodiae, Scorpio, Rhizoma seu Radix Notopterygii, Rhizoma Arisaematis, Radix Aucklandiae and Radix Glycyrrhizae.

(313) Decoction of Seven Treasured Drugs for Relieving Malaria (from *Yang's Family Prescriptions*):

Radix Dichroae, Fructus Tsaoko, Cortex Magnoliae Officinalis, Semen Arecae, Pericarpium Citri Reticulatae Viride, Pericarpium Citri Reticulatae and Radix Glycyrrhizae Preparata.

(314) Powder of Sophorae (from *Prescriptions of Universal Benevolence for Curing All People*):

Flos Sophorae, Cacumen Platycladi, Spica Schizonepetae and Fructus Aurantii (stir-baked).

(315) Decoction of Ziziphi Spinosae (from *Synopsis of Prescriptions of the Golden Chamber*):

Semen Ziziphi Spinosae, Rhizoma Anemarrhenae, Rhizoma Chuanxiong, Poria and Radix Glycyrrhizae.

(316) Semen Arecae and Semen Cucurbitae (from proved formula):

Take 60-120 grams of Semen Cucurbitae in the form of powder or decoction first, 60-120 grams of Semen Arecae two hours later, and 15 grams of Natrii Sulfas (or magnesium sulfate) another half an hour later to induce diarrhea, thus dispelling parasites from the body.

(317) Decoction of Arecae (from proved formula):

Semen Arecae, Cortex Phellodendri, Rhizoma Coptidis and Omphalia.

(318) Decoction for Removing Blood Stasis Under Diaphragm (from *Correction of Medical Classics*):

Faeces Trogopterori, Radix Angelicae Sinensis, Rhizoma Chuanxiong, Semen Persicae, Cortex Moutan, Radix Paeoniae Rubra, Radix Linderae, Rhizoma Corydalis, Radix Glycyrrhizae, Rhizoma Cyperi, Flos Carthami and Fructus Aurantii.

(319) Decoction of Coicis (from *Diagnosis and Treatment of Classified Syndromes*):

Semen Coicis, Rhizoma Chuanxiong, Radix Angelicae Sinensis, Herba Ephedrae, Ramulus Cinnamomi, Rhizoma seu Radix Notopterygii, Radix Angelicae Pubescentis, Radix Ledebouriellae, Radix Aconiti Preparata, Rhizoma Atractylodis, Radix Glycyrrhizae and Rhizoma Zingiberis Recens.

(320) Pill for Impotence (from *A Complete Collection of Jingyue's Treatise*):

Radix Rehmanniae Preparata, Radix Angelicae Sinensis, Cortex Eucommiae, Radix Morindae Officinalis, Herba Cistanches, Herba Epimedii, Fructus Cnidii, Cortex Cinnamomi, Rhizoma Atractylodis Macrocephalae, Fructus Lycii, Rhizoma Curculiginis, Fructus Corni, Semen Allii Tuberosi, Radix Aconiti Lateralis Preparata; or add Radix Ginseng, and Cornu Cervi Pantotrichum.

(321) Powder of Indigo Naturalis and Concha Meretricis seu Cyclinae (from proved formula):

Indigo Naturalis and Concha Meretricis seu Cyclinae.

(322) Powder of Agastaches for Restoring Anti-Pathogenic *Qi* (from *Benevolent Prescriptions from the Pharmaceutical Bureau of Taiping Period*):

Herba Agastaches, Folium Perillae, Radix Angelicae Dahuricae, Radix Platycodi, Rhizoma Atractylodis Macrocephalae, Cortex Magnoliae Officinalis, Massa Pinelliae Rhizomatis, Pericarpium Arecae, Poria, Pericarpium Citri Reticulatae (fresh), Radix Glycyrrhizae and Fructus Jujubae.

(323) Pill of Lapis Chloriti Usta for Expelling Phlegm (from *Treatise on Health Preserving*):

Lapis Chloriti Usta, Lignum Aquilariae Resinatum, Radix et Rhizoma Rhei, Radix Scutellariae and Natrii Sulfas.

(324) Powder of Sargassum and Dioscoreae Bulbiferae (from *Standard for Diagnosis and Treatment*):

Sargassum and Rhizoma Dioscoreae Bulbiferae.

(325) Bolus of Carapax Trionycis (from *Synopsis of Prescriptions of the Golden Chamber*):

Carapax Trionycis, Rhizoma Belamcandae, Radix Scutellariae, Radix Bupleuri, Armadillidium

Vulgare, Rhizoma Zingiberis, Radix et Rhizoma Rhei, Radix Paeoniae, Ramulus Cinnamomi, Semen Lepidii seu Descurainiae, Folium Pyrrosiae, Cortex Magnoliae Officinalis, Cortex Moutan, Herba Dianthi, Flos Campsis, Rhizoma Pinelliae, Radix Ginseng, Eupolyphaga seu Steleophaga, Colla Corii Asini, Nidus Vespae, Natrii Sulfas, Catharsius Molossus and Semen Persicae.

(326) Decoction for Relieving Manic-Depressive Syndromes (from *Correction of Medical Classics*):

Semen Persicae, Radix Bupleuri, Rhizoma Cyperi, Caulis Aristolochiae Manshuriensis, Radix Paeoniae Rubra, Rhizoma Pinelliae, Pericarpium Arecae, Pericarpium Citri Reticulatae Viride, Pericarpium Citri Reticulatae, Cortex Mori, Fructus Perillae and Radix Glycyrrhizae.

(327) Pill of Dioscoreae (from *Synopsis of Prescriptions of the Golden Chamber*):

Rhizoma Dioscoreae, Radix Ginseng, Rhizoma Atractylodis Macrocephalae, Poria, Radix Glycyrrhizae, Radix Angelicae Sinensis, Radix Paeoniae, Rhizoma Chuanxiong, Radix Rehmanniae, Colla Corii Asini, Radix Ophiopogonis, Semen Armeniacae Amarum, Radix Platycodi, Semen Sojae Germinatum, Radix Ledebouriellae, Radix Bupleuri, Ramulus Cinnamomi, Massa Medicata Fermentata, Rhizoma Zingiberis, Radix Ampelopsis and Fructus Jujubae.

(328) Decoction for Calming Liver-Wind (from *Discourse on Medical Problems Interpreted by Combined Chinese and Western Medicine*):

Radix Achyranthis Bidentatae, Os Draconis, Radix Paeoniae Alba, Radix Asparagi, Fructus Hordei Germinatus, Haematitum, Concha Ostreae, Radix Scrophulariae, Fructus Toosendan, Herba Artemisiae Scopariae, Radix Glycyrrhizae and Carapax et Plastrum Testudinis.

(329) Decoction for Relieving *Bi*-Syndromes (from *Insight into Medicine*):

Rhizoma seu Radix Notopterygii, Radix Angelicae Pubescentis, Lignum Cinnamomi, Radix Gentianae Macrophyllae, Radix Angelicae Sinensis, Rhizoma Chuanxiong, Radix Glycyrrhizae Preparata, Caulis Piperis Kadsurae, Ramulus Mori, Olibanum and Radix Aucklandiae.

(330) Detoxification Pill (from *The Medical Secrets for Effective Treatment*):

Talcum, Herba Artemisiae Scopariae, Radix Scutellariae, Rhizoma Acori Tatarinowii, Caulis Aristolochiae Manshuriensis, Bulbus Fritillariae Cirrhosae, Rhizoma Belamcandae, Fructus Forsythiae, Herba Menthae, Fructus Amomi Rotundus and Herba Agastaches.

(331) Powder for Regulating the Function of Stomach (from *Benevolent Prescriptions from the Pharmaceutical Bureau of Taiping Period*):

Radix Atractylodis, Cortex Magnoliae Officinalis, Pericarpium Citri Reticulatae, Radix Glycyrrhizae, Rhizoma Zingiberis Recens and Fructus Jujubae.

(332) Decoction of Stephaniae Tetrandrae and Astragali (from *Synopsis of Prescriptions of the Golden Chamber*):

Radix Stephaniae Tetrandrae, Radix Astragali, Radix Glycyrrhizae, Rhizoma Atractylodis Macrocephalae, Rhizoma Zingiberis Recens and Fructus Jujubae.

(333) Decoction of Stephaniae Tetrandrae and Poria (from *Synopsis of Prescriptions of the Golden Chamber*):

Radix Stephaniae Tetrandrae, Radix Astragali, Ramulus Cinnamomi, Poria and Radix Glycyrrhizae.

(334) Pill of Rhei and Eupolyphaga seu Steleophaga (from *Synopsis of Prescriptions of the Golden Chamber*):

Radix et Rhizoma Rhei, Radix Scutellariae, Radix Glycyrrhizae, Semen Persicae, Semen Armeniacae Amarum, Radix Paeoniae Alba, Radix Rehmanniae, Lacca Sinica Exsiccatae, Tabanus, Hirudo, Holotrichia Diomphalia, Eupolyphaga seu Steleophaga and Mel.

(335) Decoction for Relieving *Yin*-Deficiency Syndrome (from *An Essential Medical Manual*):

Radix Rehmanniae, Cortex Moutan, Radix Angelicae Sinensis (treated in wine), Radix

Ophiopogonis, Exocarpium Citri Rubrum, Semen Coicis, Semen Nelumbinis, Radix Paeoniae Alba, Radix Ginseng, Radix Glycyrrhizae Preparata, Fructus Schisandrae and Fructus Jujubae.

(336) Powder for Invigorating Heart-*Qi* (from *Benevolent Prescriptions from the Pharmaceutical Bureau of Taiping Period*):

Moschus, Radix Aucklandiae (roasted), Rhizoma Dioscoreae, Lignum Pini Poriaferum, Radix Astragali, Radix Polygalae, Radix Ginseng, Radix Platycodi, Radix Glycyrrhizae Preparata and Cinnabaris.

Additional Formulae:

Decoction for Benefiting *Yin*
Decoction for Clearing Away Spleen-Heat
Decoction for Purging Stagnant Blood
Decoction for Regulating Middle *Jiao*
Decoction of Acori Tatarinowii and Curcumae
Decoction of Adenophorae and Ophiopogonis
Decoction of Angelicae Sinensis and Astragali
Decoction of Angelicae Sinensis and Astragali for Reinforcing Middle *Jiao*
Decoction of Angelicae Sinensis for Strengthening Middle *Jiao*
Decoction of Ginseng and Haematitum for Nourishing *Qi*
Decoction of Notopterygii for Eliminating Dampness
Decoction of Pericarpium Citri Reticulatae
Decoction of Pericarpium Citri Reticulatae and Caulis Bambusae in Taeniam
Decoction of Scutellariae for Clearing Away Heat in Lung
Decoction of Three Kinds of Seed
Decoction of Toosendan
Detoxification Pill
Didang Pill
Dongyuan Decoction for Eliminating Retained Fire
Pill for Debility
Pill for Relaxing the Muscles and Tendons and Activating Blood Circulation
Pill of Aconiti Lateralis Preparata, Cinnamomi and Rehmanniae
Pill of Aucklandiae and Coptidis
Powder for Clearing Away Summer-Heat and Dampness
Powder for Promoting Diuresis
Powder for Regulating Gastric Function
Powder for Regulating the Liver and Spleen
White Tiger Decoction
Xiaojin Pill
Yueju Pill
Zijin Pill

图书在版编目(CIP)数据

中医中药教材　第三卷：英文／国家中医药管理局编.
—北京：新世界出版社，1996．3
ISBN 7-80005-296-6

Ⅰ．中…
Ⅱ．国…
Ⅲ．中国医药学-教材-英文
Ⅳ．R2

中医中药教材（第三册）
国家中医药管理局　编
*
新世界出版社出版
（北京百万庄路24号）
北京大学印刷厂印刷
中国国际图书贸易总公司发行
（中国北京车公庄西路35号）
北京邮政信箱第399号　邮政编码100044
1996年（英文）第一版
ISBN 7-80005-296-6
04200
14-E-2838SC